Recent Advances in Clinical Oncology

ANNALS OF THE NEW YORK ACADEMY OF SCIENCES
Volume 1138

Recent Advances in Clinical Oncology

Editors
FRANK JAMES BRANICKI, ABDU ADEM, SAAD GHAZAL-ASWAD,
AND FAWAZ CHIKH TORAB

Published by Blackwell Publishing on behalf of the New York Academy of Sciences
Boston, Massachusetts
2008

Library of Congress Cataloging-in-Publication Data

Recent advances in clinical oncology / editors, Frank James Branicki ... [et al.].
      p. ; cm. – (Annals of the New York Academy of Sciences, ISSN 0077-8923;
v. 1138)
      Includes bibliographical references and index.

      ISBN-13: 978-1-57331-700-9
      ISBN-10: 1-57331-700-4

      1. Cancer. I. Branicki, Frank J. II. New York Academy of Sciences. III. Series.
      [DNLM: 1. Neoplasms–therapy. 2. Biomedical Research–trends. W1 AN626YL
v.1138 2008 / QZ 266 R2953 2008]
      RC261.R365 2008
      616.99'4–dc22

1005721229   2008014272

The *Annals of the New York Academy of Sciences* (ISSN: 0077-8923 [print]; ISSN: 1749-6632 [online]) is published 28 times a year on behalf of the New York Academy of Sciences by Blackwell Publishing with offices at (US) 350 Main St., Malden, MA 02148-5020, (UK) 9600 Garsington Road, Oxford, OX4 2ZG, and (Asia) 165 Cremorne St., Richmond VIC 3121, Australia. Blackwell Publishing was acquired by John Wiley & Sons in February 2007. Blackwell's program has been merged with Wiley's global Scientific, Technical, and Medical business to form Wiley-Blackwell.

MAILING: The *Annals* is mailed standard rate. Mailing to rest of world by IMEX (International Mail Express). Canadian mail is sent by Canadian publications mail agreement number 40573520. POSTMAS-TER: Send all address changes to *Annals of the New York Academy of Sciences*, Blackwell Publishing Inc., Journals Subscription Department, 350 Main St., Malden, MA 02148-5020.

Disclaimer: The publisher, the New York Academy of Sciences and editors cannot be held responsible for errors or any consequences arising from the use of information contained in this publication; the views and opinions expressed do not necessarily reflect those of the publisher, the New York Academy of Sciences and editors.

Blackwell Publishing is now part of Wiley-Blackwell.

Information for subscribers: For ordering information, claims, and any inquiry concerning your subscription, please contact your nearest office:

UK: Tel: +44 (0)1865 778315; Fax: +44 (0) 1865 471775
USA: Tel: +1 781 388 8599 or 1 800 835 6770 (toll free in the USA & Canada); Fax: +1 781 388 8232 or Fax: +44 (0) 1865 471775
Asia: Tel: +65 6511 8000; Fax: +44 (0)1865 471775,
Email: customerservices@blackwellpublishing.com
Subscription prices for 2008: Premium Institutional: US$4265 (The Americas), £2370 (Rest of World). Customers in the UK should add VAT at 7%; customers in the EU should also add VAT at 7%, or provide a VAT registration number or evidence of entitlement to exemption. Customers in Canada should add 5% GST or provide evidence of entitlement to exemption. The Premium institutional price also includes online access to the current and all online back files to January 1, 1997, where available. For other pricing options, including access information and terms and conditions, please visit www.blackwellpublishing.com/nyas.

Delivery Terms and Legal Title: Prices include delivery of print publications to the recipient's address. Delivery terms are Delivered Duty Unpaid (DDU); the recipient is responsible for paying any import duty or taxes. Legal title passes to the customer on despatch by our distributors.

Membership information: Members may order copies of *Annals* volumes directly from the Academy by visiting www.nyas.org/annals, emailing membership@nyas.org, faxing +1 212 298 3650, or calling 1 800 843 6927 (toll free in the USA), or +1 212 298 8640. For more information on becoming a member of the New York Academy of Sciences, please visit www.nyas.org/membership. Claims and inquiries on member orders should be directed to the Academy at email: membership@nyas.org or Tel: 1 800 843 6927 (toll free in the USA) or +1 212 298 8640.

Printed in the USA. Printed on acid-free paper.

The *Annals* is available to subscribers online at Blackwell Synergy and the New York Academy of Sciences Web site. Visit www.blackwell-synergy.com or www.annalsnyas.org to search the articles and register for table of contents e-mail alerts.

The paper used in this publication meets the minimum requirements of the National Standard for Information Sciences Permanence of Paper for Printed Library Materials, ANSI Z39.48 1984.

ISSN: 0077-8923 (print); 1749-6632 (online)
ISBN-10: 1-57331-700-4 ISBN-13: 978-1-57331-700-9

A catalogue record for this title is available from the British Library.

ANNALS OF THE NEW YORK ACADEMY OF SCIENCES

Volume 1138

Recent Advances in Clinical Oncology

Editors

FRANK JAMES BRANICKI, ABDU ADEM, SAAD GHAZAL-ASWAD,
AND FAWAZ CHIKH TORAB

This volume is the result of a conference entitled **Recent Advances in Clinical Oncology,** organized by the Faculty of Medicine and Health Sciences, United Arab Emirates University, in association with Tawam Hospital and Johns Hopkins Medicine, and the General Authority for Health Services for the Emirate of Abu Dhabi, and held on February 19–22, 2007 at Intercontinental Resort, Al Ain, United Arab Emirates.

CONTENTS

Part III. Head and Neck Cancer

Part IV. Soft Tissue/Bone and Thoracic Cancer

Part V. Breast Cancer

Part VI. Gastrointestinal Malignancies

Part VII. Gynecological and Prostate Cancer

Part VIII. Pain Control, Palliative, and Other Therapies

Part IX. Molecular Oncology and Cell Signaling in Cancer

Preface

This volume of the *Annals of the New York Academy of Sciences* is based on the proceedings of the international conference entitled Recent Advances in Clinical Oncology, held in Al Ain, United Arab Emirates, on February 19–22, 2007. The meeting was organized by the Oncology Research Group, an initiative of the Faculty of Medicine and Health Sciences at the United Arab Emirates University. The group comprises those with a particular interest in oncology, and membership includes basic scientists and clinical faculty at the Faculty of Medicine and Health Sciences (FMHS) and clinicians from Tawam Hospital in affiliation with Johns Hopkins Medicine.

Cancer has become a major global health problem, particularly as populations are aging in many parts of the world. Cancer is the third leading cause of mortality in the UAE, responsible for 11% of all deaths. In some fields, significant advances have been evident, with the introduction of new treatment modalities, but this has been overshadowed somewhat by the need for further progress in screening, early diagnosis, and cost-effective therapies. We can no longer be solely preoccupied with survival data alone; there is now a greater understanding of the need to ensure an optimal quality of life and to meet the many and varied needs of patients requiring palliative or end-of-life care. In this regard, better communication skills and ethical issues also merit earnest consideration.

This international conference provided a forum for the exchange of ideas and knowledge concerning cancer prevention and patient education, as well as strategies for optimization of clinical care. The meeting focused on recent advances and controversies through interaction with renowned international speakers. The conference was a full four-day program, structured in the form of workshops, plenary and parallel lectures in symposia, as well as short oral and poster presentations. It provided a welcome opportunity to further continuing education in oncology and to examine the latest reviews. Issues addressed included evidence-based oncology, molecular biology, diagnosis, staging, and treatment, encompassing chemotherapy, radiation therapy, surgery and novel experimental and therapeutic strategies, palliative care, and today's challenges in cancer care. Specific topical sessions related to such common disorders in the UAE as breast, hematological, colorectal, pediatric, upper gastrointestinal, gynecological, prostatic, and endocrine malignancy, as well as lung and bone tumors. There were sessions also focusing on ethical and moral issues for staff caring for patients.

The conference proved to be of interest to anesthetists, endocrinologists, gynecologists, hematologists, internists, pediatricians, pathologists, radiologists, respiratory physicians, and surgeons involved in various aspects of general surgery and subspecialty practice. Basic scientists from FMHS also actively participated in the conference. The FMHS Alumni Association held its annual meeting at the Intercontinental Resort coincident with the first full day of the conference. Nurses, particularly those based locally at Al Ain

Ann. N.Y. Acad. Sci. 1138: xi-xiii (2008). © 2008 New York Academy of Sciences.
doi: 10.1196/annals.1414.000

and Tawam Hospitals, also participated with two workshops arranged specifically for nursing education. One of these was entitled Oncology for Nurses, and the other dealt with setting up a breast cancer support group.

Invited faculty included eminent overseas speakers, many of whom are in the international forefront of their respective fields of interest. Those coming from North America included clinicians from Johns Hopkins Hospital (Baltimore), MD Anderson Cancer Center (Houston), Memorial Sloan-Kettering Cancer Center (New York), Case Western Reserve University (Cleveland), the Mayo Clinic (Rochester), and the University of Toronto (Canada). Invited faculty from the United Kingdom came from the University of London (St. Bartholomew's Hospital and University College), Cardiff University, and the University of Newcastle (Northern Institute for Cancer Research). Speakers from continental Europe came from Belgium (University of Leuven), France (Hospital Center of Le Havre), Germany (University of Heidelberg, University of Leipzig), Italy (University of Turin), and Spain (University of Navarra). Invited faculty also traveled from Japan (Keio University), Korea (Pohang University of Science and Technology), and Australia (University of Queensland). In all, presentations were made by 31 international faculty from Australia, Belgium, Canada, France, Germany, Italy, Spain, Japan, Korea, the United Kingdom, the United States, and regionally from Saudi Arabia and Qatar. Sixteen UAE-based speakers participated by invitation from Abu Dhabi (two), Dubai (three), and eleven FMHS faculty members based in Al Ain. This was the largest group of invited internationally distinguished clinicians with oncology interests ever to gather in the UAE; the meeting attracted 1000 delegates from around the world.

A basic sciences session featuring two presentations from eminent Korean scientist, Pann-Guill Suh, was held, with new research initiatives being highlighted in a series of presentations made by basic scientists at FMHS. This session was very well received. Two preconference plenary session workshops were held on February 19th. The morning session was oriented toward nursing staff, and the afternoon session dealt with clinical aspects of cancer diagnosis, staging, and treatment. On the morning of February 20th, HE Sheikh Nahayan Bin Mubarak Al Nahayan officiated at the opening ceremony and delivered a stimulating address identifying issues of concern in the field of oncology, encouraging the medical community to rise to the challenges encountered in the prevention, diagnosis, and treatment of cancer, including quality of life considerations. This captured the imagination of all present, and his remarks were reported nationally by the press. This was followed by a plenary session entitled Evidence-Based Oncology. Subsequently, the program included fifteen sessions held over a three-day period, culminating in a closing ceremony that took place at the end of the last afternoon of the conference on February 22nd. Nineteen abstracts were selected for oral presentations and 41 for poster display. A satellite symposium was also held. One invitee, Harold J. Burstein, from Harvard Medical School, delivered an invited lecture by video conference transmission.

Financial assistance to host the meeting came from a variety of sources. Substantial support came from the Faculty of Medicine and Health Sciences, UAE University, Tawam Hospital, in affiliation with Johns Hopkins Medicine; and the General Authority for Health Services for the Emirate of Abu Dhabi. We are most grateful for the help of many of our colleagues in the Oncology Research Group, UAE University, and Tawam/Johns Hopkins.

Interacting with the very helpful editorial department of the *Annals of the New York Academy of Sciences* has been enlightening and rewarding. Special thanks are due to Linda

Mehta, acquisitions editor, and Steven Bohall, project manager, for their advice and encouragement. The efforts of Carol DiPalermo in the production phase were greatly appreciated. Mr. Abdulla Jamal, at the Department of Surgery, UAE University, has worked tirelessly with enthusiasm; his secretarial expertise in liaising with authors has proved invaluable in bringing these submissions to print. We are delighted to have had this opportunity to highlight recent advances in the diagnosis and treatment of cancer and trust that this will be useful to those with basic science interests in oncology and those with clinical involvement in caring for patients with malignant disease.

FRANK JAMES BRANICKI
United Arab Emirates University

SAAD GHAZAL-ASWAD
Tawam Hospital, United Arab Emirates University

FAWAZ CHIKH TORAB
United Arab Emirates University

ABDU ADEM
United Arab Emirates University

Prognostic Significance of New Immunohistochemistry Scoring of p53 Protein Expression in Cutaneous Squamous Cell Carcinoma of Mice

Mulazim Hussain Bukhari,[a] Shahida Niazi,[a] Muhammad Anwar,[b] Naseer Ahmed Chaudhry,[a] and Samina Naeem[a]

[a]Department of Pathology and [b]Department of Community Medicine, King Edward Medical University, Lahore, Pakistan

This study was conducted to investigate the prognostic value and therapeutic response of treatment modalities on p53 protein expression and AgNOR index in squamous cell carcinoma (SCC). Furthermore, based on data, we proposed a new p53 immunohistochemistry (IHC) scoring system. Sixty albino mice were given 7,12-dimethylbenz[a]anthracine (DMBA) and 12-O-tetradecanoly Phorbol-13-acetate (TPA) to produce skin tumors. The retinoids were given after the development of tumors. p53 immunohistochemical and AgNOR staining was performed on the sections taken before and after the retinoid administration. p53 protein was expressed in 31 of the lesions (60.8%). AgNOR index was high in all 51 (100%) of the pretreated lesions. There was a marked decrease in the expression of p53 protein in 16/51 (31.4%) and AgNOR index in 36/51 (70.6%) in post-treated mice. There was no decrease in the expression of both markers in mice harboring malignant neoplasms. p53 IHC scores were 0, I, and II in epidermal hyperplasia, papilloma, and dysplasia, respectively, while they were II, III, IV, and V in SCC *in situ*, well-differentiated, moderately differentiated, and poorly differentiated SCCs, respectively. Alteration of p53 and AgNOR index occured during the development of SCC. The p53 IHC scores are directly related to the grades of malignancy. Both markers might be used as a supportive tool with routinely performed Hematoxylin and Eosin staining and may help in the diagnosis of SCC. The newly proposed p53 IHC scoring system will help histopathologists in making their differential diagnosis among benign, premalignant, and malignant lesions. It will also help the oncologists to assess the prognosis and effectiveness of their chemotherapy.

Key words: immunohistochemistry; p53; squamous cell carcinoma

Introduction

p53 is a tumor suppressor gene that is located on chromosome 17 p 13.1 and it is the single most common target for genetic alteration in human tumors.[1] It is a phosphoprotein that is activated by DNA damage and involved in the process to determine whether the cells should stop replication or die by apoptosis.[2] Weak expression of p53 in papilloma of the skin is due to an early mutation similar to any premalignant lesion.[3] The expression of this protein has also of prognostic significance because as it increases, so does the grade and stage of skin and breast cancer.[4]

A variety of studies have shown that vitamin A is necessary for normal growth and development through control of gene

Address for correspondence: Dr. Mulazim Hussain Bukhari, MBBS, DCP, FCPS, PhD, Associate Prof Pathology, 26-MOF, GOR III, Shadman, Lahore, Pakistan. drmhbukhari@yahoo.com

Ann. N.Y. Acad. Sci. 1138: 1–9 (2008). © 2008 New York Academy of Sciences.
doi: 10.1196/annals.1414.001

expression.[5–10] Vitamin A has other important effects; it can function as a pro-oxidant or as an antioxidant. The antioxidant properties of vitamin A have been shown both *in vitro* and *in vivo*.[11] Vitamin A deficiency causes oxidative damage to the liver mitochondria in rats that can be reversed by vitamin A supplementation.[12] However, the addition of retinol and retinal to cultures of HL-60 cells causes cellular DNA cleavage and an increased formation of 8-oxo-7, 8-dihydro-2′-deoxyguanosine via superoxide generation;[13] moreover, *in vitro*, it has been shown that β-carotene cleavage products induce oxidative stress by impairing mitochondrial respiration.[14] Therefore, maintaining vitamin A concentration within the physiological range is critical to normal cell function because either a deficiency or an excess of vitamin A induces oxidative stress.[15]

In various studies it has been observed that vitamin A deficiency causes an increase in the expression p53 protein, enhances the effects of carcinogenesis, and causes mutation of p53,[3] whereas vitamin A treatment decreases the expression of p53, decreases the effect of chemical carcinogenesis, and repairs the mutation.[16,17]

Some treatment modalities, such as topical application of vitamin A, have an effect on the expression of p53. These changes in the expression of p53 may play a role in mediating the effects of therapy on the epidermis, as well as prevention of actinic neoplasia. This is achieved by adjusting any disturbance in the proliferation/apoptosis balance observed in photo-aged facial skin.[2,4]

Clinical, epidemiological, and experimental findings have provided evidence supporting a role of free radicals in the etiology of cancer. Free radical production is enhanced in many disease states, by carcinogen exposure, and under conditions of stress contributing widely to cancer development in humans. Vitamin A (all-trans-retinol) reduces free radical production and decreases the expression of the p53 protein. This has also been seen in an experimental study in breast cancer.[18]

Nucleolar organizer regions (NORs) are segments of DNA associated with argyrophilic proteins. The NORs are chromosomal loops of DNA involved in ribosomal synthesis. Associated with NORs are some nucleolar proteins which are stained with silver methods (AgNOR proteins or AgNORs). AgNORs can be identified as black dots in the nuclei. Their size and number reflect nucleolar and cell proliferative activity of tumors.[19,20]

Tumor growth is controlled by growth rate and cell cycle. The proliferative activity of tumor cells can influence the growth rate of the primary cancer and account for their aggressiveness. Variations in growth rate, cell cycle control, and proliferative activity could, in part, explain differences in invasive and metastatic properties. This can be easily studied by a simple silver staining technique.[21,22]

This study was conducted to investigate the prognostic and therapeutic response of treatment modalities on p53 protein expression and AgNOR index in squamous cell carcinoma (SCC). Additionally, it was done to introduce a new p53 immunohistochemistry (IHC) scoring system.

Materials and Methods

This study was carried out on 60 albino mice, 5–7 weeks in age for 30 weeks. All the mice were given 100 µg/mL 7, 12-dimethylbenz [a]anthracine (DMBA) and 10 µg/mL 12, O, tetradecanyol Phorbol-13-acetate (TPA) topically to produce tumors for 15 weeks (Table 1). After 15 weeks, the mice were treated with retinoids for another 15 weeks. Before starting treatment, punch biopsies were taken from the lesions to see the pretreated status of p53. All animals were sacrificed after 30 weeks according to ethical considerations for experimental animal models by giving anesthesia in a glass jar. The skin biopsies and lesions were retaken to compare the post-treated status of p53.[23]

TABLE 1. Distribution of p53 Expression in Benign and Malignant Lesions of Pretreated Mice

Mice n = 60	Benign lesions n = 36				Malignant lesions n = 15					Total
	EPH	Pap	Dys	Total	SCC-IS	SCC	MFH	IDC	Total	Total
Pre-treated biopsies	20	9	7	36 (60%)	8	5	1	1	15 (25%)	51 (85%)
Scores of p53 in pre-treated biopsies	0	I	II	I	III	IV	IV	IV	–	–
p53 expression	0	9	7	16	8	5	1	1	15	31 (60.8%)
mAgNOR in pre-treated biopsies	0.90 ± 0.05	2.27 ± 0.27	3.37 ± 0.34	36	7.05 ± 1.17	8.97 ± 2.36	8.01 ± 3.56	8.47 ± 1.56	51	51 (100%)
pAgNOR in pre-treated biopsies	8%	18%	28%	36%	39%	57%	50%	63%	51	51 (100%)

Key: EPH, epidermal hyperplasia; Pap, papilloma; Dys, dysplasia; SCC-IS, squamous cell carcinoma *in situ;* SCC, squamous cell carcinoma; MFH, malignant fibrous histiocytoma; IDC, invasive ductal carcinoma.

p53 Immunohistochemistry Staining

For each biopsy, 4-μm-thick sections were placed on glass slides and deparaffinized with Histoclear. Sections were then rehydrated through decreasing concentrations of alcohol (100%, 95%). They were then immersed in 0.01 M citric acid (pH 6.0) in a microwave oven for 20 min to enhance antigen retrieval (positive and negative controls were also used). In some cases, microwaving was repeated for two additional cycles of 5 min each.

The avidin-biotin peroxidase method was used employing an Immunotech 500 (Leica, Deerfield, IL) automated immunostainer according to the manufacturer's instructions. Briefly, the automated steps included blockage of endogenous peroxidase with 3% hydrogen peroxide and reaction with monoclonal antibodies against human p53 (clone D07; DAKO, Lahore, Pakistan) diluted 1:200. After extensive washing, sections were incubated at room temperature for 30 min with biotinylated goat anti-mouse IgG antibody and then for 30 min with avidin-biotin peroxidase complexes (1:25 final dilution). Chromogen diaminobenzidine was used for all reactions. Diaminobenzidine (0.06%) was used as the final chromogen, and cells were counterstained with 0.4% methyl green in 0.1 mol/L sodium acetate buffer (pH 4.0) followed by three washes each of water, 1-butanol, and histoclear.[4]

Positive Control: Specimens consisting of invasive ductal carcinoma breast were used as positive controls for p53.

Negative Control: Parallel running additional sections in PBS, not treated with antibody were used as negative control.

Semiquantitation of p53

IHC reactivity for p53 was read by our newly adopted scoring system, based on the quantity and quality of brown pigmentation in the nuclei of cells. Cells having a positive nuclear reaction among each 500–1000 cells revealing a positive nuclear reaction in 5–10 high power fields were counted and the percentages were calculated for scoring the p53 protein expression. We also assessed the quality of staining of IHC in the nuclei of the keratinocytes on the basis of the granularity (color, shape, and size) of IHC stains in the nuclei of epithelial cells.

To evaluate p53 staining, two expert surgical pathologists performed the p53 counts. The observers independently evaluated the stained slides without knowledge of the clinicopathological profiles of these lesions. The presence of cells with clear and unequivocal nuclear staining were identified as positive cases. The count was based on a HPF of $0.159 \, mm^2$, which is defined as a field resulting from use of an ocular with an $18 \, mm^2$ field of view at $10\times$ magnification and $40\times$ objective (with appropriate correction factors to compensate if different field oculars are used). The p53 protein-expression values were then compared with those in the controls.[24]

The AgNOR Silver Stain

AgNOR index was detected by modified method of AgNOR staining on paraffin-embedded tissue taken from all lesions of the mice in all groups.[25]

Statistical Analysis

Scoring of p53 was made on the percentage of reactive cells in any lesion, while mean AgNOR count and standard deviation of each mean were calculated (as mAgNOR). The AgNOR proliferative index (pAgNOR) was calculated by counting the cells having five or more AgNOR granules per nucleus, in 100 nuclei.[24] The Student's t-test was applied to investigate difference between the different groups. Fisher's exact test was used to compare the p53 status in different grades of SCC and control groups, and a comparison of the two methods of IHC for p53 and AgNORs.

Results

Of 60 mice, 51 (85%) animals showed positive lesions comprising 36 (70.6%) benign or premalignant lesions and 15 (29.4%) malignant cases, while p53 protein was expressed in 31 (60.8%) lesions (Table 1).

p53 expression was mild (Score I) in nine papillomas and seven dysplastic lesions (Score II) and high (Score III–IV) in 15 malignant tumors, comprising eight SCC *in situ* (Score III), five SCCs (Score III–IV), one malignant fibrous histiocytoma (MFH) (Score IV), and one invasive ductal carcinoma breast (Score IV) (Tables 1 and 2).

The AgNORs appeared as black discrete dots in a pale yellow stained nucleus of epidermal cells. The AgNOR counts were high in papillomas and dysplasias. The mAgNOR was 2.27 ± 0.27 and pAgNOR was 18% in papillomas. In contrast the mAgNOR was 3.37 ± 0.34 and pAgNOR was 31% in dysplasia. Only mAgNOR was slightly increased in epidermal hyperplasia (mAgNOR 0.90 ± 0.05). There was a mild variation in the size of AgNOR dots in papillomas and a moderate variation in dysplasia. The mean dispersion of AgNOR per cell in normal epidermal cells and epidermal hyperplasia was normal. It was low in papilloma and high in dysplasia. The AgNOR index was high in all malignant lesions (Table 1).

Only 15 lesions were observed in post-treated sacrificed mice. In mice taking retinoids, 36 benign and premalignant lesions recovered, and the p53 protein expression score was 0 in these recovered mice skin biopsies. The AgNOR index also became normal in the biopsies of these animals. Fifteen animals bearing malignant lesions did not show any response to retinoids, and p53 immunoreactivity and AgNOR index remained the same. There was no significant difference in the reactivity of both markers in pretreated and post-treated mice (Tables 2 and 3; Figs. 1–5).

TABLE 2. Distribution of p53 Expression and AgNOR Index in Benign and Malignant Lesions of Post-treated Mice

Mice n = 60	Benign lesions n = 36				Malignant lesions n = 15					
	EPH	Pap	Dys	Total	SCC-IS	SCC	MFH	IDC	Total	Total
Post-treated biopsies	Nil	Nil	Nil	Nil	8	5	1	1	15 (25%)	15 (25%)
Scores of p53 in post-treated biopsies	0	0	0	0	III	IV	IV	IV		
Decline in p53 expression	0	100%	100%	16 (31.37%)	0	0	0	0	0	0
mAgNOR in post-treated biopsies	0.36 ± 0.07	0.36 ± 0.07	0.36 ± 0.07	0	7.05 ± 1.17	8.97 ± 2.36	8.01 ± 3.56	8.47 ± 1.56	15	15 (29.4%)
PAgNOR in post-treated biopsies	8%	18%	28%	0	39%	57%	50%	63%	15	15 (29.4%)
Improved AgNOR index	20	09	7	36 (60%)	0	0	0	0	0	0

key: EPH, epidermal hyperplasia; Pap, papilloma; Dys, dysplasia; SCC-IS, squamous cell carcinoma *in situ*; SCC, squamous cell carcinoma; MFH, malignant fibrous histiocytoma; IDC, invasive ductal carcinoma.

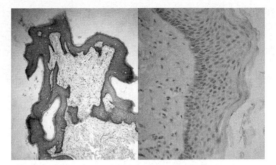

Figure 1. Photomicrograph of **(right)** squamous cell papilloma (10×; IHC staining score I), showing p53 IHC score I; and **(left)** photomicrograph of squamous cell papilloma (10×; H&E).

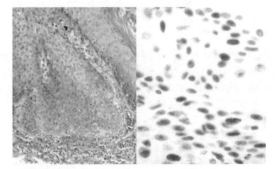

Figure 2. Photomicrograph of **(right)** SCC *in situ* (20×; IHC), showing p53 IHC score II; and **(left)** photomicrograph of SCC (40×; H&E).

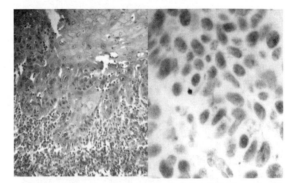

Figure 3. Photomicrograph of **(right)** well differentiated (Grade I) SCC (20×; IHC), showing p53 IHC score III; and **(left)** photomicrograph of SCC (40×; H&E).

Discussion

The running scoring system of p53 is complex, heterogeneous, and cumbersome because its results are described either in a positive or negative values and cannot describe higher

TABLE 3. Comparison of Adopted and Other Systems of Scoring for p53

Adopted score	Running scores Qin *et al.* (2002)[26]	Immunoreactivity of p53 proteins in the nuclei of tumor cell, percentage	Description
0	0	0–5%	When no or very few tumor cells Show immunoreactivity (fine and light brown staining in the nuclei) for p53 proteins expression
I	not mentioned	6–10%	When 6–10% number of tumor cells show immunoreactivity (fine to coarse light brown staining in the nuclei) for p53 proteins expression
II	+	11–30%	When 11–3-% number of tumor cells (clusters or dispersed) show immunoreactivity (coarse, light to dark staining in nuclei) for p53 protein expression. The positive cells are sparsely dispersed showing areas of heterogeneous positivity
III	++	31–50%	When 31–50% number of tumor cells show heterogeneous and homogenous immunoreactivity for (coarse and dark brown pigmentation in nuclei) for p53 protein expression
IV	not mentioned	31–50%	When 31–50% number of tumor cells show homogenous immunoreactivity for (coarse and dark brown staining in nuclei) for p53 protein expression
V	+++	>50%	When there >50% numbers of tumor cells show homogenous immunoreactivity for (course and dark brown staining in nuclei) for p53 protein expression

grades of malignancy. We, therefore, introduced a new method of p53 scoring that is easier, convenient, and reproducible when compared to previous methods. To develop the new method of p53 scoring we used AgNOR for its validation. The principle of this system is that whenever there is an increase in the proliferative index of any cell, the level of p53

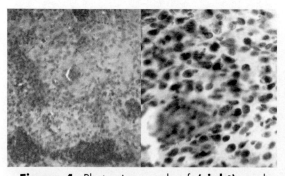

Figure 4. Photomicrograph of **(right)** moderately differentiated (Grade II) SCC (40×; IHC), showing p53 IHC score IV; and **(left)** photomicrograph of moderately differentiated (Grade II) SCC (40×; H&E).

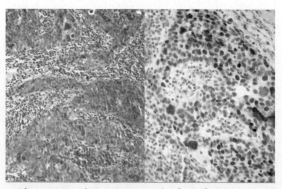

Figure 5. Photomicrograph of **(right)** poorly differentiated (Grade III) SCC (40×; IHC), showing p53 IHC score IV; and **(left)** photomicrograph of poorly differentiated (Grade III) SCC (40×; H&E).

immunoreactivity will not be at a 0 score and when there is no change in proliferative index, the level of p53 expression will not be monitored as significant. Therefore, we departed from previous reports on scoring of p53. Our scoring system departs from p53 scoring by Qin et al.,[26] who overlooked the immunoreactive cells with p53 expression levels below 10% and used a difficult and nonreproducible method of assessing IHC reaction in reactive cells. Previously, the percentage of p53 immunoreactive tumor cells was scored as 0 to 3+ in p53-positive regions (<10%, −; 10–30%, +; 31–50%, ++; >50%, +++).[26]

We agree that a semiquantitative scoring method that evaluates the percentage of positive tumor cells (0–100%) may provide a better understanding of the prognostic or predictive significance of these markers as described by Zlobec et al.[27]

Our scoring system is not in accordance with Lal et al.,[28] wherein the method of calculating the index is cumbersome and do not describe the quality of positivity of p53 IHC. Our pattern is not comparable with that of Quinn et al.,[29] whose method of evaluating the clustering level is also contradictory because most malignant neoplasms lack such features. Their method confuses the observer when there are more active areas of tumor showing a positive IHC reaction.

In our study chemical carcinogens resulted in step-wise changes in the mutation of p53 according to the development of lesions. There was no mutation in p53 in epidermal hyperplasia and the p53 IHC score was 0.

The increased number of epidermal cells and basal mitoses and a slight increase in Ag-NOR count in epidermal hyperplasia could be due to an early stress on the tumor suppressor gene. These early changes in cell cycle–controlling genes are reversible, controllable, and reparable if the abnormal stimulus is removed or the condition is treated with a suitable modality. We observed this repair by treating the lesions with retinoids.

There was weak expression of p53 in papillomas and dysplasia and a moderate increase in AgNOR index. These changes could be due to early or partial alteration in p53 genes. These lesions were completely recovered by retinoid treatment with a considerable decline in p53 protein expression and normalization of AgNOR. We suggest that the above levels of p53 expression and proliferative index should not be ignored because these conditions may be lead to cancer in the future.

In dysplasia, p53 immunoreactivity was higher when compared with papillomas. These changes may be due to rise in alteration of p53. The prognosis of these lesions was also good because retinoids have shown a tremendous improvement in these conditions. The message to dermatologists is that vitamin A prevents premalignant skin conditions and a message for molecular biologists is that repair of early or partially mutated p53 is possible and that the prognosis of such lesions is good (Table 4).

In this study the other lesions were 15 malignant tumors. There was no response to retinoids in these conditions. In these lesions the expression of p53 and AgNOR was high. We suggested a score of p53 from III–V. This semi-quantitative measurement of p53 is a good investigation for complete mutation of the p53 gene.

In our study, the IHC staining scores of p53 expression for SCC were upregulated as II, III, IV, and V in SCC *in situ*, well-differentiated SCC, moderately differentiated SCC, and poorly differentiated SCC, respectively. The increase in IHC scores of p53 were directly related to the grade of SCC, while poor relation was seen with the stages of carcinoma.

We have seen in this study that the grade of SCC does not depend upon the stage of the tumor because SCC sometimes changes its grade as it invades the tissues and at other times does not change grade even in presence of distant metastasis. This is another message—that

TABLE 4. Relationship between p53 Scores and mAgNORs in Different Benign and Malignant Skin Tumors

Scores of p53	EPH (n = 20)	Papilloma (n = 9)	Dysplasia (n = 7)	SCC-IS (n = 8)	SCC Grade I (n = 4)	SCC Grade II (n = 2)	SCC Grade III (n = 2)
0	29	–	–	–			
I	–	12	–	–			
II	–		9				
IIIa	–			10			
IIIb	–				4		
IV						2	2
mAgNOR	0.36 ± 0.07	0.36 ± 0.07	0.36 ± 0.07	7.05 ± 1.17	8.97 ± 2.36	8.97 ± 2.36	8.97 ± 2.36
pAgNOR	8%	18%	28%	39%	57%	57%	57%
Prognosis	Excellent	Good	Good	Satisfactory	Poor	Poorer	Poorest
Future Plan	Preventive	Preventive or Surgery	Preventive or Surgery	Surgery & Radiation	Poor even after Surgery & Radiation	Future Research	Future Research

tumors that do not change their grade have a good prognosis and that their metastasis is amenable to appropriate therapy.

With these observations, we can say that recovery of mutated p53 is the best indicator of therapeutic response of any treatment modality and the prognosis of such malignant lesions. It also emphasizes that premalignant conditions have partial or early mutation of p53 (cell cycle–controlling genes) that cannot be retrieved even after the stimulus is withdrawn. Suitable early treatment modalities are required to control such conditions. In our experiment, vitamin A therapy in papilloma and dysplasia resulted in recovery of early affected p53 tumor suppressor gene. Retinoids help to recover the early stages of p53 mutation by repairing the cell cycle. The newly developed p53 IHC scoring system is easy, homogeneous, and reproducible. It may help oncologists and surgeons to monitor the therapeutic response of different treatment modalities and the status of surgical margins.

Conclusion

Alteration of p53 and AgNOR index occured during the development of SCC. Retinoids may help to repair the alteration of p53 at early stages. Both markers might be used as a supportive tool with routinely performed Hematoxylin and Eosin staining. The newly developed p53 IHC scoring system will help in assessing the prognosis and effectiveness of therapeutic regime for SCC. This scoring system will also help histopathologists to make differential diagnoses among benign, premalignant, and malignant lesions.

Acknowledgments

We are thankful to Dr. M. Tarik Mehmood, Mr. Tahseen Ahmed, and Dr. Farah Rasheed, Department of Pathology and Research, Shaukat Khanum Memorial Cancer Hospital and Research Center, for providing their laboratory for detection of p53 mutation. The authors would like to acknowledge critical review and suggestions from Aejaz Nasir, MD, MPhil, FCAP and help in editing the manuscript from Elizabeth Byron, Moffitt Cancer Center Tamap, FL, USA, for their help in editing our manuscript.

Conflicts of Interest

The authors declare no conflicts of interest.

References

1. Kumar, V., A.K. Abbas & N.T. Fausto. 2004. *Robbins and Cotran. Pathologic Basis of Disease*, 6th edn.: 302–319. Elsevier. Philadelphia.

2. El-Domyati, M.M., S.K. Attia, F.Y. Saleh, *et al.* 2003. Effect of topical tretinoin, chemical peeling and dermabrasion on p53 expression in facial skin. *Eur. J. Dermatol.* **13:** 433–438.

3. Bukhari, M.H., S.M. Salaria, Z. Niaz, *et al.* 2006. Mutation of p53 in skin papilloma and tubular breast adenoma of albino mice. *J. Coll. Phys. Surg. Pak.* **16:** 280–283.

4. Bukhari, M.H., A. Iqbal, M.N. Iqbal, *et al.* 2004. Role of bioenergy of specific soil (SiO_2) of Madinah Munawwrah on chemically induced carcinogenesis in albino mice by protecting mutation of p53. *Annals KEMC* **10:** 236–240.

5. Chambon, P. 1996. A decade of molecular biology of retinoic acid receptors. *FASEB J.* **10:** 940–954.

6. Chen, Y., F, Derguini & J. Buck. 1997. Vitamin "A" in serum is a survival factor for fibroblasts. *Proc. Natl. Acad. Sci. USA* **94:** 10205–10208.

7. Evans, T.R.J. & S.B. Kayne. 1999. Retinoids; present role and future potential. *Br. J. Cancer* **80:** 1–8.

8. Niederreither, K., V. Subbarayan, P. Dollé & P. Chambon. 1999. Embryonic retinoic acid synthesis is essential for early mouse post-implantation development. *Nat. Genet.* **21:** 444–448.

9. Zile, M.H. 2001. Function of vitamin A in vertebrate embryonic development. *J. Nutr.* **31:** 705–708.

10. Batourina, E., S. Gim, N. Bello, *et al.* 2001. Vitamin A controls epithelium/mesenchymal interactions through Ret expression. *Nat. Genet.* **27:** 74–78.

11. Page, K.C., D.A. Heitzman & M.I. Chernin. 1996. Stimulation of c-jun and c-myb in rat Sertoli cells following exposure to retinoids. *Biochem. Biophys. Res. Comm.* **225:** 595–600.

12. Palacios, A., V.A. Piergiacomi & A. Catalá. 1996. Vitamin A supplementation inhibits chemiluminescence and lipid peroxidation in isolated rat liver micrososmes and mitochondria. *Mol. Cell Biochem.* **154:** 77–82.

13. Barber, T., E. Borrás, L. Torres, *et al.* 2000. Vitamin A deficiency causes oxidative damage to liver mitochondria in rats. *Free Rad. Biol. Med.* **29:** 1–7.

14. Murata, M. & S. Kawanishi. 2000. Oxidative DNA damage by vitamin A and its derivate via superoxide generation. *J. Biol. Chem.* **275:** 2003–2008.

15. Siaems, W., O. Sommerburg, L. Schild, *et al.* 2002. β-Carotene cleavage products induce oxidative stress *in vitro* by impairing mitochondrial respiration. *FASEB J.* **16:** 1289–1291.

16. Bukhari, S.M.H., R. Bajwa, S.A. Khan & C.N.A. Tayyab. 1998. Vitamin "A" deficiency enhances the effect of 7–12 Dimethyl-Benz-a-Anthracene (DMBA) induced skin carcinogenesis. *J. Coll. Phys. Surg. Pak.* **8:** 101–105.

17. Borrás, E., R. Zaragozá, M. Morante, *et al.* 2003. In vivo studies of altered expression patterns of p53 and proliferative control genes in chronic vitamin A deficiency and hypervitaminosis. *Eur. J. Biochem.* **270:** 1493–1501.

18. Calaf, G.M., N.J. Emenaker & T.K. Hei. 2005. Effect of retinol on radiation- and estrogen-induced neoplastic transformation of human breast epithelial cells. *Oncol. Rep.* **13:** 1017–1027.

19. Klencki, M., I. Kurnatowska, D. Slowinska-Klencka, *et al.* 2001. Correlation between PCNA expression and AgNOR dots in pituitary adenomas. *Endocr. Pathol.* **12:** 163–169.

20. Romão-Corrêa, R.F., D.A. Maria, M. Soma, *et al.* 2005. Nucleolar organizer region staining patterns in paraffin-embedded tissue cells from human skin cancers. *J. Cutan. Pathol.* **32:** 323–328.

21. Pich, A., L. Chiusa, F. Marmont, *et al.* 1992. Argyrophilic nucleolar organizer region counts in multiple myeloma: a histopathological study on bone marrow trephine biopsies. *Virchows Archiv.* **421:** 143–147.

22. Rosai, J. 2004. *The Breast. Rosai and Ackerman's Surgical Pathology*, 9th edn.: 1763–1776. Mosby. St Louis, Missouri.

23. Bukhari, M.H., S.S. Qureshi, S. Niazi, *et al.* 2007. Chemotherapeutic/chemopreventive role of retinoids in chemically induced skin carcinogenesis in albino mice. *Int. J. Dermatol.* **46:** 1160–1165.

24. Hussein, M.R. 2005. Alterations of p53 and Bcl-2 protein expression in the laryngeal intraepithelial neoplasia. *Cancer Biol. Ther.* **4:** 213–217.

25. Bukhari, M.H., S. Niazi, S.A. Khan, *et al.* 2007. Modified method of AgNOR staining for tissue and interpretation in histopathology. *Int. J. Exp. Path.* **88:** 47–53.

26. Qin, L.X., Z.Y. Tang, Z.C. Ma, *et al.* 2002. p53 immunohistochemical scoring: an independent prognostic marker for patients after hepatocellular carcinoma resection. *World J Gastroenterol.* **8:** 459–463.

27. Zlobec, I., R. Steele, R.P. Michel, *et al.* 2006. Scoring of p53, VEGF, Bcl-2 and APAF-1 immunohistochemistry and interobserver reliability in colorectal cancer. *Modern Pathol.* **19:** 1236–1242.

28. Lal, P., L. Pal, S. Kumar, *et al.* 2007. Implications of p53 over-expression in the outcome with radiation in head and neck cancers. *J. Can. Res. Ther.* **3:** 17–22.

29. Quinn, D.I., S.M. Henshall, D.R. Head, *et al.* 2000. Prognostic significance of p53 nuclear accumulation in localized prostate cancer treated with radical prostatectomy. *Cancer Res.* **60:** 1585–1594.

Intra-operative Echographic Localization for Radioactive Ophthalmic Plaques in Choroidal Melanoma

Tahra Al Mahmoud,[a] Magdi Mansour,[a] Jean Deschênes,[a] Chaim Edelstein,[a] Miguel Burnier,[a] Michel Marcil,[b] George Shenouda,[c] Christine Corriveau,[e] and Michael Evans[d]

[a]*Department of Ophthalmology,* [b]*Department of Medicine,* [c]*Department of Radiation Oncology,* and [d]*Medical Physics Unit, McGill University, Montréal, Québec, Canada*

[e]*Department of Ophthalmology, Notre Dame Hospital, Montréal, Québec, Canada*

The objectives were to evaluate the beneficial effect of intra-operative echographic plaque site localization and to assess the rate of complications of postplaque insertion. This paper is a descriptive study of 48 patients with choroidal melanoma who underwent iodine-125 (I^{125}) or ruthenium-106 (Ru^{106}) plaque radiotherapy with intra-operative echographic confirmation of plaque placement with the aid of a nonradioactive plaque (dummy) at McGill University Health Centre from 1997 to 2003. Patients' mean age was 63.7 years; 52% (25/48) male, 48% (23/48) female. Twenty-seven percent (13/48) of the tumors were confined to the right eye and 73% (35/48) to the left eye. Forty-eight percent (23/48) of the tumors were located posterior to the equator, 14.6% (7/48) were anterior to the equator, 18.7% (9/48) in posterior pole, and 18.7% (9/48) at equator. Sixty-nine percent (33/48) received I^{125} and 31% (15/48) had Ru^{106} treatment. Ninety percent of the dummy plaques were initially positioned suboptimally and required repositioning under echographic guidance. At mean follow-up of 18.8 months, there was no tumor-related death or metastasis, but one patient required enucleation. The dummy plaque technique under echographic visualization resulted in reduction of radioactive exposure time during surgery of up to 50%. Intra-operative echographic utilization has the ability to localize precisely the tumor–plaque relationship, thereby optimizing the radiation delivered to the choroidal melanoma, while minimizing the surgeon's exposure time.

Key words: echography; choroidal melanoma; radioactive plaque

Introduction

Malignant uveal melanoma is the most common primary intraocular malignancy and is the only potentially fatal primary intraocular tumor in adults.[1] Radioactive episcleral plaque therapy is the most common form of radiotherapy used for uveal melanoma.[2–4] It is a modality that offers an equal survival rate when compared with enucleation, with the possibility of preserving the affected eye as well as the patient's vision.[5] Consequently, patients have a better quality of life. In recent years, echography has become an essential component in the clinical practice of ophthalmology and, in particular, of ocular oncology.

Patients and Methods

Clinical records and echographic data of patients with choroidal melanoma who were

Address for correspondence: Tahra AlMahmoud, MBBS, United Arab Emirates University, Faculty of Medicine and Health Sciences, P.O. Box 17666, Al Ain, United Arab Emirates. Voice: +971-3-7137580; fax: +971-3-7672067. uaeye27@hotmail.com

Ann. N.Y. Acad. Sci. 1138: 10–14 (2008). © 2008 New York Academy of Sciences.
doi: 10.1196/annals.1414.002

treated with iodine-125 (I^{125}) (33 patients) or ruthenium-106 (Ru^{106}) (15 patients) plaque irradiation and intra-operative echographic plaque localization at McGill University Health Centre (MUHC) between January 1997 and December 2003 were reviewed. Diagnosis of uveal melanoma was made prior to the treatment in all patients based on the clinical characteristics of the tumor, as well as B-scan and A-scan findings. Age, gender, eye involved, tumor diameter (transverse or base, longitudinal, and depth or height), and location (anterior, posterior, or at the equator and posterior pole) were also recorded. Collaborative Ocular Melanoma Study (COMS) protocol was followed for categorization of tumor size. The tumor is classified as small if the height is less than 2.5 mm and/or the base diameter is less than or equal to 8.0 mm. The tumor is considered medium in size if the height is equal to or greater than 2.5 mm and less than or equal to 10.0 mm and/or the base diameter is greater than or equal to 8.1 and less than or equal to 16.0 mm. Large tumors are those of height greater than or equal to 10.1 mm and/or base diameter greater or equal to 16.1 mm.[6] Tumors were classified according to their location being anterior to the equator, posterior to the equator, equatorial, or in a posterior pole location. A tumor was considered anteriorly located if more than 50% of its diameter was anterior to the equator, posterior if 50% or more of the tumor diameter was located posterior to the equator including the posterior pole tumors, equatorial if 50% or more of the diameter was located within the equator area, and close to the optic nerve if it was within 5 degrees from the optic nerve head.

Patients were followed up twice a year for 5 years postoperatively and once a year thereafter. At each visit, besides the full ophthalmic and B-scan ultrasound exam, a complete systemic evaluation, chest X-ray, and liver function tests were performed at the time of diagnosis and annually thereafter.

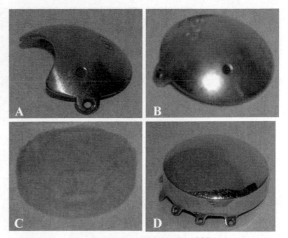

Figure 1. Plaque models: **(D)** I^{125} 20 mm; **(C)** 20 mm silastic insert for I^{125}; **(A)** notched nonradioactive Ruthenium-type plaque (dummy); **(B)** Ru^{106} 20 mm plaque.

Surgical Procedures

COMS dosimetry protocol was followed for all patients.[7,8] A 360-degree conjunctival priotomy was performed. A 2-0 cotton suture was placed around the insertion of each rectus muscle. An indirect ophthalmoscope was used, when indicated, to identify the tumor margin. The nonradioactive Ru-plaque (notched plaque for tumors near the optic nerve [Fig. 1A] or non-notched Ru-plaque [Fig. 1B] in any other location) was applied at the tumor site with a 2 mm border using two temporary 5-0 nylon sutures. Echographic localization of the plaque was performed by the same physician for all patients so as to view the tumor border in relation to the dummy plaque prior to actual radioactive plaque insertion. After confirming a suitable tumor–dummy relationship, the dummy plaque was removed leaving the sutures in place. The radioactive I^{125} plaque, which consisted of the plastic carrier (Fig. 1C) with radioactive iodine pellets inside the gold cover (Fig. 1D), was inserted at the predetermined location. Plaque type has been chosen, since 2001, according to the tumor height. Ru^{106} was given for tumors with apical height less than

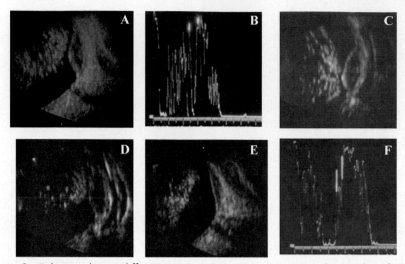

Figure 2. Echography at different stages: **(A)** intra-operative echography of choroidal melanoma; **(B)** A-scan with medium–high reflectivity prior to treatment; **(C)** nonradioactive plaque at the tumor site required readjustment of posterior margin; **(D)** plaque is adjusted with good coverage of borders; **(E)** melanoma regression 3 years post treatment; **(F)** A-scan with low–medium internal reflectivity post plaque radiotherapy.

or equal to 5 mm, otherwise I^{125} was administered. Reconfirmation of the exact plaque–tumor relationship by using echography was done prior to conjunctival closure. Figure 2 shows the B-scan and A-scan of a 53-year-old woman who was followed up since 1992 for left choroidal melanoma. Plaque insertion was performed in 1997 when evidence of growth was first noticed. Intra-operative echography (Fig. 2A) shows the tumor size to be $14 \times 13 \times 4.7$ mm, and the A-scan (Fig. 2B) shows the low-to-medium internal reflectivity pre-operatively. Intra-operative echography shows that the non-radioactive plaque is not covering the tumor margins well (Fig. 2C). Readjustment was done and the tumor margin was well covered with the radioactive plaque (Fig. 2D). Figure 2E shows an A-scan with high internal reflectivity post plaque radiotherapy, and in (Fig. 2F) the B-scan demonstrates a reduction in the tumor size to $11 \times 12.5 \times 2.7$ mm, 3 years post treatment.

Results

Mean follow-up was 26.8 months (I^{125} 35 months and Ru^{106} 8.6 months). The median

follow-up was 24 months (I^{125} 24 months and Ru^{106} 6 months). Prior to the plaque insertion 37.5% (18/48) of patients had retinal detachment, 2% (1/48) had vitreous hemorrhage, 2% (1/48) had age-related macular degeneration, and 8% (4/48) had cataracts. One patient had interstitial keratitis secondary to syphilis, 14.6% (7/48) had systemic hypertension, 20.8% (10/48) had diabetes mellitus, and 10.4% (5/48) had one or more other systemic cancers (including colon, breast, head and neck, prostate, and basal cell carcinoma). One patient was lost during follow-up and one patient had enucleation 3 months post plaque insertion due to poor local control, but no metastases were discovered during follow-up visits. Post radiation, 6% (3/48) of patients had dry eye and 16.7% (8/48) had radiation retinopathy. One patient (2%) developed cataract. No neovascular glaucoma was observed.

Placement of episcleral plaque is critical for accurate treatment delivery. We found that nearly 90% of the time (with at least one tumor margin uncovered) the dummy plaque needed readjustment on insertion under echographic visualization (Fig. 2C, D). Total time for the procedure, including the dummy plaque on insertion, echography, and radioactive plaque insertion, ranged from 10–30 min. However, the radioactive exposure time was 5–15 min, which may represent a reduction of up to 50%. Periodic finger dosimetry measurement of the surgeons' exposure time has been found to be minimal (approximately 0.2 mSv per procedure).

Discussion

The results of this study are consistent with the report by Tabandeh and colleagues[4] of 117 patients who underwent intra-operative ultrasound for I^{125} episcleral plaque localization. A 370-month follow-up showed no metastatic disease or mortality.[4] In contrast, Packer and colleagues[9] found that 17.2% of patients died of metastasis, 7.8% had local recurrence, 45.3% developed cataract, 3.1% had keratitis, 10.9% were found to have neovascular glaucoma, 23.4% had radiation retinopathy, and 17.2% required enucleation. In the present study, we experienced postradiation complications less frequently: 6% had dry eye, 16.7% had radiation retinopathy, and 2% developed cataract. No neovascular glaucoma or mortalities were detected during our follow-up period. This could be due to the smaller sample size and shorter follow-up period in our study. Raivio[10] reported 359 patients diagnosed with uveal melanoma between 1923 and 1966 in Finland, and the 5-, 10-, and 15-year survival rates based on melanoma-related deaths were 65%, 52%, and 46% respectively.

In our study, intra-operative echography showed that 90% of the nonradioactive plaques were found to be malpositioned, that is either noncoverage of one or more of the tumor margins of more than or equal to 0.5 mm or suboptimal centration of the plaque despite coverage of all the tumor margins. Fifteen percent of the malpositioned plaques were greater than 2 mm off center. A similar frequency (14%) of suboptimal positioning of plaques was reported by Harbour and co-workers[11] Finger[12]

remarked in his study that intra-operative ultrasound aids in making plaque radiation therapy more accurate, but may add time to plaque insertion and greater exposure to radiation for the surgeons and healthcare personnel. Laube and colleagues[13] remarked that radioactive plaque operations are safe but the time for plaque handling should be minimized. Surgeon dose exposure is dependent on the duration of the surgery, distance from plaque, and plaque activity. Intra-operative ultrasound without the use of a dummy aids in making plaque radiation therapy more accurate but may also add time to plaque insertion and greater radiation exposure to the surgeon and healthcare personnel.[7]

Laube and colleagues[13] found that the duration of an eye plaque operation is approximately 30 min but extend to 50 min in 10–15% of cases. This is consistent with our study, in which the total time for the procedure including the dummy plaque, echography, and radioactive plaque insertion ranged from 10–30 min. Ultrasound imaging time ranged from 1–4 min. The surgeon exposure time ranged between 5–10 min; a reduction of 50%, since the exact location is predetermined by the control plaque and prefixation of the sutures at the tumor site prior to handling of the radioactive plaque. There was a trend toward I^{125} plaque insertion taking longer than Ru^{106}. As Ru^{106} plaques are thinner (1 mm) than I^{125} (4.5 mm), they are technically easier to insert. Another consideration is that more I^{125} plaques were used for posteriorly located tumors, which are more time consuming. The periodic ring dosimetry initial results estimated that the surgeon radiation exposure is approximately 0.2 mSv per procedure. The yearly limit to extremities (finger, hands, etc.) is 500 mSv for nuclear energy workers and 50 mSv for the general public.[14] This indicates that the current technique of localizing the exact site of plaque insertion through use of the dummy plaque prior to radioactive plaque exposure is well within the safety limits if the "plaquing" surgeon is considered to be a member of the general public.

Conclusion

Echographic localization can be used to localize precisely the tumor–plaque relationship allowing for immediate repositioning of the plaque if required. Intraoperative echography improves localization in choroidal melanoma, enhances treatment success, and may reduce complication rates. In addition, the use of the dummy plaque technique in localizing the insertion site may reduce exposure time and reduce the risk of the radiation exposure for surgeons and healthcare personnel. Longer follow-up of plaque-irradiated patients with the aid of intraoperative echography is needed.

Conflicts of Interest

The authors declare no conflicts of interest.

References

1. Egan, K.M., J.M. Seddon, R.J. Glynn, *et al*. 1988. Epidemiologic aspects of uveal melanoma. *Surv. Ophthalmol*. **32:** 239–251.
2. Augsburger, J.J. 1993. Diagnosis and management of posterior uveal tumors. In *Practical Atlas of Retinal Disease and Therapy*. W.R. Freeman, Ed. 103–124. Raven Press. New York.
3. Shields, J.A., C.L. Shields, P. De Potter, *et al*. 1993. Plaque radiotherapy for uveal melanoma. *Int. Ophthalmol. Clin*. **33:** 129–135.
4. Tabandeh, H., N.A. Chaudhry, T.G. Murray, *et al*. 2000. Intraoperative echographic localization of iodine-125 episcleral plaque for brachytherapy of choroidal melanoma. *Am. J. Ophthalmol*. **129:** 199–204.
5. Finger, P.T. 1997. Radiation therapy for choroidal melanoma. *Surv. Ophthalmol*. **42:** 215–232.
6. Collaborative Ocular Melanoma Group. 1993. Design and methods of clinical trial for rare condition: the collaborative ocular melanoma study. *Controlled Clinical Trials* **3:** 362–391.
7. Earle, J., R.W. Kline & D.M. Robertson. 1987. Selection of iodine 125 for the Collaborative Ocular Melanoma Study. *Arch. Ophthalmol*. **105:** 763–764.
8. Evans, M.D., M.A. Astrahan & R. Bate. 1993. Tumor localization using fundus view photography for episcleral plaque therapy. *Med. Phys*. **20:** 769–775.
9. Packer, S., S. Stoller, M.L. Lesser, *et al*. 1992. Long-term results of iodine 125 irradiation of uveal melanoma. *Ophthalmology* **99:** 767–773.
10. Raivio, I. 1977. Uveal melanoma in Finland. An epidemiological, clinical, histological and prognostic study. *Acta Ophthalmol*. Suppl: 1–64.
11. Harbour, J.W., T.G. Murray, S.F. Byrne, *et al*. 1996. Intraoperative echographic localization of iodine 125 episcleral radioactive plaques for posterior uveal melanoma. *Retina* **16:** 129–134.
12. Finger, P.T. 2000. Intraoperative echographic localization of iodine-125 episcleral plaque for brachytherapy of choroidal melanoma. *Am. J. Ophthalmol*. **130:** 539–540.
13. Laube, T., D. Fluhs, C. Kessler, *et al*. 2000. Determination of surgeon's absorbed dose in iodine 125 and ruthenium 106 ophthalmic plaque surgery. *Ophthalmology* **107:** 366–368.
14. Canadian Nuclear Safety Commission. 2000. Radiation protection regulation. Part 2[134], 1128. Canada Gazette.

Iodine-125 Radiotherapy for Choroidal Melanoma

Tahra Al Mahmoud,[a] Magdi Mansour,[a] Jean Deschênes,[a] Chaim Edelstein,[a] Miguel Burnier,[a] Michel Marcil,[b] George Shenouda,[c] Christine Corriveau,[e] and Michael Evans[d]

[a]*Department of Ophthalmology,* [b]*Department of Medicine,* [c]*Department of Radiation Oncology,* [d]*Medical Physics Unit, McGill University, Montréal, Québec, Canada*

[e]*Department of Ophthalmology, Notre Dame Hospital, Montréal, Québec, Canada*

The objective was to evaluate the effect of the gender, size, and tumor location at the time of the diagnosis on the regression response of choroidal melanoma following plaque radiotherapy treatment. The paper is a longitudinal prospective study of 28 patients diagnosed with choroidal melanoma at McGill University Health Centre from 1997 to 2002. All patients were treated with episcleral iodine-125 (I^{125}) plaque radiotherapy. Plaques were inserted at the tumor site under echographic visualization. All patients had medium-size tumors, except for three. Patients had periodic ophthalmic evaluation at 3 and 6 months post radiation treatment, followed by 6-month intervals thereafter. Patients' mean age was 62 ± 15 years, 16 males and 12 females. Fifty percent of the tumors were located posterior to the equator with significant reduction in size at 12 months post plaque radiotherapy treatment. Significant regression was observed in all the tumor diameters at 5 years post treatment follow-up. Reduction in the depth diameter was significant ($P < 0.01$) in both male and female groups post treatment. There was a 25% ($P < 0.001$) reduction in the medium size of tumors at 5-year follow-up. Tumors located posterior to the equator responded best to I^{125} plaque radiotherapy. Male patients responded better than females to treatment. Medium-size melanoma responded well to plaque radiotherapy.

Key words: choroidal melanoma; I^{125}; radiotherapy

Introduction

Choroidal melanoma is the most common primary intraocular malignancy and is the only primary ocular tumor that can be fatal in adults.[1] Approximately half of patients die from the disease within 10 to 15 years of enucleation.[2,3] Despite diagnostic advances and introduction of new treatment modalities, the rate of metastasis has not been substantially reduced,[2] with highest rates of metastasis occurring within the first 5 years after enucleation.[1] Plaque radiotherapy is an important treatment alternative for patients with intraocular tumor. It is the most common form of radiotherapy used for choroidal melanoma.[4–6] It offers patients the possibility of eye preservation and possible useful vision.[7] However it is associated with a 4–18% rate of tumor recurrence.[6,8–13] In addition, the effects of irradiation on healthy tissues surrounding the radioactive plaque with iodine-125 (I^{125}) and ruthenium-106 (Ru^{106}) have been found to be less damaging to normal ocular structures when compared with other radioactive materials, such as cobalt-60 (Co^{60}).[14,15]

Address for correspondence: Tahra AlMahmoud, MBBS, United Arab Emirates University, Faculty of Medicine and Health Sciences, P. O. Box: 17666, Al Ain, United Arab Emirates. Voice: +971-3-7137580; fax: +971-3-7672067. uaecyc27@hotmail.com

Ann. N.Y. Acad. Sci. 1138: 15–18 (2008). © 2008 New York Academy of Sciences.
doi: 10.1196/annals.1414.003

TABLE 1. Patients' Demographic Data and Number of Patients at Each Follow-up Visit

	Total patients[†]		Months after intervention							
	n	Mean age	3	6	12	18	24	36	48	60
Male	16	62 ± 13	16	15	14	13	11	9	4	0
Female	12	63 ± 18	12	11	10	10	9	8	6	3

[†]At the beginning of the study.

Patients and Methods

Clinical records and echographic data of all patients with choroidal melanoma who were treated with I^{125} plaque irradiation along with intra-operative echographic plaque localization at McGill University Health Centre (MUHC) between January 1997 and December 2002 were reviewed. Diagnosis of choroidal melanoma was made prior to the treatment. The Collaborative Ocular Melanoma Study (COMS) protocol was followed for categorization of tumor size. A tumor was classified as small if the height (depth) was less than 2.5 mm and/or base (transverse) diameter was less than or equal to 8 mm. The tumor was considered medium in size if the height was equal to or greater than 2.5 mm and less than or equal to 10.0 mm and/or its base diameter was greater than or equal to 8.1 and less than or equal to 16.0 mm. Large tumors were those of height greater than or equal to 10.1 and/or base diameter greater or equal to 16.1 mm.[16] Tumors were also classified according to their location in the eye. Tumors were considered in location *I* (equatorial), if 50% or more of the diameter was located within the equator area; location *II* (posterior to the equator), if 50% or more of the tumor diameter was posterior to the equator; location *III* (anterior), if more than 50% of the diameter of the tumor was anterior to equator; and location *IV* (close to optic nerve), if it was centered within 5° from the optic nerve. Patients were followed-up at a mean interval of 6 months for 5 years postoperatively and once a year thereafter. Age, sex, eye involved, and tumor diameters (transverse, height, and depth) were recorded prior to and

after plaque radiotherapy. During these follow-up visits; visual acuity, intraocular pressure, slit lamp, and dilated fundal exam were performed for both eyes, in addition to echographic examinations for the involved eye. Complete systemic evaluation, chest X-ray, and liver function tests were performed upon diagnosis and annually thereafter. Forty-eight eyes in 48 patients underwent plaque radiotherapy insertion during the study period. Exclusion criteria were follow-up of less than 3 months post plaque insertion (3 patients), loss of follow-up of 3 or more consecutive visits (1 patient), enucleation (1 patient required enucleation at 3 months post radioactive plaque insertion due to failure of local control and continued growth of the tumor), and Ru^{106} plaque insertion (15 patients). Inclusion criteria were at least 3 months follow-up post radioactive plaque insertion and I^{125} plaque radiotherapy use as the treatment modality. A total of 28 patients were included in this study. Student's *t*-tests, one-way analysis of variance (ANOVA), and polynomial regression analysis were performed with the Prism Instat program.

Results

Twenty-eight eyes of 28 patients, 16 males (57%) and 12 females (43%) with mean age of 62 ± 15 years, were included in the analysis (Table 1). With at least 1 year follow-up in all patients, no metastasis was detected. Retinal detachment was present in nine eyes (32%), additional nonmelanoma tumor was present in four (14%) patients. All patients had medium-size tumors based on the COMS classification,

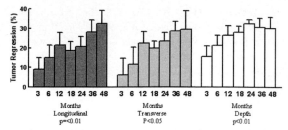

Figure 1. Tumor response to plaque radiotherapy in the male group. The different diameters (longitudinal, transverse, or depth) were measured over a 4-year follow-up period.

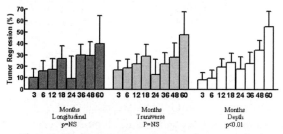

Figure 2. Tumor response to plaque radiotherapy in the female group. The different diameters (longitudinal, transverse or depth) were measured over 5-year follow-up period.

except for three lesions, which were 0.25 mm out of the range, two of these fell in the large-size group and one in the small-size group. Tumors at the equator accounted for 18% (5/28) and anterior to the equator 18% (5/28); 14% (4/28) were near the optic nerve, and 50% (14/28) posterior to the equator. During a mean of 5 years follow-up there was a significant reduction in size of 25% ($P < 0.001$) in the medium-size tumor group, 43% in the small-size, and 8% in the large-size group. However, there the numbers of patients in the latter two groups were too small for detection of statistical significance. Figure 1 shows a reduction of the tumor size—statistically significant in the longitudinal, transverse, and depth diameters—in the male group, while in the female group a significant reduction was observed in the depth diameter only (Fig. 2). Tumors located posterior and anterior to the equator responded well to the plaque radioactive treatment, with 31% and 30% reductions in size respectively at 5 years follow-up.

Discussion

In this study males were predominant; this is consistent with the study of Yanoff and Zimmerman who reported a 6:4 male-to-female ratio in a group of 100 eyes referred to the Armed Forces Institute of Pathology.[17] The male group responded better than the female group in terms of regression in all tumor diameters, while females showed a significant reduction only in depth. However, studies showed similar long-term survival rates in both groups. This supports the view that tumor depth is the main parameter to monitor melanoma growth, or it may implicate some other differences between the two genders that deserve further investigation.

Medium-size tumors responded well to plaque radiotherapy. The other groups were of small sample size, which made comment on the treatment response difficult.

Conclusion

In our study population tumors located posterior to the equator responded best to the treatment. Despite the differences observed in the effects of the plaque radiotherapy on the transverse and longitudinal diameters in the male and female groups, the only common similar response has been shown to be in the depth variable. Taking into consideration the similar long term survival rate, this might be an adequate indicator for monitoring tumor size during follow up. Plaque radiotherapy is an effective treatment in controlling the growth of choroidal melanoma. In total, tumor diameters regressed by 25–54% depending on the variable measured (longitudinal, transverse, or depth).

Future Research

1. Longer follow-up of plaque-irradiated patients is needed to determine the metastasis rate in the long-term post treatment.

2. Despite previous studies indicating that overall survival of patients treated with plaque radiotherapy is comparable to other management techniques,[18,19] would incorporating intra-operative echographic localization of plaque for choroidal melanoma improve patient care by enabling the delivery of radiation precisely to the tumor?

3. Why did tumors in the male group respond significantly better in more than one diameter compared to the female group? This needs to be investigated in larger study group.

4. Should plaque radiotherapy be used for choroidal melanoma in locations anterior and posterior to equator tumors, since these tumors responded the best of all to the radioactive plaque treatment? Further studies are required before one can recommend this treatment approach as the "standard of care."

Conflicts of Interest

The authors declare no conflicts of interest.

References

1. Egan, K.M., J.M. Seddon, R.J. Glynn, *et al.* 1988. Epidemiologic aspect of uveal melanoma. *Surv. Ophthalmol.* **32:** 239–251.

2. Jensen, O.A. 1982. Malignant melanomas of the human uvea: 25-year follow-up of cases in Denmark, 1943–1952. *Acta Ophthalmol.* **60:** 161–182.

3. Ravio, I. 1977. Uveal melanoma in Finland: an epidemiological, clinical, histological and prognostic study. *Acta Ophthalmol.* **133:** 3–64.

4. Augsburger, J.J. 1993. Diagnosis and management of posterior uveal tumors. In *Practical Atlas of Retinal Disease and Therapy.* W.R. Freeman, Ed.: 103–124. Raven Press. New York.

5. Shields, J.A., C.L. Shield, P. De Potter, *et al.* 1993. Plaque radiotherapy for uveal melanoma. *Int. Ophthalmol. Clin.* **33:** 129–135.

6. Tabandeh, H., N.A. Chaudhry, T.G. Murry, *et al.* 2000. Intraoperative echographic localization of iodine-[125] episcleral plaque for brachytherapy of choroidal melanoma. *Am. J. Ophthalmol.* **129:** 199–204.

7. Finger, P.T. 1997. Radiation therapy for choroidal melanoma. *Surv. Ophthalmol.* **42:** 215–232.

8. Char, D.H., J.M. Quivery, J.R. Castro, *et al.* 1993. Helium ions versus iodine[125] brachytherapy in the management of uveal melanoma. A prospective, randomized, dynamically balanced trial. *Ophthalmology* **100:** 1547–1554.

9. Karlsson, U.L., J.J. Augsburger, J.A. Shields, *et al.* 1989. Recurrence of posterior uveal melanoma after Co[60] episcleral plaque therapy. *Ophthalmology* **96:** 382–388.

10. Garreston, B.R., D.M. Roberston & J.D. Earle. 1987. Choroidal melanoma treatment with iodine[125] brachytherapy. *Arch. Ophthalmol.* **105:** 1394–1397.

11. Packer, S., M. Rotman, P. Salantro. 1984. Iodine-[125] irradiation of choroidal melanoma: clinical experience. *Ophthalmology* **91:** 1700–1708.

12. Gass, J.D.M. 1985. Comparison of prognosis after enucleation vs cobalt[60] irradiation of melanomas. *Arch. Ophthalmol.* **103:** 916–923.

13. Lommatzch, P.K. 1983. B-irradiation of choroidal melanoma with Ru[106]/Rh[106] application. *Arch. Ophthalmol.* **101:** 713–717.

14. Lommatzsch, P.K. & I.H. Kirsch. 1988. Ru[106]/Rh[106] plaque radiotherapy for malignant melanomas of the choroid: with follow-up results more than 5 years. *Doc. Ophthalmol.* **68:** 225–238.

15. Earle, J.D., W.K. Robert, M.R. Dennis, *et al.* 1987. Selection of Iodine[125] for the collaborative ocular melanoma study. *Arch. Ophthalmol.* **105:** 763–764.

16. Collaborative Ocular Melanoma Group. 1993. Design and methods of clinical trial for rare condition: the collaborative ocular melanoma study. *Controlled Trials* **3:** 362–391.

17. Yanoff, M., Zimmerman L.E. 1967. Histogenesis of malignant melanoma of uvea. II. Relation of uveal nevi to malignant melanomas. Cancer. 77:493–507.

18. Augsburger, J.J., J.W. Gamel, K. Lauritzen, *et al.* 1990. Cobalt[60] plaque radiotherapy vs enucleation for posterior uveal melanoma. *Am. J. Ophthalmol.* **109:** 585–592.

19. Augsburger, J.J., Z.M. Correa, J. Friere & L.W. Brady. 1998. Long term survival in choroidal and ciliary body melanoma after enucleation versus plaque radiation therapy. *Ophthalmology* **105:** 1670–1678.

Update on Recent Developments for Patients with Newly Diagnosed Multiple Myeloma

Antonio Palumbo, Valeria Magarotto, Francesca Gay, Patrizia Falco, Sara Bringhen, and Mario Boccadoro

Divisione di Ematologia dell'Università di Torino, Torino, Italy

Recent studies have demonstrated that novel therapeutic combinations are challenging melphalan and prednisone (MP) as the standard of care in elderly patients with multiple myeloma. Combination regimens containing bortezomib or thalidomide can achieve response rates, especially complete response rates, which are superior to those seen with standard MP alone, and offer new possibilities for this patient population.

Key words: multiple myeloma; bortezomib; thalidomide; lenalidomide

With a median age at diagnosis of 63 years, multiple myeloma (MM) is a disease of the elderly and any new treatment must demonstrate efficacy and tolerability in this patient population.

The Phase III APEX trial, which investigated bortezomib treatment in patients with relapsed MM, included patients aged >65 years (of 333 bortezomib-treated patients, 125 were aged ≥65 years). Bortezomib was found to be equally effective in elderly and younger patients; the response rate and time to progression did not differ substantially between the two groups.[1] In addition, the overall incidence of grade 3/4 adverse events was comparable in elderly and younger patients, indicating that bortezomib is equally well tolerated across all age groups.[1]

The success of bortezomib in the treatment of relapsed and refractory MM provides the rationale for its use in the treatment of newly diagnosed disease, both as single agent and in combination with conventional chemotherapy and autologous stem cell transplantation. In a Phase II study in patients with previously untreated MM, an overall response rate (ORR) of 90%, with a complete response (CR) plus near CR (nCR) rate of 19%, was achieved in 48 evaluable patients receiving bortezomib plus dexamethasone.[2] Dexamethasone was added in patients with less than a partial response (PR) after two cycles or less than a CR after four cycles. Typically, responses were rapid and increased cumulatively over the first six treatment cycles. Best response was achieved after two cycles in 40%, after four cycles in 79%, and after six cycles in 90% of patients. An improved response was seen after the addition of dexamethasone in 23 patients. The most common adverse events were neuropathy, fatigue, constipation, nausea, and neutropenia. Overall, adverse events were found to be predictable and manageable.[2]

Bortezomib is also undergoing investigation in the first-line setting for elderly patients. Mateos[3] conducted a Phase I/II study to evaluate the effect of adding bortezomib to melphalan and prednisone (MP) in elderly patients (aged >65 years) with untreated MM. The median age of the 60 enrolled patients was 74 years (range 65–85 years), with almost half of all patients (47%) aged >75 years. Analysis of response rates after cycle 1 revealed an ORR of 70% (6% CR, 2% nCR, and 64% PR rates), demonstrating that response rates

Address for correspondence: Antonio Palumbo, MD, Divisione di Ematologia dell'Università di Torino, Azienda Ospedaliera S. Giovanni Battista, Via Genova 3, 10126 Torino, Italy. Voice: +390116635814; fax: +390116963737. appalumbo@yahoo.com

Ann. N.Y. Acad. Sci. 1138: 19–21 (2008). © 2008 New York Academy of Sciences.
doi: 10.1196/annals.1414.004

with a combination of bortezomib and MP (MPV) after only one cycle of therapy were significantly higher than those typically observed after six cycles of treatment with MP alone.[4] Best-response analysis with MPV after a median of five cycles revealed an ORR of 86% (30% CR, 13% nCR, 43% PR rates); efficacy of MPV was comparable across all age groups (i.e., in patients aged <75 and >75 years). With a median follow-up of 10.5 months, event-free survival (EFS) and progression-free survival (PFS) were 85% and 93%, respectively.

Toxicity was manageable and similar to that previously observed in other bortezomib studies. The most common grade 3/4 toxicities included thrombocytopenia (52%), neutropenia (43%), infection (17%), diarrhea (17%), and anemia (10%). Thirty-five percent of patients required bortezomib dose reduction, mostly due to neuropathy. Peripheral neuropathy was found to be more common in patients aged >75 years than in those aged <75 years, possibly due to the generally more frail physical condition of the older patients. Overall, toxicities were found to decrease after cycle 3.

Based on the positive results of the Phase I/II MPV study, a Phase III, multicenter, international trial of bortezomib in combination with MP versus MP alone is currently ongoing in patients with newly diagnosed disease who are not transplant candidates. The study will assess the efficacy, overall safety, and tolerability of MPV versus MP alone and will examine whether MPV is superior to MP, the current standard of care in elderly patients with MM.

Thalidomide is also undergoing investigation in the first-line treatment of MM. Two studies that examined the addition of thalidomide to standard MP therapy (MPT) for the treatment of elderly patients with newly diagnosed MM were presented at the 2005 meeting of the American Society of Hematology.[5–7] In both studies, the MPT regimen was associated with higher ORR and CR rates. In addition, PFS and EFS were found to be prolonged with MPT treatment compared with MP,[5–7] which translated into a significant improvement in overall survival in one of the studies.[5]

Not unexpectedly, MPT was associated with more toxicities than the MP regimen. Grade 3/4 adverse events were reported in 48% of patients receiving MPT, compared with 25% of patients treated with MP.[7] Deep vein thrombosis (DVT) occurred in 12% of patients receiving MPT and in 5% receiving MP in the study by Facon.[5] Similarly, in the Palumbo study, grade 3/4 thromboembolic events were noted in 12% and 2% of patients treated with MPT and MP, respectively.[7] Neuropathy was observed in 30% of patients receiving MPT in one study, and this was grade 3/4 in 8% of patients treated with MPT in the second study.[5,7] Dose modification was required in a large number of thalidomide-treated patients. In 29% of patients, the dose had to be reduced to 50 mg/day, and thalidomide treatment had to be discontinued in 33% of patients.[7]

Lenalidomide is another novel agent that is being evaluated in the relapsed/refractory setting and has also been studied in combination with MP in a trial in elderly patients with newly diagnosed MM.[8] An ORR of 70% (10% CR rate) was observed with the combination of lenalidomide and MP as first-line therapy; however, the regimen was associated with toxicities, notably grade 3/4 neutropenia in 58% of patients. Thromboembolism occurred in 3% of patients, with all patients receiving aspirin to reduce the risk.

Acknowledgments

We thank the patients, physicians, data managing (Maria Josè Fornaro, Tiziana Marangon), and nursing staff (Tiziana De Lazzer, Ornella Tresoldi, Manuela Grasso, Michela Verbale).

Conflicts of Interest

The authors declare no conflicts of interest.

References

1. Richardson, P.G. 2005. Safety and efficacy of bortezomib in high-risk and elderly patients with relapsed myeloma. *J. Clin. Oncol.* **23:** 568s (Abstract 6533).
2. Jagannath, S. 2005. Bortezomib therapy alone and in combination with dexamethasone for patients with previously untreated multiple myeloma. *Blood* **106** (Abstract 783).
3. Mateos, M. 2005. A phase I/II national, multicenter, open-label study of bortezomib plus melphalan and prednisone (V-MP) in elderly untreated multiple myeloma (MM) patients. *Blood* **106** (Abstract 786).
4. Hernandez, J.M. 2004. Randomized comparison of dexamethasone combined with melphalan versus melphalan with prednisone in the treatment of elderly patients with multiple myeloma. *Br. J. Haematol.* **127:** 159–164.
5. Facon, T. 2005. Major superiority of melphalan – prednisone (MP) + thalidomide (THAL) over MP and autologous stem cell transplantation in the treatment of newly diagnosed elderly patients with multiple myeloma. *Blood* **106** (Abstract 780).
6. Palumbo, A. 2005. Oral melphalan, prednisone and thalidomide for multiple myeloma. *Blood* **106** (Abstract 779).
7. Palumbo, A. 2006. Oral melphalan and prednisone chemotherapy plus thalidomide compared with melphalan and prednisone alone in elderly patients with multiple myeloma: randomised controlled trial. *Lancet* **367:** 825–831.
8. Palumbo, A. 2005. Oral Revlimid® Plus melphalan and prednisone (R-MP) for newly diagnosed multiple myeloma. *Blood* **106** (Abstract 785).

Advances in the Management of Pediatric Central Nervous System Tumors

Shaker Abdullah,[a] Ibrahim Qaddoumi,[b] and Eric Bouffet[c]

[a]*Department of Oncology, King Abdulaziz Medical City-Jeddah, Jeddah, Kingdom of Saudi Arabia*

[b]*International Outreach Program, St. Jude Children's Research Hospital, Memphis, Tennessee, USA*

[c]*Paediatric Brain Tumour Program, Division of Haematology/Oncology, Hospital for Sick Children, Toronto, Ontario, Canada*

Central nervous system tumors are the most common pediatric solid tumors and a leading cause of cancer-related mortality and morbidity in this age group. Survival rates have improved significantly over the last decades for most of the tumor types, as a consequence of improvements in neuroimaging, neurosurgery and neuroanesthesia, radiation oncology, and medical oncology. The complexity of the management of these patients requires a multidisciplinary approach and has led to the emergence of a new subspecialty of pediatric neuro-oncologists who are dedicated to the management and follow-up of this population. This review highlights the most critical advances in the diagnostic and treatment modalities of pediatric brain tumors. A specific review of the most common tumor types discusses treatment options, controversies, and ongoing developments, with an emphasis on cooperative trials.

Key words: **brain tumor; children; medulloblastoma; glioma; ependymoma; cooperative trials**

Over the last decade, increasing awareness has emerged concerning the specific place of central nervous system (CNS) tumors in pediatric oncology. CNS tumors are the most common childhood solid tumors and a leading cause of cancer-related mortality and morbidity in this age group. Several factors affect the management of these tumors, and one of the main challenges, which increases the complexity of the management of childhood brain tumors, is the immaturity of the CNS in children. Treatment choices in pediatric CNS tumors are guided by histological diagnosis, stage of disease, and the patient's individual characteristics, particularly age, which may influence treatment deci-

sions and subsequent outcomes. The increasing complexity of this discipline has led to the emergence of a new subspecialty of pediatric neuro-oncologists who are dedicated to the management and follow-up of this population.[1] Still, few pediatric oncology units have a dedicated pediatric neuro-oncologist, and many places still lack multidisciplinary coordination and cooperation in the management of pediatric brain tumors. This review addresses some of the current issues concerning the care of the most common pediatric brain tumors, with an emphasis on recent developments and new perspectives in clinical research.

Diagnosis and Diagnostic Imaging

Many reports have pointed out the difficulty in establishing a timely diagnosis of brain tumor in children. The delay in the diagnosis of pediatric brain tumors is certainly

Address for correspondence: Dr Eric Bouffet, Director of the Paediatric Brain Tumour Program, Professor of Paediatrics, Division of Haematology/Oncology, The Hospital for Sick Children, 555 University Avenue, Toronto M5G 1X8, Canada. Voice: +1-416-813-7457; fax: +416-813-8024. eric.bouffet@sickkids.ca

Ann. N.Y. Acad. Sci. 1138: 22–31 (2008). © 2008 New York Academy of Sciences.
doi: 10.1196/annals.1414.005

multifactorial.[2] Infants and young children might not be able to voice complaints, such as headaches, decreased visual acuity, or other neurological symptoms. The heterogeneity of initial neurological features and the lack of specificity of the most commons signs and symptoms (such as headaches and vomiting), which may mimic other more common diagnoses often contribute to delays in the diagnosis of brain tumors in this age group. Recent reports have drawn attention to the importance of behavioral symptoms, which account for up to one-fifth of initial symptoms in children.[2,3] Contrary to expectations, the introduction of modern imaging techniques has not influenced the delay between the first symptoms and the diagnosis, which appears unchanged in the literature since the 1980s.[4–6] Increasing awareness of the issues associated with the diagnosis of brain tumors in children among community healthcare professionals may contribute to limiting delays in diagnosis. However, whether this may translate into improved outcome is still unknown. Once the diagnosis is suspected, modern imaging techniques, especially computed tomography (CT) and magnetic resonance imaging (MRI) scans, undoubtedly facilitate the diagnostic process by providing information, such as tumor location, tumor extent, enhancing patterns, and resectability.[7] Although many children may have an initial CT as a screening imaging, the use of diagnostic MRI has now become standard in most institutions. Some tumors may show typical MRI characteristics, which allow precise diagnosis and initiation of treatment without the need for histological confirmation. This is particularly the case for diffuse pontine gliomas, tectal plate glioma and chiasmatic/hypothalamic gliomas.[8] Attempts at radiologically predicting histological diagnosis have been only marginally successful, and the use of magnetic resonance spectroscopy (MRS) remains investigational.[8–10] Therefore, most tumors will require histological confirmation. When radiological characteristics are in favor of malignant tumor, the use of preoperative MRI scan of the spine is highly recommended, particularly in the presence of a posterior fossa tumor. This allows detection of leptomeningeal spread. The use of preoperative MRI staging prevents false positive signals due postsurgical artifacts secondary to inflammation, edema, or scarring particularly in the upper cervical spine and in the lower spine.[11]

Surgery

Surgery is the mainstay of treatment for the majority of pediatric brain tumors. Surgery is curative in most low-grade tumors located in accessible areas. This is particularly the case of cerebellar astrocytomas, which account for nearly 10% of all pediatric CNS tumors.[12] In most malignant brain tumors, the role of surgery is also critical, although additional postoperative treatment is required. The extent of resection is a major prognostic factor in medulloblastoma, ependymoma, choroid plexus carcinoma, atypical rhabdoid teratoid tumors, and even in high-grade gliomas (HGG).[13–17] Technical advances have made neurosurgery safer and have reduced the complication rate.[18] This includes preoperative assessment of the surgical risk and resectability using functional MRI, magnetoencephalography, or more recently tractography.[19] Depending on the tumor type and location, surgeons may use image-guided stereotactic techniques, intraoperative electophysiologic monitoring, or electrocorticography. Because of the paramount importance of resection on outcome in some pediatric brain tumors, a second operation may be advocated when resection is incomplete. This may be considered immediately or after chemotherapy.

Radiation Treatment

Although there is a general reluctance among pediatricians to use radiation in children, the role of this treatment modality is still critical in the management of many pediatric brain tumors, particularly for malignant lesions.

The role of radiation has evolved during the last three decades, particularly in the management of young children. Radiation was used widely in the 1970s, including in the very young, and early medulloblastoma protocols used standard doses of craniospinal radiation in children from the age of 18 months.[20,21] Following significant concerns over the intellectual outcome of irradiated infants, the next generation of protocols recommended delaying radiation until the age of 3 years.[22] During the 1990s and more recently, several cooperative studies were developed with the aim of avoiding radiation therapy in young children. However, major advances in radiation techniques explain the recent reintroduction of radiation in the therapeutic arsenal of infant brain tumors.[23] Newer focal radiation techniques are able to limit the highest dose to the tumor bed and, therefore, to reduce the side effects of the treatment to the surrounding structures. Pilot studies have demonstrated the short-term safety of these new techniques and as a consequence, radiation has been reintroduced recently in the management of some malignant brain tumors in infants, especially for ependymoma and medulloblastoma.[24] The role of proton therapy is still under investigation, but the main limitation of this technique is its cost, which precludes its availability and use as a standard treatment.[25]

Chemotherapy

Disappointingly, only a limited number of new antineoplastic agents have emerged in the field of pediatric neuro-oncology over the last decade, and most agents currently used in the management of pediatric brain tumors were already available two or three decades ago. Temozolomide (TMZ), a promising agent in the treatment of HGG in adults, has given disappointing results in pediatric neuro-oncology.[26,27] Other agents, such as irinotecan, are still under investigation in phase II studies, and their role in the management of newly diagnosed or recurrent brain tumors is still unclear. However, advances in the chemotherapeutic management of childhood brain tumors have been significant, with the development of high-dose chemotherapy protocols followed by progenitor cell rescue, or more recently of sequential high-dose chemotherapy, which may achieve a higher dose exposure with less toxic morbidity.[28] Other chemotherapeutic approaches have been explored, such as low-dose schedules or concomitant chemoradiotherapeutic strategies.

Common Pediatric CNS Tumors

Low-Grade Gliomas

Low-grade gliomas (LGG) represent the largest group of CNS tumors in childhood, accounting for one-third of all brain tumors in this age group. LGG can arise in any part of the CNS. The term LGG includes all World Health Organization (WHO) grade I and grade II gliomas. In children, the most common histological type by far is the juvenile pilocytic astrocytoma (grade I). The behavior of LGG can be erratic. Most LGG have an indolent course, but some tumors may present with aggressive behavior and can even disseminate to the neuraxis.[29] Dissemination is more specific of hypothalamic LGG and more common in younger children who seem to present with more aggressive tumors. The recent identification of a pilomyxoid subtype of pilocytic astrocytoma may in part explain differences in the behavior of these tumors in younger children.[30]

Surgery is the treatment of choice of pediatric LGG, when the tumor can be safely removed with an acceptable risk of neurological morbidity.[18] This is the case for cerebellar LGG, which are often cured by surgical resection and associated with an excellent outcome.[12] However, some LGG are located in areas that are not amenable to radical resection or are associated with a significant risk of permanent neurological damage following aggressive surgery. This is particularly so for tumors arising in the diencephalon, in the hypothalamic/chiasmatic region, or in the basal ganglia. For these lesions, the role of surgery is limited and other forms of treatment should be considered. Both radiation and chemotherapy have shown activity in pediatric LGG, but the respective role of each treatment modality is still a matter of debate.[31]

Chemotherapy can produce significant tumor shrinkage or tumor stabilization. Several agents and combinations have been evaluated. The choice of the chemotherapeutic agents should take into account the activity of the drugs and their short- and long-term side effects.[32] The ideal agent or combination should have a good activity profile and no, or very moderate, short- and long-term toxicity. For this reason, the vincristine–carboplatin combination is favored by many oncologists.[33,34] Its main limitation is the risk of allergic reaction, which occurs in up to 40% of patients.[35] Alternative regimens are currently being explored.

Radiation is increasingly considered as a salvage option, in the case of tumor progression despite chemotherapy. Some institutions still consider radiation as the first-line treatment for older children, with different thresholds for defining "older" (e.g., 5 years or 10 years). In the absence of randomized studies, comparisons between radiation and chemotherapy are difficult. There is a growing body of evidence that chemotherapy can delay progression of LGG and may obviate the need of radiation in some patients. For this reason, there is currently a trend toward using chemotherapy as a first option and even to use chemotherapy for subsequent progression. As a consequence, the respective role of chemotherapy and radiation is evolving. Radiation has been held responsible for several long-term side effects, such as strokes, endocrine and cognitive deficits, and secondary tumors, which makes this technique less appealing in the context of a benign tumor, particularly in young children.[36] In addition, the risk of radiation-induced vascular complications and secondary tumors appears to be greater in children with neurofibromatosis type 1, an autosomal dominant disorder associ-

ated with a high prevalence of LGG of the optic pathways.[37] However, the role of the tumor itself in these long-term complications cannot be excluded, and children treated with chemotherapy only can also develop vascular complications and endocrine or cognitive deficits, particularly for tumors involving the hypothalamic region. Advances in radiation techniques may allow the use of reduced volume radiation fields, thereby minimizing the risk of late sequelae, and clinical trials are ongoing to evaluate the efficacy and toxicity of these new techniques of radiation.[38]

Medulloblastoma and Primitive Neuro-ectodermal Tumors

Medulloblastoma is the most common malignant CNS tumor in children. Major advances in the management of medulloblastoma have been achieved since the first cooperative studies took place in the late 1970s.[20,21] At that time the standard treatment of medulloblastoma was based on surgery followed by craniospinal radiation. Pilot and randomized studies have contributed to refine the staging system, to identify risk groups, and to better tailor treatment according to risk factors. With the introduction of chemotherapy and improvement in surgical and radiotherapy techniques, 5-year survival rates in patients with average-risk medulloblastoma treated with craniospinal radiation and chemotherapy exceed 80%.[39,40] Improvements in survival have led to attempts to reduce the dose of craniospinal irradiation in average-risk patients, and the standard dose of craniospinal irradiation has dropped from 36 Gy in the 1980s and early 1990s to 23.4 Gy currently. The Children's Oncology Group is currently conducting a randomized study to determine whether it is possible to reduce further the craniospinal dose of radiation therapy to 18 Gy in children 3–7 years of age.[41] Other attempts are currently under way to minimize the high dose of radiation to the cochlea, the hypothalamus, the pituitary axis, and the supratentorial brain by delivering the boost to the tumor bed rather than to the whole posterior fossa.[42] Similar trends of improved outcome are observed in high-risk medulloblastoma patients, however, the interpretation of this trend is complex and should take into account advances in imaging techniques that have allowed better detection of metastatic disease. Therefore comparisons of series of high-risk medulloblastoma patients treated in the pre-MRI and MRI era are questionable. Results of recent prospective protocols using a combination of high doses of radiation (between 36 and 40 Gy to the neuraxis) and multiagent chemotherapy have shown promising survival rates above 60% at 5 years in patients with metastases.[40]

Major advances in the understanding of the molecular biology of medulloblastoma are expected to lead to the development of new protocols based on new stratification systems taking into account clinical staging, histology, and molecular markers. Recently, a pilot study has demonstrated the feasibility of rapid molecular analysis of medulloblastoma samples from multiple institutions. Potential molecular markers for stratification are TrkC, ERBB2, C-Myc, N-MYC, and nuclear beta-catenin.[43,44] In addition, some histopathologic features have been correlated with aggressive behavior, and patients with large-cell and anaplastic medulloblastoma are currently excluded from average risk protocols.[45]

Ependymoma

Ependymoma is most commonly seen in infants and young children. Not surprisingly, the majority of ependymoma studies conducted in recent decades were related to the development of so called "baby-brain" strategies. However, major advances in surgical and radiation techniques have dramatically influenced the management of intracranial ependymoma in recent years with a consequent effect on survival.

Ependymoma can occur anywhere in the CNS, and usually arises in paraventricular locations. In children, the majority of ependymomas are located in the posterior fossa. The WHO classification describes three grades: grade I (myxopapillary) ependymomas are usually located at the spinal level and observed in adults; grade II (with the cellular, papillary, clear cell, tanycytic variants); and grade III lesions (also called anaplastic or malignant ependymoma) can be distinguished on morphological characteristics. However, the histological grading of ependymomas and its prognostic value is still uncertain. Differences in the proportion of grade II and grade III ependymoma in series are considerable and this constitutes a major obstacle toward the development of protocols tailored according to histological grading.[17]

There is a large consensus that optimal treatment of nonmetastatic ependymoma is based on maximal surgery followed by focal radiation. Results obtained with this approach depend on the extent of resection, with 5-year event survival rates in the range of 50 to 70% after complete resection.[46,47] Tumor resection may require a two-stage approach in some cases, and the role of second-look surgery is increasingly recognized as a way to achieve maximal resection in this disease.[48] Two international studies are built on the same design and recommend second-look surgery after chemotherapy for children with incomplete initial resection.[49,50] In these protocols, radiation is given immediately after initial surgery in children with complete resection, and after chemotherapy +/− second-look surgery in children with incomplete resection. Because of concerns about long-term side effects of treatment, the use of radiation in young children has been discouraged until recently. Infants and young children have been classically treated with surgery followed by adjuvant chemotherapy. However, the results of this approach are disappointing, with 5-year event-free survival rates in the range of 9 to 37%.[51] Strategies aimed at avoiding radiotherapy have been recently challenged by the results of a pilot study in which children with nonmetastatic intracranial ependymoma aged 12 months and above were treated with postoperative conformal radiation.[24] In this study the progression-free survival at 3 years for children younger than 3 years was 69.5%. At a median follow-up of 38 months all neurocognitive outcomes were within normal limits. Children younger than 3 years had a significantly lower Intelligence Quotient (IQ) compared with older children; however, this difference was already present at the time of the first evaluation and serial assessments showed a gradual increase in IQ levels over time. The result of this study has largely influenced North American practice, and postoperative conformal radiotherapy is considered the best standard of care for all children with intracranial ependymoma from the age of 12 months onwards.

The role of chemotherapy in ependymoma remains ill defined. Results of phase II studies have been disappointing, and so far, there is no evidence that the addition of chemotherapy is associated with a survival benefit.[17,52] The only recognized role of chemotherapy concerns children with incomplete initial resection. There is some suggestion that chemotherapy may facilitate second-look surgery in these patients.[48]

Better understanding of the molecular biology of ependymoma may influence the design of future protocols. Recently, retrospective studies have correlated hTERT expression and high expression of ERBB2 and ERBB4 with poorer survival.[53,54] Additional studies are ongoing to confirm these results. This may not only influence treatment strategies with the development of new stratification tools, but may also open the way to new strategies, as telomerase or tyrosine kinase inhibitors are currently available or under investigation.

High-Grade Gliomas

Malignant gliomas are among the most devastating brain tumors, leading to death in most cases. Although pediatric HGG manifest properties that clearly distinguish them from their adult counterparts, their prognosis remains disappointing. Extensive resection improves outcome, and the current recommendation is to consider aggressive debulking.[15] However, this may not always be possible because of an unacceptable risk of neurological deficit, and there is evidence that the extent of resection is site dependant. Postoperative radiation is routinely employed, except in infants and young children. Although children with HGG appear to benefit from adjuvant chemotherapy, the extent of this benefit is unclear. Two randomized studies were conducted by the Children's Cancer Group. The first study, CCG-943, demonstrated a significant difference in event-free and overall survival in the group of children treated with adjuvant chemotherapy (Lomustine, vincristine, and prednisone), particularly in children with glioblastoma.[55] The second study, CCG-945, compared two chemotherapy regimens—Lomustine-vincristine-prednisone and the eight-drugs-in-one-day combination, which had shown promising activity in phase II studies.[56] This study accrued a large number of patients, and despite the lack of difference in event-free and overall survival between the two arms, this CCG-945 protocol remains a pivotal study for the understanding of pediatric HGG. In particular, it emphasized the role of central pathology review in pediatric HGG, provided important insight into the diagnostic difficulties involving these tumors, and contributed to a better knowledge of the biology of pediatric HGG.[57-60] Several other phase II studies using single agents or combinations have demonstrated modest activity. TMZ has shown little benefit in the pediatric setting. In a phase II study for patients with recurrent HGG, the response rate was only 12%.[27] The Children's Oncology Group ACNS0126 study single-arm phase II trial of chemoradiotherapy with TMZ (90 mg/m^2/day $\times$ 42 days during X-ray therapy) followed by 10 cycles of adjuvant chemotherapy with TMZ (200 mg/m^2/day $\times$ 5 days every 28 days) accrued 107 patients.[61] Historic control cohorts from CCG-945 served as the comparative group, and no difference in survival was observed between the two cohorts. Other studies combining various agents are ongoing or in development in European and North American groups.

Diffuse Pontine Glioma

Advances in neuroimaging have resulted in a better understanding of brain stem gliomas, which are currently stratified in two categories: 20% are low grade, arising in the midbrain, medulla, or dorsal pons, radiologically often focal and dorsally exophytic, and amenable to surgical resection with a relatively good prognosis.[8] The remaining 80% of tumors are diffuse in nature, involve the majority of the pons, and have a dismal prognosis. At present, surgery has no role in the diagnosis or treatment of diffuse pontine gliomas. Although focal radiation improves symptoms in 70% of patients, this treatment is only palliative and most patients will succumb within a year of diagnosis. Numerous chemotherapy studies have been conducted over the last three decades; however, there is little, if any, evidence that chemotherapy affects the outcome of these tumors.[62] New hope is rising with the development of new targeted biological agents, such as epidermal growth factor receptor signal inhibitors, antiangiogenesis agents, and farnesyl transferase inhibitors, and several clinical trials are currently ongoing or in development.[63]

Brain Tumors in Young Children

The survival of infants and young children with CNS tumors is significantly worse than that of older children. Several factors account for this difference in prognosis. Tumor types are different, and some tumors, which are more specific to infancy, are associated with aggressive biological behavior. In addition, treatment options are limited, due to the extreme vulnerability of the developing brain, in particular to radiation. Due to these limitations, protocols were designed in the 1980s for infants and young children. The main principle of this first

generation of protocols was to use postoperative chemotherapy to delay or even to avoid radiation.[22] The results of these first experiences of prolonged postoperative chemotherapy have offered mixed results. Efforts to defer radiation had limited success, particularly in embryonal tumors, and most infants were experiencing early progression. In addition, the use of delayed radiation until the age of 3 years was still associated with major intellectual impairment and subsequent protocols tried to intensify chemotherapy in order to improve outcomes and eliminate radiotherapy.

The conclusions of most recent trials are that intensive or high-dose chemotherapy alone can be used successfully to cure infants and young children with good risk features. The identification of good risk and poor risk patients has allowed stratification, as has been done with older children. This has been particularly important in medulloblastoma protocols wherein good risk patients—patients with completely resected nonmetastatic tumors and desmoplastic histology—have achieved excellent outcomes without the use of radiation.[64] Results in patients with metastatic medulloblastoma and supratentorial primitive neuro-ectodermal tumors are still unsatisfactory, despite promising reports of high-dose chemotherapy.[65]

Utilization of radiation for local tumor control is being reconsidered for this age group, in view of the possibility of improved targeting through the use of conformal methods. This is particularly important in ependymoma, where the use of adjuvant chemotherapy has proven generally to be disappointing.[66] The use of conformal radiation has also been investigated in infants and young children with medulloblastoma and rhabdoid tumors.[14,23,24]

Conclusions

This brief overview summarizes the most significant advances that together have contributed to improve the outcome of pediatric CNS tumors. Most important is the fact that these advances have been achieved through the development of collaborative national and international trials.[67] The coming years are expected to see many critical advances: the application of improved knowledge of the molecular biology of these tumors to new biology-based stratification systems to optimize treatment, the introduction of targeted therapies into the therapeutic arsenal, and the refinement of drug delivery strategies.

Finally, as a result of increasing complexity, there an obvious risk to confining the benefit of these breakthroughs to a limited number of children worldwide. Although the development and the organization of clinical trials have been essentially limited to high-income countries, significant efforts are currently being developed to facilitate and promote the organization of pediatric neuro-oncology services and the implementation of protocols in low-income countries.[68] Ultimately, these advances should benefit all children, including those who currently live in countries where access to treatments that can save life is currently very limited or nonexistent.

Conflicts of Interest

The authors declare no conflicts of interest.

References

1. Cohen, M.E. 1993. Why a neuro-oncologist? *J. Child Neurol.* **8:** 287–291.
2. Wilne, S.H. *et al.* 2006. The presenting features of brain tumours: a review of 200 cases. *Arch. Dis. Child.* **91:** 502–506.
3. Wilne, S. *et al.* 2007. Presentation of childhood CNS tumours: a systematic review and meta-analysis. *Lancet Oncol.* **8:** 685–695.
4. Flores, L.E. *et al.* 1986. Delay in the diagnosis of pediatric brain tumors. *Am. J. Dis. Child.* **140:** 684–686.
5. Pollock, B.H., J.P. Krischer & T.J. Vietti. 1991. Interval between symptom onset and diagnosis of pediatric solid tumors. *J. Pediatr.* **119:** 725–732.
6. Mehta, V. *et al.* 2002. Latency between symptom onset and diagnosis of pediatric brain tumors: an Eastern Canadian geographic study. *Neurosurgery* **51:** 365–372; discussion 372–373.
7. Barkovich, A.J. 1992. Neuroimaging of pediatric brain tumors. *Neurosurg. Clin. North Am.* **3:** 739–769.
8. Zimmerman, R.A. 1996. Neuroimaging of pediatric brain stem diseases other than brain stem glioma. *Pediatr. Neurosurg.* **25:** 83–92.
9. Peet, A.C. *et al.* 2007. Short echo time 1 H magnetic resonance spectroscopy of childhood brain tumours. *Childs Nerv. Syst.* **23:** 163–169.
10. Peet, A.C. *et al.* 2007. Magnetic resonance spectroscopy suggests key differences in the metastatic behaviour of medulloblastoma. *Eur. J. Cancer* **43:** 1037–1044.
11. Cronqvist, S., D. Greitz & P. Maeder. 1993. Spread of blood in cerebrospinal fluid following craniotomy simulates spinal metastases. *Neuroradiology* **35:** 592–595.
12. Pencalet, P. *et al.* 1999. Benign cerebellar astrocytomas in children. *J. Neurosurg.* **90:** 265–273.
13. Zeltzer, P.M. *et al.* 1999. Metastasis stage, adjuvant treatment, and residual tumor are prognostic factors for medulloblastoma in children: conclusions from the Children's Cancer Group 921 randomized phase III study. *J. Clin. Oncol.* **17:** 832–845.
14. Hilden, J.M. *et al.* 2004. Central nervous system atypical teratoid/rhabdoid tumor: results of therapy in children enrolled in a registry. *J. Clin. Oncol.* **22:** 2877–2884.
15. Finlay, J.L. & J.H. Wisoff. 1999. The impact of extent of resection in the management of malignant gliomas of childhood. *Childs Nerv. Syst.* **15:** 786–788.
16. Berger, C. *et al.* 1998. Choroid plexus carcinomas in childhood: clinical features and prognostic factors. *Neurosurgery* **42:** 470–475.
17. Bouffet, E. *et al.* 1998. Intracranial ependymomas in children: a critical review of prognostic factors and a plea for cooperation. *Med. Pediatr. Oncol.* **30:** 319–329; discussion 329–331.
18. Rutka, J.T. *et al.* 2004. Advances in the treatment of pediatric brain tumors. *Expert Rev. Neurother.* **4:** 879–893.
19. Gupta, N. & M.S. Berger. 2003. Brain mapping for hemispheric tumors in children. *Pediatr. Neurosurg.* **38:** 302–306.
20. Evans, A.E. *et al.* 1990. The treatment of medulloblastoma. Results of a prospective randomized trial of radiation therapy with and without CCNU, vincristine, and prednisone. *J. Neurosurg.* **72:** 572–582.
21. Tait, D.M. *et al.* 1990. Adjuvant chemotherapy for medulloblastoma: the first multi-centre control trial of the International Society of Paediatric Oncology (SIOP I). *Eur. J. Cancer* **26:** 464–469.
22. Duffner, P. *et al.* 1993. Postoperative chemotherapy and delayed radiation in children less than three years of age with malignant brain tumors. *N. Engl. J. Med.* **328:** 1725–1731.

23. Kirsch, D.G. & N.J. Tarbell. 2004. New technologies in radiation therapy for pediatric brain tumors: the rationale for proton radiation therapy. *Pediatr. Blood Cancer* **42:** 461–464.

24. Merchant, T.E. *et al*. 2004. Preliminary results from a phase II trial of conformal radiation therapy and evaluation of radiation-related CNS effects for pediatric patients with localized ependymoma. *J. Clin. Oncol.* **22:** 3156–3162.

25. Yock, T.I. and N.J. Tarbell. 2004. Technology insight: proton beam radiotherapy for treatment in pediatric brain tumors. *Nat. Clin. Pract. Oncol.* **1:** 97–103; quiz 1 p following 111.

26. Nicholson, H.S. *et al*. 2007. Phase 2 study of temozolomide in children and adolescents with recurrent central nervous system tumors: a report from the Children's Oncology Group. *Cancer* **110:** 1542–1550.

27. Lashford, L.S. *et al*. 2002. Temozolomide in malignant gliomas of childhood: a United Kingdom Children's Cancer Study Group and French Society for Pediatric Oncology Intergroup Study. *J. Clin. Oncol.* **20:** 4684–4691.

28. Dunkel, I.J. 2000. High-dose chemotherapy with autologous stem cell rescue for malignant brain tumors. *Cancer Invest.* **18:** 492–493.

29. Perilongo, G. *et al*. 1997. Diencephalic syndrome and disseminated juvenile pilocytic astrocytomas of the hypothalamic-optic chiasm region. *Cancer* **80:** 142–146.

30. Tihan, T. *et al*. 1999. Pediatric astrocytomas with monomorphous pilomyxoid features and a less favorable outcome. *J. Neuropathol. Exp. Neurol.* **58:** 1061–1068.

31. Schmandt, S.M. & R.J. Packer. 2000. Treatment of low-grade pediatric gliomas. *Curr. Opin. Oncol.* **12:** 194–198.

32. Reddy, A.T. & R.J. Packer. 1999. Chemotherapy for low-grade gliomas. *Childs Nerv. Syst.* **15:** 506–513.

33. Packer, R.J. *et al*. 1993. Carboplatin and vincristine for recurrent and newly diagnosed low-grade gliomas of childhood. *J. Clin. Oncol.* **11:** 850–856.

34. Packer, R.J. *et al*. 1997. Carboplatin and vincristine chemotherapy for children with newly diagnosed progressive low-grade gliomas. *J. Neurosurg.* **86:** 747–754.

35. Gnekow, A.K. *et al*. 2000. [HIT-LGG: effectiveness of carboplatin-vincristine in progressive low-grade gliomas of childhood—an interim report]. *Klin Padiatr.* **212:** 177–184.

36. Bowers, D.C. *et al*. 2006. Late-occurring stroke among long-term survivors of childhood leukemia and brain tumors: a report from the Childhood Cancer Survivor Study. *J. Clin. Oncol.* **24:** 5277–5282.

37. Grill, J. *et al*. 1999. Radiation-induced cerebral vasculopathy in children with neurofibromatosis and optic pathway glioma. *Ann. Neurol.* **45:** 393–396.

38. COG-ACNS0221. http://www.cancer.gov/search/ViewClinicalTrials.aspx?cdrid=445095&version=patient&protocolsearchid=3754892 (accessed June 24, 2008).

39. Packer, R.J. *et al*. 2006. Phase III study of craniospinal radiation therapy followed by adjuvant chemotherapy for newly diagnosed average-risk medulloblastoma. *J. Clin. Oncol.* 24: 4202–4208.

40. Gajjar, A. *et al*. 2006. Risk-adapted craniospinal radiotherapy followed by high-dose chemotherapy and stem-cell rescue in children with newly diagnosed medulloblastoma (St Jude Medulloblastoma-96): long-term results from a prospective, multicentre trial. *Lancet Oncol.* **7:** 813–820.

41. COG-ACNS0331. http://www.cancer.gov/search/ViewClinicalTrials.aspx?cdrid=365506&version=patient&protocolsearchid=3755853 (accessed June 24, 2008).

42. Huang, E. *et al*. 2002. Intensity-modulated radiation therapy for pediatric medulloblastoma: early report on the reduction of ototoxicity. *Int. J. Radiat. Oncol. Biol. Phys.* **52:** 599–605.

43. Gilbertson, R.J. & A. Gajjar. 2005. Molecular biology of medulloblastoma: will it ever make a difference to clinical management? *J. Neurooncol.* **75:** 273–278.

44. Gajjar, A. *et al*. 2004. Clinical, histopathologic, and molecular markers of prognosis: toward a new disease risk stratification system for medulloblastoma. *J. Clin. Oncol.* **22:** 984–993.

45. Eberhart, C.G. *et al*. 2004. Histopathological and molecular prognostic markers in medulloblastoma: c-myc, N-myc, TrkC, and anaplasia. *J. Neuropathol. Exp. Neurol.* **63:** 441–449.

46. Pollack, I.F. *et al*. 1995. Intracranial ependymomas of childhood: long-term outcome and prognostic factors. *Neurosurgery* **37:** 655–666; discussion 666–667.

47. Foreman, N.K. & E. Bouffet. 1999. Ependymomas in children. *J. Neurosurg.* **90:** 605.

48. Foreman, N.K. *et al*. 1997. Second-look surgery for incompletely resected fourth ventricle ependymomas: technical case report. *Neurosurgery* **40:** 856–860; discussion 860.

49. SIOP-EPENDYMOMA-99. http://www.cancer.gov/search/ViewClinicalTrials.aspx?cdrid=67465&version=patient&protocolsearchid=3755071 (accessed June 24, 2008).

50. COG-ACNS0121. http://clinicaltrials.gov/ct/show/NCT00027846;jsessionid=96902B85E1A46E688C0E24EF667C25FD?order=3 (accessed June 24, 2008).

51. Grundy, R.G. *et al*. 2007. Primary postoperative chemotherapy without radiotherapy for

intracranial ependymoma in children: the UKCCSG/SIOP prospective study. *Lancet Oncol.* **8:** 696–705.

52. Bouffet, E. & N. Foreman. 1999. Chemotherapy for intracranial ependymomas. *Childs Nerv. Syst.* **15:** 563–570.

53. Gilbertson, R.J. *et al.* 2002. ERBB receptor signaling promotes ependymoma cell proliferation and represents a potential novel therapeutic target for this disease. *Clin. Cancer Res.* **8:** 3054–3064.

54. Tabori, U. *et al.* 2006. Human telomere reverse transcriptase expression predicts progression and survival in pediatric intracranial ependymoma. *J. Clin. Oncol.* **24:** 1522–1528.

55. Sposto, R. *et al.* 1989. The effectiveness of chemotherapy for treatment of high grade astrocytoma in children: results of a randomized trial. A report from the Childrens Cancer Study Group. *J. Neurooncol.* **7:** 165–177.

56. Finlay, J.L. *et al.* 1995. Randomized phase III trial in childhood high-grade astrocytoma comparing vincristine, lomustine, and prednisone with the eight-drugs-in-1-day regimen. Childrens Cancer Group. *J. Clin. Oncol.* **13:** 112–123.

57. Pollack, I.F. *et al.* 2006. O6-methylguanine-DNA methyltransferase expression strongly correlates with outcome in childhood malignant gliomas: results from the CCG-945 Cohort. *J. Clin. Oncol.* **24:** 3431–3437.

58. Pollack, I.F. *et al.* 2002. Expression of p53 and prognosis in children with malignant gliomas. *N. Engl. J. Med.* **346:** 420–427.

59. Pollack, I.F. *et al.* 2003. The influence of central review on outcome associations in childhood malignant gliomas: results from the CCG-945 experience. *Neuro. Oncol.* **5:** 197–207.

60. Fouladi, M. *et al.* 2003. Outcome of children with centrally reviewed low-grade gliomas treated with chemotherapy with or without radiotherapy on Children's Cancer Group high-grade glioma study CCG-945. *Cancer* **98:** 1243–1252.

61. Cohen, K. *et al.* 2007. Should temozolomide be the standard of care for children with newly diagnosed high-grade gliomas? Results of the Children's Oncology Group ACNS0126 Study. *Neuro-oncology* **9:** 188.

62. Hargrave, D., U. Bartels & E. Bouffet. 2006. Diffuse brainstem glioma in children: critical review of clinical trials. *Lancet Oncol.* **7:** 241–248.

63. Bode, U. *et al.* 2007. Phase II trial of nimotuzumab in the treatment of refratory and relapsed high-grade gliomas in children and adolescents—Final report. *Pediatr. Blood Cancer* **49:** 435.

64. Rutkowski, S. *et al.* 2005. Treatment of early childhood medulloblastoma by postoperative chemotherapy alone. *N. Engl. J. Med.* **352:** 978–986.

65. Chi, S.N. *et al.* 2004. Feasibility and response to induction chemotherapy intensified with high-dose methotrexate for young children with newly diagnosed high-risk disseminated medulloblastoma. *J. Clin. Oncol.* **22:** 4881–4887.

66. Bouffet, E., U. Tabori & U. Bartels. 2007. Paediatric ependymomas: should we avoid radiotherapy? *Lancet Oncol.* **8:** 665–666.

67. Murphy, S. 1995. The national impact of clinical cooperative group trials for pediatric cancer. *Med. Pediatr. Oncol.* **24:** 279–280.

68. Qaddoumi, I. *et al.* 2007. Impact of telemedicine on pediatric neuro-oncology in a developing country: the Jordanian-Canadian experience. *Pediatr Blood Cancer* **48:** 39–43.

Role of Prognostic Factors in the Management of Pediatric Solid Tumors

Takaaki Yanagisawa,[a] Ute Bartels,[b] and Eric Bouffet[b]

[a]*Division of Paediatric Neuro-Oncology, Department of Neuro-Oncology, Saitama Medical University International Medical Center, Saitama, Japan*

[b]*Paediatric Brain Tumour Program, Division of Haematology/Oncology, Hospital for Sick Children, Toronto, Ontario, Canada*

The importance of prognostic factors in predicting outcome in pediatric oncology is largely recognized, and most current protocols tailor treatment based on risk stratification. Further refinements of classical staging systems are ongoing, and the future of pediatric oncology is in the development of strategies based on individual tumor characteristics. This review details significant advances in our understanding of prognostic factors in the most common pediatric solid tumors and potential applications for clinical management.

Key words: **children; solid tumors; prognostic factors**

Introduction

Progress in the treatment of childhood cancers is a true success story, and survival rates are currently approaching 80% in countries where children have access to high-quality care. Advances in diagnostic imaging, surgery, anesthesia, radiation oncology, medical oncology, and supportive care have contributed equally to this success. Along with this improvement in survival, a step-by-step refinement of the understanding of each neoplastic process has led to the development of specific and sophisticated stratification systems.[37] These systems are based on prognostic factors derived from studies in which patients were initially treated without any risk stratification. Over time, the identification of specific prognostic factors shed new light on the behavior of pediatric malignancies and gave rise to new protocols tailored to the specific condition of each individual patient. The use of prognostic factors is not unique to pediatric oncology. Prognostic factors are widely used in the treatment of multiple medical conditions. They help identify patients with different risks of specific outcomes and guide treatment options. In oncology, they may be simple measures such as stage of disease or tumor size.[20,36,39] However, prognostic factors have evolved during the recent decades, particularly since the emergence of cooperative clinical trials, which have allowed the inclusion of large numbers of patients and the conduct of additional studies using radiology, pathology, or biology data. Prognostic marker studies are becoming increasingly complex, and often multiple variables have been correlated with event-free or overall survival.

Pediatric malignancies demonstrate diversity in their clinical behavior and multiple prognostic factors have been identified in each tumor type.[37] The aim of this review is to summarize the current knowledge on prognostic factors in pediatric solid tumors, with a specific focus on Wilms tumors, sarcoma, neuroblastoma, liver, germ cell, and central nervous system (CNS) tumors.

Address for correspondence: Dr. Eric Bouffet, Director of the Paediatric Brain Tumour Program, Professor of Paediatrics, Division of Haematology/Oncology, The Hospital for Sick Children, 555 University Avenue, Toronto M5G 1X8, Canada. Voice: +1-416-813-7457; fax: +1-416-813-8024. eric.bouffet@sickkids.ca

Ann. N.Y. Acad. Sci. 1138: 32–42 (2008). © 2008 New York Academy of Sciences.
doi: 10.1196/annals.1414.006

Wilms Tumor

Wilms tumor is the most common malignant renal tumor in children. The International Society of Pediatric Oncology (SIOP) and the National Wilms Tumor Study (NWTS) have conducted several clinical trials, which have resulted in an increase in the survival rate of children with Wilms tumor from 20% before the chemoradiotherapy era to 90% currently.[40,53] These results have been achieved while using shorter duration and total dosage of chemotherapy. In addition, the use of radiotherapy has been drastically reduced over time and doses of radiation significantly diminished.[44] Therapy for patients with Wilms tumor is based on the risk of relapse, using such variables as histology, stage (based on lymph node involvement, local or intravascular tumor extension, and presence of metastatic disease), and age at diagnosis. There is a different approach in the treatment of Wilms tumor between the North American (NWTS) and the European (SIOP) groups and this has a significant influence on the respective staging systems.[84] The SIOP strategy gives preoperative chemotherapy, based on the premise that preoperative therapy reduces the risk of surgical spillage of the tumor, and thereby reduces the likelihood of local and distant recurrence. In contrast, the NWTS protocols consider that the first step in the treatment of Wilms tumor is surgical staging followed by radical nephrectomy, if possible. One of the consequences of preoperative chemotherapy is an increase in the number of lower-stage tumors at surgery, leading to a decrease in the intensity of postoperative chemotherapy and in some case to radiotherapy avoidance. This certainly explains the higher rate of irradiated patients in NWTS trials. However, results of SIOP-6 showed a higher rate of local relapse in patients with stage II tumors who were not given radiation.[44,80] This suggests that some of these patients might have been true stage III patients who were downstaged following preoperative chemotherapy.

Several studies have been conducted in order to include new prognostic factors in the decision-making process. Histology has been identified as the other major prognostic factor in Wilms tumors. Five to ten percent of Wilms tumors show anaplastic features, characterized by nuclear enlargement, nuclear atypia, and irregular mitotic figures.[40] Anaplasia is associated with a poor prognosis due to the putative chemoresistance of the tumor cells, which are associated with tumor-specific mutations and high p53 protein expression.[26] In addition, a retrospective analysis of the protocol SIOP 93–01 showed that postoperative histological classification was more important than tumor stage. The use of preoperative chemotherapy appears to change the distribution pattern as well as the prognostic value of the different histological subtypes compared to tumors treated with immediate surgery. Based on this review, the SIOP group concluded that the response to preoperative chemotherapy could be used to stratify the postoperative treatment according to the individual risk of the patient. The new SIOP classification only applies to patients treated with preoperative chemotherapy and is based on the observation that tumors with persistent viable cells occupying more than two-thirds of the lesion and composed predominantly of blastema have a relapse risk similar to that of anaplastic tumors.[83]

Older age at diagnosis has been shown to be associated with poorer outcome in low-stage patients with favorable histology both in the NWTS-1 and United Kingdom Children's Cancer Study Group (UKW2 and UKW3) trials, and in patients with stage II and III tumors in the NWTS-3 trial.[14,69] Because of differences in the statistical analyses between studies, the reported cutoffs were different in the NWTS ($\geq$2 years) and the UK ($\geq$4 years) trials. This prompted warnings regarding treatment reductions for these age groups.

Although the outcome of patients with favorable histology is excellent, further studies have been conducted to better identify patients who are at higher risk of relapse. A recent study from NWTS has identified a biologically distinct group with loss of heterozygosity for chromosome 1p and 16q have who have a poorer event-free survival and might be considered for treatment intensification, especially for patients with advanced-stage disease.[38] The same study demonstrated a positive correlation between risk of recurrence and telomerase expression in the tumor.[25] Although these results were statistically significant in their context, they have not yet been adopted for treatment stratification.

Neuroblastoma

Neuroblastoma is the most common extracranial solid tumor in children, and one of the most enigmatic with regard to its behavior. Stage and age are the most important clinical factors predictive of outcome. Cooperative studies conducted in Europe and North America have shown a survival rate in stage I patients of nearly 100%; stage II, 90%; stage II, 30–40%; stage IV, 10–15%; and stage IV-S, 80–90%.[79] There is evidence that older age is associated with worse outcome, particularly in advanced-stage neuroblastoma. Based on the work conducted by Breslow in the early 1970s,[13] age has been used as a prognostic variable. For many years, 1 year has been chosen as a convenient age cutoff, and patients >1 year of age with advanced disease were treated with more intensive therapy including megatherapy and stem cell rescue. Several studies have since confirmed the significant impact of this age cutoff. However, recent work has revisited this issue and suggested, based on a review of several large cooperative studies that this cutoff should be increased to a value in the range of 15–19 months.[48,49] At the other end of the age spectrum, there is increasing evidence that neuroblastomas that occur during adolescence and adulthood have a number of peculiarities that should be taken into account when designing therapeutic protocols.[21] Tumor site is an additional clinical factor of prognostic relevance, and patients with primary

tumors in the adrenal gland seem to do worse than patients with tumors originating at other sites.

A number of genetic and biological features have been investigated in recent years in an effort to improve the understanding of the behavior of neuroblastoma. Many prognostic studies have identified genetic characteristics associated with outcome, including *MYCN* copy number, ploidy, deletion or loss of heterozygosity of chromosome 1p, and gain of chromosome 17q.[15] However, it has proved difficult to identify which prognostic markers are the most useful for clinical purposes. Riley and colleagues conducted a systematic review of the literature and identified 195 different prognostic factors studied in relation to screening, diagnosis, prognosis, and monitoring of neuroblastoma in the 428 papers that were selected for their review.[70,71] This systematic review identified *MYCN*, chromosome 1p, DNA index, VMA:HVA ratio, CD44, Trk-A, NSE, lactate dehydrogenase (LDH), ferritin, and multidrug resistance as potentially important prognostic tools. In these reviews, the authors acknowledge that they did not include more recent data on 17q gains, which is associated with more aggressive behavior.

Most current studies for the treatment of neuroblastoma patients are based on risk groups that take into account these biological factors in addition to patient's age and stage. Tumor histopathology, determined by the Shimada classification, takes into consideration the quantity of Schwann cells in the stroma, mitotic figures, and degeneration of nuclei and divides tumors into favorable and unfavorable histological types. This classification is another important independent prognostic factor, at least for certain subsets of patients.[77]

The risk stratification of neuroblastoma is likely to evolve with the results of ongoing studies of genetic and molecular profiling using microarray, serial analysis of gene expression, or other techniques.[15,57] These studies will not only improve understanding of the behavior of this complex disease, but also help to identify genes, pathways, or proteins that could be targeted using biologically based therapies.

Sarcomas

Rhabdomyosarcoma

Several studies have identified prognostic factors in soft-tissue sarcoma, and particularly in rhabdomyosarcoma (RMS), the most common soft-tissue sarcoma in childhood. These studies have shown that the two major subsets of RMS, embryonal and alveolar RMS, have differing prognostic factors and clinical outcomes.[37] In addition to the major influence of histological subtypes, the combination of stage, group, site, size, age, and the presence or absence of regional nodes or distant metastases are used to stratify patients into one of four "risk-groups" (low A, low B, intermediate, and high risk).

Five-year survival rate for patients without metastases currently exceeds 75%. In a recent analysis of the North American Intergroup Rhabdomyosarcoma Studies (IRS) III and IV, the estimated 5-year failure-free survival rate was 81% for patients with non-metastatic embryonal RMS, compared to 65% for patients with alveolar or undifferentiated histology.[9,56,59,63] Patients with low-risk tumors (group low A and low B) identified as embryonal RMS developing at favorable sites (orbit and eyelid, genitourinary except prostate and bladder, or head and neck except parameningeal) or as embryonal RMS at unfavorable sites (bladder, prostate, extremity, parameningeal, or others such as trunk and retroperitoneal), that were grossly resected had a 5-year event-free survival rate above 85%. Complete resection was also associated with excellent outcome in patients with stage 1 and 2 alveolar RMS. Patients with embryonal RMS located in unfavorable sites with gross tumor remaining after definitive surgery (intermediate risk group) had, overall, a less favorable prognosis. Patients with stage 3 alveolar tumors located at unfavorable sites that were either incompletely resected or associated with lymph node involvement were

doing poorly, with an estimated 5-year survival rate of 34%.

Approximately 15% of children with RMS present with metastatic disease, which is the strongest predictor of clinical outcome. These children fare poorly and only 25% are expected to be free of disease 3 years after diagnosis. However, analyses of European patients with metastatic RMS have found age older than 1 year and younger than 10 years, the absence of bone or bone marrow metastases, and a primary tumor in head and neck or genitourinary sites to be independently favorable factors for both overall and event-free survival.[18] Histology was not an independent prognostic in metastatic patients, but this may be related to the close association between alveolar histology and other adverse factors, such as bone marrow involvement and unfavorable tumor sites. In the retrospective analysis of the North American studies IRS III and IV, results were slightly different and did not identify age as a significant prognostic factor.[12] Patients with embryonal histology and those with two or fewer sites of metastatic disease had a significantly better 5-year failure-free and overall survival.

Local/regional recurrence is the most common cause of treatment failure in RMS, accounting for 70% of all failures. Among prognostic variables at recurrence, the type and time of recurrence and its relation with therapy are strongly associated with outcome. A retrospective analysis of the Italian protocols RMS79, RMS88, and RMS96 identified four prognostic factors that were associated with longer survival: histology, primary tumor site, type of recurrence, and its relation with therapy.[52] Patients who had tumors with nonalveolar histology, a primary tumor site different from parameningeal or "other" sites, local recurrence, and recurrence off therapy had a better prognosis.

Nearly 60% of cases of alveolar RMS have a characteristic t(2;13) translocation, which generates a chimeric gene, fusing PAX3 on chromosome 2 to FKHR on chromosome 13. A variant t(1;13) translocation fuses PAX7 on chromosome 1 to FKHR and is found in 20%

of alveolar RMS.[64] A recent analysis of alveolar RMS based on their gene expression profile showed that a PAX–FKHR expression signature can be used to predict tumor behavior.[24] This study used a model representing 25 genes and identified three distinct groups with striking differences in survival (7% versus 48% versus 93% 5-year survival). This suggests that molecular genetic analysis might be able to refine further the identification of prognostic indicators in subgroups of RMS patients.

Ewing Sarcoma

Like most other pediatric malignancies, the outcome of patients with Ewing sarcoma (ES) has improved considerably over the past two decades, and at least two-thirds of patients with localized ES currently achieve long-term survival through a multidisciplinary approach combining intensive chemotherapy and local control by surgery and/or radiation. By contrast, the outcome of patients with metastatic disease remains poor and the key prognostic factor in Ewing's tumor is the presence of detectable metastases at diagnosis.[54] For patients with localized disease, several studies of prognostic factors have shown different and slightly inconsistent results. In the analysis conducted by the European Intergroup Cooperative Ewing's Sarcoma Study group on 975 patients, site, age group, and study period were the most significant predictors of outcome in patients with localized disease.[22] In a retrospective analysis of 220 patients treated between 1979 and 2004 at St. Jude Children's Research Hospital, older age, pelvic primary tumor, large tumors, and metastatic disease were associated with worse outcome, but only stage and tumor size remained significant in the multivariate analysis.[72] For patients with localized disease, local control with both surgery and irradiation was found to result in the best outcome. By contrast, the strongest prognostic factors in the French study for localized ES were the histological response to chemotherapy in patients who underwent surgery and the size of the tumor in

patients who did not.[60,61] Age and site were not significant. In a single-institution review of 579 patients, male gender, age, serum levels of LDH, tumor volume, number of chemotherapy drugs, type of local treatment, and histological grade of response to preoperative treatment each had an independent influence on outcome in patients with nonmetastatic ES.[3] In the German Cooperative Ewing Sarcoma Study CESS, tumor volume was the most significant prognostic factor.[1] This analysis pointed out the influence of treatment on prognostic factors. Comparison between the two consecutive studies CESS 81 and CESS 86 showed a shift in the cutoff of tumor volume from 100 mL in CESS 81 to 200 mL in CESS 86 and the loss of prognostic significance of histological response to chemotherapy in CESS 86 compared to the CESS 81 trial. For patients with metastatic disease, although the overall survival is poor, patients with pulmonary metastases only have a better prognosis than patients who have bone metastases at diagnosis (with or without lung metastases).[65]

Molecular prognostic parameters have been extensively studied in ES. Homozygous deletion of *p16/p14ARF* and *p53* alteration, detected in approximately 20% and 10% of ES tumor samples, respectively, are prognostically unfavorable.[42,43] In a recent study, telomere length in tumor cells at diagnosis was the most significant predictor of outcome.[2] This suggests that some molecular markers of clinical outcome in ES could be used to tailor treatment, particularly in patients with localized disease, before initial chemotherapy. Recent work on detection of bone marrow micrometastases and circulating tumor cells by reverse transcriptase polymerase chain reaction reveals that patients with localized ES who show peripheral or bone marrow occult tumor cells harbor a pejorative prognostic.[75,81]

Osteosarcoma

In osteosarcoma, tumor stage is also a major prognostic indicator, and patients with metastatic disease have a dismal survival rate.

Numerous prognostic factors have been investigated in nonmetastatic osteosarcoma. In a literature review, Bentzen identified 47 papers published between 1975 and 1998 in which more than 20 different potential prognostic factors were studied, including age, gender, stage, number of positive nodes, tumor site and size, differentiation, fracture at presentation, symptom duration, inadequate surgical margin, type of chemotherapy, dose of chemotherapy, radiotherapy, serum alkaline phosphatase, erythrocyte sedimentation rate, serum LDH, and S-phase fraction.[6] The author notes that the conclusions of many papers were speculative and largely influenced by the low power of the studies. The Cooperative Osteosarcoma Study (COSS) Group reported an analysis based on 1702 patients enrolled in sequential studies from 1980 through 1998 and identified primary metastatic disease and axial primary site as unfavorable prognostic features.[8] For patients presenting with osteosarcoma of the extremity, this study identified proximal tumors and primary metastasis as unfavorable features. Two other major prognostic factors identified by the COSS Group were histological necrosis after initial chemotherapy and macroscopic residual tumor after surgical resection, and in this experience, long-term survival without complete surgical resection the primary tumor—and if present, metastatic disease—was the rare exception. In a review of 789 patients with osteosarcoma of the extremity, Bacci and colleagues found an increased risk of recurrence when the following characteristics were present: age >14 years, elevated serum alkaline phosphatase at presentation, tumor volume >200 mL, inadequate surgical margins, and poor histological response to preoperative chemotherapy.[4] In the Brazilian Osteosarcoma Group Treatment Studies III and IV, although survival rates were lower than the rates reported in other cooperative studies (50 and 39% overall survival and event-free survival at 5 years, respectively), the multivariate analysis was consistent with previous reports from North American and European groups and showed that the presence of metastases, tumor size more than 12 cm, and postchemotherapy necrosis grades 1 and 2 were independent prognostic factors.[67] A study from the French group analyzed factors influencing survival in a series of 78 patients with metastatic osteosarcoma. In the multivariate analysis, pretreatment features associated with a shorter event-free survival were metastasis to at least two organs and high alkaline phosphatase levels. Prognostic factors were also studied in patients with recurrent osteosarcoma. A short time to relapse, recurrences involving more than one lesion, and, in the case of lung metastases, bilateral disease and pleural disruption, were negative prognostic factors. Among treatment-related variables, surgery and a second surgical complete remission were correlated with improved overall survival.

In addition to these clinical factors, potential biological prognostic factors have been investigated in osteosarcoma. Recently, retrospective studies have identified multidrug resistance status, loss of heterozygosity of the RB gene, and *HER2*/erbB-2 expression as potential factors.[29,35,76] These results have yet to be substantiated by large-scale prospective studies.

Extracranial Germ Cell Tumors

Cooperative studies have clearly emphasized the specificity of extracranial germ cell tumors (GCT) in infancy and childhood, and prognostic factors are different from those reported in adult studies.[34] In this group of tumors, prognostic factors seem to be largely influenced by treatment-related variables, and in particular the use of carboplatin versus cisplatin based regimens. The French group analyzed the outcome of children with localized GCT treated with carboplatin.[5] Age younger than 10 years, sacrococcygeal or mediastinal primary site, and elevated alpha fetoprotein (AFP) values were associated with poorer event-free survival, but were not significant for overall survival. A level of AFP >10,000 ng/mL was associated with a higher risk of treatment failure. In the United Kingdom Children's Cancer Study Group experience with carboplatin-based regimens, AFP level >10,000 ku/L and stage III/IV disease were the strongest predictors of treatment failure.[50] By contrast, the analysis of the Pediatric Intergroup Study (POG 9049/CCG 8882) did not identify AFP as a significant prognostic factor.[51] In this protocol, chemotherapy regimens were cisplatin-based and this may account for the differences observed. Only age was found to be significant, with a statistically significant higher risk of relapse for patients >12 years old. In the multivariate regression model used, the combination of age >12 years and thoracic primary site resulted in six times the risk of death compared with patients younger than 12 years with tumors at other sites. The German Cooperative group Maligne Keimzelltumoren (MAKEI) analyzed factors influencing outcome in sacrococcygeal region tumors, the most common GCTs in infants.[17] In their cisplatin-based strategy, high AFP levels at diagnosis did not indicate poor outcome. In addition, neither the occurrence of metastases nor bone metastases or extension of tumor into bone had a significant effect on prognosis. Patients with tumor size >5 cm and visceral metastases had a significantly poorer outcome. In order to better identify patients who may benefit from treatment intensification, a meta-analysis evaluating all patients with GCT treated by the different cooperative groups is being considered.

Hepatoblastoma and Hepatocarcinoma

International cooperative studies have contributed to identifying factors influencing outcome in these exceptionally rare liver neoplasms. Both in hepatoblastoma and in hepatocarcinoma, the major factor identified to date is the completeness of the surgical resection.[55] There is evidence that pretreatment characteristics influence tumor resectability. However, comparisons between different cooperative groups are difficult because different staging systems are used.[16,45] The SIOP group uses the Pre Treatment Extent of Disease grouping system (PRETEXT), which divides the liver in four sectors[16,23] and defines four surgical PRETEXT groups (I to IV) according to operability. In the SIOP experience with hepatoblastoma, both PRETEXT grouping and presence of metastasis at diagnosis were identified as independent predictors of event-free survival. In the Pediatric Oncology Group experience, extent of resection and presence of metastasis are the most significant predictors of outcome.[46,62] In hepatocarcinoma, children with initially resectable tumors have a good prognosis. Outcome is uniformly poor for children with advanced-stage disease.[23,45] The role of AFP in hepatoblastoma is controversial in the literature. Initial AFP serum levels, as well as the timing and slope of AFP decline under chemotherapy, have been suggested to indicate clinical outcome. Patients with a low AFP level seem to have a poor outcome. A relationship between low AFP levels and unfavorable histological features is possible.[30,55,82]

Other Extracranial Solid Tumors

In the majority of other pediatric solid tumors, tumor stage is the most important prognostic factor of outcome. Additional prognostic factors have been investigated in nearly every tumor type. One major problem is that many studies are too small, and therefore underpowered, to identify even quite strong prognostic factors.

Brain Tumors

Similarly to extracranial tumors, stage is the strongest predictor of outcome in most pediatric brain tumors. The most common staging system in use for pediatric CNS tumors is the Chang system, initially developed for medulloblastoma.[19] Metastatic spread is not specific for malignant tumors, as dissemination can also be observed in benign tumors, such as low-grade gliomas or myxopapillary ependymomas.[28,66] The diversity of pediatric CNS brain tumors precludes any generalization regarding prognostic factors. For example, although metastatic disease predicts poorer survival, the influence of tumor stage is not demonstrated in germinomas; the outcome is excellent in patients with either localized or metastatic germinomas.[10] Age is often identified as a prognostic factor, but the reason for this worse outcome is not clear and may be related to more aggressive tumor biology, treatment-related parameters, such as reluctance to give postoperative radiation therapy, or use of lower doses of radiation.[47] The extent of resection is the strongest prognostic factor most nonmetastatic tumors, particularly in medulloblastoma, ependymoma, choroid plexus carcinoma, and rhabdoid tumors.[7,11,41,85] There are also some exceptions, such as germinoma, for which the degree of resection has no influence on outcome.[10] Recognition that the clinical outcome in some pediatric CNS tumors varies according to prognostic indicators has led to the development of risk-stratified treatments, in particular for medulloblastoma and ependymoma.[73]

Recent studies have pointed out the prognostic value of molecular markers, particularly in medulloblastoma, ependymoma, and high-grade gliomas.[33,68,78] In medulloblastoma, a number of potential molecular markers, such as TrkC, ERBB2, C-Myc and N-MYC, and nuclear beta-catenin have been identified.[27,31-33] In addition, some histopathological features in medulloblastoma have been correlated with aggressive behavior, and patients with large-cell and anaplastic medulloblastoma are currently excluded from average risk protocols.[27] Conversely, desmoplasia has been associated with better survival in infants.[74] However, this information is not yet used for a molecular disease risk-stratification system to guide treatment selection.

Conclusions

Identification of prognostic factors is becoming increasingly important to more effectively tailor treatment to individual patient characteristics. Over the last three decades, identification of prognostic factors in pediatric solid tumors through cooperative trials has been critical, and tremendous progress has been made in the refinement of the stratification of pediatric malignancies. It is unlikely that the clinical and radiological staging system will significantly change over time. Further refinement of therapy and improvements in outcome will depend on more accurate stratification of patients using novel prognostic factors. Identification of specific molecular alterations now appears critical to discriminate tumors according to their behavior and not only according to their clinico-radiological staging. This emphasizes two critical aspects of clinical research in pediatric oncology: the crucial role of cooperative protocols[58] and the importance of tissue banking.

Conflicts of Interest

The authors declare no conflicts of interest.

References

1. Ahrens, S., C. Hoffmann, S. Jabar, *et al.* 1999. Evaluation of prognostic factors in a tumor volume adapted treatment strategy for localized Ewing sarcoma of bone: the CESS 86 experience. Cooperative Ewing Sarcoma Study. *Med. Pediatr. Oncol.* **32:** 186.

2. Avigad, S., I. Naumov, A. Ohali, *et al.* 2007. Short telomeres: a novel potential predictor of relapse in Ewing sarcoma. *Clin. Cancer Res.* **13:** 5777.

3. Bacci, G., A. Longhi, S. Ferrari, *et al.* 2006. Prognostic factors in non-metastatic Ewing's sarcoma tumor of bone: an analysis of 579 patients treated at a single institution with adjuvant or neoadjuvant chemotherapy between 1972 and 1998. *Acta Oncol.* **45:** 469.

4. Bacci, G., A. Longhi, M. Versari, *et al.* 2006. Prognostic factors for osteosarcoma of the extremity treated with neoadjuvant chemotherapy: 15-year experience in 789 patients treated at a single institution. *Cancer* **106:** 1154.

5. Baranzelli, M.C., A. Kramar, E. Bouffet, *et al*. 1999. Prognostic factors in children with localized malignant nonseminomatous germ cell tumors. *J. Clin. Oncol.* **17:** 1212.

6. Bentzen, S.M. 2001. Prognostic factor studies in oncology: osteosarcoma as a clinical example. *Int. J. Radiat. Oncol. Biol. Phys.* **49:** 513.

7. Berger, C., P. Thiesse, A. Lellouch-Tubiana, *et al*. 1998. Choroid plexus carcinomas in childhood: clinical features and prognostic factors. *Neurosurgery* **42:** 470.

8. Bielack, S.S., B. Kempf-Bielack, G. Delling, *et al*. 2002. Prognostic factors in high-grade osteosarcoma of the extremities or trunk: an analysis of 1,702 patients treated on neoadjuvant cooperative osteosarcoma study group protocols. *J. Clin. Oncol.* **20:** 776.

9. Blakely, M.L., R.J. Andrassy, R.B. Raney, *et al*. 2003. Prognostic factors and surgical treatment guidelines for children with rhabdomyosarcoma of the perineum or anus: a report of Intergroup Rhabdomyosarcoma Studies I through IV, 1972 through 1997. *J. Pediatr. Surg.* **38:** 347.

10. Bouffet, E., M.C. Baranzelli, C. Patte, *et al*. 1999. Combined treatment modality for intracranial germinomas: results of a multicentre SFOP experience. Societe Francaise d'Oncologie Pediatrique. *Br. J. Cancer* **79:** 1199.

11. Bouffet, E., G. Perilongo, A. Canete, *et al*. 1998. Intracranial ependymomas in children: a critical review of prognostic factors and a plea for cooperation. *Med. Pediatr. Oncol.* **30:** 319.

12. Breneman, J.C., E. Lyden, A.S. Pappo, *et al*. 2003. Prognostic factors and clinical outcomes in children and adolescents with metastatic rhabdomyosarcoma–a report from the Intergroup Rhabdomyosarcoma Study IV. *J. Clin. Oncol.* **21:** 78.

13. Breslow, N. & B. McCann. 1971. Statistical estimation of prognosis for children with neuroblastoma. *Cancer Res.* **31:** 2098.

14. Breslow, N., K. Sharples, J. Beckwith, *et al*. 1991. Prognostic factors in nonmetastatic, favorable histology Wilms' tumor. Results of the Third National Wilms' Tumor Study. *Cancer* **68:** 2345.

15. Brodeur, G.M. 2003. Neuroblastoma: biological insights into a clinical enigma. *Nat. Rev. Cancer* **3:** 203.

16. Brown, J., G. Perilongo, E. Shafford, *et al*. 2000. Pretreatment prognostic factors for children with hepatoblastoma—results from the International Society of Paediatric Oncology (SIOP) study SIOPEL 1. *Eur. J. Cancer* **36:** 1418.

17. Calaminus, G., D.T. Schneider, J.P. Bokkerink, *et al*. 2003. Prognostic value of tumor size, metastases, extension into bone, and increased tumor marker in children with malignant sacrococcygeal germ cell tumors: a prospective evaluation of 71 patients treated in the German cooperative protocols Maligne Keimzelltumoren (MAKEI) 83/86 and MAKEI 89. *J. Clin. Oncol.* **21:** 781.

18. Carli, M., R. Colombatti, O. Oberlin, *et al*. 2004. European intergroup studies (MMT4-89 and MMT4-91) on childhood metastatic rhabdomyosarcoma: final results and analysis of prognostic factors. *J. Clin. Oncol.* **22:** 4787.

19. Chang, C., E. Housepian & C.J. Herbert. 1969. An operative staging system and a megavoltage radiotherapeutic technic for cerebellar medulloblastomas. *Radiology* **93:** 1351.

20. Conley, B. & S. Taube. 2004. Prognostic and predictive markers in cancer. *Dis. Markers* **20:** 35.

21. Conte, M., B. De Bernardi, C. Milanaccio, *et al*. 2005. Malignant neuroblastic tumors in adolescents. *Cancer Lett.* **228:** 271.

22. Cotterill, S.J., S. Ahrens, M. Paulussen, *et al*. 2000. Prognostic factors in Ewing's tumor of bone: analysis of 975 patients from the European Intergroup Cooperative Ewing's Sarcoma Study Group. *J. Clin. Oncol.* **18:** 3108.

23. Czauderna, P., G. Mackinlay, G. Perilongo, *et al*. 2002. Hepatocellular carcinoma in children: results of the first prospective study of the International Society of Pediatric Oncology group. *J. Clin. Oncol.* **20:** 2798.

24. Davicioni, E., F.G. Finckenstein, V. Shahbazian, *et al*. 2006. Identification of a PAX-FKHR gene expression signature that defines molecular classes and determines the prognosis of alveolar rhabdomyosarcomas. *Cancer Res.* **66:** 6936.

25. Dome, J.S., C.A. Bockhold, S.M. Li, *et al*. 2005. High telomerase RNA expression level is an adverse prognostic factor for favorable-histology Wilms' tumor. *J. Clin. Oncol.* **23:** 9138.

26. Dome, J.S., C.A. Cotton, E.J. Perlman, *et al*. 2006. Treatment of anaplastic histology Wilms' tumor: results from the fifth National Wilms' Tumor Study. *J. Clin. Oncol.* **24:** 2352.

27. Eberhart, C.G., J. Kratz, Y. Wang, *et al*. 2004. Histopathological and molecular prognostic markers in medulloblastoma: c-myc, N-myc, TrkC, and anaplasia. *J. Neuropathol. Exp. Neurol.* **63:** 441.

28. Fassett, D., J. Pingree & J. Kestle. 2005. The high incidence of tumor dissemination in myxopapillary ependymoma in pediatric patients. Report of five cases and review of the literature. *J. Neurosurg.* **102:** 59.

29. Feugeas, O., N. Guriec, A. Babin-Boilletot, *et al*. 1996. Loss of heterozygosity of the RB gene is a poor prognostic factor in patients with osteosarcoma. *J. Clin. Oncol.* **14:** 467.

30. Fuchs, J., J. Rydzynski, D. Von Schweinitz, *et al*. 2002. Pretreatment prognostic factors and treatment results in children with hepatoblastoma: a report from the

German Cooperative Pediatric Liver Tumor Study HB 94. *Cancer* **95:** 172.

31. Gajjar, A., M. Chintagumpala, D. Ashley, *et al*. 2006. Risk-adapted craniospinal radiotherapy followed by high-dose chemotherapy and stem-cell rescue in children with newly diagnosed medulloblastoma (St Jude Medulloblastoma-96): long-term results from a prospective, multicentre trial. *Lancet Oncol.* **7:** 813.

32. Gajjar, A., R. Hernan, M. Kocak, *et al*. 2004. Clinical, histopathologic, and molecular markers of prognosis: toward a new disease risk stratification system for medulloblastoma. *J. Clin. Oncol.* **22:** 984.

33. Gilbertson, R.J. & A. Gajjar. 2005. Molecular biology of medulloblastoma: will it ever make a difference to clinical management? *J. Neurooncol.* **75:** 273.

34. Gobel, U., G. Calaminus, D.T. Schneider, *et al*. 2002. Management of germ cell tumors in children: approaches to cure. *Onkologie* **25:** 14.

35. Gorlick, R., A. Huvos, G. Heller, *et al*. 1999. Expression of HER2/erbB-2 correlates with survival in osteosarcoma. *J. Clin. Oncol.* **17:** 2781.

36. Gospodarowicz, M. & B. O'Sullivan. 2003. Prognostic factors in cancer. *Semin. Surg. Oncol.* **21:** 13.

37. Grosfeld, J.L. 1999. Risk-based management: current concepts of treating malignant solid tumors of childhood. *J. Am. Coll. Surg.* **189:** 407.

38. Grundy, P.E., N.E. Breslow, S. Li, *et al*. 2005. Loss of heterozygosity for chromosomes 1p and 16q is an adverse prognostic factor in favorable-histology Wilms tumor: a report from the National Wilms Tumor Study Group. *J. Clin. Oncol.* **23:** 7312.

39. Hermanek, P. 1999. Prognostic factor research in oncology. *J. Clin. Epidemiol.* **52:** 317.

40. Herz, D., D. McLellan, K. Garrels, *et al*. 2000. Pediatric genitourinary tumors. *Curr. Opin. Oncol.* **12:** 273.

41. Hilden, J.M., S. Meerbaum, P. Burger, *et al*. 2004. Central nervous system atypical teratoid/rhabdoid tumor: results of therapy in children enrolled in a registry. *J. Clin. Oncol.* **22:** 2877.

42. Honoki, K., E. Stojanovski, M. McEvoy, *et al*. 2007. Prognostic significance of p16 INK4a alteration for Ewing sarcoma: a meta-analysis. *Cancer* **110:** 1351.

43. Huang, H.Y., P.B. Illei, Z. Zhao, *et al*. 2005. Ewing sarcomas with p53 mutation or p16/p14ARF homozygous deletion: a highly lethal subset associated with poor chemoresponse. *J. Clin. Oncol.* **23:** 548.

44. Jereb, B., J. Burgers, M. Tournade, *et al*. 1994. Radiotherapy in the SIOP (International Society of Pediatric Oncology) nephroblastoma studies: a review. *Med. Pediatr. Oncol.* **22:** 221.

45. Katzenstein, H.M., M.D. Krailo, M.H. Malogolowkin, *et al*. 2002. Hepatocellular carcinoma in children and adolescents: results from the Pediatric

Oncology Group and the Children's Cancer Group Intergroup study. *J. Clin. Oncol.* **20:** 2789.

46. Katzenstein, H.M., W.B. London, E.C. Douglass, *et al*. 2002. Treatment of unresectable and metastatic hepatoblastoma: a pediatric oncology group phase II study. *J. Clin. Oncol.* **20:** 3438.

47. Kellie, S. 1999. Chemotherapy of central nervous system tumours in infants. *Childs Nerv. Syst.* **15:** 592.

48. London, W.B., L. Boni, T. Simon, *et al*. 2005. The role of age in neuroblastoma risk stratification: the German, Italian, and children's oncology group perspectives. *Cancer Lett.* **228:** 257.

49. London, W.B., R.P. Castleberry, K.K. Matthay, *et al*. 2005. Evidence for an age cutoff greater than 365 days for neuroblastoma risk group stratification in the Children's Oncology Group. *J. Clin. Oncol.* **23:** 6459.

50. Mann, J.R., F. Raafat, K. Robinson, *et al*. 2000. The United Kingdom Children's Cancer Study Group's second germ cell tumor study: carboplatin, etoposide, and bleomycin are effective treatment for children with malignant extracranial germ cell tumors, with acceptable toxicity. *J. Clin. Oncol.* **18:** 3809.

51. Marina, N., W.B. London, A.L. Frazier, *et al*. 2006. Prognostic factors in children with extragonadal malignant germ cell tumors: a pediatric intergroup study. *J. Clin. Oncol.* **24:** 2544.

52. Mazzoleni, S., G. Bisogno, A. Garaventa, *et al*. 2005. Outcomes and prognostic factors after recurrence in children and adolescents with nonmetastatic rhabdomyosarcoma. *Cancer* **104:** 183.

53. Merguerian, P.A. 2003. Pediatric genitourinary tumors. *Curr. Opin. Oncol.* **15:** 222.

54. Meyers, P. & A. Levy. 2000. Ewing's sarcoma. *Curr. Treat Options Oncol.* **1:** 247.

55. Meyers, R.L. 2007. Tumors of the liver in children. *Surg. Oncol.* **16:** 195–203.

56. Meza, J.L., J. Anderson, A.S. Pappo, *et al*. 2006. Analysis of prognostic factors in patients with nonmetastatic rhabdomyosarcoma treated on Intergroup Rhabdomyosarcoma Studies III and IV: the Children's Oncology Group. *J. Clin. Oncol.* **24:** 3844.

57. Mora, J., W.L. Gerald, N.K. Cheung 2003. Evolving significance of prognostic markers associated with new treatment strategies in neuroblastoma. *Cancer Lett.* **197:** 119.

58. Murphy, S.B. 1995. The national impact of clinical cooperative group trials for pediatric cancer. *Med. Pediatr. Oncol.* **24:** 279.

59. Neville, H.L., R.J. Andrassy, T.E. Lobe, *et al*. 2000. Preoperative staging, prognostic factors, and outcome for extremity rhabdomyosarcoma: a preliminary report from the Intergroup Rhabdomyosarcoma Study IV (1991–1997). *J. Pediatr. Surg.* **35:** 317.

60. Oberlin, O., M.C. Deley, B.N. Bui, *et al*. 2001. Prognostic factors in localized Ewing's tumours and peripheral neuroectodermal tumours: the third study of the French Society of Paediatric Oncology (EW88 study). *Br. J. Cancer* **85:** 1646.

61. Oberlin, O., C. Patte, F. Demeocq, *et al*. 1985. The response to initial chemotherapy as a prognostic factor in localized Ewing's sarcoma. *Eur. J. Cancer Clin. Oncol.* **21:** 463.

62. Ortega, J.A., E.C. Douglass, J.H. Feusner, *et al*. 2000. Randomized comparison of cisplatin/vincristine/fluorouracil and cisplatin/continuous infusion doxorubicin for treatment of pediatric hepatoblastoma: a report from the Children's Cancer Group and the Pediatric Oncology Group. *J. Clin. Oncol.* **18:** 2665.

63. Pappo, A.S., J.L. Meza, S.S. Donaldson, *et al*. 2003. Treatment of localized nonorbital, nonparameningeal head and neck rhabdomyosarcoma: lessons learned from Intergroup Rhabdomyosarcoma Studies III and IV. *J. Clin. Oncol.* **21:** 638.

64. Pappo, A.S., D.N. Shapiro, W.M. Crist, *et al*. 1995. Biology and therapy of pediatric rhabdomyosarcoma. *J. Clin. Oncol.* **13:** 2123.

65. Paulussen, M., S. Ahrens, S. Burdach, *et al*. 1998. Primary metastatic (stage IV) Ewing tumor: survival analysis of 171 patients from the EICESS studies. European Intergroup Cooperative Ewing Sarcoma Studies. *Ann. Oncol.* **9:** 275.

66. Perilongo, G., C. Carollo, L. Salviati, *et al*. 1997. Diencephalic syndrome and disseminated juvenile pilocytic astrocytomas of the hypothalamic-optic chiasm region. *Cancer* **80:** 142.

67. Petrilli, A.S., B. de Camargo, V.O. Filho, *et al*. 2006. Results of the Brazilian Osteosarcoma Treatment Group Studies III and IV: prognostic factors and impact on survival. *J. Clin. Oncol.* **24:** 1161.

68. Pollack, I.F., S.D. Finkelstein, J. Woods, *et al*. 2002. Expression of p53 and prognosis in children with malignant gliomas. *N. Engl. J. Med.* **346:** 420.

69. Pritchard-Jones, K., A. Kelsey, G. Vujanic, *et al*. 2003. Older age is an adverse prognostic factor in stage I, favorable histology Wilms' tumor treated with vincristine monochemotherapy: a study by the United Kingdom Children's Cancer Study Group, Wilm's Tumor Working Group. *J. Clin. Oncol.* **21:** 3269.

70. Riley, R.D., S.A. Burchill, K.R. Abrams, *et al*. 2003. A systematic review and evaluation of the use of tumour markers in paediatric oncology: Ewing's sarcoma and neuroblastoma. *Health Technol. Assess.* **7:** 1.

71. Riley, R.D., D. Heney, D.R. Jones, *et al*. 2004. A systematic review of molecular and biological tumor markers in neuroblastoma. *Clin. Cancer Res.* **10:** 4.

72. Rodriguez-Galindo, C., T. Liu, M.J. Krasin, *et al*. 2007. Analysis of prognostic factors in Ewing sarcoma family of tumors: review of St. Jude Children's Research Hospital studies. *Cancer* **110:** 375.

73. Rutka, J.T., J.S. Kuo, M. Carter, *et al*. 2004. Advances in the treatment of pediatric brain tumors. *Expert Rev. Neurother.* **4:** 879.

74. Rutkowski, S., U. Bode, F. Deinlein, *et al*. 2005. Treatment of early childhood medulloblastoma by postoperative chemotherapy alone. *N. Engl. J. Med.* **352:** 978.

75. Schleiermacher, G., M. Peter, O. Oberlin, *et al*. 2003. Increased risk of systemic relapses associated with bone marrow micrometastasis and circulating tumor cells in localized Ewing tumor. *J. Clin. Oncol.* **21:** 85.

76. Serra, M., K. Scotlandi, M.C. Manara, *et al*. 1995. Analysis of P-glycoprotein expression in osteosarcoma. *Eur. J. Cancer* **31A:** 1998.

77. Shimada, H., I. Ambros, L. Dehner, *et al*. 1999. The International Neuroblastoma Pathology Classification (the Shimada system). *Cancer* **86:** 364.

78. Tabori, U., J. Ma, M. Carter, *et al*. 2006. Human telomere reverse transcriptase expression predicts progression and survival in pediatric intracranial ependymoma. *J. Clin. Oncol.* **24:** 1522.

79. Tanaka, T., T. Iehara, T. Sugimoto, *et al*. 2005. Diversity in neuroblastomas and discrimination of the risk to progress. *Cancer Lett.* **228:** 267.

80. Tournade, M., C. Com-Nougue, P. Voute, *et al*. 1993. Results of the Sixth International Study of Pediatric Oncology Wilms' Tumor Trial and Study: a risk-adapted therapeutic approach in Wilm's tumor. *J. Clin. Oncol.* **11:** 1014.

81. Vermeulen, J., S. Ballet, O. Oberlin, *et al*. 2006. Incidence and prognostic value of tumour cells detected by RT-PCR in peripheral blood stem cell collections from patients with Ewing tumour. *Br. J. Cancer* **95:** 1326.

82. von Schweinitz, D. 2000. Identification of risk groups in hepatoblastoma—another step in optimising therapy. *Eur. J. Cancer* **36:** 1343.

83. Vujanic, G.M., B. Sandstedt, D. Harms, *et al*. 2002. Revised International Society of Paediatric Oncology (SIOP) working classification of renal tumors of childhood. *Med. Pediatr. Oncol.* **38:** 79.

84. Wu, H.Y., H.M. Snyder, 3rd & G.J. D'Angio. 2005. Wilms' tumor management. *Curr. Opin. Urol.* **15:** 273.

85. Zeltzer, P.M., J.M. Boyett, J.L. Finlay, *et al*. 1999. Metastasis stage, adjuvant treatment, and residual tumor are prognostic factors for medulloblastoma in children: conclusions from the Children's Cancer Group 921 randomized phase III study. *J. Clin. Oncol.* **17:** 832.

Implantable Port Devices Are Catheters of Choice for Administration of Chemotherapy in Pediatric Oncology Patients—A Clinical Experience in Pakistan

Barkat Hooda, Gulrose Lalani, Zehra Fadoo, and Ghaffar Billoo

The Aga Khan University, Karachi, Pakistan

Phlebitis and cellulitis are commonly encountered problems in oncology patients receiving chemotherapy through peripherally inserted intravenous catheters. Use of central venous access devices (CVAD) is desirable. We have seen a steady increase in the use of CVADs in our oncology service with frequent use of indwelling ports, particularly during the last 2 years. In this study we have attempted to elucidate advantages of CVAD and compared them to peripheral catheters. This is a retrospective study with chart review of all oncology patients admitted in our oncology service at the Aga Khan University Hospital from March 2003 to March 2005. A survey was also conducted from a randomly selected sample of parents of children with cancer to elicit parental views regarding their choice of a particular catheter. Catheter-related infections were quite common (over 50%) in patients with peripheral lines, resulting in increased costs and prolonged hospitalization. Externalized CVADs were found difficult to care for, carried a risk of being accidentally pulled out or punctured, and were deemed undesirable for older female patients for cosmetic reasons. We found that the internalized CVADs (portacath) were superior to the externalized or peripheral lines and resulted in better patient and family satisfaction. Use of peripheral lines must be gradually phased out of pediatric oncology practice in Pakistan. Indwelling CVADs have become the standard of care internationally and should be considered for most patients in developing countries whenever resources are available.

Key words: pediatric oncology; acute lymphocytic leukemia; vascular access; portacath

Introduction

Administration of chemotherapy in children through a peripheral line is associated with multiple discomforting problems. Insertion usually requires multiple attempts that could potentially result in the introduction of infection in an immunocompromised host.[1] The procedure itself is often painful and time consuming and results in poor psychosocial well-being of the patient. Integrity of the peripheral veins may be compromised by pro-inflammatory chemotherapeutic agents and the trauma related to repetitive blood sampling.[2] Accordingly, reliable peripheral venous access becomes progressively more difficult to obtain and even harder to maintain in a patient requiring ongoing care.[3]

Acute lymphocytic leukemia (ALL) accounts for approximately one-third of the total oncology practice in pediatrics in most parts of the world, including Pakistan. Treatment for ALL lasts from 2–3 years in most protocols. A majority of patients with solid tumors also require prolonged therapy and multiple admissions to

Address for correspondence: Barkat Hooda, The Aga Khan University, Stadium Road, P.O. Box 3500, Karachi, Pakistan. barakaat@fastmail.fm

Ann. N.Y. Acad. Sci. 1138: 43–46 (2008). © 2008 New York Academy of Sciences.
doi: 10.1196/annals.1414.007

the hospital. A reliable and less complication-prone alternative to peripheral lines is essential for such patients.[4]

Indwelling, tunneled, externalized central venous catheters of the Hickman or Broviac type and totally implantable central venous access port systems (portacath) have been advocated to improve reliability of venous access and reduce the discomfort associated with repetitive peripheral venous cannulation.[5] Obvious advantages of indwelling lines are better compliance and improved overall quality of life.[6]

Use of an implantable venous access device (portacath) has revolutionized contemporary oncology care for children by providing a better alternative. These semipermanent, indwelling ports require a heparin flush at 4–6 week intervals to maintain patency for long-term use and provide highly reliable venous access whenever required.[7] Ports have the advantage of providing minimal restrictions of daily routines including bathing or sporting activities.[8] They are associated with lower risk of infection and malfunction.[9] A single port may last for the total duration of therapy for most patients.

The Aga Khan University Hospital, Karachi, is a tertiary-care private academic medical center in Pakistan. We currently see approximately 45 new pediatric oncology cases per year. This study was conducted to evaluate advantages and disadvantages of various modes of chemotherapy administration in a third world country.

Patients and Methods

This is a retrospective chart review study performed at The Aga Khan University Hospital Karachi. Medical records of each episode for 92 pediatric oncology patients, aged under 15 years, undergoing therapy admitted and readmitted between April 2003 and April 2005 were reviewed. There were a total of 660 admissions in 2003 and 675 in 2004. Study patients received either standard peripheral venous access, a Hickman catheter, or an implantable

venous access port system. Criteria for catheter failure included documentation of irreversible mechanical malfunction, including occlusion, or complication, including infection of the port pocket/tunnel and persistent positive growth despite adequate therapy including fungal infections.[10] Peripheral lines were deemed ineffective if integrity of the venous access site was compromised resulting in local pain, cellulitis, swelling, or extravasation.

A separate survey was conducted with 52 available parents of the patients to determine their views regarding their preference for a particular venous access modality. The following questions were asked:

1. What would be your choice for venous access for your child peripheral line? semi permanent central line?
2. Please specify reason/s for your selection?
3. There are two kinds of semi permanent central lines used in our service; which one would you prefer: Hickman line? Portacath?
4. Please specify reason/s for your selection?

Results

All patients in the year 2003–2004 had peripheral venous catheterization except two who had a portacath inserted and four who had a Hickman line inserted. Patients with peripheral lines developed multiple complications, including infection, extravasation with chemical burns, leakage, and pain.[11] Two patients with Hickman lines developed resistant infection, one had rupture of the lumen, and one suffered significant accidental hemorrhage due to detachment of tubing connections. Regular use of portacath insertion was implemented during 2004–2005, and a total of 40 ports were inserted during that time. Complications, including infection, rupture, and reinsertion, occurred less frequently with ports when compared to other types of venous access (Figs. 1–3). Fifty-two parents participated in the

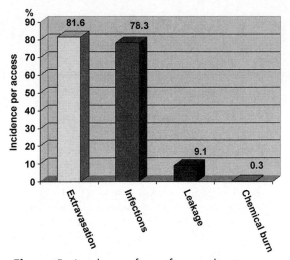

Figure 1. Incidence of specific complications per 100 access attempts—peripheral lines.

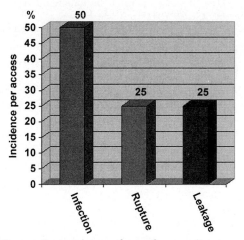

Figure 2. Incidence of specific complications per 100 access attempts—Hickman lines. Please note that extravasations and chemical burns were not encountered.

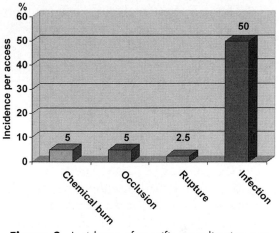

Figure 3. Incidence of specific complication per 100 access attempts—portacath.

survey. All of them showed clear preference for portacath even if their child had been treated via peripheral lines during times when ports were not in routine use at our hospital.[10]

Discussion

Maintaining long-term venous access for patients requiring cytotoxic chemotherapy is one of the challenging tasks for the healthcare team looking after children with cancer.[12]

The overall safety of port systems was demonstrated by the low complication rate observed in this study, although the infection rate was high but significantly less than with peripheral venous access devices. McLean and colleagues have shown that neutropenia is an independent risk factor for infection related to catheters and for sepsis of unknown origin.[13] In our study only two ports needed to be removed because of infection. Most infections were due to gram positive organisms. *Staphylococcus epidermidis* was found to be the most commonly isolated organism in our study, confirming trends of catheter infections all over the world.[14] This study confirms that the use of ports for the administration of chemotherapy preserves venous integrity and avoids pain and trauma associated with repetitive needle pricks. Accidental catheter withdrawal or hemorrhagic complications usually associated with Hickman lines are rarely seen since ports do not extrude from the chest.[15] In our study, patients suffered reduced anxiety with port access procedures knowing that access is always available, and that, in our opinion, resulted in improved compliance with the therapy.

In a typical third-world setting, it is generally more convenient for untrained staff to use peripheral lines for patients with cancer. When ports are available in a tertiary care facility, access procedures after hours often requires provision of competent nursing personnel.[16] Training of support staff for adequate coverage of oncology patients having such devices is thus particularly important.

Conclusion

During times of economic constraints and availability of limited healthcare resources, our findings have important implications for healthcare planners of cancer care services in developing countries. We conclude that implantable ports are a safe and effective method of venous access in patients with cancer when compared to other alternatives.[17] It is not clear though if the obvious advantages of ports outweigh their additional costs. Further studies of economic considerations are required to address this issue.

Conflicts of Interest

The authors declare no conflicts of interest.

References

1. Greene, F.L., W. Moore, G. Strickland, *et al*. 1988. Comparison of a totally implantable access device for chemotherapy (Port-a-Cath) and long-term percutaneous catheterization (Broviac). *South Med. J.* **81:** 580–583.

2. Groeger, J.S., A.B. Lucas, H.T. Thaler, *et al*. 1993. Infectious morbidity associated with long-term use of venous access devices in patients with cancer. *Ann. Intern. Med.* **119:** 1168–1174.

3. Harvey, W.H., T.E. Pick & R.I. Solenberger. 1989. A prospective evaluation of the Port-a-Cath implantable venous access system in chronically ill adults and children. *Surg. Gynecol. Obstet.* **169:** 495–500.

4. Brothers, T.E., L.K. Von Moll, J.E. Niederhuber, *et al*. 1988. Experience with subcutaneous infusion ports in three hundred patients. *Surg. Gynecol. Obstet.* **166:** 295–301.

5. Guenier, C., J. Ferreira & J.C. Pector. 1989. Prolonged venous access in cancer patients. *Eur. J. Surg. Oncol.* **15:** 553–555.

6. Becton, D.L., M. Kletzel, E.S. Gollady, *et al*. 1988. An experience with an implanted port system in 66 children with cancer. *Cancer* **61:** 376–378.

7. Lokich, J.J., A. Bothe, Jr., P. Benotti, *et al*. 1985. Complications and management of implanted venous access catheters. *J. Clin. Oncol.* **3:** 710–717.

8. Gves, J., W. Ensminger & J. Niederhuber. 1982. Totally implanted system for intravenous chemotherapy in patients with cancer. *Am. J. Med.* **73:** 841–846.

9. Brincker, H. & G. Saeter. 1986. Fifty-five patient years' experience with a totally implanted system for intravenous chemotherapy. *Cancer* **57:** 1124–1129.

10. Carde, P., M.F. Cosset-Delaigue, A. LaPlanche, *et al*. 1989. Classical external indwelling central venous catheter versus totally implanted venous access systems for chemotherapy administration: a randomized trial in 100 patients with solid tumours. *Eur. J. Clin. Oncol.* **25:** 939–944.

11. Mirro, J. Jr., B.N. Rao, D.C. Stokes, *et al*. 1989. A prospective study of Hickman/Broviac catheters and implantable ports in pediatric oncology patients. *J. Clin. Oncol.* **7:** 214–222.

12. Kappers-Klunne, M.C., J.E. Degener, T. Stijnen, *et al*. 1989. Complications from long-term indwelling central venous catheters in hematologic patients with special reference to infection. *Cancer* **64:** 1747–1752.

13. McLean, T.W., C.J. Fisher, B.M. Snively & A.R. Chauvenet. 2005. Central venous lines in children with lesser risk. Acute lymphoblastic leukemia: optimal type and timing of placement. *J. Clin. Oncol.* **23:** 3024–3029.

14. Mueller, B.U., J. Skelton, D.P.E. Callender, *et al*. 1992. A prospective randomized trial comparing the infectious and non-infectious complications of an externalized catheter versus a subcutaneously implanted device in cancer patients. *J. Clin. Oncol.* **10:** 1943–1948.

15. Stanislav, G., R.J. Fitzgibbons, R.T. Bailey, *et al*. 1987. Reliability of implantable central venous access devices in patients with cancer. *Arch. Surg.* **122:** 1280–1283.

16. Ingram *et al*. 1991. Complications of indwelling venous access lines in the pediatric hematology patient: a prospective comparison of external catheters and subcutaneous ports. *Am. J. Pediatr. Hematol. Oncol.* **13:** 130–136.

17. Strum, S., J. McDermed, A. Korn, *et al*. 1986. Improved methods for venous access: the Port-a-Cath, a totally implanted catheter system. *J. Clin. Oncol.* **4:** 596–603.

Attitudes, Perceptions, and Family Coping in Pediatric Cancer and Childhood Diabetes

Valsamma Eapen,[a] **AbdelAzim Mabrouk,**[b] **and Salem Bin-Othman**[b]

[a]*Faculty of Medicine and Health Sciences,*

[b]*School Health Services, UAE University, Al Ain, United Arab Emirates*

The importance of psychosocial factors in psychological adjustment and coping in children with cancer and their families is well recognized. In this study, parental attitudes, children's self-perceptions, and families' coping were studied in 38 children with leukemia, 30 children with juvenile diabetes, and 30 control subjects. Children with cancer scored themselves more negatively than their parents on all the subscales except scholastic competence, while children with diabetes scored negatively in the area of athletic competence. With regard to family coping, parental hope as well as social and family communication were the most important factors that contributed to better coping in children with leukemia, while parental education and health awareness were integral to better coping in children with diabetes. Awareness of family coping and understanding the domains of self-competence and self-worth, which are vulnerable in children with cancer, can help healthcare providers to target these issues and to offer appropriate psychosocial intervention.

Key words: childhood cancer; diabetes mellitus; psychosocial factors; self-perceptions; family coping

Introduction

Psychosocial research in recent decades has significantly advanced our understanding of the psychosocial issues in the context of pediatric cancer[1] and diabetes.[2] Survival rates of children with cancer have improved dramatically over the last two decades. In keeping with this remarkable medical achievement, psychosocial research has changed from helping patients and families deal with issues related to death and dying to issues of health promotion intervention for cancer survivors. In an international comparison of contributions to psychosocial research and survivors, Last and colleagues[3] showed significant descriptive differences depending on the place of origin of the study. This and other reports suggest that these issues vary from one culture to another, hence the need to study these factors locally in each community.

Subjects and Methods

The subjects were ascertained through a tertiary referral pediatric cancer unit (children with leukemia) and the Central School Health Clinic (children with diabetes and control subjects) in Al Ain, United Arab Emirates (UAE). They were evaluated using the Arabic version of the Harter's Self Perception Profile for Children (SPPC)[4] and the parallel parent version. SPPC, a self-report inventory for measuring perceived competence in children consists of a subscale of global self-worth indicating the general sense of self-esteem as well as five specific domains, namely scholastic competence, social acceptance, athletic competence, physical

Address for correspondence: Valsamma Eapen, PhD., FRCPsych, FRANZCP, Professor and Chair of Infant, Child & Adolescent Psychiatry, University of New South Wales, ICAMHS—Mental Health Centre, L1, Liverpool Hospital, Elizabeth Street, NSW 2170, Australia. Voice: +61 2 9616 4245; fax: +61 2 9601 2773. v.eapen@unsw.edu.au appearance, and behavioral conduct. Other relevant individual, family, and psychosocial variables were explored using a semistructured interview schedule.

Results

On Harter's SPPC, children with leukemia and diabetes scored themselves significantly lower on the total score as compared to control subjects (leukemia $P < 0.0001$; diabetes $P = 0.014$). On the subscales, significantly lower scores were noted in the areas of physical appearance ($P = 0.02$) and social acceptance ($P = 0.01$) for children with leukemia, while children with diabetes scored significantly lower than the control group on global self-worth ($P = 0.01$). Children with cancer scored themselves more negatively than their parents on all the subscales (social acceptance, athletic competence, physical appearance, and behavioral conduct) except that of scholastic competence. Children with diabetes, on the other hand, scored themselves more negatively than did their their parents only in the area of athletic competence ($P = 0.023$).

With regard to family coping, we found that parental hope ($P = 0.001$) as well as social and family communication in the form of opportunities for sharing and expression of emotions ($P = 0.005$) were the most important factors that contributed to better coping in children with leukemia, while parental education and health awareness ($P < 0.0001$) were integral to better coping in patients with diabetes.

Discussion

Our findings that physical appearance and social acceptance are particularly affected in children with cancer is interesting. These findings are significant since these two domains are particularly vulnerable in children with cancer and can be explained as resulting from the effects of chemotherapy on physical appearance and a self-perception that they are socially undesirable or a burden to others. Perceived physical appearance seems to be of special importance to children with cancer, with direct effects on psychological adjustment and indirect effects mediated through self-esteem. With regard to children with diabetes, it may be that some of these children are also obese, which may have a direct link to their athletic competence and an indirect link to global self-worth. While children with cancer had a more negative view of themselves than their parents in all the other domains, there was agreement with regard to the domain of scholastic performance, which may be due to the fact that this is a relatively more objective construct than the other domains. Indeed self-esteem and self-confidence are important determinants in the psychosocial development and adaptation of young people suffering from chronic physical illnesses, and other studies have suggested that psychosocial adjustment and coping in these situations may be enhanced through social skills training and other cognitive behavioral methods.[5]

Patenaude and Kupst[6] and Kazak[7] recently reviewed the advances made in psycho-oncology and highlighted the shift in research toward the concerns of long-term survivors. Several studies in this regard have shown that children with cancer do exceptionally well, and several variables including optimism, hardiness, and repressive adaptation have all been described as important in the multiple pathways to resilience.[8] Our finding that parental hope and better family sharing and communication are associated with better coping supports this view. Similarly, the association between better coping and higher parental education and health awareness in diabetes may be mediated through better self-care and well being in these children as a result of the involvement of parents in their children's health issues and their role in instilling positive personal model beliefs[9] in their children about the need and the effectiveness of diabetes treatment regimens. These findings lend further support to the need and the importance of parent and family partnerships in the care of children with chronic physical illnesses. Thus, although there are certain differences between children with cancer and diabetes in relation to their attitudes and self-perceptions, and in relation to the factors that contribute to adjustment and coping, there are also parallels and similarities in the general principles related to the value of parental and family involvement and support. Understanding the differential effects of psychosocial issues in cancer versus diabetes will also no doubt help psychosocial teams to differentially target and intervene as part of the comprehensive treatment regimen that would help restore the life of young persons with chronic physical illness to the best of their capacities.

Conclusion

While ongoing research at basic science and clinical levels is continuing to make advances in the treatment of both cancer and diabetes, clinicians working in this field are becoming increasingly aware of the importance of psychosocial intervention as part of the overall management. This is not surprising given the fact that life stresses and families' adjustments and coping with these stressors play a crucial role in determining compliance to treatment programs as well as treatment response in these young patients. It is hoped that a better understanding of these variables in this sociocultural setting will help clinicians to incorporate appropriate psychosocial interventions and thus facilitate better quality of life in these children.

Conflicts of Interest

The authors declare no conflicts of interest.

References

1. Patenaude, A.F. & B. Last. 2001. Cancer and children: where are we coming from? Where are we going? *Psychooncology* **10:** 281–283.
2. Wysocki, T., L.M. Buckloh, A.S. Lochrie & H. Antal. 2005. The psychologic context of pediatric diabetes. *Pediatr. Clin. North Am.* **52:** 1755–1778.
3. Last, B.F., M.A. Grootenhuis & C. Eiser. 2005. International comparison of contributions to psychosocial research on survivors of childhood cancer: past and future considerations. *J. Pediatr. Psychol.* **30:** 99–113.
4. Eapen, V., A. Naqvi & A.S. Al-Dhaheri. 2000. Cross cultural validation of Harter's Self Perception Profile in the United Arab Emirates. *Ann. Saudi Med.* **20:** 8–11.
5. Varni, J.W., E.R. Katz, R. Colegrove, Jr. & M. Dolgin. 1993. The impact of social skills training on the adjustment of children with newly diagnosed cancer. *J. Pediatr. Psychol.* **18:** 751–767.
6. Patenaude, A.F. & M.J. Kupst. 2005. Psychosocial functioning in pediatric cancer. *J. Pediatr. Psychol.* **30:** 9–27.
7. Kazak, A.E. 2005. Evidence-based interventions for survivors of childhood cancer and their families. *J. Pediatr. Psychol.* **30:** 29–39.
8. Phipps, S. 2005. Commentary: contexts and challenges in pediatric psychosocial oncology research: chasing moving targets and embracing "good news" outcomes. *J. Pediatr. Psychol.* **30:** 41–45.
9. Skinner, T.C., M. John & S.E. Hampson. 2000. Social support and personal models of diabetes as predictors of self-care and well-being: a longitudinal study of adolescents with diabetes. *J. Pediatr. Psychol.* **25:** 257–267.

Role of Tc^{99m} MIBI SPECT in the Assessment of Treatment Response in Pharyngeal Carcinoma

Ambreen Khawar,[a] **Muhammad Asif Rafique,**[b] **Rafaqat Ali Jafri,**[b] **and Shabana Saeed**[a]

[a]*Department of Medical Sciences, Pakistan Institute of Engineering and Applied Sciences (PIEAS), Islamabad, Pakistan*

[b]*Nuclear Medicine, Oncology and Radiotherapy Institute (NORI), Islamabad, Pakistan*

The purpose of this study was to compare Tc^{99m} MIBI SPECT imaging with computed tomography (CT) for assessment of post-radiotherapy treatment response in pharyngeal carcinoma. Twenty-two subjects took part in this study, which included six patients with nasopharyngeal carcinoma (Group I), three patients with oropharyngeal carcinoma and eight patients with hypopharyngeal carcinoma (Group II), and five control patients (Group III). All scans were analyzed qualitatively and quantitatively and correlated with findings on local examination and biopsy. Various indices such as ratios of nasopharynx, oropharynx, and hypopharynx to scalp (NSR, OSR, HSR), to nuchal muscles (NNR, ONR, HNR), and parotid glands (NPR, OPR, HPR) were calculated. The mean values of these above mentioned ratios calculated in the control group (Group III) were used as cutoff values to determine the presence or absence of tumor tissue in the patient groups (Groups I and II). The cutoff values calculated were 2.89 (NSR), 1.39 (NNR), 0.57 (NPR), 3.83 (OSR), 1.81 (ONR), 0.83 (OPR), 2.86 (HSR), 1.73 (HNR), and 0.59 (HPR). The results revealed 100% sensitivity for primary nasopharyngeal tumors but less sensitivity for primary oropharyngeal and hypopharyngeal tumors (63.6%). Based on a relative decrease in tracer uptake, Tc^{99m} MIBI SPECT scan was able to predict partial remission, complete remission, and no response on post-therapy scans. There were three false-negative results of disease progression in addition to evidence of disease eradication on CT scan. Thus Tc^{99m} MIBI SPECT imaging has shown promising results in the detection of primary tumors and evaluation of treatment response much earlier than CT scan, which needs further exploration and large-scale studies.

Key words: Tc^{99m} MIBI SPECT; CT; pharyngeal carcinoma

Introduction

Among extracranial head and neck carcinomas, more than 90% are squamous cell carcinomas of the oral, pharyngeal, or laryngeal regions.[1] The annual incidence of nasopharyngeal carcinoma has been reported to be highest in China and South East Asia, amounting to 5–10/100,000 in females and 10–20/100,000 in males.[2] The world incidence of oropharyngeal and hypopharyngeal cancer of 0.9 in females to 4.9 in males/year/100,000 is noted.[1] Despite the fact that anatomical imaging modalities like computed tomography (CT) and magnetic resonance imaging (MRI), a priori, in this region of complex anatomy leave little scope for functional imaging in diagnosis of primary tumors, in post-therapeutic settings (i.e., after surgery or radio or chemotherapy) they still pose a dilemma for the diagnosis of residual or

Address for correspondence: Dr. Ambreen Khawar, Department of Medical Sciences, PIEAS, P.O. Nilore, Islamabad, Pakistan. ambreen_khawar@hotmail.com, fac053@pieas.edu.pk

Ann. N.Y. Acad. Sci. 1138: 50–57 (2008). © 2008 New York Academy of Sciences. doi: 10.1196/annals.1414.009

TABLE 1. Demographic Profile of Patients

Groups	Total patients	M:F	Mean Age ± S.E.M.	Primary site of lesion	Presence of lymph nodes on on C/F[a] or CT[b] scan
Group I	6	5:1	29 ± 19.0	Nasopharynx	5
Group II	11	2:9	49 ± 12.6	Oro/Hypopharynx	3
Group III (Controls)[c]	5	3:2	51 ± 1.10	None	none

[a]Clinical features.
[b]Computed tomography.
[c]Those without any pharyngeal lesion who had come to the center for cardiac rest scans.

recurrent tumor. The diagnosis of residual or recurrent tumor as both CT and MR diagnostic criteria depend upon structural alterations. Moreover, the histopathologic diagnosis from blind biopsies of these sites for suspected residual disease proves to be inconclusive owing to the ensuing fibrosis or edema at these sites.[3] It has been advised radiobiologically to treat persistent tumors within a relatively brief period, as both the target volume and the required dose will be smaller.[1] Therefore, it is very important to assess the treatment response, and functional imaging, such as radionuclide scintigraphy, can prove very helpful and beneficial in this regard.

Among the radionuclide studies for pharyngeal carcinoma considerable experience has been accrued with Tc^{99m} methoxyisobutylisonitrile (MIBI), thallium (Tl-201), and fluorodeoxyglucose (FDG-18) positron emission tomography (PET) studies of nasopharyngeal carcinoma pre- and post-therapeutically,[5–12] but no studies have been carried out in a Pakistani population. To our knowledge, only one or two studies have been conducted regarding oropharyngeal and hypopharyngeal carcinoma pretherapeutically[1] but no study has explored the role of Tc^{99m} MIBI in the assessment of treatment response. The purpose of the current study was to evaluate the role of Tc^{99m} MIBI single photon emission computed tomography (SPECT) scan for detecting primary tumors and assessing treatment response, as measured by residual tissue, in pharyngeal carcinoma and compare these findings with the efficacy of CT scan imaging.

Patients and Methods

Patients

Between September 2003 and March 2004, a total of 22 consecutive patients, including six diagnosed with nasopharyngeal carcinoma (Group I, 5 males, 1 female, mean age 29 ± 19.0), 11 suffering from histologically confirmed carcinoma of the hypopharynx ($n = 8$) or oropharynx ($n = 3$) (Group II, 2 males, 9 females, mean age 49 ± 12.6), and five control patients (Group III, 3 males and 2 females, mean age 51 ± 7.4) were enrolled in this study. The demographic profile is given in Table 1. The study was approved by the Ethics Committee of the Pakistan Institute of Engineering and Applied Sciences, Nilore, Islamabad, Pakistan. All patients and controls gave their informed consent prior to their participation in the study. In the pretherapy group, all patients in Groups I and II were included. Post-therapy assessment was done by Tc^{99m} MIBI SPECT scans and CT scans in two patients in Group I and six patients in Group II 4 weeks after radiotherapy.

Tc^{99m} MIBI SPECT

The preparation of Tc^{99m} MIBI (MIBI PINSCAN produced by RIPG, PINSTECH, Islamabad) was performed according to the manufacturer's instructions. Tc^{99m} MIBI SPECT acquisition was started 10 min after intravenous injection of 650–800 MBq Tc^{99m} MIBI. The SPECT scintigraphy was performed using the

ADAC single-head rotating gamma camera interfaced with an online Pegasus computer equipped with a low-energy high resolution collimator. Sixty-four splash views around 360°, 30 s each with a zoom factor of 1 were recorded in a $128 \times 128 \times 16$ matrix. Images were reconstructed by a filtered back projection technique using a Butterworth filter ($f_c = 2.5$, order $= 15$) and analytic y-axis filter. Patient motion was ruled out on sinograms and cinedisplay. The attenuation correction was applied to transverse slices by drawing an ellipse around the mid-transverse slice and using an attenuation coefficient of 0.12 and pixel calibration factor of 0.592. The slices were reoriented, mid-sagittal and coronal slices were generated, and volume images and 3D display were analyzed to locate the lesion as shown in Figure 1.

CT Imaging

CT starting from the skull base to the thoracic inlet was performed without contrast followed by 20 min postcontrast (100 mg injectate of Urografin or Ultravist as a bolus). Axial and coronal slices, 10 mm in the case of large lesions and 5 mm for small lesions, were made. Images were analyzed by a radiologist blinded to Tc^{99m} MIBI scan findings. Tumor extent was assessed visually by taking into account the presence of mass, asymmetry in regional wall thickness of the pharynx, and contrast enhancement, as shown in Figure 2.

Data Analysis

Qualitative assessment of Tc^{99m} MIBI SPECT images was compared with CT scan, nasoscopy, and laryngoscopy/histopathology findings by two nuclear medicine physicians. Any uptake other than the normal sites seen in images in the control group (Group III), as shown in Figure 3 and Table 2, was considered abnormal. For semiquantitative analysis, a composite of midsagittal slices was used to calculate the ratios of nasopharynx to scalp

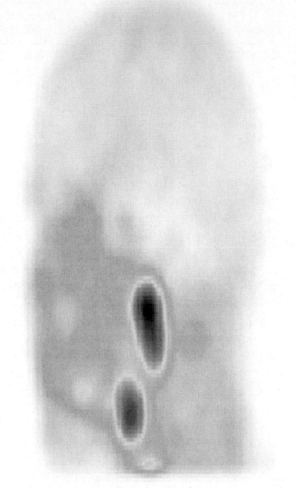

Figure 1. 3D volume image of patient in control group representing the tracer distribution in head and neck region according to metabolic status of tissue as found highest in thyroid and parotid glands.

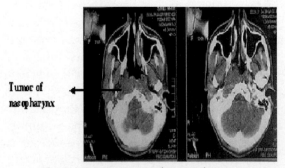

Figure 2. CT image showing lesion in nasopharynx.

TABLE 2. Radiopharmaceutical Distribution in Control Group

Grades of radio-pharmaceutical uptake	Low/mild intensity	Medium intensity	High intensity
Sites of uptake	Scalp, neck, muscles, nasal cavity, oral cavity, pharyngeal region, lateral ventricles in brain, and pituitary gland	Posteromedial part of orbits bilaterally, tongue, and sometimes nasal cavity	Thyroid, parotid, submandibular glands, and sometimes lacrimal glands

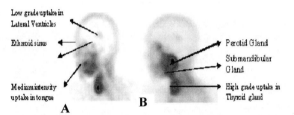

Figure 3. (A) Composite midsagittal slices to show the normal distribution of Tc⁹⁹ᵐ MIBI in head and neck region and **(B)** composite of all sagittal slices to show normal tracer distribution in the salivary and thyroid glands.

(NSR) and to nuchal muscles (NNR), oropharynx to scalp (OSR) and to nuchal muscles (ONR), and hypopharynx to scalp (HSR) and to nuchal muscles (HNR). Regions of interest were drawn on respective sites of nasopharynx, oropharynx, hypopharynx, scalp, and parotid glands on a composite of midcoronal slices to calculate the ratios of Naso-, Oro-, and Hypopharynx to parotid glands (NPR, OPR, HPR) respectively as shown in Figure 4. The mean values of all these ratios—NSR, NNR, NPR, OSR, ONR, OPR, HSR, HNR, and HPR—from the control group subject scans were taken as cutoff values for comparison with the patient groups. The cutoff values calculated are given in Table 3.

Statistical analysis of the data was done using Microsoft Excel statistical tools. The mean and standard error of the mean (S.E.) were calculated for the demographic data, for the indices mentioned above, and for the presence or absence of lesion. The sensitivity and false-negative values were calculated for each group.

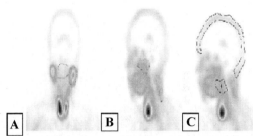

Figure 4. Diagram showing regions of interest for calculation of **(A)** nasopharynx to parotid gland ratio (NPR) in midcoronal slices composite, **(B)** nasopharynx to nuchal muscle ratio (NNR) in midsagittal slice composite, and **(C)** oropharynx to scalp ratio (OSR) in midsagittal slices composite.

TABLE 3. Cutoff Values for Nasopharynx, Oropharynx, and Hypopharynx

Ratios (abbreviations described in text)	Cutoff values
NSR	2.98
NNR	1.39
NPR	0.57
OSR	3.83
ONR	1.81
OPR	0.83
HSR	2.86
HNR	1.73
HPR	0.59

Results

Primary Tumor Detection

The Tc⁹⁹ᵐ MIBI SPECT scans proved to be 100% sensitive for primary disease of the nasopharynx but showed only 63.6% sensitivity for Group II, oro/hypopharyngeal carcinoma (Table 4). However, much lower sensitivity, 20% in the case of nasopharyngeal

TABLE 4. Qualitative Analysis Data for Primary Lesion and Lymph Nodes

Group No.	Lesion	Modality	n	TP	Sensitivity (%)
I	Primary	Tc[99m] MIBI SPECT	6	6	100%
		CT	6	5	90%
	L. Nodes	Tc[99m] MIBI SPECT	5	1	20
		CT	5	5	100
II	Primary	Tc[99m] MIBI SPECT	11	7	63.6
		CT	11	11	100
	L. Nodes	Tc[99m] MIBI SPECT	3	0	0

TABLE 5. Results of Semiquantitative Analysis in Pretherapy Imaging of Groups I and II

Group No.	Modality used	Ratios	n	TP	Sensitivity(%)
I	CT	None	6	6	100%
	Tc[99m] MIBI SPECT	Nasopharynx/scalp ratio	6	6	100%
		Nasopharynx/nuchal muscle ratio	6	5	83
		Nasopharynx/parotid gland ratio	6	3	50
II	CT	None	11	11	100
	Tc[99m] MIBI SPECT	Tumor/scalp ratio	11	8	73
		Tumor/nuchal muscle ratio	11	6	54
		Tumor/parotid gland ratio	11	10	91

TABLE 6. Results of Post-therapy Comparison of CT and Tc[99m] MIBI Scans

Group No.	Modality used	No. of pts followed	No change	Partial remission	Complete remission	Disease has increased
I	CT	2	2	None	None	None
	Tc[99m] MIBI SPECT	2	None	1	None	1
II	CT	6	3	2	1	None
	Tc[99m] MIBI SPECT	6	2	2	None	2

carcinoma and zero for oro/hypopharyngeal carcinoma patients, was seen for lymph node metastasis. The mean ± S.E. value of nasopharynx to scalp ratio (NSR) was 4.5 ± 1.45, nasopharynx to nuchal muscle ratio (NNR) = 1.88 ± 0.74, and nasopharynx to parotid gland ratio (NPR) = 0.38 ± 0.26 for Group I.

In the case of hypopharyngeal carcinoma patients, the following values were determined. The mean ± S.E. value of hypopharynx to scalp ratio (HSR) was 3.72 ± 0.81; hypopharynx to nuchal muscles ratio (HNR) had a range of (1.18–2.23) and a mean of 1.67 ± 0.35; and hypopharynx to parotid gland ratio (HPR) had a range (0.53–1.27) and a mean of (0.85 ± 0.24). For patients with oropharyn-

geal carcinoma, the ranges and mean values were: oropharynx to scalp ratio (OSR) 2–7.07 and 4.52 ± 2.53, oropharynx to nuchal muscles ratio (ONR) 1.13–3.45 and 2.25 ± 2.98), and oropharynx to parotid gland ratio (OPR) 0.73–1.67 and 1.1 ± 1.37). The sensitivities of various semiquantitative indices are given in Table 5.

Treatment Response

The results of post-therapy comparisons of Tc[99m] MIBI SPECT scans and CT scans are given in Table 6. The Tc[99m] In Group I patients, MIBI SPECT scans showed one patient with partial remission (Fig. 5) and one with disease aggravation (Fig. 6), in contrast to two

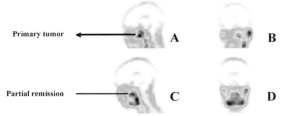

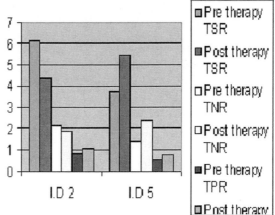

Primary tumor ← **A**   **B**

Partial remission ——— **C**   **D**

Figure 5. Partial remission in post-therapy scans as shown by reduction of tracer uptake in post-therapy scans **(C, D)** in comparison with pretherapy scans **(A, B)** in patient Group I.

Figure 7. Comparison of pretherapy and post-therapy semiquantitation in two patients of Group I.

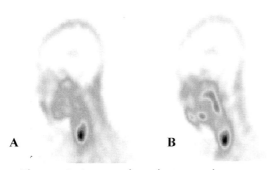

A   **B**

Figure 6. Increased uptake in post-therapy scans **(B)** in comparison with initial lesion in pretherapy scan **(A)** of patient of Group I.

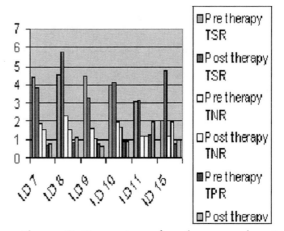

Figure 8. Comparison of pretherapy and post-therapy semiquantitation in five patients of Group IIA and one patient of Group IIB.

with no change The same outcome was evident on semiquantitative analysis, as shown in Figure 7 for two representative patients. In the case of the six patients of Group II who were followed by Tc^{99m} MIBI SPECT, the scan revealed two with no change, two with partial remission, and two with disease aggravation,. In contrast, CT scans indicated three patients with no change, two with partial remission, and one with complete remission, as shown in Table 6 and Figure 8. No histopathological confirmation could be obtained in these patients because of the risk of bleeding.

Discussion

The role of functional imaging for diagnosis and management of malignant disease is still evolving.[13] Most important is the decision regarding residual tissue in the post-treatment tumor bed, as prompt detection and early salvage therapy helps in reducing morbidity and mortality.[14] To date no promising results have been obtained by the various anatomical imaging modalities (CT and MRI). These modalities are able to detect the abnormal masses but are unable to distinguish viable malignant disease from inflammatory changes, edema, fibrosis, and scarring that may ensue after surgery, chemotherapy, or radiotherapy.[15,16]

Many radiopharmaceuticals have been tried in the setting of malignancy. One of these, Tc^{99m} MIBI, is taken up in tumor cells in proportion to its mitochondrial content (driven by negative inner mitochondrial potential) and

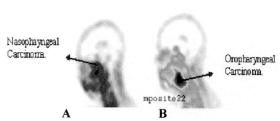

Figure 9. Increased tracer uptake in **(A)** the region of nasopharynx in a positive case of nasopharyngeal carcinoma and **(B)** the region of base of tongue in a positive case of oropharyngeal carcinoma.

hence reflecting its metabolic activity. Its uptake is also directly proportional to increased blood flow to tumor. Tc^{99m} MIBI has been utilized for detection of various primary and residual tumors,[17] but data on Tc^{99m} MIBI for the detection and staging of primary and residual pharyngeal carcinoma are scarce. In this study, the role of this agent for the detection of primary or residual pharyngeal disease has been analyzed.

The study revealed mild, moderate, and gross physiological uptake of Tc^{99m} MIBI in various head and neck structures. The uptake conformed to the passive influx due to the negative potential of plasma membrane and the mitochondrial inner membrane, as well as reversible accumulation within mitochondria of both malignant cells (Fig. 9) and normal cells (Fig. 3).

Tc^{99m} MIBI was found to be 100% sensitive for primary nasopharyngeal carcinoma, similar to that of CT in concurrence with the findings of Chiewit and colleagues[10] and Kostakoglu and colleagues.[4] These authors also reported 100% sensitivity, compared with Leitha and colleagues,[11] who documented a sensitivity of 90%. However, the index calculated for NSR in our study was found to be 2.98, compared to 1.3 in the study by Pui and colleagues[5] and 1.5 by Kostakoglu and colleagues.[4] The NSR (nasopharynx to scalp ratio) cutoff was the best way to detect nasopharyngeal carcinoma in comparison to the lower sensitivity of NNR (nasopharynx to nuchal muscle ratio) and NPR (nasopharynx to parotid gland ratio). The sensitivity of Tc^{99m} MIBI for oro/hypopharyngeal patients (Group II) was found to be low—only 63.6% for the primary mass, as compared to 100% sensitivity of CT scan—which was in concurrence with the reported sensitivity of 68% by Henze and co-workers.[1] This low tumor-detection rate could be due to the masking effect of intense physiological uptake in the salivary glands, thyroid gland, and larynx, which makes delineation of tumor difficult and may be attributable to the small tumor size.[1] The HNR (hypopharynx to nuchal muscle ratio) was found to be 1.39, as compared to value of 2.2 given by Henze and colleagues.[1] This difference in ratio again may be related to the above-mentioned high uptake in the surrounding areas, and, secondly, the difference may be because Henze and colleagues had used perchlorate suppression of salivary glands, which was not done in this study.[1]

Regarding the low sensitivity of the Tc^{99m} MIBI scans for lymph node detection, the small size of lymph nodes, less than the inherent spatial resolution of the gamma camera system, as well as masking due to the surrounding structures, could be responsible.[18]

The comparison of post-therapy scans of Tc^{99m} MIBI with post-therapy CT and pretherapy Tc^{99m} MIBI and CT scans gave varied results in terms of partial remission, no change, disease aggravation, and complete remission. Due to lack of histopathology, owing to the risk of bleeding at this post-therapy interval, in the post-therapy settings confirmation of these findings could not be obtained. It is important to note that before the anatomical changes occur, prediction of disease could be made with functional imaging, as evident by the post-therapy comparison of scans in the Group I patients who had no evidence of partial remission or disease aggravation on CT scans; the same observation was encountered in Group II patients. In addition, it was noted that inflammatory changes, increased blood supply, blood flow in the healing tissues, and irreversible cell death related to changes in membrane potentials that set in after radiotherapy in these patients also contribute to the false-negative results of the disease interpretation[18] at 4 weeks post-therapy. Hence, post-therapy scans should be performed at a later stage.

Again, regarding semi-quantitative results, the NSR, OSR, and HSR were found to be better predictors of disease status than NNR, NPR, HNR, HPR, ONR, and OPR. The findings regarding NPR ratio, which increases post-therapy due to radiation-induced damage to parotid glands, were not observed consistently in all patients, which could be due to the difference in radiation dose administered to the patient or perhaps to unresolved parotitis that may have ensued in these patients.

Despite the small number of patients included in this study, the role of Tc⁹⁹ᵐ MIBI is commendable. Validation of its results and decisions regarding incorporation of this functional scan in the management regimens of pharyngeal tumors now require large-scale studies.

Conflicts of Interest

The authors declare no conflicts of interest.

References

1. Henze, M., A. Mohammed, W. Mier, *et al.* 2002. Pretreatment evaluation of carcinoma of hypopharynx and larynx with 18F flourodeoxyglucose, I¹²³ I-methyl L-tyrosine and Tc99m-hexakis 2-methoxyisobytylisonitrile. *Eur. J. Nuclear Med. Mol. Imaging* **29:** 324–330.

2. Ho, J.H. 1976. Epidemiology of nasopharyngeal carcinoma. In *Cancer in Asia*. T. Hirayama, Ed.: 49. Baltimore University Press. Baltimore, MD.

3. Chisin, R. 1999. Nuclear medicine in head and neck oncology: reality and perspectives. *J. Nucl. Med.* **40:** 91–95.

4. Kostakoglu, L., U. Uysal, E. Ozyar, *et al.* 1997. A comparative study of technetium-99m sestamibi and technetium-99m tetrofosmin single photon tomography in the detection of nasopharyngeal carcinoma. *Eur. J. Nucl. Med.* **24:** 621–628.

5. Pui, M.H., J.Q. Du, T.C. Yueh & S.Q. Zeng. 1998. Imaging of nasopharyngeal carcinoma with Tc-99m MIBI. *Clin. Nucl. Med.* **1:** 29–32.

6. Sun, S.S., S.C. Tsai, Y.J. Ho, *et al.* 2001. Detection of cervical lymph node metastases in nasopharyngeal carcinoma: comparison between Tc-9m methoxyisobutylisonitrile single photon emission computed tomography and computer tomography. *Anticancer Res.* **21:** 1307–1310.

7. Tai, C.G., Y.C. Shiau, M.H. Tsai, *et al.* 2002. Detection of cervical lymph node metastases in nasopharyngeal carcinomas: comparison between Tc-99m methoxyisobutyl isonitrile single photon emission computed tomography with magnetic resonance imaging. *Neoplasma* **49:** 251–254.

8. Shiau, Y.C., S.C. Tsai, Y.J. Ho, *et al.* 2001. Comparison of Tc-99m methoxyisobutyl isonitrile single photon computed tomography and to detect recurrent or residual nasopharyngeal carcinomas after radiotherapy. *Anticancer Res.* **21:** 2213–2217.

9. Kao, C.H., Y.C. Shiau, Y.Y. Shen, *et al.* 2002. Detection of recurrent or persistent nasopharyngeeal carcinomas after radiotherapy with Tc-99mMIBI SPECT and CT: comparison with F-18 FDG PET. *Cancer* **94:** 1981–1986.

10. Chiewit, S., S. Sangruchi, V. Veerasan, *et al.* 2000. Tc99m sestamibi single photon emission computerized tomography in the detection of nasopharyngeal carcinoma. *AJR* **6:** 91–100.

11. Leitha, T., C. Glaser, M. Pruckmayer, *et al.* 1998. Technetium-99m-MIBI in primary and recurrent head and neck tumors: contribution of bone SPECT image fusion. *J. Nucl. Med.* **39:** 1166–1171.

12. Tomura, N., O. Watanabe, S. Takahashi, *et al.* Comparison of Tl-201 Chloride SPECT with Tc-99m MIBI SPECT in the depiction of malignant head and neck tumors. *Ann. Nuclear Med.* **20:** 107–114.

13. Müller, S.T., B. Guth-Tougelides & H. Creutzig. 1987. Imaging of malignant tumours with Tc99m MIBI (abstract). *J. Nucl. Med.* **28:** 562.

14. Anzai, Y., W.R. Carroll, D.J. Quint, *et al.* 1996. Recurrence of head and neck cancer after surgery or irradiation: prospective comparison of 2-deoxy-2-[F-18] fluoro-D-glucose PET and MR imaging diagnoses. *Radiology* **200:** 135–141.

15. Bronstein, A.D., A.N. Nyberg Schwartz, W.P. Shuman & B.R. Griffen. 1989. Soft tissue changes after head and neck radiation: CT findings. *Am. J. Neuroradiol.* **10:** 171–175.

16. Glazer, H.S., J.H. Niemeyer, N.M. Balfe, *et al.* 1986. Neck neoplasms: mr imaging. II. posttreatment evaluation. *Radiology* **160:** 349–354.

17. Fukumoto, M. 2004. Single photon agents for tumor imaging: ²⁰¹Tl, ⁹⁹ᵐTc-MIBI, ⁹⁹ᵐTc-tetrofosmin. *Ann. Nuclear Med.* **18:** 79–95.

18. Kostakoglu, L., U. Uysal, E. Ozyar, *et al.* 1996. Pre-and post-therapy thallium-201 and technetium-99m-sestamibi SPECT in nasopharyngeal carcinoma. *J. Nucl. Med.* **37:** 1956–1962.

Selective Surgical Management of Well-Differentiated Thyroid Cancer

Ashok Shaha

Attending Surgeon, Memorial Sloan-Kettering Cancer Center, Head and Neck Service, New York, New York, USA

Professor of Surgery, Cornell University Medical Center, New York, New York, USA

There has been a rapid rise in the incidence of thyroid cancer in the United States, along with more incidentalomas of the thyroid. Treatment of thyroid cancer revolves around appropriate surgical intervention, minimizing complications, and the use of adjuvant therapy in select circumstances. Prognostic features and risk-group analysis are crucial in determining the appropriate treatment. Thyroid cancers are divided into low-, intermediate-, and high-risk groups. Surgical treatment should adhere to the risk-group analysis. The prognostic features in thyroid cancer are age, gender, size and grade of the tumor, extrathyroidal extension, and completeness of resection. The patient presenting with extrathyroidal extension needs extra attention in the operating room to remove all gross tumor during the initial surgical procedure to avoid future recurrences. Nodal metastasis generally has minimal implications; however, in older patients and those with poorly differentiated histology, it has major implications. Grading of the tumor is important, especially for understanding the poorly differentiated varieties of thyroid cancer, such as tall cell and insular. These patients do not respond well to RAI and are best followed with a PET scan. Overall survival in patients with well-differentiated thyroid cancer exceeds 95%.

Key words: thyroid cancer; incidentaloma; prognostic features; risk groups in thyroid cancer; surgical treatment of thyroid cancer

Introduction

There appears to be a rapid rise in the incidence of thyroid cancer over the last two decades. Approximately 32,000 new patients with thyroid cancer were expected to be seen in the year 2007 in the United States.[1] A large number of these appear to be incidental findings. Whether this rapid rise is due to increasing diagnostic utilization or a true rise in the incidence of thyroid cancer remains unclear. Another tumor with such a rapid rise is cutaneous malignant melanoma. Even though the incidence of thyroid cancer has tripled in the United States, mortality from thyroid cancer has remained essentially unchanged (Fig. 1). The majority of deaths from thyroid cancer are related to anaplastic or medullary thyroid cancer. Recently, pathologists have been able to distinguish poorly differentiated thyroid carcinoma where the incidence of local recurrence and distant metastasis is quite high with a high mortality rates. The prognostic factors in thyroid cancer have been well described in recent years from Mayo Clinic, Lahey Clinic, and Memorial Sloan-Kettering Cancer Center.[2-5] These prognostic factors include age, sex, grade of tumor, extrathyroidal extension, size of tumor, and distant metastasis. Gender, multicentricity, and lymph node metastasis do not have a major prognostic bearing on thyroid cancer. Memorial Sloan-Kettering Cancer Center has divided its thyroid cancer patients into low-, intermediate-,

Address for correspondence: Ashok Shaha, MD, FACS, 1275 York Avenue, New York, NY 10021. Voice: +212-639-7649; fax: +212-717-3302. shahaa@mskcc.org

Ann. N.Y. Acad. Sci. 1138: 58–64 (2008). © 2008 New York Academy of Sciences.
doi: 10.1196/annals.1414.010

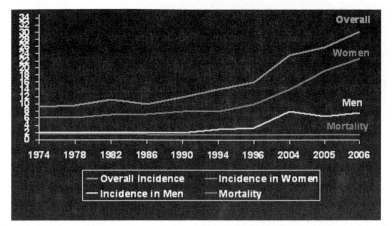

Figure 1. Thyroid cancer: incidence & mortality, 1974–2006. (In color in *Annals* online.)

TABLE 1. Risk-Group Definitions in Differentiated Carcinoma of the Thyroid

	Low risk	Intermediate risk	Intermediate risk	High risk
Age (years)	<45	<45	>45	>45
Distant metastasis	M0	M+	M0	M+
Tumor size	T1, T2 (<4 cm)	T3, T4 (>4 cm)	T1, T2 (<4 cm)	T3, T4 (>4 cm)
Histology and grade	Papillary	Follicular and/ or high-grade	Papillary	Follicular and/ or high-grade
5-year survival	100%	96%	96%	72%
20-year survival	99%	85%	85%	57%

and high-risk groups (Table 1). This risk stratification is critical in understanding the biology of thyroid cancer, its prognosis, and the appropriate treatment modalities, including adequate surgical extirpation.[6]

Low-risk thyroid cancers are generally in young patients (low-risk patients) and are small tumors (less than 4 cm) without extrathyroidal extension and with well-differentiated histology. High-risk thyroid cancers include high-risk patients (above the age of 45) and high-risk tumors (larger than 4 cm) with extrathyroidal extension or poor histology. The intermediate-risk group includes young patients with aggressive thyroid cancer or older patients with small tumors. This risk stratification appears to be consistent in various published series. The treatment decisions and the role of adjuvant therapy, such as radioactive iodine and external radiation therapy, are well defined based on this risk stratification. The subject of thy-

roid cancer has generated considerable debate, with a large volume of published literature and continued controversy among surgeons and endocrinologists.[7] There are strong proponents and opponents of total versus less-than-total thyroidectomy. What is important is to identify the risk groups and apply appropriate surgical treatment based on patient and tumor characteristics. The entire idea of selective surgical treatment rests on understanding the biology of the tumor, applying the appropriate surgical procedure based on the aggressiveness of the cancer, not over-treating every patient with thyroid cancer, and using adjuvant therapy selectively.

Surgical Treatment of Thyroid Cancer

The surgical treatment of thyroid cancer can be divided into treatment of primary tumor, treatment of regional nodes, and treatment of distant metastasis.

Surgical Treatment of Primary Thyroid Tumor

A patient presenting with a thyroid nodule and suspected to have thyroid cancer needs either a thyroid lobectomy or total thyroidectomy, depending upon the extent of the disease. Patients in the high-risk group, or those with aggressive thyroid cancer, will require a total thyroidectomy. This is mainly because total thyroidectomy will allow the patients to receive adjuvant radioactive iodine. Patients who are likely to require radioactive iodine treatment should undergo total thyroidectomy to facilitate postoperative radioactive iodine ablation. The advantages of thyroid lobectomy include minimizing over-treatment and the high incidence of complications in total thyroidectomy. These include nerve injury and temporary or permanent hypoparathyroidism. Also a selected group of patients do not require thyroid supplementation in follow-up. The pros of total thyroidectomy include: the complication rate in the hands of good thyroid surgeons is not higher than that in thyroid lobectomy, the ease of radioactive iodine scanning and ablation and the ease of follow-up of patients with thyroglobulin.

Both thyroid lobectomy and total thyroidectomy appear to render similar long-term results in low- and selected intermediate-risk group patients.[8] There are no randomized prospective trials in patients presenting with low-risk thyroid cancer with total or less-than-total thyroidectomy. Obviously, the philosophy of extent of thyroidectomy will depend on the surgical center, the approach taken by individual surgeons, and the patient's preference. However, a Google search will convince the majority of patients with thyroid cancer to undergo total thyroidectomy so that they can get radioactive iodine ablation and thyroglobulin follow-up. Unfortunately, the thyroglobulin follow-up is

TABLE 2. Thyroid Cancer: A Unique Human Neoplasm

- Age is the most important prognostic factor
- No stage III & IV cancers in patients < 45
- Multicentricity of thyroid cancer is frequent, though without prognostic impact
- No prognostic impact of microscopic tumor – "laboratory cancer"
- Nodal metastasis has no impact on outcome
- Impact of extrathyroidal spread is high with local recurrence
- Grade of the tumor & histologic poorly differentiated features have impact on outcome

likely to show an incidental lymph node metastasis, the treatment of which continues to be most debatable.

Obviously, if the preoperative ultrasound shows thyroid nodularity involving the contralateral lobe, patients should undergo total thyroidectomy. Subtotal and near-total thyroidectomy should be abandoned for patients with suspected or known thyroid cancer. There is always a small amount of thyroid tissue left behind after these procedures, which can be seen on radioactive iodine scanning in the postoperative period. Recently, postoperative dosimetry and ablation have been performed with recombinant thyroid stimulating hormone (TSH), which has helped improve quality of life for patients who otherwise would have undergone approximately 6 weeks of hypothyroidism (Table 2).

Management of Neck Nodes in Thyroid Cancer

Many series reported in the literature have shown that regional nodal metastasis in well-differentiated thyroid cancer has no major prognostic implications.[9–11] However, with the recent increasing use of preoperative ultrasound, a large number of patients with well-differentiated thyroid cancer are noted to have nodal metastasis.[12] Obviously, these patients will require appropriate nodal clearance.

TABLE 3. Surgical Decisions for Metastatic Cervical Nodes from Thyroid

- Modified neck dissection for palpable nodes
- Evaluate jugular and superior mediastinal nodes at the time of surgery
- Modified neck dissection
  - "Berry picking"
  - Preserve sternocleidomastoid (SCM), internal jugular vein (IJV), XI (accessory) nerve
  - Submandibular gland
  - Selective or compartment-oriented neck dissection

Standard radical neck dissection is rarely performed for well-differentiated thyroid carcinoma. The berry picking operation, which was a popular operation approximately two decades ago, is rarely used today. There was a high incidence of multiple positive nodes in the neck, and berry picking will allow further recurrence of nodal metastasis, requiring additional neck surgery. The standard surgical procedure utilized now is a modified neck dissection, with the removal of lymph nodes at levels II, III, IV, and V. The incidence of nodal metastasis at level I from well-differentiated thyroid carcinoma is quite low, and generally, the region is not dissected routinely, as there may be a high incidence of injury to the lower division of the facial nerve (ramus mandibularis). Some authors use the terms, "compartment oriented dissection" or "selective nodal dissection," for removal of the selected groups of lymph nodes[12] (Table 3). The incidence of nodal metastasis above the accessory nerve is quite low, and skeletonization of the accessory nerve is not necessary in all patients with cervical nodal metastasis.

The most important aspect of neck dissection is central compartment clearance. Again, there continues to be considerable controversy as to routine use of central compartment clearance. Practically every patient undergoing surgery for thyroid cancer should have a thorough and complete central compartment evaluation. This is generally a clinical evaluation at the time of surgery. If the nodes appear to be enlarged or suspicious, they should be removed with appropriate central compartment clearance. A frozen section may be of help in patients with Hashimoto's thyroiditis to see if these are benign or metastatic lymph nodes. Routine paratracheal clearance is likely to result in a high incidence of temporary and permanent hypoparathyroidism and is best avoided, unless there is a strong suspicion of nodal metastasis. However, it is important to undertake appropriate paratracheal clearance in individuals with locally aggressive, large thyroid cancers, or suspected paratracheal lymph node metastasis. In patients undergoing surgery for medullary carcinoma of the thyroid, routine central compartment clearance is a standard procedure, as there appears to be a high incidence of nodal metastasis in patients with medullary thyroid carcinoma. The superior mediastinal lymph nodes should also be dissected in these individuals. However, superior mediastinal clearance is generally not indicated in well-differentiated thyroid carcinoma unless there is an obvious clinical suspicion of superior mediastinal lymph nodes during surgery.

Management of Locally Aggressive Thyroid Cancer

One of the most important prognostic features in well-differentiated thyroid cancer is the presence of extrathyroidal extension.[13] This has been shown to be the most important prognostic feature in various series around the world. When the thyroid tumor is intrathyroidal, the outcome is excellent. However, once the tumor comes out of the thyroid gland and invades the surrounding structures, the incidence of local recurrence is high (Fig. 2). The majority of these tumors happen to be in older individuals and generally with a more aggressive histology, such as tall cell, insular, or poorly differentiated thyroid cancer. It is very important for the pathologist to differentiate these various types of poorly differentiated thyroid cancers.

The structures that are commonly involved in locally aggressive thyroid cancer are the anterior structures and the posterior structures.

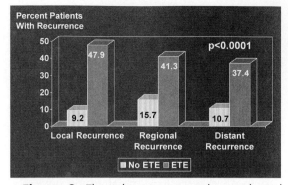

Figure 2. Thyroid carcinoma with extrathyroid extension (ETE) treatment failure. (Memorial Sloan-Kettering data.) (In color in *Annals* online.)

The anterior structures include the sternohyoid and sternothyroid muscles. These generally do not have major prognostic implications, as they can be easily resected. However, when the tumor invades the posterior structures, such as the recurrent laryngeal nerve, esophageal musculature, and tracheal wall, the overall outcome is quite poor, and surgical resection may be quite difficult. If the tumor invades the recurrent laryngeal nerve and the recurrent laryngeal nerve is known to be paralyzed preoperatively, it should be resected at the time of surgery for better resection of locally aggressive thyroid cancer. Preoperative evaluation of the vocal cords is essential. When the tumor is adherent to the esophageal musculature, it can be easily resected. However, when the tumor is adherent to the tracheal wall, it is important to evaluate the exact extent of the tumor invasion into the trachea.[14–16] If the tumor is adherent to the tracheal wall, it can be easily shaved off. It is vitally important to leave no gross tumor behind. Obviously, the microscopic tumor in these individuals requires adjuvant therapy, such as radioactive iodine or external radiation therapy. However, if the tumor is invading the trachea with submucosal or intraluminal extension, tracheal resection is generally recommended. A sleeve resection is advisable with end-to-end anastomosis.[15] Obviously, the radicality of surgery changes with tracheal resection, and when such findings are noted intra-

operatively, the decision making may be quite difficult, unless the surgeon has considerable experience in these procedures.

Occasionally, secondary surgical intervention may be necessary, if the primary surgeon is not prepared for radical resection. However, the extent of the radicalness should depend upon the extent of the locally aggressive thyroid cancer. The basic oncologic principle that should be adhered to is the removal of all gross tumor at the time of the first surgical procedure. Preoperative evaluation in these individuals is crucial, including evaluation of the vocal cord function. Extent of the disease in the central compartment should be evaluated with imaging studies, such as CT scan or MRI of the neck. If the CT scan is to be performed, the contrast dye may interfere with postoperative radioactive iodine ablation, and MRI or CT without contrast should be considered. If the tumor is minimally invading the trachea, a partial tracheal resection can be performed. However, reconstructing partial defects may be more difficult than classical sleeve resection. If the tumor invades the cricothyroid junction or the laryngeal structure, the treatment becomes extremely complex, as primary total laryngectomy is rarely indicated in well-differentiated thyroid carcinoma. However, occasionally, the larynx is considerably destroyed, and if there is extensive involvement of the laryngeal framework, total laryngectomy may be required. A partial laryngectomy may be attempted in selected patients if all gross tumor could be removed, and the laryngeal function can still be maintained.

The involvement of the carotid artery and prevertebral fascia are generally considered to present an inoperable situation, and such individuals are best considered for palliative treatment. Postoperative radioactive iodine ablation is routinely considered in these individuals. However, it must be remembered that the effectiveness of radioactive iodine ablation is much inferior in poorly differentiated thyroid carcinoma. Such individuals are best followed with a PET scan, since these tumors are 18 Fluorodeoxy Glucose (FDG) avid. External radiation therapy is used in selected individuals, especially with poor histologic features. External radiation therapy has been shown to improve local control in patients with locally aggressive thyroid carcinoma. There is clearly a high incidence of distant metastases in these individuals. Total thyroidectomy should be routinely performed in these patients to facilitate radioactive iodine ablation. Appropriate neck evaluation should be considered at the time of primary surgery, since there is generally a higher incidence of regional recurrence in patients with locally aggressive thyroid carcinoma (Fig. 2).

Management of Distant Metastases in Well-Differentiated Thyroid Carcinoma

Although rare, the most frequent areas where the tumor generally metastasizes include the lungs, bones, and the brain.[17] Pulmonary metastases are fairly common in young individuals, in patients with locally aggressive or advanced primary tumor. It is also well known in patients with bulky nodal metastases. The chest x-ray may be normal, and even the CT scan of the chest may be normal; however, the best way to identify pulmonary metastases is radioactive iodine ablation. The majority of these patients present miliary diffuse pulmonary metastases. In patients with diffuse pulmonary metastases, there is no role for surgical intervention. However, if the patient has developed massive pleural effusion, pleurodesis or sclerotherapy may be considered in selected individuals.

The bony metastases, though rare, are seen most commonly in patients with follicular carcinoma or Hurthle cell carcinoma. These individuals generally present with backache or hip pain. Occasionally, they may present with pathological fracture. It is not uncommon to see a patient presenting with bony metastasis as an initial sign of thyroid cancer. These individuals

are best treated with total thyroidectomy and radioactive iodine ablation. External radiation therapy may be used for pain control from bony metastases.

Brain metastases are fairly rare in patients with well-differentiated thyroid carcinoma. However, they may be part of a diffuse metastatic process. Brain metastases are best evaluated with an imaging study, such as a CT, MRI, or PET scan. Occasionally, a craniotomy may be necessary for diagnostic purposes for a space-occupying lesion. These patients are best treated with radioactive iodine ablation, or with external radiation therapy. During external radiation therapy, patients may develop brain edema and may need steroid supplementation. Overall prognosis in patients with bone and brain metastases is quite poor. The highest thyroglobulin levels are generally seen in bony metastases.

Conclusion

There continues to be considerable controversy regarding the optimal extent of thyroidectomy in patients presenting with low-risk well differentiated thyroid carcinoma. The debate continues primarily due to varying philosophies of the individual treating physicians, the consideration of use of radioactive iodine ablation, and concerns about the complications of total thyroidectomy. In low-risk patients, generally there is hardly any difference in the overall outcome, whether the patient has undergone total versus less-than-total thyroidectomy. The decisions regarding the extent of thyroidectomy should be made in the operating room, based on a variety of factors, including risk-group stratification, extent of the disease, condition of the opposite lobe, involvement of the central compartment lymph nodes, and opportunities for long-term follow-up of these patients.

In patients with locally aggressive thyroid cancer, one needs to be aggressive for removal of the entire gross tumor. The first surgical procedure should be the most appropriate and adequate with the use of adjuvant therapy, such as radioactive iodine ablation and external radiation therapy, in selected individuals. Most of these patients may have aggressive histology, such as tall cell or poorly differentiated thyroid carcinoma. The treatment of nodal metastases should include appropriate nodal clearance by modified neck dissection. Follow-up in these individuals includes radioactive iodine ablation, thyroglobulin monitoring, and ultrasound evaluation of the neck. If the ultrasound reveals obvious metastatic disease, appropriate neck dissection should be considered. However, resection of subcentimeter lymph nodes should be considered against the complications of surgery and the need for further surgeries. The management of distant metastases generally is palliative, including radioactive iodine ablation and external radiation therapy in select circumstances. Bony metastases pose the worst prognosis. Patients with advanced, well-differentiated thyroid carcinoma should be treated in a multidisciplinary fashion, with appropriate involvement of thyroid surgeons, endocrinologists involved in thyroid cancer management, and nuclear physicians.

Thyroid cancer continues to be a unique human neoplasm, different from other human cancers, generally with an excellent prognosis and unique biological behavior (Table 2).

Conflicts of Interest

The author declares no conflicts of interest.

References

1. Jemal, A., R. Siegel, E. Ward, *et al.* 2007. Cancer statistics, 2006. *CA Cancer J. Clin.* **56:** 106–130.
2. Hay, I.D., C.S. Grant, W.F. Taylor, *et al.* 1987. Ipsilateral lobectomy versus bilateral lobar resection in papillary thyroid carcinoma: a retrospective analysis of surgical outcome using a novel prognostic scoring system. *Surgery* 1088–1095.
3. Hay, I.D., E.J. Bergstralh, J.R. Goellner, *et al.* 1993. Predicting outcome in papillary thyroid carcinoma: development of a reliable prognostic scoring system in a cohort of 1779 patients surgically treated at one institution during 1940 through 1989. *Surgery* **102**(6): 947–953.
4. Cady, B. 1997. Hayes Martin Lecture. Our AMES is true: how an old concept still hits the mark, or risk group assignment points the arrow to rational therapy selection in differentiated thyroid cancer. *Am. J. Surg.* **174**(5): 462–468.
5. Shaha, A.R. 2004. Implications of prognostic factors and risk groups in the management of differentiated thyroid cancer. *Laryngoscope* **114:** 393–402.
6. Shaha, A. 2006. Treatment of thyroid cancer based on risk groups. *J. Surg. Oncol.* **94:** 683–691.
7. Mazzaferri, E.L. & S.M. Jhiang. 1994. Long-term impact of initial surgical and medical therapy on papillary and follicular thyroid cancer. *Am. J. Med.* **97**(5): 418–428.
8. Shaha, A.R., J.P. Shah & T.R. Loree. 1997. Low-risk differentiated thyroid cancer: the need for selective treatment. *Ann. Surg. Oncol.* **4:** 328–333.
9. Noguchi, M. *et al.* 1993. Multivariate study of prognostic factors of differentiated thyroid carcinoma: The significance of histologic subtype. *Int. Surg.* **78**(1): 10–15.
10. Sugitani, I., N. Kasai, Y. Fujimoto & A. Yanagisawa. 2004. A novel classification system for patients with PTC: addition of the new variables of large (3 cm or greater) nodal metastases and reclassification during the follow-up period. *Surgery* **135:** 139–148.
11. Sherman, S.I., J.D. Brierley, M. Sperling, *et al.* 1998. Prospective multicenter study of thyroid carcinoma treatment: initial analysis of staging and outcome. National Thyroid Cancer Treatment Cooperative Study Registry Group. *Cancer* **83**(5): 1012–1021.
12. Grubbs, E.G. & D.B. Evans. 2007. Role of lymph node dissection in primary surgery for thyroid cancer. *J. Natl. Compr. Canc. Netw.* **5:** 623–630.
13. Patel, K.N. & A.R. Shaha. 2005. Locally advanced thyroid cancer. *Curr. Opin. Otolaryngol. Head Neck Surg.* **13:** 112–116.
14. Shaha, A.R. 2000. Controversies in the management of thyroid nodule. *Laryngoscope* **110**(2 Pt 1): 183–193.
14. Czaja, J.M. & T.V. McCaffrey. 1997. The surgical management of laryngotracheal invasion by well-differentiated papillary thyroid carcinoma. *Arch. Otolaryngol. Head Neck. Surg.* **123**(5): 484–490.
15. Grillo, H.C. & P. Zannini. 1986. Resectional management of airway invasion by thyroid carcinoma. *Ann. Thorac. Surg.* **42**(3): 287–298.
16. Anderson, P.E. *et al.* 1995. Differentiated carcinoma of the thyroid with extrathyroidal extension. *Am. J. Surg.* **170**(5): 467–470.
17. Cohen, E.G., R.M. Tuttle & D.H. Kraus. 2003. Postoperative management of differentiated thyroid cancer. *Otolaryngol. Clin. North Am.* **36:** 129–157.

Captopril as a Potential Inhibitor of Lung Tumor Growth and Metastasis

Samir Attoub,[a] **Anne Marie Gaben,**[d] **Suhail Al-Salam,**[b]
M.A.H. Al Sultan,[a] **Anne John,**[b] **M. Gary Nicholls,**[c]
Jan Mester,[d] **and Georg Petroianu**[a]

Departments of [a]Pharmacology, [b]Pathology, and [c]Internal Medicine, Faculty of Medicine and Health Sciences, UAE University, Al Ain, United Arab Emirates

[d]INSERM U 673, Molecular and Clinical Oncology of Solid Tumors, University Pierre et Marie Curie Paris VI, Hospital Saint-Antoine, Paris, France

Lung cancer is the most common form of cancer in the world, and 90% of patients die from their disease. The angiotensin converting enzyme (ACE) inhibitors are used widely as antihypertensive agents, and it has been suggested that they decrease the risk of some cancers, although available data are conflicting. Accordingly, we investigated the anticancer activity of the ACE inhibitor, captopril, in athymic mice injected with highly tumorigenic LNM35 human lung cells as xenografts. Using this model, we demonstrated that daily IP administration of captopril (2.8 mg/mouse) for 3 weeks resulted in a remarkable reduction of tumor growth (58%, $P < 0.01$) and lymph node metastasis (50%, $P = 0.088$). There were no undesirable effects of captopril treatment on animal behavior and body weight. In order to determine the mechanism by which captopril inhibited tumor growth, we investigated the impact of this drug on cell proliferation, apoptosis, and angiogenesis. Immunohistochemical analysis demonstrated that captopril treatment significantly reduced the number of proliferating cells (*Ki*-67) in the tumor samples but was not associated with inhibition of tumor angiogenesis (CD31). Using cell viability and fluorescent activated cell sorting analysis tests, we demonstrated that captopril inhibited the viability of LNM35 cells by inducing apoptosis, providing insight about the mechanisms underlying its antitumorigenic activities. In view of these experimental findings, we conclude that captopril could be a promising option for the treatment of lung cancer.

Key words: captopril; lung tumor; metastasis

Introduction

The angiotensin converting enzyme (ACE), or kininase II, is a dipeptidyl carboxy metalolpeptidase that plays a major role in blood pressure, volume, and electrolyte regulation. ACE is present as a membrane-bound enzyme in endothelial and epithelial cells in the lung, kidney, intestine, testes, and brain and as a soluble form in blood.[2] Endothelial and circulating ACE converts inactive angiotensin I into the vasoactive octapeptide, angiotensin II (Ang II), and also inactivates the vasodilator peptide bradykinin.

Ang II via its type 1 receptor promotes angiogenesis through activation of vascular endothelial growth factor (VEGF) and VEGF receptor type 2 (KDR) expression in endothelial cells.[3-6] The Ang II type 2 receptor is a 7-transmembrane G-protein coupled receptor that regulates signal transducer and activator of transcription-3 (STAT3).[7] We recently established heterotrimeric G-proteins and STAT3 as new therapeutic targets in lung and colon cancer.[8,9] Ang II acts as an anti-apoptotic agent

Address for correspondence: Dr. Samir Attoub, Department of Pharmacology, Faculty of Medicine and Health Sciences, UAE University, P.O. Box 17666, Al Ain, United Arab Emirates. Voice: +9713-7137-219; fax: +9713-767-2033. samir.attoub@uacu.ac.ae

Ann. N.Y. Acad. Sci. 1138: 65–72 (2008). © 2008 New York Academy of Sciences.
doi: 10.1196/annals.1414.011

and as a growth factor acting through the epidermal growth factor receptor transactivation-ERK signaling pathway.[10,11,12]

Lever and colleagues (1998) have suggested that long-term use of ACE inhibitors protects against some cancers.[1] In this regard, we demonstrated that some of the long-term beneficial effects of ACE inhibitors could be mediated by a peroxisome proliferator activator receptor (PPAR).[13] Activators of PPAR alpha and gamma inhibit colorectal tumor progression, possibly via inhibition of proliferation and, remarkably, inhibit the growth of human lung cancer cells through induction of apoptosis.[14,15]

In this context, ACE inhibition with captopril, an ACE inhibitor widely used in the management of hypertension, has been shown experimentally to inhibit tumor angiogenesis and to induce apoptosis.[16,17] In contrast, ACE inhibition with quinaprilat or perindopril reportedly promotes angiogenesis in a rabbit model of hindlimb ischemia.[18,19] In agreement with these results, Ebrahimian and co-workers demonstrated that ACE inhibition promoted neovascularization through activation of bradykinin B2 receptor signaling independently of VEGF expression, whereas it reduced blood vessel growth through inhibition of the Ang II pathway.[19,20] Thus, ACE inhibitors with high tissue affinity appear to have proangiogenic effects. In another report, perindopril inhibited angiogenesis and metastasis of hepatocellular carcinoma.[21] In conclusion, the effect of ACE inhibitors on angiogenesis and tumor growth remains controversial.

In the present study, we investigated the impact of the ACE inhibitor, captopril, on human lung tumor growth, angiogenesis, and metastasis *in vivo* and on cell viability and apoptosis *in vitro*.

Methods

Cell Culture and Reagents

Human non-small cell lung cancer cells LNM35 were maintained in Roswell Park Memorial Institute (RPMI) 1640 (Invitrogen,

Cergy Pontoise, France) supplemented with 10% fetal bovine serum (FBS) (Roche Molecular Biochemicals, Meylan, France) and antibiotics. The pharmacological inhibitor of ACE (captopril) was purchased from Sigma (Saint-Quentin Fallavier, France). Primary antibodies were purchased from the following manufacturers: monoclonal rat antimouse CD31 antibody (BD PharMingen, San Jose, CA), monoclonal mouse antihuman Ki-67 antibody (Dako, Copenhagen, Denmark). The secondary antibodies were goat antirat antibody (Sigma, St. Louis, MO) and rabbit antimouse antibody (Dako, Copenhagen, Denmark).

Cell Viability

LNM35 cells were seeded at a density of 5000 cells/well onto 96-well plates in RPMI plus 10% FBS. After 24 h, cells were treated for 24 h with increasing concentrations of captopril (0.01–10 mM), in triplicate assays. The effect of captopril on cell viability was determined using a CellTiter-Glo Luminescent Cell Viability assay (Promega Corporation, Madison, WI), which is based on quantification of the ATP level, which signals the presence of metabolically active cells. Luminescent signal was measured in the GLOMAX Luminometer system (Promega, Corp.). The data are presented as proportional viability (%) by comparing the treated group with the untreated cells, the viability of which was assumed to be 100%.

Cell Apoptosis

LNM35 cells (1×10^6) were plated and cultured at 37°C on 100-mm Petri dishes in RPMI supplemented with 10% FBS. After 24 h, cells were treated or not (controls) with increasing concentrations of captopril (0.001–10 mM) for 24–48 h in RPMI 0.5% FBS. For flow cytometric analysis, adherent and floating cells were combined, washed once with phosphate-buffered saline (PBS), and fixed overnight at 4°C in 70% ethanol. Subsequently cells were washed with PBS, incubated for 30 min at 37°C with 1 μg/mL RNase

A, and stained with propidium iodide. The stained cells were analyzed on a FACScan flow cytometer for relative DNA content (FACSCalibur; Becton Dickinson, Le Pont de Claix, France). About 10,000 cells were recorded per assay.

Tumor Growth Assays

Six-week-old athymic NMRI female nude mice (nu/nu; Elevage Janvier, Le Genest Saint Isle, France) were housed in filtered-air laminar flow cabinets and handled under aseptic conditions. Procedures involving animals and their care were conducted in conformity with Institutional guidelines that are in compliance with Faculty of Medicine and Health Sciences, UAE University, national and international laws and policies (EEC Council Directive 86/609, OJ L 358, 1, December 12, 1987; and NIH Guide for Care and Use of Laboratory Animals, NIH Publication No. 85-23, 1985). Human Pulmonary LNM35 cells (1×10^6 cells) were injected subcutaneously into the lateral flank of the nude mice. One week after inoculation, when tumors had reached the volume of approximately 100 mm^3, animals (six in each group) were treated with captopril (2.8 mg/mouse) or control (carrier solution alone) during three cycles of 6 days and one rest day for a total of 21 days. Tumor dimensions were measured with calipers every 3 days. Tumor volume (V) was calculated using the formula: $V = 0.4 \times a \times b^2$, with a being the length and b the width of the tumor. The animals were sacrificed 21 days after treatment initiation, and the tumors excised, weighed, and fixed for immunohistochemical analysis.

Immunohistochemical Determination of Proliferating Cell Nuclear Antigen *Ki*-67 and CD31/Platelet-endothelial Cell Adhesion Molecule 1 for Microvessel Density

Five micrometer paraffin-embedded tissue sections were deparaffinized, microwaved for 5 min for antigen retrieval, and then incubated with a monoclonal mouse antihuman antibody against *Ki*-67 (DAKO, clone MIB-1, 1:50) for 1 h at room temperature. The samples were then washed and incubated with secondary antibody for 1 h at room temperature, followed by incubation with the streptavidin-peroxidase complex. Ten high-power fields (0.159 mm^2) per section of four to five tumors per treatment group were examined microscopically, and the average number of cells that stained positive for *Ki*-67 per treatment group was evaluated.

The effect of captopril on angiogenesis was evaluated by CD31 immunostaining. The tumor tissues were quickly frozen in isopentane at $-130°C$ and stored at $-70°C$ until further processing. Frozen sections (8 μm) were fixed in acetone and incubated overnight with a CD31 antibody (1:400). Slides were then washed three times in PBS and incubated with secondary antibody (goat antirat 1:200) for 1 h at room temperature. The sections were then stained with 3,3'-diaminobenzidine (DAB) and counterstained with hematoxylin. Vessel density was determined by counting the number of microvessels. The area occupied by CD31-positive microvessels and total tissue area per section were quantified and compared between treated and control mice. For individual tumors, the microvessel count was scored by averaging the counts from all fields. All analyses were performed in a blind fashion.

Statistical Analysis

Results are expressed as the mean $\pm$ SEM of the number of experiments indicated. The difference between experimental and control values were assessed by the Independent Samples Test and ANOVA and $P < 0.05$ was considered as a statistically significant difference.

Results

Impact of Captopril on Tumor Growth and Metastasis

The anticancer activity of captopril was investigated in athymic mice inoculated with

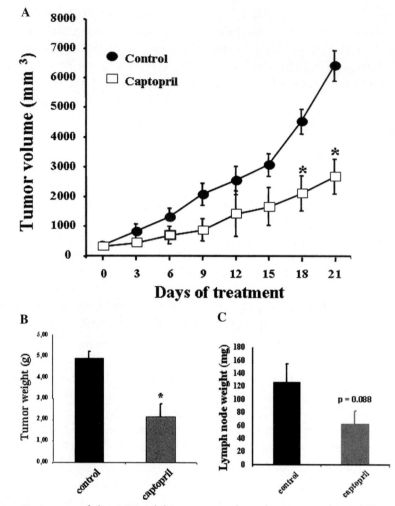

Figure 1. Impact of the ACE inhibitor captopril on the tumor volume **(A)**, weight **(B)**, and lymph node metastasis weight **(C)** of established human lung cancer xenografts. Nude mice were xenografted s.c. with human lung LNM35 cancer cells (10^6 cells per animal) and treated with captopril (2.8 mg/mouse during three cycles of 6 days and one rest day for a total of 21 days) or with saline solution alone. Data points represent the mean ± SEM of four to five mice per group. Statistically significant differences are indicated in **A** for tumor volume (*, $P < 0.01$ versus control) and in **B** for tumor weight (*, $P < 0.01$ versus control).

highly tumorigenic LNM35 human lung cells as xenografts. The IP administration of captopril (2.8 mg/mouse) significantly reduced the growth of LNM35 human tumor xenografts by 52% at day 18 and 58% at day 21 (*, $P < 0.01$ versus control) (Fig. 1A). A similar difference between captopril-treated and control animals was also found in tumor weight (4.92 ± 0.33 g versus 2.13 ± 0.63 g) (Fig. 1B). There was no loss of body weight or other sign of toxicity from captopril administration.

The metastatic dissemination of human cancer cells constitutes the most aggressive aspect of the neoplastic progression leading to a fatal outcome. In order to determine whether inhibition of ACE by captopril affects the dissemination of human cancer cells, we assessed the metastatic behavior of the human pulmonary cell line LNM35 by examining axillary lymph nodes. In the captopril-treated group, the mean lymph node weight was 63.5 mg compared with 127 mg in the vehicle-treated

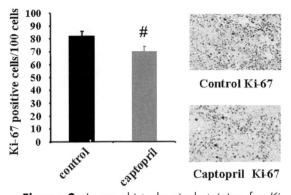

Figure 2. Immunohistochemical staining for *Ki-67* in LNM35 human lung cancer growing in nude mice treated with saline (control) or captopril. #*P* < 0.05 versus control.

control group. This difference, though sizable, was in a small group of animals and failed to reach conventional levels of statistical significance ($P = 0.088$) (Fig. 1C).

Effect of Captopril on Tumor Angiogenesis and Cell Proliferation *In Vivo*

The effect of captopril on tumor angiogenesis *in vivo* was assessed by CD31-immunostaining of LNM35 tumor tissue xenografts. CD31 is specifically expressed on the surface of endothelial cells and is weakly expressed on lymphoid cells and platelets. Immunohistochemical analysis indicated that when the CD31-positive areas or number of microvessels were normalized to tumor area, captopril versus control caused nonsignificant vascular regression in the tumors (data not shown).

Next, we analyzed the effect of captopril on tumor-cell proliferation *in vivo* by assessing the levels of the nuclear antigen *Ki*-67, which is present in all phases of the cell cycle except G0. There was a significant decrease in the mean number of *Ki*-67-positive cells in the captopril-treated group in comparison with the control group (Fig. 2, $P < 0.05$). Thus, the highly significant inhibition of tumor growth by captopril appears to be due, at least in part, to a direct effect on the proliferation of tumor cells.

Effect of Captopril on Cell Viability and Apoptosis *In Vitro*

To determine the mechanism by which captopril reduced tumor growth, we investigated the effect of captopril on cellular viability. Proliferating LNM35 cells were incubated in the absence or presence of various concentrations (0.01, 0.1, 1, and 10 mM) of captopril for 24 h. At all these concentrations, captopril had an inhibitory impact on the LNM35 cell viability at 24 h (#, $P < 0.05$; *, $P < 0.01$ versus control) (Fig. 3A).

Fluorescent activated cell sorting (FACS) analysis assays were performed to determine whether the antitumor effect of captopril was due to cell death. We demonstrated that treatment of LNM35 cells for 48 h with high concentrations of captopril (1 and 10 mM) was associated with induction of apoptosis from 2.5% for control to 9% and 15.5%, respectively, for captopril-treated cells (Fig. 3B). These results suggest that upon treatment with captopril, LNM35 cells underwent apoptosis, and that there is a good correspondence between apoptosis rate and inhibition of cell viability.

Discussion and Conclusion

Lung cancer is the most common form of cancer in the world, with the highest mortality rate (90% of lung cancer patients die from their disease). A retrospective study of 5207 patients showed that long-term use of ACE inhibitors may protect against cancer.[1] This observation, however, is contrary to a somewhat similar study in elderly people who participated in a Swedish trial of antihypertensive drugs in which ACE inhibitors reportedly had no effect on the risk of developing cancer.[22] ACE inhibitors are widely used as antihypertensive agents and, in general, are not associated with serious side effects. The present study using the non-small cell lung carcinoma LNM35 preclinical model revealed that the ACE inhibitor, captopril, significantly inhibited tumor growth. Our findings

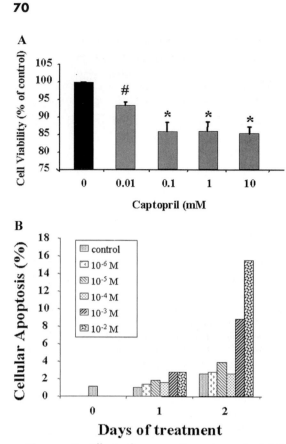

Figure 3. Effect of captopril on the cell viability and apoptosis of LNM35 cancer cells. **(A)** The data are presented as proportional viability (%) by comparing the treated group with the untreated cells, the viability of which was assumed to be 100%. Statistical significance was evaluated with Independent Samples Test and ANOVA ($^#$, $P < 0.05$ versus control; *, $P < 0.01$ versus control). **(B)** Flow cytometry analysis of captopril-induced apoptosis. LNM35 cells were cultured for 24–48 h in the presence or absence of graded concentrations of captopril and analyzed at the sub-G1 fraction.

are in agreement with other studies showing that captopril and other ACE inhibitors inhibit tumor growth of human renal cell carcinoma and head and neck squamous carcinoma.[23,24] In this context, Chisi and colleagues reported that captopril (100 mg/kg or 2.8 mg/mouse) may be of use in protecting primitive hematopoietic cells against the toxicity of anticancer therapeutic regimens.[25] The acquisition of metastatic ability leads to clinically incurable disease. Our data demonstrate that captopril also inhibited the LNM35 lymph

node metastasis in nude mice, although this inhibition, while apparently substantial, failed to reach conventional levels of statistical significance. These results are in agreement with evidence that captopril inhibits human glioma cell migration and invasion related to a reduction in matrix metalloproteinase activity.[26]

Tumor invasion and metastasis are critical events in cancer progression, and angiogenic factors are now considered to play a major role in metastasis. In this context, Ang II reportedly promoted the invasive potency of cervical carcinoma cells by increasing the secretion of VEGF.[27] These results are in agreement with our recent work showing that VEGF induces colon cancer cell invasion.[28] In this regard, we demonstrate here that captopril treatment resulted in a weak and non significant decrease of angiogenesis in the LNM35 tumors. In contrast, the Sukhatme group demonstrated that treatment with captopril induced anti-angiogenic activity *in vitro* and *in vivo*.[29] In conclusion, the effect of ACE inhibitors on angiogenesis remains controversial.

To explain the antitumor effect of captopril, we considered two theories: first, that captopril directly inhibits the proliferation of LNM35 tumor cells. To address this theory, we performed immunohistochemical analysis of proliferating cells (Ki-67) in the tumor samples treated with captopril. Quantification of the Ki-67-positive cells showed a decreased number of dividing tumor cells after treatment with captopril. However, the *in vitro* proliferation assay for LNM35 cells revealed no antiproliferative effect as a result of ACE inhibition. These results are in agreement with the earlier observation that captopril was ineffective in preventing cell proliferation in several neoplastic cell lines (K562, HeLa, and MDA-MB-361).[30]

The effect of captopril on tumor growth appears to be due, at least in part, to direct inhibition of the survival of tumor cells. There was a significant difference in the percentage of viable cells after incubation with captopril (0.01–10 mM) versus control. It was confirmed by FACS assay that the inhibition of cell viability observed after treatment with captopril was due to therapy-induced cell death. Then, exposure of LNM35 cells to increasing concentrations of captopril resulted in an inhibition of cell viability accompanied by induction of apoptosis.

In conclusion, we report an antitumor effect of captopril in a highly aggressive human lung cancer xenograft in nude mice. In view of the available experimental findings, we contend that captopril may have clinical potential as an anticancer agent. The first line chemotherapeutic protocol in non-small cell lung cancer is cisplatin in combination with paclitaxel, docetaxel, vinorelbine, gemcitabine, or irinotecan. It is possible that captopril will turn out to be a therapeutic option in the management of lung cancer, perhaps in combination with standard anticancer drugs, such as cisplatin.

Acknowledgments

This work was financially supported by the Research Affairs at the UAE University under a contract no. 01-04-8-11/06. This work was also supported by INSERM, France. We thank Ms. K. Arafat, Ms. D. Catala, Mr. Chandranath, and Mr. S.M. Nurulain for their technical assistance.

Conflicts of Interest

The authors declare no conflicts of interest.

References

1. Lever, A.F., D.J. Hole, C.R. Gillis, *et al.* 1998. Do inhibitors of angiotensin-I-converting enzyme protect against risk of cancer? *Lancet* **352:** 179–184.

2. Bader, M., J. Peters, O. Baltatu, *et al.* 2001. Tissue renin-angiotensin systems: new insights from experimental animal models in hypertension research. *J. Mol. Med.* **79:** 76–102.

3. Otani, A., H. Takagi, K. Suzuma & Y. Honda. 1998. Angiotensin II potentiates vascular endothelial growth factor-induced angiogenic activity in retinal microcapillary endothelial cells. *Circ. Res.* **82:** 619–628.

4. Tamarat, R., J.S. Silvestre, M. Durie & B.I. Levy. 2002. Angiotensin II angiogenic effect in vivo involves vascular endothelial growth factor- and inflammation-related pathways. *Lab. Invest.* **82:** 747–756.

5. Egami, K., T. Murohara, T. Shimada, *et al.* 2003. Role of host angiotensin II type 1 receptor in tumor angiogenesis and growth. *J. Clin. Invest.* **112:** 67–75.

6. Fujita, M., I. Hayashi, S. Yamashina, *et al.* 2005. Angiotensin type 1a receptor signaling-dependent induction of vascular endothelial growth factor in stroma is relevant to tumor-associated angiogenesis and tumor growth. *Carcinogenesis* **26:** 271–279.

7. Horiuchi, M., W. Hayashida, M. Akishita, *et al.* 1999. Stimulation of different subtypes of angiotensin II receptors, AT1 and AT2 receptors, regulates STAT activation by negative crosstalk. *Circ. Res.* **84:** 876–882.

8. Rivat, C., S. Rodrigues, E. Bruyneel, *et al.* 2005. Implication of STAT3 signaling in human colonic cancer cells during Intestinal Trefoil Factor (TFF3) and VEGF-mediated cellular invasion and tumor growth. *Cancer Res.* **65:** 195–202.

9. Prevost, G.P., M.O. Lonchampt, S. Holbeck, *et al.* 2006. The novel inhibitor of heterotrimeric G-protein signaling BIM-46174, enhances the anticancer activity of cisplatin in human NSCLC lung tumor xenografts. *Cancer Res.* **66:** 9227–9234.

10. Wolf, G. & U.O. Wenzel. 2004. Angiotensin II and cell cycle regulation. *Hypertension* **43:** 693–698.

11. Escobar, E., T.S. Rodriguez-Reyna, O. Arrieta & J. Sotelo. 2004. Angiotensin II, cell proliferation and angiogenesis regulator: biologic and therapeutic implications in cancer. *Curr. Vasc. Pharmacol.* **2:** 385–399.

12. Hama, K., H. Ohnishi, H. Yasuda, *et al.* 2004. Angiotensin II stimulates DNA synthesis of rat pancreatic stellate cells by activating ERK through EGF receptor transactivation. *Biochem. Biophys. Res. Commun.* **315:** 905–911.

13. Petroianu, G., E Adeghate, Mohd Hassan, *et al.* 2004. Intraperitoneal exposure to captopril but not to lisinopril activates the peroxisome proliferator activated receptor (PPAR). *Clin. Exp. Pharmacol. Physiol.* **31**(Suppl 1): A100.

14. Jackson, L., W. Wahli, L. Michalik, *et al.* 2003. Potential role for peroxisome proliferator activated receptor (PPAR) in preventing colon cancer. *Gut* **52:** 1317–1322.

15. Zhang, M., P. Zou, M. Bai, *et al.* 2003. Apoptosis of human lung cancer cells induced by activated peroxisome proliferator-activated receptor-gamma and its mechanism. *Zhonghua Yi Xue Za Zhi* **83:** 1169–1172.

16. Volpert, O.V., W.F. Ward, M.W. Lingen, *et al.* 1996. Captopril inhibits angiogenesis and slows the growth

of experimental tumors in rats. *J. Clin. Invest.* **98:** 671–679.

17. Buemi, M., A. Allegra, D. Marino, *et al.* 1999. Does captopril have a direct pro-apoptotic effect? *Nephron* **81:** 99–101.

18. Fabre, J.E., A. Rivard, M. Magner, *et al.* 1999. Tissue inhibition of angiotensin-converting enzyme activity stimulates angiogenesis in vivo. *Circulation* **99:** 3043–3049.

19. Silvestre, J.S., S. Bergaya, R. Tamarat, *et al.* 2001. Proangiogenic effect of angiotensin-converting enzyme inhibition is mediated by the bradykinin B(2) receptor pathway. *Circ. Res.* **89:** 678–683.

20. Ebrahimian, T.G., R. Tamarat, M. Clergue, *et al.* 2005. Dual effect of angiotensin-converting enzyme inhibition on angiogenesis in type 1 diabetic mice. *Arterioscler Thromb. Vasc. Biol.* **25:** 65–70.

21. Yoshiji, H., S. Kuriyama, M. Kawata, *et al.* 2001. The angiotensin-I-converting enzyme inhibitor perindopril suppresses tumor growth and angiogenesis: possible role of the vascular endothelial growth factor. *Clin. Cancer Res.* **7:** 1073–1078.

22. Lindholm, L.H., H. Anderson, T. Ekbom, *et al.* 2001. Relation between drug treatment and cancer in hypertensives in the Swedish Trial in Old Patients with Hypertension 2: a 5-year, prospective, randomised, controlled trial. *Lancet* **358:** 539–544.

23. Hii, S.I., D.L. Nicol, D.C. Gotley, *et al.* 1998. Captopril inhibits tumour growth in a xenograft model of human renal cell carcinoma. *Br. J. Cancer* **77:** 880–883.

24. Yasumatsu, R., T. Nakashima, M. Masuda, *et al.* 2004. Effects of the angiotensin-I converting enzyme inhibitor perindopril on tumor growth and angiogenesis in head and neck squamous cell carcinoma cells. *J. Cancer Res. Clin. Oncol.* **130:** 567–573.

25. Chisi, J.E., C.V. Briscoe, E. Ezan, *et al.* 2000. Captopril inhibits in vitro and in vivo the proliferation of primitive haematopoietic cells induced into cell cycle by cytotoxic drug administration or irradiation but has no effect on myeloid leukaemia cell proliferation. *Br. J. Haematol.* **109:** 563–570.

26. Nakagawa, T., T. Kubota, M. Kabuto & T. Kodera. 1995. Captopril inhibits glioma cell invasion in vitro: involvement of matrix metalloproteinases. *Anticancer Res.* **15:** 1985–1989.

27. Kikkawa, F., M. Mizuno, K. Shibata, *et al.* 2004. Activation of invasiveness of cervical carcinoma cells by angiotensin II. *Am. J. Obstet. Gynecol.* **190:** 1258–1263.

28. Nguyen, Q.D., S. Rodrigues, C. Rodrigue, *et al.* 2006. Inhibition of VEGF-165 and Semaphorin 3A-mediated cellular invasion and tumor growth by the VEGF signaling inhibitor ZD4190 in human colon cancer cells and xenografts. *Mol. Cancer Ther.* **5:** 2070–2077.

29. Merchan, J.R., B. Chan, S. Kale, *et al.* 2003. *In vitro* and *in vivo* induction of antiangiogenic activity by plasminogen activators and captopril. *J. Natl. Cancer Inst.* **95:** 388–399.

30. Stanojkovic, T.P., Z. Zizak, N. Mihailovic-Stanojevic, *et al.* 2005. Inhibition of proliferation on some neoplastic cell lines-act of carvedilol and captopril. *J. Exp. Clin. Cancer Res.* **24:** 387–395.

Mesothelioma and Environmental Exposure

A Newly Developed Animal Model for Fiber Exposure

Csaba Varga and Katalin Szendi

Department of Environmental Health, Institue of Public Health Medicine,
University of Pecs, Pecs, Hungary

A novel animal model was developed to study the direct exposure of mesothelial cells to crocidolite and chrysotile asbestos fibers. Chemically pure and pretreated Union Internationale Centre le Cancer (UICC) samples were implanted into a peritoneal envelope (Kertai's fold) of Wistar rats. Following the 12-month exposure, lack of mesothelioma induction was detected in all groups. Results suggest that the mechanism of mesothelioma formation is not a consequence of peritoneal physical exposure to the fibers.

Key words: asbestos; mesothelioma; rat model; Kertai's fold

Introduction

Highly persistent asbestos fibers and fibrils will be present in the human environment even after asbestos products have been completely banned. This fact emphasizes the importance of further preventive measures for handling this permanent problem. Beside the classical *occupational*, *para-occupational* and *neighborhood (inhalation)* exposures, *ingestion* as an alternative way of absorption should also be considered.[1] Long-term exposure to asbestos fibers can initiate asbestosis, bronchial carcinoma, and pleural or peritoneal mesothelioma.[2] Crocidolite (an amphibole) and chrysotile (serpentine) asbestos are studied intensively, and the former is considered the most carcinogenic type inducing malignant mesothelioma. Asbestos fibers can be considered as archetypes of toxic mineral fibers. Oxidative damage caused by the fibers has been studied in *in vitro* genotoxicity tests involving comet assay, analyses of bacterial mutagenicity, and cytogenetic alterations in cultured cells.[3–5] But the crucial endpoint (mesothelioma) is very difficult to study in an *in vitro* system. Human peritoneal mesothelial cell cultures have a very short proliferative lifespan. Cells of the aging cultures generate more reactive oxygen species and display increased quantities of oxidatively modified DNA. Therefore they are not suitable for testing similar induced effects by fibers and long-term exposures.[6] We developed an *in vivo* mesothelioma-induction test for research on fibrous materials. The test involves a single treatment and simple surgical methods using a minimal number of rats. Pure Union Internationale Centre le Cancer (UICC; Geneva, Switzerland) amphibole (crocidolite) and serpentine (Rhodesian chrysotile) asbestos were used as exposing agents. As a model of environmental exposure, the experiments were repeated with fibers pretreated with nitroarene (1-nitropyrene (NP)), a potent carcinogen and genotoxicant.[7]

Materials and Methods

UICC asbestos samples—crocidolite and Rhodesian chrysotile—were prepared by Rendall and Timbrell (SPI Supplies, Glamorgan, UK).[8] Chemically pure and NP-pretreated samples were used for the experiments. Pretreatment involved an overnight shaking of portions of 10 mg fibers in saturated aqueous NP solution. Five groups of six inbred Wistar

Address for correspondence: Csaba Varga, Szigeti u. 12., Pécs, Hungary, H-7643. Voice: +36-72-536-394; fax: +36-72-536-395. chemsafety@freemail.hu

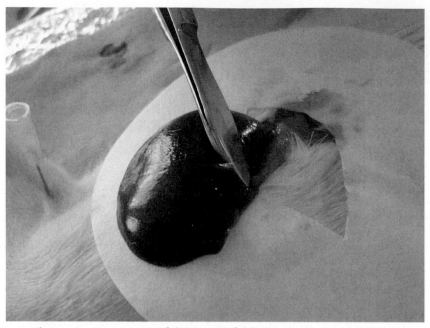

Figure 1. Preparation of the Kertai's fold. (In color in *Annals* online.)

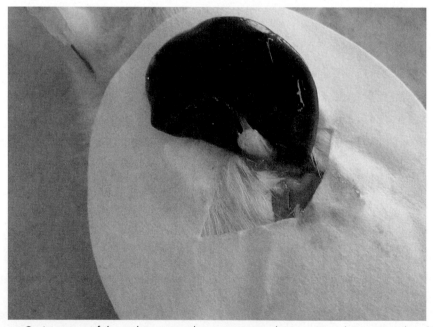

Figure 2. Location of the gelatin capsule containing asbestos. (In color in *Annals* online.)

rats were used, in each with approximate body weights of 400 g. Ligament of the minor omentum attached to the concave inner surface of the big liver lobe (Kertai's fold) was prepared for the exposure. Pharmaceutical hard gelatin capsules were filled with 10 mg of the tested asbestos species and implanted into this peritoneal envelope, lined with mesothelial cells (Figs. 1 and 2).

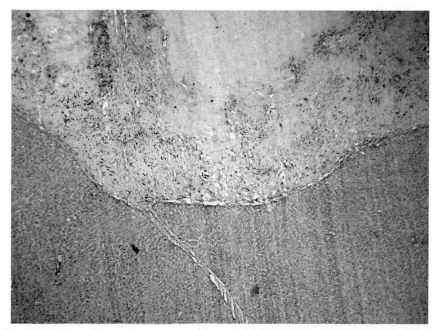

Figure 3. Granulomatous reaction of foreign body type. (In color in *Annals* online.)

Zinc-oxide was used as a negative control. Autopsies of the animals were performed after 12 months.

Results

Upon autopsy, gray/blue bulks of asbestos fibers were detected in the peritoneal cavity: in the Kertai's fold and on the surface of near organs (omentum, peritoneum). Thickening of the gastric wall was also observed. The histological evaluation of tissue samples showed only unchanged structure of the liver tissue and granulomatous reaction of foreign body type with multinucleated giant cells (Figs. 3 and 4). Signs of mesothelioma were not detected either macroscopically or microscopically in either the exposed or control groups.

Discussion

Active iron ions carried by amphiboles cause a continuous generation of reactive oxygen species that are related to fiber toxicity and effects on DNA and proteins.[9] Iron can also

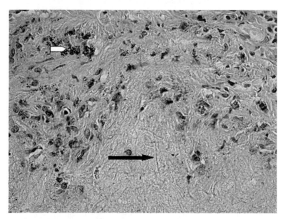

Figure 4. With condenser switched off, asbestos fibers (black arrow) can be seen together with foreign body type multinucleated giant cells. The black granules are pigments of formalin (white arrow). (In color in *Annals* online.)

be present as a substituent of magnesium in chrysotile fibers. The carcinogenicity of asbestos may be based on DNA damage and changes in proliferation and differentiation in the target cells. In several mesotheliomas, chromosomal deletions and loss of tumor suppressor genes have also been reported. Several signaling pathways (NK-kappaB, PKC, and

MAPK-ERK 1/2) are activated upon asbestos exposure.[10–12]

Human mesothelial cells in culture are not transformed by asbestos fibers, probably because of marked cytotoxic effects. Release of TNF-alpha of human mesothelial cells upon crocidolite exposure may provide a possible explanation of *in vivo* transformation phenomenon. TNF-alpha mediates NK-kappaB activation, reducing cytotoxicity of the fibers and providing proliferation of damaged mesothelial cells.[10] In previous studies we demonstrated that arene-pretreated crocidolite and anthophyllite fibers caused cytogenetic action in rats, that is, significant enhancement in the sister chromatid exchange frequencies of bone barrow cells. Chemically pure fibers were not genotoxic in this test.[3,4] Following oral exposure, cells prepared from omentum and intestine of rats showed a high level of DNA strand breaks. Pretreatment of fibers increased this effect significantly.[13]

In our present *in vivo* study, however, even the long-term direct exposure of mesothelial cells to asbestos fibers was not able to induce peritoneal mesothelioma. This was completely unexpected, especially in the case of pretreated fibers showing cogenotoxicity in separate studies. This observation suggests the possibility that the mechanism of mesothelioma formation is independent of the physical contact among fibers and mesothelial cells. We should rather look for a remote effect in the background.

Acknowledgments

The authors wish to thank Prof. P. Kertai for methodological help. Research was supported by a grant from the Hungarian Ministry of Health (No. ETT 50188). Csaba Varga was a Bolyai-fellow of the Hungarian Academy of Science.

Conflicts of Interest

The authors declare no conflicts of interest.

References

1. Varga, C. 2005. Can one assess genotoxic and carcinogenic risk of asbestos without mentioning ingested fibres? *Mutat. Res.* **572:** 173–174.
2. IARC. 1977. *IARC Monographs on the Evaluation of Carcinogenic Risk to Chemicals on Man*, Vol. 14. Asbestos, pp. 1–106. IARC. Lyon.
3. Varga, C., G. Horváth & V. Timbrell. 1996. In vivo studies on genotoxicity and cogenotoxicity of ingested UICC anthophyllite asbestos. *Cancer Lett.* **105:** 181–185.
4. Varga, C., Z. Pocsai, G. Horváth & V. Timbrell. 1996. Studies on genotoxicity of orally administered crocidolite asbestos in rats: implications for ingested asbestos induced carcinogenesis. *Anticancer Res.* **16:** 811–814.
5. Varga, C., G. Horváth, Z. Pocsai & V. Timbrell. 1998. On the mechanism of cogenotoxic action between ingested amphibole asbestos fibres and benzo[a]pyrene: I. Urinary and serum mutagenicity studies with rats. *Cancer Lett.* **128:** 165–169.
6. Varga, C. & K. Szendi. 2006. Relevance of the in vitro and in vivo studies in genotoxicological research on fibres. *ALTEX* **23:** 133.
7. Varga, C., K. Szendi & I. Ember. 2006. An in vivo model for testing genotoxicity of environmental fibre-associated nitroarenes. *In Vivo* **20:** 539–542.
8. Timbrell, V. & R.E.D. Rendall. 1971/72. Preparation of the UICC standard reference samples of asbestos. *Powder Technol.* **5:** 279–287.
9. Shulka, A., M. Gulumian, T.K. Hei, *et al.* 2003. Multiple roles of oxidants in the pathogenesis of asbestos-induced diseases. *Free Rad. Biol. Med.* **34:** 1117–1129.
10. Mossman, B.T., P.J. Borm, V. Castranova, *et al.* 2007. Mechanisms of action of inhaled fibers, particles and nanoparticles in lung and cardiovascular diseases. *Particle Fiber Toxicol.* **4:** 4.
11. Nádasi, E., I. Ember & I. Arany. 2005. Extracellular signal-regulated kinase as biomarker in the molecular epidemiology of human carcinogenesis. I. Molecular mechanisms. *Hung. Epidemiol.* **2:** 297–304.
12. Nádasi, E., I. Ember & I. Arany. 2006. Extracellular signal-regulated kinase as biomarker in the molecular epidemiology of human carcinogenesis. II. Clinical implications. *Hung. Epidemiol.* **3:** 53–58.
13. Varga, C., G. Horváth & V. Timbrell. 1999. On the mechanism of cogenotoxic action between ingested amphibole asbestos fibres and benzo[a]pyrene: II. Tissue specificity studies using comet assay. *Cancer Lett.* **139:** 173–176.

Surgical Management of Very Large Musculoskeletal Sarcomas

Rafiq Abed[a] and Derek Younge[b]

[a]*Department of Orthopaedics, Tawam Hospital and*

[b]*Department of Surgery, Faculty of Medicine and Health Sciences, UAE University, Al Ain, United Arab Emirates*

The management of almost all sarcomas in the musculoskeletal system includes surgery, although chemotherapy and radiotherapy also may play an important role in the treatment. The surgical treatment comprises complete resection of the tumor with a margin of normal tissue. This can be accomplished by local resection and then reconstruction of the resultant deficit, or amputation. Resection of the tumor without amputation, that is, limb-salvage surgery, can be accomplished in 80% of cases and is generally preferred by the patient. The very large, neglected, or aggressive tumor, however, can make resection with a wide margin impossible or very difficult. Many large tumors will require amputation in order to be sure that the entire tumor is removed, as the priority is saving the patient's life, with limb preservation secondary. Even an amputation may be very difficult when the pelvic or shoulder girdle is involved. Sometimes the surgeon may agree to do a marginal resection when the patient or family absolutely refuses amputation, but they must be made to understand that this may compromise survival. In cases where there is circumferential skin involvement or projected loss, some unusual techniques, such as amputation-replantation can be done, especially in the upper limb, where in spite of gross shortening, function can be much better than any prosthesis. Even if there are metastases present, sometimes amputation or even local resection is offered as palliation if the patient's life is made miserable by a large fungating tumor. Local resection of a huge tumor can be a formidable challenge to the surgeon, and the margin may consist of a few millimeters of compressed muscle. Good skin cover may be a major problem, and free tissue transfer may be necessary if local flaps are not possible. In all cases, one must ask if the resection-reconstruction with all its complications and risk to the patient of recurrence is really better than an amputation.

Key words: musculoskeletal sarcomas; large sarcomas; surgery of sarcomas; limb-salvage surgery

Introduction

Although chemotherapy and radiotherapy play an increasingly important role in the treatment of musculoskeletal sarcomas, surgery still has an essential part to play in the removal of the primary tumor. The surgical treatment comprises complete resection of the tumor with a margin of normal tissue. This can be accomplished by local resection and then reconstruction of the resultant deficit, or by amputation. Resection of the tumor without amputation (known as limb-salvage surgery) can be accomplished in over 80% of cases and is generally preferred by the patient for both psychological and functional reasons. The role of amputation in extremity sarcomas has been decreasing over the past 15–20 years.[1]

The very large tumor can make resection with a wide margin impossible or very difficult. The decision to perform an amputation rather than attempt local resection can be problematic for the surgeon and depends on several factors,

Address for correspondence: Professor Derek Younge, Faculty of Medicine, Box 17666, Al Ain, UAE. dyounge@gmail.com including survival of the patient, whether or not the neurovascular structures can be preserved, soft-tissue coverage, ability to achieve a so-called wide margin, and presence of distant metastases.[2]

The goals for limb-salvage surgery for malignant tumors remain resection with tumor-free margins and a viable functional limb.

The factors that we will discuss herein are: survival of the patient, size of the tumor, how wide is a wide margin, reconstruction, and the limits of limb salvage.

Survival of the Patient

Most large centers undertaking limb-salvage surgery have found that postoperative survival is only marginally less than that after very proximal amputation. Amputation just above the tumor has a similar recurrence rate to limb-salvage surgery.[3]

Many large tumors will require amputation in order to be sure that the entire tumor is removed, as the priority is to save the patient's life, with limb preservation as a secondary consideration. For some large tumors even an amputation may be very difficult, such as when the pelvic or shoulder girdle is involved and not enough skin is available for closure. Because of the need for wide resection, local muscle flaps are often not available.

Faced with a very large tumor, the surgeon has to decide whether his refusal to attempt limb salvage will provoke the patient into "going home to die," or force him or her to accept the inevitable. Sometimes the surgeon may reluctantly accept doing a marginal resection when the patient or family absolutely refuses amputation, but in this case the patient and family must understand that this may compromise survival. On the other hand, the surgeon may not want to attempt an extremely difficult resection with a high chance of failure. The surgeon may also feel that he or she is likely to be blamed for the failure and subsequent loss of the limb.

Even if metastases are present, sometimes amputation or even local resection is offered as palliation if the patient's life is made miserable by a large fungating tumor. If the local resection and reconstruction is relatively easy and complications are unlikely, for instance in the case of a distal femur resection, then it may well be the procedure of choice. The distal femur would usually be replaced by a nail-cement construction and walking could be nearly immediate.

Size of the Tumor

We all know a large tumor when we see one, but it is not easy to define what a large tumor is.

The American Joint Commission on Cancer categorizes bone tumors and soft-tissue tumors by size.[2] Stage T1 bone tumors are <8 cm, whereas stage T2 bone tumors are larger than 8 cm. Stage T1 soft-tissue tumors are <5 cm, whereas stage T2 soft-tissue tumors are larger than 5 cm. These classifications are useful as they are based on data showing a difference in prognosis. Some authors have used volume as calculated on MRI or CT as an indication of size.

How do tumors get so large? The cause of the large size is either long neglect by the patient or family or aggression of the tumor. Patients typically do not have pain until the late stages of the disease, and swelling without pain typically does not provoke patients to seek medical attention. This is especially true for soft-tissue sarcomas, which can be missed by obese patients for some time. Bone tumors cause pain and usually will present sooner. Pelvic and sacral tumors are often neglected for a long period, even in the West, as low back pain is so common, and the tumors can become quite large before they cause any obstructive symptoms or are apparent.

Another important reason for late presentation is that traditional, alternative treatments are often tried before the patient visits the hospital. The patient will come to the hospital as a last resort, or sometimes disappear during treatment because of family pressure to try the traditional treatments. The traditional system of medicine used in Saudi Arabia is based on the use of cautery.

For osteosarcoma it has been shown that there is a good correlation between large size of a tumor and poor prognosis.[4] This usually means that the tumor is aggressive and is growing very rapidly. In the developed world, a very large sarcoma occurs because of an aggressive nature of the tumor rather than neglect.

Many of the tumors seen in the senior author's (DY) practice in Saudi Arabia, however, have been larger than 10 cm and some have been larger than 20 cm. In the less developed world, extremely large or giant tumors are usually slow-growing malignancies or neglected benign tumors and have become large because of neglect.

How Wide Is a Wide Margin?

A wide margin is accomplished when the tumor and its pseudocapsule and a cuff of normal tissue peripheral to the tumor are removed *en bloc* in all directions.

There is no magical number, such as 1 cm or 2 cm or 3 cm. After resection, a soft-tissue margin will shrink or retract, and the margin will appear much smaller than the surgeon thought he was taking. A bony margin however, will remain the same.

Local recurrence rates of around 30% will be seen with positive microscopic margins.[5] However, extension of the resection beyond an adequate margin (e.g., by amputation where limb salvage is possible) does not increase overall survival.[5]

Good judgment is therefore necessary to balance the competing aims of adequacy of excision and retention of function. With adjuvant management of tumors, such as chemotherapy and radiotherapy, especially before surgery, even narrow margins for high-grade sarcomas can be oncologically and functionally acceptable or desirable.[6]

Reconstruction

Joint replacement with the so-called megaprosthesis, or arthrodesis with large bone grafts are the most common surgical procedures used to treat patients with bone tumors, as most resections involve loss of a joint. Depending on the specific patient, blood vessel reconstruction can be carried out and free flaps or pedicle flaps used. Loss of a major nerve is a relative contraindication, but not absolute. For example, resection of the sciatic nerve with a large posterior thigh tumor can be done, though trophic problems of the leg or foot can be a serious drawback for the patient.

All surgeons dealing with sarcomas learn early that the vessels and nerves are "pushed aside" by the growing tumor and can be dissected free from the tumor with care. Most surgeons are willing to do this as long as the structures are not "stuck" to the tumor. This means that a very thin margin of compressed tissue remains as the tumor "margin." The deciding factor is usually the condition of the skin, and whether enough good skin and soft tissue will remain to cover the reconstruction. Because of the wide margin that needs to be taken with the tumor, there are often no muscles left in the area to be used as flaps.

Rotation-plasty is very useful for bone tumors of the distal femur or proximal tibia in the small child. Parents are often horrified at the thought, but the children accept it well and do not feel amputated.

Limits of Limb-Salvage Surgery

Most tissues can be reconstructed using modern surgical techniques; however, the limits for selecting patients for limb salvage have not yet been defined.

Who should do this kind of surgery? These large tumors continue to be inappropriately

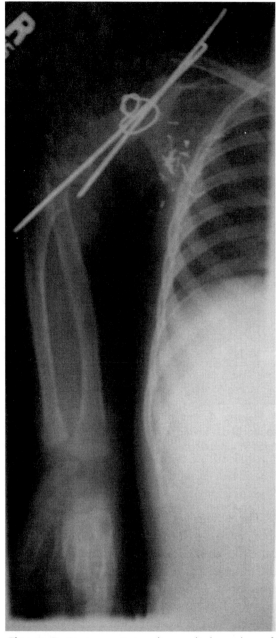

Figure 5. Postoperative radiograph shows loss of shoulder joint and a very short humerus.

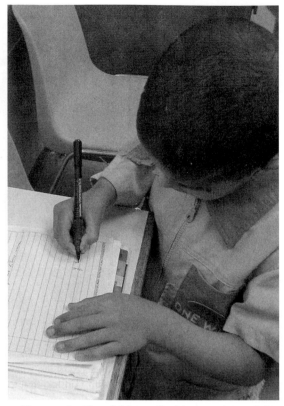

Figure 6. The child is still able to write with his right hand, in spite of having a very short humerus and no shoulder joint.

limb. Sometimes amputation will give better function than limb-salvage surgery, which sometimes leaves a limb with good vascularization but poor function.

A tumor that is too large will often require amputation. Each surgeon has to decide whether he or she has the skill to remove the tumor with an adequate margin and still preserve function of the limb. Both the surgeon and the patient need to be realistic in this decision.

Conflicts of Interest

The authors declare no conflicts of interest.

References

1. Williard, W.C., S.I. Hajdu, E.S. Casper & M.F. Brennan. 1992. Comparison of amputation with limb-sparing operations for adult soft tissue sarcoma of the extremity. *Ann. Surg.* **215:** 269–275.
2. Agarwal, M. & A. Puri. 2007. Management of Sarcomas in the Developing World, focus on Large Tumors, in American Academy of Orthopaedic Surgeons, Orthopaedic Knowledge Online, Jan 22, 2007. http://www5.aaos.org/oko/slideshowHtml.cfm?topic-ONC003 (accessed July 15, 2008).

3. Simon, M.A. 1998. General Considerations. In *Surgery for Bone and Soft-Tissue Tumors*. Vol. 20. M.A. Simon & D.S. Springfield, Eds.: 227. Lippincott-Raven. Philadelphia, New York.

4. Bieling, P., N. Rehan, P. Winkler, *et al.* 1996. Tumor size and prognosis in aggressively treated osteosarcoma. *J. Clin. Oncol.* **14:** 848–858.

5. Clark, M.A. & J.M. Thomas. 2003. Amputation for soft-tissue sarcoma. *Lancet Oncol.* **4:** 335–342.

6. Simon, M.A. 1998. Surgical Margins. In *Surgery for Bone and Soft-Tissue Tumors*. Vol. 8. M.A. Simon & D.S. Springfield, Eds.: 92. Lippincott-Raven. Philadelphia, New York.

7. Brooks, A.D., J.S. Gold, D. Graham, *et al.* 2002. Resection of the sciatic, peroneal, or tibial nerves: assessment of functional status. *Ann. Surg. Oncol.* **9:** 41–47.

8. Geller, D.S., S. David, F.J. Hornicek, *et al.* 2007. Soft tissue sarcoma resection volume associated with wound-healing complications. *Clin. Orthop. Related Res.* **459:** 182–185.

HER-2/neu Ile655Val Polymorphism and the Risk of Breast Cancer

A Case–Control Study

Awatif Siddig,[a] Abdelrahim Osman Mohamed,[b] Hammed Kamal,[c] Salma Awad,[d] Ahmed H. Hassan,[d] Erika Zilahi,[e] Mohammed Al-Haj,[e] Roos Bernsen,[f] and Abdu Adem[g]

[a]*Faculty of Medical Laboratory Technology, Sudan University for Science and Technology, Khartoum, Sudan*

[b]*Department of Biochemistry, Faculty of Medicine and Health Science, University of El Imam El-Mahdi, Kosti, Sudan*

[c]*Department of Surgery, Faculty of Medicine, Khartoum University Khartoum, Sudan*

[d]*Department of Biochemistry,* [e]*Department of Medical Microbiology,* [f]*Department of Community Medicine, and* [g]*Department of Pharmacology, Faculty of Medicine and Health Sciences, UAE University, Al Ain, United Arab Emirates*

Genetic alterations of the proto-oncogene human epidermal growth factor receptor (HER-2/neu) have been shown to induce malignant transformation and metastasis. Genotyping studies have addressed the association of codon 655 isoleucine to valine polymorphism located in the transmembrane coding region and the risk of breast cancer, but the results are inconsistent. In this study, we investigated the association of HER-2/neu Ile655Val polymorphism and the risk of breast cancer in a Sudanese population. In addition, the joint effects of HER-2/neu variants and our previously reported ESR1C325G polymorphism were tested for their association with breast cancer risk. Candidate single nucleotide polymorphism (SNP) in HER-2/neu Ile655Val [db SNP rs1136200] was genotyped in breast cancer patients and in healthy controls that were randomly selected from the same age group as the patients. Genotyping was performed using a high-throughput allelic discrimination method using real-time PCR, and data on clinical features and demographic details were collected. Associations between genotype and breast cancer were assessed by means of logistic regression. The prevalence of Val/Val genotype was similar in patients of breast cancer and control subjects. In comparison with the Ile/Ile genotype, the Ile/Val had a borderline significantly ($P = 0.06$) higher risk of breast cancer (OR = 2.95, 95% CI: 0.97–8.96). Regarding the genotypic and allelic frequencies stratified by age and menopausal status, there were no significant associations. A significantly higher risk of breast cancer was observed among homozygous carriers of ESR1325 CC genotype and heterozygous carriers of HER-2/neu655 Ile/Val genotype ($P = 0.05$; adjusted OR = 4.9, 95% CI: 1.0–24). The association of HER-2/neu Ile655Val polymorphism and the risk of breast cancer was borderline significant with the heterozygous carrier being at higher risk. However, the frequency of different polymorphic variants varies with ethnicity. The results of this

Address for correspondence: Prof. Abdu Adem, Ph.D., Department of Pharmacology, Faculty of Medicine and Health Sciences, UAE University, P.O Box 17666, Al Ain, UAE. Voice: +00971504482894; fax: +0097137672033. abdu.adem@uaeu.ac.ae study suggest that a significant gene–gene interaction between ESR1325C (previously reported) and HER-2/neu Ile655Val variants may jointly contribute to a higher risk of breast cancer.

Key words: breast cancer; HER-2/neu; polymorphism; risk

Introduction

The human epidermal growth factor receptor 2 (also known as c-erbB-2 or HER-2/neu) is a member of HER family, which includes four homologous receptors named HER-1 to HER-4.[1,2] These receptors share a similar molecular structure including an extra cellular ligand-binding domain, a single hydrophobic transmembrane domain, and a cytoplasmic tyrosine kinase domain. HER-2/neu is a proto-oncogene that is located on chromosome 17q11.2-12 and encodes a 185 kDa ($p^{185HER2}$) transmembrane glycoprotein with tyrosine kinase activity.[3,4] HER-2/neu has no identified ligand, therefore, it is considered as an orphan receptor that plays a central role in the HER family, being the preferred heterodimerization partner for the other HER family members.[5] HER-2/neu forms a more stable heterodimer than other combinations without HER-2/neu, with particularly high ligand binding and potent signaling cascade proteins.[6–8] The overexpression of HER-2/neu in epithelial cells has been shown to affect the regulation of cellular growth, apoptosis, motility, and adhesion.[9] Previous studies have indicated that HER-2/neu activation through amplification/overexpression is involved in oncogenic transformation and tumorigenesis in breast cancer.[10–13] Clinical studies have shown that HER-2/neu overexpression is observed in 60% of ductal carcinoma *in situ* and in 20–30% of infiltrating breast carcinoma, which is correlated with other parameters indicative of tumor progression, such as tumor size, nodal involvement, and the absence of hormone receptor expression.[14–16] A more recent study proposed that HER-2 contributes to angiogenesis and metastasis.[17]

Activation of HER-2/neu through point mutation in the transmembrane encoding region in animal models as well as in the NIH3T3 cell line was reported to enhance transforming ability.[18–20] Papewalis and colleagues identified a polymorphism of human HER-2/neu, at codon 655 that resulted in an isoleucine (Ile)-to-valine (Val) substitution (Ile655Val).[21] Positive association of this polymorphism with breast cancer was first reported by Xie and colleagues.[22] However, subsequent studies on Ile655Val and its relation to breast cancer remain controversial. In the present study, we aimed to evaluate the association of HER-2/neu Ile655Val polymorphism and the risk of breast cancer in a Sudanese population.

Patients and Methods

Study Population

A case–control study was conducted to assess the association between genotype frequencies and breast cancer risk. We used biospecimens to identify common low penetrance alleles. One hundred patients with primary breast cancer were studied: 98 females and 2 males, mean (SD) age: 46.4 (13.5) years, and 90 controls: 84 females and 4 males, mean (SD) age: 46.2 (13.4) were investigated in this study. Patients with pathologically confirmed disease were diagnosed between June 2004 and July 2005 in Khartoum Teaching Hospital, Soba University Hospital, and Omdurman Hospital, Sudan. Peripheral blood samples from cases as well as control subjects were obtained and kept frozen until genotyping. Control subjects were randomly selected from the general population in Khartoum State from the same age group as the

TABLE 1. Demographic and Clinical Characteristics of 100 Breast Cancer Patients and 90 Controls

| | Patients ($N = 100$) | | Controls ($N = 90$) | |
Characteristics	N (%)	N^*	N (%)	N^*
Age		94		88
≤50 years	67 (71.3)		60 (69.0)	
Gender		100		88
female	98 (98.0)		84 (95.5)	
Marital status		100		88
married	95 (95.0)		71 (80.7)	
Parity		92		88
nulliparous	30 (32.6)		24 (27.9)	
State		88		88
Khartoum	28 (32.4)		39 (45.1)	
North	9 (10.3)		13 (15.6)	
Central	24 (27.9)		17 (20.4)	
West	15 (17.6)		13 (15.5)	
East/South/White Nile	10 (11.8)		3 (3.4)	
Menopausal status		92		88
Premenopausal	65 (70.7)		63 (71.6)	
Histology		100		N.A.**
Ductal	97 (97.0)			
Fibroadenoma	3 (3.0)			

All participants were nonsmokers and nonalcohol users and none exercised on a regular basis.
*Number of individuals for whom this characteristic is known.
**Not applicable.

patients. In addition a structured questionnaire was completed to elucidate information on demographic factors, menstruation, reproductive history, dietary habits, prior diseases, physical activities, and tobacco and alcohol use. Written informed consent regarding the usage of samples for genetic experiments was obtained from all subjects, and the study protocol was approved by the Research Board of the College of Medical Laboratory Sciences, University of Sudan for Science and Technology, Khartoum, Sudan.

Genomic DNA Extraction

Genomic DNA for genotyping was extracted from peripheral blood samples. DNA was extracted using a QiaAmp DNA Blood Mini Kit (Qiagen GmbH, Duesseldorf, Germany) according to the manufacturer's recommendations. Concentration and purity of the genomic DNA samples were determined by mea-

suring the absorbance at 260 nm (A_{260}) and the ratio of the absorbance at 260 nm and 280 nm ($A_{260nm/280nm}$). The genomic DNA samples were prepared to a final concentration of 10 ng/μL of DNA and stored at $-20°$C.

Genotyping by Real-time PCR

An allelic discrimination assay was employed using a real-time PCR method that proves to be a faster, more reliable, and more accurate than conventional methods based on restriction enzyme digestion. Genotyping of codon 655 Ile-to-Val single nucleotide polymorphism (SNP) missense mutations [db SNP rs1136200] was carried out. PCR primers and TaqMan probes specific for the HER-2/neu Ile655Val polymorphism were purchased from Applied Biosystems. The labeled primer/probe set was selected from the Applied Biosystems Assays-on-Demand™ product (Applied Biosystems, Foster City, CA). All details of the target gene

TABLE 2. Genotypic and Allelic Frequencies of HER-2/neu Ile655Val in the Sudanese Population: Breast Cancer Group Compared to Control Group (Odds Ratios (OR) with 95% Confidence Intervals (95% CI))

	Genotyping frequencies				Allele freq.		
	Ile/Ile	Ile/Val	Val/Val	OR (95% CI)* (*P*-value)	Ile	Val	OR(95%CI)** (*P*-value)
Patients	56 (82.4)	11 (16.2)	1 (1.5)		155 (92.3)	13 (7.7)	
Controls	75 (92.6)	5 (6.2)	1 (1.2)	2.95 (0.97–8.96) *P* = 0.06	155 (95.7)	7 (4.3)	1.86 (0.72–4.78) *P* = 0.29

*OR (Ile/Val versus Ile/Ile) for being a case.
**OR (Ile versus Val) for being a case.

and the SNP (location in the genome, reference sequence number, length of the amplicon) were available from the Applied Biosystems web site (http://appliedbiosystems.com). TaqMan SNP Genotyping products consist of a 40X mix of unlabeled PCR primers and TaqMan MGB probe. The assay enables scoring of the wild-type allele as well as a variant allele in a single well.

Assays were performed in 96-Well Optical Plates (4306737; Applied Biosystems). Real-time PCR was performed in an ABI Prism 7500 Sequence Detection System (Applied Biosystem). The PCR reaction was carried out in a 6 μL reaction volume containing TaqMan Universal Master Mix (2X, 4331182; Applied Biosystems), TaqMan Genotyping Assay (40X), and optimized quantities of genomic DNA. The Universal Master Mix contained AmpliTaq Gold DNA Polymerase, AmpErase UNG, dNTPs with dUTP, Passive Reference, and optimized buffer components. The PCR samples

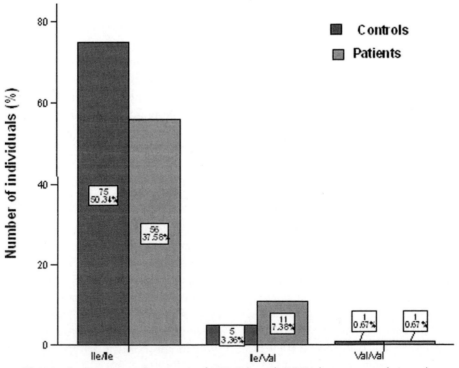

Figure 1. Genotypic frequency of HER-2/neu Ile655Val in cases and controls.

TABLE 3. Genotypic and Allelic Frequencies Stratified by Age and Menopausal Status (pre and post)

	Genotyping frequencies					Allele freq.		
	Ile/Ile N (%)	Ile/Val N (%)	Val/Val N (%)	OR (95% CI)* (*P*-value)		Ile N (%)	Val) N (%)	OR (95% CI)* (*P*-value)
Patients ≤50 controls	43 (82.7)	8 (15.4)	1 (1.9)	2.48 (0.62–10.01) (*P* = 0.20)	≤50	94 (98.4)	10 (9.6)	2.94 (0.78–11.06) (*P* = 0.15)
	40 (93.0)	3 (7.0)	0 (0.0)			83 (96.5)	3 (3.5)	
Patients ≤50 controls	12 (80.0)	3 (20.0)	0 (0.0)	2.25 (0.33–15.54) (*P* = 0.41)	≤50	27 (90.0)	3 (10.0)	2.11 (0.33–13.51) (*P* = 0.65)
Patients pre controls	41 (82.0)	8 (16.0)	1 (2.0)	1.90 (0.53–6.83) (*P* = 0.32)	pre	90 (90.0)	10 (10.0)	
	39 (90.7)	4 (9.3)	0 (0.0)			82 (95.3)	4 (4.7)	
Patients post controls	13 (81.3)	3 (18.8)	0 (0.0)	3.69 (0.34–39.84) (*P* = 0.28)	post	92 (90.6)	3 (9.4)	3.41 (0.34–34.7) (*P* = 0.35)
	16 (94.1)	1 (5.9)	0 (0.0)			33 (97.1)	1 (2.9)	

*OR (Il/Val versus Ile/Ile) for being a case.

were placed in the machine, which was set to detect FAM (to detect the variant allele) and VIC (to detect the wild-type allele) reporter dyes simultaneously. Reactions were set up in duplicates. Thermal cycling was initiated by incubation at 95°C for 10 min for optimal AmpErase UNG activity and activation of Ampli-Taq Gold DNA Polymerase, respectively. After this initial step, 50 cycles of PCR were performed. Each PCR cycle consisted of heating to 92°C for 15 s for melting, and to 60°C for 1 min for annealing and extension.

Statistical Analysis

The Hardy–Weinberg equilibrium was tested among patients and controls separately with the χ^2-test. We computed odds ratios (OR) with 95% confidence intervals (95% CI) for being a case (Ile/Ile genotyping compared to Ile/Val genotyping) by means of logistic regression. The Val/Val group was excluded from these computations because this group was too small to yield any meaningful results. The same logistic regression analysis was applied to subgroups according to menopausal status, and age (≤50 and >50 years). For the test of symmetry of the disagreement distribution regarding genotype of normal tissue and malignant tissue, the McNemar–Bowker test was used. Symme-

try of disagreement regarding allele typing was tested with McNemar's test.

Results

We found that patients with breast cancer and control groups were comparable in the major known risk factors that were studied together with demographic features. Although the response rate for participating in this study was high, some of the participants refused to provide their blood, other data were missed, and some of the DNA samples were not genotyped. Demographic and clinical characteristics of breast cancer patients compared with control subjects are shown in Table 1.

Detection of the HER-2/neu Ile655Val Polymorphism by Real-time PCR

Table 2 shows the genotypic and allelic frequencies of HER-2/neu Ile655Val of peripheral blood. Statistical analysis revealed a nearly significant difference ($P = 0.06$) between genotyped breast cancer patients and control subjects, the heterozygous Ile/Val frequency being higher in the case group (16.2%) than in the control group (6.2%) (OR: 2.95, 95% CI: 0.97–8.96) (Fig. 1). The overall prevalence of the Val allele among Sudanese healthy

TABLE 4. Stratified Analyses between HER-2/neu Polymorphisms and Breast Cancer risk by ESR1 Genotypes

	ESR1 CC				ESR1 CG				ESR1 GG			
	Cases n(%)	Controls n(%)	OR*	95% CI (P)	Cases n(%)	Controls n(%)	OR*	95% CI (P)	Cases n(%)	Controls n(%)	OR*	95% CI (P)
Ile/Ile (ref)	42 (93.9)	46 (93.9)	-	-	14 (82.4)	22 (88.0)	-	-	0 (0.0)	2 (100.0)	-	-
Ile/Val	9 (17.6)	2 (4.1)	4.9	1.0–24.1 (0.05)	2 (11.8)	3 (12.0)	1.0	0.2–7.1 (0.96)	0 (0.0)	0 (0.0)	**	**
Val/Val	0 (0.0)	1 (2.0)	**	**	1 (5.9)	0 (0.0)	**	**	0 (0.0)	0 (0.0)	**	**
Ile/Val+Val/Val	9 (17.6)	3 (6.1)	3.3	0.8–13.0 (0.08)	3 (17.6)	3 (12.0)	1.6	0.3–8.9 (0.61)	0 (0.0)	0 (0.0)	**	**

*OR of being a case (Ile/Ile is the reference group).

**Not estimable because of empty cells.

control subjects is much lower compared with those reported in Asians (Chinese and Taiwanese, 52.1%) and compared with Americans and European populations (approximately 20%) (Table 2). The analyses stratified by age (Table 3) and according to menopausal status (Table 4) yielded similar, nonsignificant associations. Comparison of the genotype of the tumor tissue to that of its matched normal adjacent tissue (Table 5), shows that 80% (95% CI: 69%–89%) had genotype Ile/Ile in both tissues, 12% (95% CI: 5%–22%) of both tissues had Ile/Val heterozygous, and only 1% (95% CI: 0%–8%) of studied tissues was carrying the rare homozygous Val/Val in both tumor and normal adjacent tissue, the nonmatching tissue comprising 7% of the 67 tested tissue samples.

Combined Effect of ESR1 C325G and HER-2/neu Ile655Val

We found that the SNPs of ESR1 C325G and HER-2/neu Ile655Val were associated with a significantly increased risk of breast cancer. Carriers of ESR1325CC and heterozygous carrier of HER-2/neu 655Ile/Val were more common among patients compared to control groups $P = 0.05$ [adjusted OR (95% CI) = 4.9 (1.0–24) (Table 4).

Discussion

A wide range of molecular biomarkers involved in breast carcinogenesis have been studied as potential prognostic markers. These include markers of proliferation (e.g., Ki-67) of the estrogen and progesterone receptors and the human epidermal growth factor receptor 2.[23] HER-2/neu is the one of the most important proto-oncogenes in invasive breast cancer and is believed to have a central role in the HER family.

Oncogenic amplification of HER-2/neu gene occurs in about 30% of early-stage breast cancers, and significant correlation has

TABLE 5. Previously Published Studies of HER-2/neu Ile655Val Polymorphism and Risk of Breast Cancer

Population	Subjects	Ile/Ile	Ile/Val	Val/Val	OR (95% CI)	P-value
Ghanaian	Total (200)	100	0	0	(0–0.01)	N.A.
African-American	Total (90)	56.7	38.9	4.4	(0.18–0.30)	N.A.
Caucasian	Total (257)	65.4	29.2	5.4	(0.17–0.24)	N.A.
Ameyaw et al. (2000)						
Chinese (Shanghai)	Case (339)	71.7	25.1	3.2	1.4 (1.0–2.0)	0.005
Xie et al. (2000)	Control (361)	78.0	21.7	0.3		
Japanese	Case (263)	77.7	21.6	1.3	0.3 (0.08–1.24)	N.S.
Hishida et al. (2002)	Control (184)	73.9	22.3	3.8		
Filipino	Control (73)	83.7	15.0	1.3	0.09 (0.02–0.16)	N.A.
Saudi	Control (101)	80.2	17.8	0.2	0.11 (0.06–0.19)	N.A.
Sudanese	Control (52)	82.7	17.3	0	0.09 (0.01–0.16)	N.A.
Kenyan	Control (114)	97.4	26.0	0	0.01 (0–0.03)	N.A.
Ghanaian	Control (200)	100	0	0	0 (0–0.01)	N.A.
Ameyaw et al. (2002)						
Korean	Case (177)	78.5	18.6	2.8	1.79 (0.46–6.99)	N.S.
Jung An et al. (2005)	Control (126)	76.2	23.0	0.8		
Iranian	Case (204)	71.1	27.9	1.0	1.16 (0.67–2.03)	N.S.
Kamali-Sarvestani et al. (2004)	Control (138)	74.0	23.2	2.8		
Iowa	Case (154)	58.4	38.3	3.3	0.9 (0.6–1.4)	N.S.
Zheng et al. (2001)	Control (325)	56.9	38.8	4.3		
U.S.A. (midwestern)	Case (1094)	58.2	36.2	5.6	0.71 (0.49–1.04)	N.S.
Nelson et al. (2005)	Control (976)	56.5	36.5	7.1		
U.S.A.	Case (754)	87.2	11.7	1.1	N.A.	0.06
African American	Control (676)	89.6	10.4	0.0		
White	Case (1261)	59.7	34.0	6.3	N.A.	N.S.
Millikan et al. (2003)	Control (1132)	60.4	33.1	6.5		
Hawaii & Los Angeles Multiethnic	Case (675)	73	27	Δ	1.27 (0.96–1.68)	0.09
McKean-Cowdin et al. (2001)	Control (545)	79	21			
Portugal	Case (152)	N.A	N.A	N.A	2.0 (1.23–3.25)	0.005
Pinto et al. (2004)	Control (146)					
Ashkenasim, Washington DC	Case (1375)	76	22.4	1.5	(0.9–2.2)	N.A.
Israeli	Case (193)	73	24	3	(2.6–3.4)	
Rutter et al. (2003)						
U.S radiologic technologist	Cases	57.9	42.1	Δ	1.51(0.83–2.49)	N.S.
Hauptmann et al. (2003)						
British	Case (315)	60.3	34.6	5.1	N.A.	N.S.
Baxter and Campbell (2001)	Control (256)	53.9	39.4	6.6		
	Over (314)	58.3	34.1	7.1		
German	Case (615)	69	36	6	1.1 (0.7–1.8)	N.S.
Caucasian	Control (1078)	60	35	5		
Wang-Gohrke and Chang-Claude (2001)						
German	Case (960)	53.6	38.0	8.4	1.05 (0.82–1.34)	N.S.
Frank et al. (2005)	Control (347)	54.7	39.3	6.0		
Caucasian	Case (1272)	N.A.	N.A.	N.A.	0.68 (0.47–0.98)	N.A.
Cox et al. (2005)	Control (1667)					
Australian	Case (409)	58.7	33.7	7.6	3 (1.4–6.8)	0.01

Continued

TABLE 5. *Continued*

Population	Subjects	Ile/Ile	Ile/Val	Val/Val	OR (95% CI)	*P*-value
Montgomery *et al.* (2003)	Control (299)	65.6	31.4	3.0		
Present study Sudanese	Case (68)	82.4	16.2	1.5	2.95 (0.97–8.96)	0.06
Siddig *et al.* (2008)[48]	Control (81)	92.6	6.2	1.2		

N.S. Not significant

N.A. Not available

Δ Computed with Ile/Val genotype due to small number of Val/Val genotype

been reported between HER-2/neu overexpression and conditions, such as steroid hormone receptor-negative status, higher histological grades, higher rate of proliferation, reduced response to chemotherapy and hormone therapy, and reduced survival of breast cancer patients.[2,11] The isoleucine to valine polymorphism of codon 655 of the HER-2/neu gene has been repeatedly investigated for an association with breast cancer[23–43] and other solid tumors.[36,42] These studies show either increased risk, decreased effect, or no overall association, possibly depending on ethnic variation.[24] Assuming that gene activation through missense mutation might affect individual susceptibility to breast cancer risk, we analyzed the prevalence of Ile655Val polymorphism located in the transmembrane domain of HER-2/neu.

We found that being a heterozygous Ile/Val carrier was associated with a modestly increased risk of breast cancer. The rare homozygous Val/Val genotype was detected in patients (1.5%) as well as in controls (1.2%), in contrast to the study by Ameywa and colleagues[24] in a Ghanaian healthy population, where the Val allele was not detected. In another study conducted by the same researcher, the Val allele was detected in Sudanese, Kenyan, Saudi, and Filipino populations.[25] Highly significant increases in the risk of breast cancer $(P = 0.005)$ and $(P = 0.01)$ and of being a carrier of the Val allele were reported in a European population.[37,39] In contrast to our results, Nelson and colleagues and Cox and colleagues found the Val allele to have a lesser effect on the risk of the breast cancer, although an increased risk of

disease progression was observed.[31,43] On the other hand, some studies did not find evidence of association between the Val allele and risk of breast cancer.[26–29,36,38,40] These contradictory results may be attributed to different genetic backgrounds in different ethnic groups or differences in diet, body size, physical activity, and reproductive pattern, which may correlate with ethnicity.

In this study, the association of genotypic and allelic frequencies in relation to age and risk of breast cancer revealed no significant association, although Xie and co-workers demonstrated that the Val allele was linked to an increased risk of breast cancer among women in Shanghai, China,[22] particularly among women younger than 45 years of age $(P = 0.005)$. In a similar study among Ashkenazim,[34] the same association was reported, particularly among women 50 years and younger and in women with a family history of breast cancer. Moreover, homozygosity of Val/Val655 has been associated with an increased risk of early-onset breast cancer in Australian women diagnosed before the age of 45 and 40.[41] Other data on early-onset cases show no significant association with the Val allele, yet a trend toward an increased risk has been observed. Hauptmann and colleagues concluded that the association of the Val allele might be real by age 70 years.[33]

In addition, menopausal status had no effect in our studied SNPs; the variant displayed similar distribution among patients and controls. Functional analysis of this SNP is not yet well established. However, isoleucine-to-valine changes are known to affect stabilization of hydrophobic protein domains, such as transmembrane domains, by altering hydrophobicity.[44] Another study has shown that this Val655 SNP is linked to another polymorphic site, Val654, and that this linkage mediates dimerization of HER-2/neu in the cell membrane.[45] Thus, polymorphism in these two loci results in two consecutive valine residues instead of two isoleucine residues in the transmembrane domain. Based on the knowledge that a substitution of Ile654 by a valine residue would stabilize the formation of active HER-2/neu dimers,[38] this active form may increase autophosphorylation, tyrosine kinase activity, and cell transformation.

Joint Effect of ESR1C325G and HER-2/neu Ile655Val and Risk of Breast Cancer

We have found a significant gene–gene interaction between ESR1C325G and HER-2/neu Ile655Val variants in relation to risk of breast cancer. Patients who are carrying the CC genotype of ESR1 as well as heterozygous for Ile/Val at 655 of HER-2/neu are at higher risk compared to control group ($P = 0.05$). These loci were suggested as susceptible alleles when each locus was consider alone in our study, therefore, the joint effects of SNPs in ESR1and HER-2/neu further confirm our suggestion that ESR1CC and HER-2/neu Ile/Val were susceptible alleles. Numerous hypotheses have been put forward to explain the clinically observed inverse proportion of breast cancer that overexpresses estrogen receptor (ER) and HER family members.[46] In particular, the existence of multiple cross-talk mechanisms between the activated receptor tyrosine kinases and ER signaling pathways is now commonly implicated as a mechanism accounting for the endocrine resistance of some ER positive breast cancers.[47] However, how this crosstalk signaling happens between ER and HER-2/neu is still poorly understood, and the joint effects of these SNPs could be one of the underlying causes of hormonal resistance that is observed in HER-2/neu–positive breast cancer, the major cause of treatment failure and cancer death. Obviously, the biological evidence for this gene–gene interaction needs further in-depth investigation.

In conclusion, our results show that the HER-2/neu Ile655Val polymorphism may contribute to breast cancer risk. A somewhat increased overall breast cancer risk was seen among women with the HER-2/neu Ile/Val655 heterozygosity. The frequency of different polymorphic variants of this gene varies with ethnicity. Our study demonstrated, for the first time, a significant gene–gene interaction between the ESR1 gene and the HER-2/neu gene, mainly, that the ESR1325CC variant and HER-2/neu Ile655Val variant may contribute to risk of breast cancer.

Conflicts of Interest

The authors declare no conflicts of interest.

References

1. Stern, D.F., P.A. Heffman & R.A. Weinbeg. 1986. p185 a product of the neu proto-oncogene is a receptorlike protein associated with tyrosine kinas activity. *Mol. Cell Biol.* **6:** 1729–1740.

2. Stern, D.F. 2000. Tyrosine kinase signaling in breast cancer: ErbB family receptor tyrosine kinases. *Breast Cancer Res.* **2:** 176–183.

3. Akiyama, T., C. Sudo, H. Oguwara, *et al.* 1986. The product of the c-erbB-2 gene: a 185-kilodalton glycoprotein with tyrosine kinase activity. *Science* **232:** 1644–1646.

4. Callahan, R. 1989. Genetic alteration in primary breast cancer. *Breast Cancer Res. Treat.* **13:** 191–203.

5. Graus-Porta, D., R.R. Beerli, J.M. Daly & N.E. Hynes. 1997. ErbB-2, the preferred heterodimerization partner of all ErbB receptors, is a mediator of lateral signaling. *Eur. Med. Biol. Org. J.* **16:** 1647–1655.

6. Sliwkowsk, M.X., G. Schaefer, R.W. Akita, *et al.* 1994. Co expression of erbB-2 and erbB-3 proteins reconstitutes a high affinity receptor for hergulin. *J. Biol. Chem.* **269:** 14661–14665.

7. Tzahar, E., H. Waterman, X. Chen, *et al.* 1996. A hierarchial network of interreceptor interactions

determines signal transduction by Neu differentia-tion factor/neuregulin and epidermal growth factor. *Mol. Cell Biol.* **16:** 5276–5287.

8. Karunagaran, D., E. Tzahar, R.R. Beerli *et al.* 1996. ErbB-2 is a common auxiliary subunit of NDF and EGF receptor: implications for breast cancer. *EMBO J.* **15:** 254–264.

9. Eccles, S.A. 2001. The role of c-erbB/HER/neu in breast cancer progression and metastasis. *J. Mammary Gland Biol. Neoplasia* **6:** 393–406.

10. Di Fiore, P.P., J.H. Pierce, T.P. Fleming, *et al.* 1987. Overexpression of the human EGF receptor confers an EGF-dependent transformed phenotype to NIH 3T3 cells. *Cell* **51:** 1063–1070.

11. Di Fiore, P.P., J.H. Pierce, M.H. Kraus, *et al.* 1987. erbB-2 is a potent oncogene when overexpressed in NIH/3T3 cells. *Science* **237:** 178–182.

12. Liu, A., M. Thor, M. He, *et al.* 1992. The HER-2 (c-erbB-2) oncogene is frequently amplified in situ carcinomas of the breast. *Oncogene* **7:** 1027–1032.

13. Salmon, D.J., G.M. Clark, S.G. Wong, *et al.* 1987. Hu-man breast cancer: correlation of relapse and survival with amplification of HER-2/neu oncogene. *Science* **235:** 177–182. I.

14. Schonborn, W., E. Zschiesche, C. Spitzer, *et al.* 1994. C-erbB-2 overexpression in primary breast cancer: independent prognostic factor in patients at high risk. *Breast Cancer Res. Treat.* **29:** 287–295.

15. Hartmann, L.C., J.N. Ingle, L.E. Wold, *et al.* 1994. Prognostic value of c-erbB-2 overexpression in axil-lary lymph node positive breast cancers: results from a randomized adjuvant treatment protocol. *Cancer* **74:** 2956–2963.

16. Tetu, B. & J. Brisson. 1994. Prognostic significance of HER-2/neu oncoprotein expression in node positive breast cancer. *Cancer* **73:** 2359–2365.

17. Niu, G. & W. Bradford Carter. 2007. Human epider-mal growth factor receptor 2 regulates angiopoietin-2 expression in breast cancer via AKT and mitogin-activated protein kinase pathways. *Cancer Res.* **67:** 1487–1493.

18. Barmann, C.L., M.C. Hung & R.A. Weinberg. 1986. Multiple independent activation of the neu oncogene by a point mutation altering transmembrane domain of p185. *Cell* **45:** 649–657.

19. Barmann, C.L., R.A. Weinberg. 1988. Oncogenic activation of the neu- encoded receptor protein by point mutation and deletion. *EMBO J.* **7:** 2043–2052.

20. Segatto, O., C.R. King, J.H. Pierce, *et al.* 1988. Dif-ferent structural alteration upregulate in vitro tyro-sine kinase activity and transforming potency of the ErbB-2. *Mol. Cell Biol.* **8:** 5570–5574.

21. Papewalis, J., A.Y. Nikitin & M.F. Rajewsky. 1991. G to A polymorphism at amino acid codon 655 of the human erbB-2/HER-2 gene. *Nucleic Acids Res.* **19:** 5452.

22. Xie, D., X.O. Shu, Z. Deng, *et al.* 2000. Population-based, case-control study of HER2 genetic polymor-phism and breast cancer risk. *J. Natl Cancer Inst.* **92:** 412–417.

23. Esteva, F.J. & G.N. Hortobagyi. 2004. Prognostic molecular markers in early breast cancer. *Breast Cancer Res.* **6:** 109–118.

24. Ameywa, M.M., N. Thornton & H.L. McLeod. 2000. Population based, case control study of HER2 genetic polymorphism and breast cancer risk. *J. Natl. Cancer Inst.* **92:** 1947.

25. Ameywa, M.M., M. Tayeb, N. Thornton, *et al.* 2002. Ethnic variation in the HER-2 codon 655 genetic polymorphism previously associated with breast can-cer. *J. Hum. Genet.* **47:** 172–175.

26. Hishida, N., H. Hamajima, K. Iwata, *et al.* 2002. Population-based, case-control study of HER2 ge-netic polymorphism and breast cancer risk. *J. Natl Cancer Inst.* **94:** 1807–1808.

27. Kamali-Sarvestani, A., A. Talei & A. Merat. 2004. IIe to Val polymorphism at codon 655 of HER-2 gene and breast cancer risk in Iranian women. *Cancer Lett.* **215:** 83–87.

28. Jung An, H., N.K. Kim, D. Oh, *et al.* 2005. Her2^{v655} Genotype and breast cancer progression in Korean women. *Pathol. Int.* **55:** 48–52.

29. Zheng, W., N. Kataoka, D. Xie & S.R. Young. 2001. Population-based case-control study of HER2 ge-netic polymorphism and breast cancer risk. *J. Natl. Cancer Inst.* **93:** 558–559.

30. McKean-Cowdin, R., L.N. Kolonel, M.F. Press, *et al.* 2001. Germ-line HER-2 variant and breast cancer risk by stage of disease. *Cancer Res.* **61:** 8394.

31. Nelson, S.E., M.N. Gauld, J.M. Hampton & A. Trentham-Dietz. 2005. A case-control study of the HER2 IIe655Val polymorphism in relation to risk of invasive breast cancer. *Breast Cancer Res.* **7:** R357–R364.

32. Millikan, R., A. Eaton, K. Worley, *et al.* 2003. HER2 codon 655 polymorphism and risk of breast cancer in African American and whites. *Breast Cancer Res. Treat.* **79:** 355–364.

33. Hauptmann, M., A.J. Sigurdson, N. Chatterjee, *et al.* 2003. Population-based, case-control study of HER2 genetic polymorphism and breast cancer risk. *J. Natl. Cancer Inst.* **95:** 1251–1252.

34. Rutter, J.L., N. Chatterjee, S. Wacholder & J.P. Struewing. 2003. The HER2 I655V polymorphism and breast cancer risk in Ashkenazim. *Epidemiology* **14:** 694–700.

35. Keshava, C., E.C. McCanlies, N. Keshava, *et al.* 2001. Distribution of HER2V655 genotypes in breast

cancer cases and controls in the United States. *Cancer Lett.* **173:** 37–41.

36. Baxter, S.W. & I.G. Campbell. 2001. Population-based case-control study of HER2 genetic polymorphism and breast cancer risk. *J. Natl Cancer Inst.* **93:** 557–558.

37. Zúbor, P., A. Vojvodová, J. Danko, *et al.* 2006. HER-2 [Ile655Val] polymorphism in association with breast cancer risk: a population-based case-control study in Slovakia. *Neoplasma* **53:** 49–55.

38. Frank, B., K. Hemminik, M. Wirtenberger, *et al.* 2005. The rare ERBB2 variant IIe654Val is associated with an increased familial breast cancer risk. *Carcinogenesis* **26:** 643–647.

39. Pinto, D., A. Vasconcelos, S. Costa, *et al.* 2004. HER2 polymorphism and breast cancer risk in Portugal. *Eur. J. Cancer Prev.* **13:** 177–181.

40. Wang-Gohrke, S. & J. Chang-Claude. 2001. Re: Population-based case-control study of HER2 genetic polymorphism and breast cancer risk. *J. Natl Cancer Inst.* **93:** 1657–1658.

41. Montgomery, K.G., D.M. Gertig, S.W. Baxter, *et al.* 2003. The HER2 I655V polymorphism and risk of breast cancer in women < age 40 years. *Cancer Epidemiol. Biomarkers Prev.* **12:** 1109–1111.

42. Chan, K.Y., A.Y. Cheung, S.P Yip, *et al.* 2002. Population-based case-control study of HER2 genetic polymorphism and breast cancer risk. *J. Natl. Cancer Inst.* **94:** 20.

43. Cox, D.G., S.E. Hankinson & D.J. Hunter. 2005. The erbB/HER2/neu receptor polymorphism Ile655val and breast cancer risk. *Pharmacogenetics Genomics* **15:** 447–450.

44. Amunddatottir, L.T. & P. Leder. 1998. Signal transduction pathways activated and required for mammary carcinogenesis in response to specific oncogenes. *Oncogene* **16:** 737–746.

45. Mendrola, J.M., M.B. Berger, M.C. King & M.A. Lemmon. 2002. The single transmembrane domain of ErbB receptors self associate in cell membrane. *J. Biol. Chem.* **277:** 4704–4712.

46. Benz, C. & D. Tripathy. 2000. ErbB2 overexpression in breast cancer: biology and clinical translation. *J. Woman Cancer* **2:** 33–40.

47. Sommer, S. & S.A.W. Fuqa. 2001. Estrogen receptor and breast cancer. *Cancer Biol.* **11:** 339–352.

48. Siddig, A. *et al.* 2008. Estrogen receptor α gene polymorphism and breast cancer. *Ann. N. Y. Acad. Sci.* Recent Advances in Clinical Oncology. In Press.

Estrogen Receptor α Gene Polymorphism and Breast Cancer

Awatif Siddig,[a,f] **Abdelrahim Osman Mohamed,**[b] **Salma Awad,**[c] **Ahmed H. Hassan,**[c] **Erika Zilahi,**[d] **Mohammed Al-Haj,**[d] **Roos Bernsen,**[e] **and Abdu Adem**[f]

[a]*Faculty of Medical Laboratory Technology, Sudan University for Science and Technology, Khartoum, Sudan*

[b]*Department of Biochemistry, Faculty of Medicine and Health Science, University of El Imam El-Mahdi, Kosti, Sudan*

[c]*Department of Biochemistry,* [d]*Department of Medical Microbiology,* [e]*Department of Community Medicine,* [f]*Department of Pharmacology, Faculty of Medicine and Health Sciences, UAE University, Al Ain, United Arab Emirates*

Estrogen and estrogen receptors play important roles in the proliferation and development of breast cancer. Several genetic alterations identified in the estrogen receptor α gene (ESR1) are thought to influence the expression or function of this protein, and many have been evaluated for their role in breast cancer predisposition. The aim of this study was to evaluate the role of the C325G single nucleotide polymorphism (SNP) in the ESR1 in predisposition to breast cancer. The candidate SNP C325G in ESR1, exon 4 was genotyped in breast cancer patients and in healthy controls that were age and sex matched. Genotyping was performed using both single-stranded conformational polymorphism (SSCP) and a higher throughput allelic discrimination method using real-time PCR. Data on clinical features and demographic details were collected. Significant association of breast cancer risk was shown in the subgroup of women 50 years and younger who had the C allele (OR: 2.28, 95% CI: 1.10–4.72) ($P = 0.03$). However, the overall susceptibility to breast cancer was not significant, although all estimates were in the direction of a higher risk in women with CC genotypes. This study found significant evidence that polymorphism within the low penetrance ESR1 is associated with breast cancer susceptibility in women of 50 years or younger. There is also an indication that G allele is protective (compared to C allele).

Key words: breast cancer; estrogen receptor α gene; exon 4; polymorphism

Introduction

Breast cancer is the most frequent cancer among women worldwide and it is the second leading cause of death after lung cancer.[1] In Sudan breast cancer is the most common cancer, comprising 34% of all cancer patients. It is widely believed that breast cancer re-

sults in many genetic and epigenetic changes in a population of cells[2,3] which can disrupt several molecular pathways. Functionally defective mutations in the BRCA1 and BRCA2 genes are responsible for up to 5% of all patients with breast cancer, while other genes (so-called low penetrance genes) account for the remainder of breast cancer patients.[4,5] Among the possible low-penetrance candidate genes for breast cancer, evidence points toward the estrogen receptor α gene (ESR1). ESR1 is localized on chromosome 6q25.1[6] and encodes a nuclear protein ER (estrogen receptor) that

Address for correspondence: Prof. Abdu Adem, Ph.D., Department of Pharmacology, Faculty of Medicine and Health Sciences, UAE University, P.O. Box 17666, Al Ain, UAE. Voice: +00971504482894; fax: +0097137672033. abdu.adem@uaeu.ac.ae

Ann. N.Y. Acad. Sci. 1138: 95–107 (2008). © 2008 New York Academy of Sciences.
doi: 10.1196/annals.1414.015

regulates DNA transcription upon binding estrogen or another ligand.[7,8] ER–estrogen interactions thus lead to stimulation of cell growth in various tissues including breast epithelial tissue. Single nucleotide polymorphisms (SNPs) in specific candidate genes are thought to influence expression and/or activity of encoding proteins, thereby predisposing to cancer, especially breast cancer.[9] Several SNPs in the ER gene (*ESR1*) have been identified that are associated with an increased or a decreased risk of breast cancer and other diseases.[10,11] The best-characterized SNPs of *ESR1* are the *PvuII* and *XbaI* restriction-site polymorphisms, both of which are located in the first intron.[12,13] The polymorphism investigated in this study was selected in the light of a previous report[14] showing that the ESR1 was polymorphic. The polymorphism investigated in this study is a C-to-G substitution at codon 325 causing no change to the corresponding amino acid (synonymous). As breast cancer development is dependent on estrogenic influences, we have investigated whether polymorphisms in the ESR1 are associated with breast cancer risk. The aim of the present study was to evaluate polymorphism of the ESR1 at exon 4 codon 325 CCC → CCG in a panel of breast cancer patients in an attempt to establish a genetic polymorphism database. This will allow us to correlate these polymorphisms with the distinctive clinical features of our breast cancer patients and to estimate the association between the SNP and breast cancer risk.

Patients and Methods

Study Population

A case–control study was conducted to assess the association between genotype frequencies and breast cancer risk. We used biospecimens to identify common low-penetrance alleles. One hundred patients of primary breast cancer were studied: (98 females and 2 males, mean (SD) age: 46.4 (13.5) years) and 90 controls (84 females and 4 males, mean (SD) age: 46.2 (13.4) years). Patients with pathologically confirmed

disease were diagnosed between June 2004 and July 2005 in Khartoum Teaching Hospital, Soba University Hospital, and Omdurman Hospital, Sudan. Tumor tissues and matched normal adjacent tissues were obtained sequentially in the operating room. Representative segments were excised and snap frozen in liquid nitrogen then kept at −20°C until processing. Control subjects were randomly selected from the general population in Khartoum State from the same age group as the patients. Peripheral blood samples from all subjects were obtained and kept frozen until genotyping. Pathologic data were confirmed by a senior pathologist; in addition a structured questionnaire was completed to elucidate information on demographic factors, menstruation, reproductive history, dietary habits, prior diseases, physical activities, and tobacco and alcohol use. Written informed consent regarding the use of samples for genetic experiments was obtained from all subjects, and the study protocol was approved by the Research Board of College of Medical Laboratory Sciences, University of Sudan for Science and Technology, Khartoum, Sudan.

Genomic DNA Extraction

Genomic DNA for genotyping was extracted from peripheral blood samples and tissue samples. DNA was extracted according to the manufacturer's recommendations using a QiaAmp DNA Blood Mini Kit (Qiagen GmbH, Duesseldorf, Germany). Concentration and purity of the genomic DNA samples were determined by measuring the absorbance at 260 nm (A_{260}) and the ratio of the absorbance at 260 nm and 280 nm ($A_{260nm/280nm}$) using Beckman DU 70 spectrophotometer (Beckman Coulter, Inc., Fullerton, CA). The genomic DNA samples were prepared to obtain a final concentration of 10 ng/μL of DNA and they were stored at −20°C.

PCR-SSCP Genotyping

A fragment of exon 4 of ESR1 was amplified using a forward primer (5′-ACCTGTGTT

TTCAGGGATACGA-3′) and a reverse (5′-GCTGCGGCTTCGATTCTTAC-3′) for the DNA of the tumor tissue, normal adjacent tissue, and peripheral blood samples, using Promega (Madison, WI) master mix. The PCR products were screened for the presence of mutation using single-strand conformational polymorphism (SSCP) technique. Optimal electrophoretic separation for SSCP was conducted. A mix of 3 μL each of PCR product and loading buffer (21.1 mM formamide; 9.02 M of 1% xylene cyanol; 0.58 mM bromophenol blue) was denatured at 96°C for 5 mins and immediately chilled on ice. Then the mixture was loaded onto a 12% nondenaturing polyacrylamide gel and run at 100 V for 5 h at 4°C, using a BioRad (Hercules, CA) vertical electrophoresis cell (10 × 7 cm; 0.75 mm). The silver staining kit (Amersham Buckinghamshire, UK) was used to stain DNA bands in the polyacrylamide gels according to the manufacturer's instructions. Briefly, DNA bands in the gels were fixed 30 min by benzene sulfonic acid (0.6%). The gels were incubated in silver nitrate solution provided by the kit for 30 min, DNA bands were visualized by incubating the gels in a mixture of sodium carbonate (2.5%), formaldehyde (37%), and sodium thiosulphate (2%). The developed color was stopped by using a mixture of acetic acid (1%), sodium acetate (5%), and glycerol (10%).

PCR-RFLP Genotyping

PCR products of exon 4 were digested by the endonuclease enzyme *Hinf1*, described in a pervious study.[15] Briefly, 1 unit of the enzyme was added to 50 ng of the PCR product and incubated overnight at 37°C. The reactions were then run on 2% agarose gels.

Genotyping by Real-time PCR

Allelic discrimination assay was employed using a real-time PCR method that proves to be a faster, more reliable, and more accurate than conventional methods based on restriction enzyme digestion. Genotyping of c975 C → G SNPs (codon 325 CCC → CCG, synonymous Pro, [db SNP rs1801132]) was carried out using the allelic discrimination assay. PCR primers and TaqMan probes specific for the ESR1 C325G polymorphism were purchased from Applied Biosystems (Foster City, CA). The labeled primer/probe set was selected from the applied Biosystems Assays-on-Demand™ product. All details of the target gene and the SNP (location in the genome, reference sequence number, length of the amplicon) were available from the Applied Biosystems Website (http://appliedbiosystems.com). TaqMan SNP genotyping products consist of a 40X mix of unlabeled PCR primers and TaqMan MGB probe. The assay enables scoring of both alleles in a single well.

Assays were performed in 96-Well Optical Plates (4306737, Applied Biosystems). Real-time PCR was performed in an ABI Prism 7500 Sequence Detection System (Applied Biosystems). The PCR reaction was carried out in a 6 μL reaction volume containing TaqMan Universal Master Mix (2X, 4331182, Applied Biosystems), TaqMan Genotyping Assay (40X), and optimized quantities of genomic DNA. The Universal Master Mix contained AmpliTaq Gold DNA Polymerase, AmpErase UNG, dNTPs with dUTP, passive reference, and optimized buffer components. The PCR samples were placed in the ABI Prism 7500 Sequence Detection System, which was set to detect FAM and VIC reporter dye simultaneously. Reactions were set up in duplicate. Thermal cycling was initiated by incubation at 95°C for 10 mins for optimal AmpErase UNG activity and activation of AmpliTaq Gold DNA polymerase. After this initial step, 50 cycles of PCR were performed. Each PCR cycle consisted of heating to 92°C for 15 s for melting, and to 60°C for 1 min for annealing and extension.

Statistical Analysis

The Hardy–Weinberg equilibrium was tested among patients and controls separately with the χ^2-test. We computed odds ratios

TABLE 1. Demographic and Clinical Characteristics of 100 Patients of Breast Cancer Patients and 90 Controls

Characteristic	Patients ($N = 100$)		Controls ($N = 90$)	
	n (%)	N^*	n (%)	N^*
Age		94		88
≤50 years	67 (71.3)		60 (69.0)	
Gender		100		88
female	98 (98.0)		84 (95.5)	
Marital status		100		88
married	95 (95.0)		71 (80.7)	
Parity		92		88
nulliparous	30 (32.6)		24 (27.9)	
State		88		88
Khartoum	28 (32.4)		39 (45.1)	
North	9 (10.3)		13 (15.6)	
Central	24 (27.9)		17 (20.4)	
West	15 (17.6)		13 (15.5)	
East/South/White Nile	10 (11.8)		3 (3.4)	
Education		94		N.D***
No	51 (54.3)			
Primary	27 (28.7)			
Secondary	12 (12.8)			
Higher	4 (4.3)			
Menopausal status		92		88
Premenopausal	65 (70.7)		63 (71.6)	
Histology		100		N.A.**
Ductal	97 (97.0)			
Fibroadenoma	3 (3.0)			

All participants were nonsmokers and nonalcohol users and none exercised on a regular basis.
*Number of individuals for whom this characteristic is known.
**Not applicable.
***Not determined.

(OR) with 95% confidence intervals (95% CI) for being a case (CC genotyping/CG genotyping) by means of logistic regression. The GG group was excluded from these computations because this group was too small. The same analysis was applied to subgroups according to menopausal status, parity (nulliparous and parous women), and age (≤50 and >50 years).

Results

The demographic and clinical characteristics of breast cancer patients compared to control subjects are shown in Table 1. Breast cancer patients and control groups were comparable. The associations (odds ratios) between ESR1 genotyping and breast cancer and between allelic frequency and breast cancer are shown in Table 2. In Table 3 these associations are stratified by menopausal status (3A), parity (3B), and age (3C).

Detection of ESR1 Mutation by PCR-SSCP and PCR-RFLP

Screening for mutations of exon 4 including the C325G codon by PCR-SSCP revealed abnormal migration patterns in tumor tissues and their matched normal adjacent tissue, suggesting the presence of mutation. The C325G

TABLE 2. Genotypic and Allelic Frequencies of Estrogen Receptor-1 Exon 4 C325G in the Sudanese Population: Breast Cancer Group Compared to Control Group (Odds Ratios (OR) with 95% Confidence Intervals (95% CI))

	Genotype frequencies				Allele freq.		
	CC N (%)	CG N (%)	GG N (%)	P-value (McNemar)	C N (%)	G N (%)	P-value
Patients							
malignant tissue	55 (69.6)	23 (29.1)	1 (1.3)	0.23	133 (84.2)	25 (15.8)	0.26
normal tissue	60 (75.9)	17 (21.5)	2 (2.5)		137 (86.7)	21 (13.3)	
				OR (95% CI)* (P-value)			OR(95%CI)** (P-value)
blood	59 (74.7)	20 (25.3)	0 (0)		138 (87.3)	20 (12.7)	
Controls				1.42 (0.72–2.82) (0.31)			1.54 (0.84–2.83) (0.17)
blood	56 (65.9)	27 (31.8)	2 (2.4)		139 (81.8)	31 (18.2)	

*OR (CC/CG) for being a case.
**OR (C/G) for being a case.

polymorphism with *Hinf1* endonuclease enzyme was detected in 7.26% out of 50 paired samples of tumor tissue and their matched normal tissue.

Detection of the Polymorphism by Real-time PCR

Table 2 shows the genotypic and allelic frequencies within the Sudanese group studied, indicating that the frequency of the G allele in codon 325 did not differ significantly between the malignant tissues and their matched normal adjacent tissue. With regard to genotype and allelic frequencies of peripheral blood, statistical analysis revealed no significant difference between genotyped breast cancer patients and control subjects (Table 2 and Fig. 1) (OR (patients/controls, CC/CG): 1.42, 95%CI: 0.72–2.82) (OR (patients/controls, CC/CG): 1.54, 95%CI: 0.84–2.83). The overall prevalence of allele G among the Sudanese population is much lower (12.7%) compared to those reported in Asians (Chinese and Taiwanese, 52.1%) and U.S., UK, and European populations (approximately 20%). Additionally, in the subgroup of women aged 50 years or younger,

the association between allele frequencies and breast cancer was significant (P = 0.03), and no significant differences were shown among this group and their matched tissues (Table 3C). Regarding the genotypic and allelic frequencies stratified by menopausal status (Table 3A) and by parity, no significant associations were observed between the patients and controls and between the genotype matching from tumor tissues and the normal adjacent tissues. No statistical tests were done in the (small) male subgroup, but it is interesting that the two patients in this group had the CC genotype, while all four controls had either CG or GG genotype. This observation may warrant further investigation. Comparison of the genotype of the tumor tissue to that of its matched normal adjacent tissue (see Table 4), shows that 61% (95% CI: 50%–72%) had genotype CC in both tissues, 14% (95% CI: 7%–23%) had CG heterozygosity in both tissues, and only 1% out of the 79 studied tissue pairs carried the rare homozygous GG in both tumor and normal adjacent tissue. In the remaining 24% of the 79 tested tissue-sample pairs, the tumor and normal tissues had different genotypes.

TABLE 3A. Genotypic and Allelic Frequencies Stratified by Pre- and Postmenopausal Status

Patients	CC	CG	GG	P-value (McNemar)		C	G	P-value (McNemar)
Malignant				0.26 #				0.63#
pre	39 (69.6)	16 (28.6)	1 (1.8)		pre	94 (83.9)	18 ((16.1))	
post	13 (65.0)	7 (35.0)	0 (0)		post	33 (82.5)	7 (17.5)	
Normal				1.00##				1.00##
pre	43 (76.8)	11 (19.6)	2 (3.6)		pre	97 (86.6)	15 (13.3)	
post	14 (70.0)	6 (30.0)	0 (0)		post	34 (85)	6 (15)	
				OR(95%CI)* (P-value)				OR(95%CI)** (P-value)
Patients controls Blood pre	43 (76.8)	13 (13.2)	0 (0)	1.82 (0.77–4.35) (0.17)	pre	99 (88.4)	13 (11.6)	1.64 (0.75–3.58) (0.24)
	31 (64.6)	17 (35.4)	0 (0)			79 (82.3)	17 (17.7)	
Patients controls Blood post	13 (65.0)	7 (35.0)	0 (0)	1.09 (0.29–4.00) (0.91)	post	33 (82.5)	7 (17.5)	1.07 (0.34–3.38) (1.00)
	12 (63.2)	7 (36.8)	0 (0)			31 (81.6)	7 (18.4)	

*OR (CC/CG) for being a case.
**OR (C/G) for being a case.
#Comparison between malignant tissue and normal tissue for premenopausal women.
##Comparison between malignant tissue and normal tissue for postmenopausal women.

TABLE 3B. Genotypic and Allelic Frequencies Stratified by Parity

Patients	CC	CG	GG	P-value (McNemar)		C	G	P-value (McNemar)
Malignant								
nulliparous	20 (80.0)	4 (16.0)	1 (4.0)	0.55#	nulliparous	44 (88.0)	6 (12.0)	1.00#
parous	32 (67.7)	19 (37.3)	0 (0)		parous	83 (81.4)	19 (81.6)	
Normal								
nulliparous	20 (80.0)	3 (12.0)	2 (8.0)		nulliparous	43 (86.0)	7 (14.0)	
parous	37 (72.5)	14 (27.5)	0 (0)	0.27##	parous	88 (86.3)	14 (13.7)	0.27##
				OR (95%CI)** (P-value)				OR (95%CI)* (P-value)
Patients controls								
Blood nulli	19 (76.0)	6 (24.0)	0 (0)	***	nulli	44 (88.0)	6 (12.0)	***
	10 (100)	0 (0)	0 (0)			20 (100)	0 (0)	
Patients controls								
Blood parous	37 (72.5)	14 (27.5)	0 (0)	1.92 (0.85–4.35) (0.11)	parous	88 (86.3)	14 (13.7)	1.68 (0.82–3.45) (0.21)
	33 (57.9)	24 (42.1)	0 (0)			90 (78.9)	24 (21.1)	

*OR (CC/CG) for being a case.

**OR (C/G) for being a case.

***Not estimated due to empty cells.

#Comparison between malignant tissue and normal tissue for nulliparous women.

##Comparison between malignant tissue and normal tissue for parous women.

TABLE 3C. Genotypic and Allelic Frequencies Stratified by Age

Patients		CC	CG	GG	P-value (McNemar)		C	G	P-value (McNemar)
Malignant					0.26#				0.63##
Age	≤50	41 (69.5)	17 (28.8)	1 (1.7)		≤50	99 (83.9)	19 (16.1)	
Age	>50	13 (68.4)	6 (31.6)	0 (0)		>50	32 (84.2)	6 (15.8)	
Normal					1.00##				1.00##
Age	≤50	45 (76.3)	12 (20.3)	2 (3.4%)		≤50	102 (86.4)	16 (13.6)	
Age	>50	14 (73.7)	5 (26.3)	0 (0)		>50	33 (86.8)	5 (13.2)	
					OR (95%CI)* (P-value)				OR (95%CI)** (P-value)
Patients controls									
Blood	>50	45 (76.3)	14 (23.7)	0 (0)		≤50	104 (88.1)	14 (11.9)	2.28 (1.10–4.72) (0.03)
	>50	28 (57.1)	19 (38.8)	2 (4.1)	2.17 (0.94–5.09) (0.07)	>50	75 (76.5)	23 (23.5)	
Patients controls									
Blood	>50	13 (68.4)	31 (31.6)	0 (0)		>50	32 (84.2)	6 (15.8)	1.01 (0.31–3.31) (1.00)
	>50	15 (68.2)	7 (31.8)	0 (0)	1.01 (0.27–3.85) (0.99)	>50	37 (84.1)	7 (15.9)	

*OR (CC/CG) for being a case.

**OR (C/G) for being a case.

\# Comparison between malignant tissue and normal tissue women aged 50 years or less.

\## Comparison between malignant tissue and normal tissue for women older than 50 years.

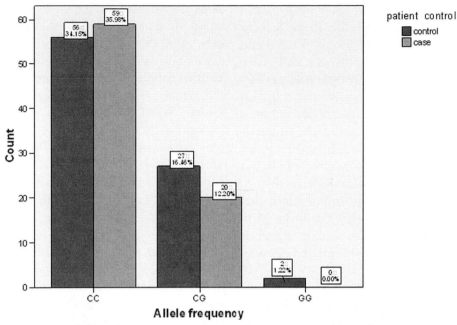

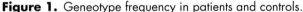

Figure 1. Geneotype frequency in patients and controls.

Discussion

The association of ESR1 genetic polymorphism with breast cancer risk has been the subject of increasing interest because the protein encoded by this gene acts as an important mediator of hormonal response in estrogen-sensitive tissues such as the breast. Therefore it is conceivable that a variation in ESR1 sequences might affect the proliferation of these tissues.[16] Several functionally important exonic and intronic loci of ESR1 polymorphisms that are associated with breast cancer and other diseases have been extensively studied. Among these, the C325G polymorphism has been evaluated for possible linkage with breast cancer[17-22] and other conditions, such as migraine[15] and stroke.[23]

In our population-based, case–control study, we found that the overall frequency of the wild type, CC, was higher in the breast cancer patients (CC = 74.7%) compared to the control individuals (CC = 65.9%), although not significantly ($P = 0.31$). However, when stratified according to age, a significant association with risk of breast cancer in control women

TABLE 4. Comparison of the Genotype of the Tumor Tissue to that of Its Matched Normal Adjacent Tissue in 79 Patients

Normal tissue	Malignant tissue			
	CC	CG	GG	Total
CC	48 (61%) (50%–72%)	12 (15%) (7%–23%)	0 (0%) -	60
CG	6 (8%) (2%–13%)	11 (14%) (6%–22%)	0 (0%) -	17
GG	1 (1%) (0%–4%)	0 (0%) -	1 (1%) (0%–4%)	2
Total	55	23	1	79

Presented are absolute numbers and percentages of total, with 95% confidence intervals.

who are 50 years and younger was evident. The prevalence of the G allele is significantly higher ($P = 0.03$) in the peripheral blood of the control group compared to that of patients, suggesting that the C allele is a susceptible allele, although it is wild type, whereas the G allele is a protective allele. This finding is in agreement with a study conducted in an Asian population,[14] which found lower frequency of G allele among patients with breast cancer compared to the control group, 52.1% and 58.2%, respectively. Although the difference was not significant ($P = 0.099$), the authors suggested that the G allele was a protective allele together with a low incidence rate of breast cancer among the Asian population. Comparing our finding with other reported data, we observed that the G allele is less frequent in our population than in Asian and Western studies, which may contribute to the high incidence of breast cancer observed in our population. In contrast to our results, a statistically significant association was found between the polymorphism of codon C325G [Pro-Pro] and a self-reported family history of breast cancer in a hospital-based study of 188 patients conducted by Roodi and colleagues.[17] (OR = 4.3, 95% CI = 1.8–10.1). The G allele frequency was 28% in 34 patients with breast cancer and a family history of the disease and 11% in 154 patients without such a family history ($P < 0.001$). Two other studies, one among the British population[18] and the other in a Portuguese population[19] demonstrated a significant correlation between the G allele and breast cancer risk ($P = 0.057$) and ($P = 0.038$) in the two studies, respectively. On the other hand, a more recent study by Onay and co-workers.[20] observed no significant association. The authors, using a dense map of SNPs including the C325G codon among the Ontario Familial Breast Cancer Registry, concluded that there was no significant association, although GG was more common in women with breast cancer (37.1%) than in the control group (31.7%) (OR = 1 with 95% CI). In line with the latter, Southey and colleagues[21] found no association between ESR1 polymorphism in codon C325G and the risk of breast cancer in a population-based, case–control study of breast cancer in younger women (<40 years). Additionally, in a cross-sectional association study in Caucasian-Australians, no association was found,[22] and the CC frequency was 83% in patients versus 77% in controls ($P = 0.14$). The same codon was studied in a Korean population with no association observed.[24] Moreover, another study reported a slight negative association between homozygosity for any of the two intron 1 SNPs and heterozygosity for the c.975C → G SNP and ductal cancer risk among Swedish women.[25] A possible explanation for these inconsistencies across studies may be that they are due to the differences among populations in which the studies were conducted. Alternatively, the reported differences might be due to differences in study design. Population history might also contribute to an explanation of the controversial results in different populations such that the causative variant might be linked to one marker allele in one population but with the other allele in another population. However, we support the view that the causality of genetic polymorphism in breast cancer is uncertain but the association is biologically plausible.[26]

The polymorphism studied is a base-pair exchange in the third codon position central to the ESR1 that does not alter the encoded amino acid (synonymous). This polymorphism could be regarded as a marker, potentiality in linkage disequilibrium with another functional locus or loci.[25] How breast cancer is affected by this silent polymorphism is not fully understood. It was reported that this polymorphism may indirectly affect the protein function through alteration of the RNA half-life or protein translation, hence indirectly affecting the level of the ER α protein. The exact mechanisms and their clinical significance remain unclear.[27] Additionally, a recent study published on line from the National Cancer Institute revealed that silent a SNP affected protein function because it forced the cell to read a different DNA codon than it usually does, while the same protein sequence eventually was made. Thus, this silent change might slow the folding rhythm resulting in an altered protein conformation, which in turn affects function. However, we suggest that this central silent polymorphism together with two other silent polymorphisms (one in exon 1, codon 10, known as S10S, and the other in exon 8, which is known as T594T) may play a role in maintaining the architecture of the gene. This gene is known to be polymorphic across the entire reading frame, thus silent mutations in these important sites can reduce the harmful effect of these mutations.

To test the field cancerization (or field effect) hypothesis, we examined genotyping frequencies in the tumor tissues and their matched normal adjacent tissues. We observed 48 (60.8%) of the tissues scoring the wild type CC/CC allele, 11 (13.9%) are heterozygote CG/CG, and only 1.3% is carrying the rare allele GG/GG (Table 4). These data indicate the concordance of the tumor tissue and their matched normal adjacent tissue, and further confirm the higher prevalence of the C allele in patients' tissues compared to the G allele, suggesting that C allele is susceptible allele. In contrast, the discordance represents 19 (24%), whether it is CC/CG, CG/CC, or CC/GG. These nonconcordances provide an estimate of the prevalence of allelic imbalance (AI) in normal breast tissue. Although AI may not be a cancer precursor, the frequency of AI in these cancer patients may be a manifestation of an aberrant ongoing malignant transformation process in an individual's breast tissue.[28] However, it has been proven that normal-appearing adjacent tissue may harbor genetic lesions, a process known as field cancerization.[29,30]

SSCP can be used alone for screening purposes, as it can detect the presence of mutations. We confirmed the presence of the C325G SNP by RFLP technique using endonuclease *Hinf1* enzyme, where we were able to detect only 7.3% (data not shown), which is a low frequency compared to high-throughput real-time PCR. RFLP for detection of polymorphism is relatively insensitive because a small amount of undigested template, which could correspond to mutant, might not be visible, and incomplete digestion of the wild-type template could lead to false results. Inappropriate cutting when digestion proceeds for more than the recommended time can give false results.[31] Finally, we analyzed the questionnaire data in the whole study

and found that the patients and controls are comparable in the major known risk factors that were studied together with demographic features. Although the response rate for participating in this study was high, some of the participants refused to provide their blood, other data were missed, and some of the DNA samples were not genotyped. To our knowledge no previous study in our population or even in the Arab region has considered the influence of this marker in ESR1 on breast cancer risk. This study has strength in being a population–based, case–control study which could reduce the selection bias, and it has been conducted in relatively homogeneous ethnic background population. In addition, selected information on life-style factors that are related to estrogen exposure allowed us to evaluate their interaction with genetic polymorphism.

To search for a strong association of the influence of this polymorphism, precise estimation of the risks associated with this gene and other genes, such as carcinogen metabolism genes (GSTPI and COMT), DNA repair genes (PTEN and HER2), cytokines and growth factor genes (IL10 and ILIa), and signal transduction and cell-cycle control genes (CCND1 and p27), as well as investigation of more risks arising from gene–gene and gene–environment interaction will be required in a much larger study.

In summary, our results indicate that the ESR1 exon 4 codon 325 CCC → CCG polymorphism is associated with breast cancer risk. The association was significantly higher in women 50 years and younger. The involvement of this polymorphism in breast cancer susceptibility and its clinical importance is not yet fully understood. Our study was based on a relatively small population size. Clearly, additional larger studies are necessary to clarify the impact of this polymorphism in breast carcinogenesis.

Acknowledgments

We thank the National Health Laboratory, Khartoum Radio Isotopes Hospital, and Khartoum Teaching Hospital, Khartoum, Sudan for their help and cooperation. Also we would like to thank Prof. Sherif Karam and Prof. Tahir Rizvi for their valuable assistance. The authors gratefully thank all the patients who participated in this study.

Conflicts of Interest

The authors declare no conflicts of interest.

References

1. Parkin, D.M., F. Bray, J. Ferlay. 2005. Global cancer statistics, 2002. *CA Cancer J .Clin.* **55:** 74–108.
2. Hanahan, D. & R.A. Weinberg. 2000. The hallmark of cancer. *Cell* **100:** 57–70.
3. Balmain, A., J. Gray & B. Ponder. 2003. The genetic and genomic of cancer. *Nat. Genet.* **33:** 238–244.
4. Weber, B.L. & K.L. Nathanson. 2000. Low penetrance genes associated with increased risk for breast cancer. *Eur. J. Cancer* **36:** 1193–1199.
5. Dunning, A.M., C.S, Healey & P.D. Pharoah, *et al.* 1999. A systematic review of genetic polymorphisms and breast cancer risk. *Cancer Epidemiol. Biomarkers Prev.* **8:** 843–854.
6. Menasce, L.P., G.R. White, C.J. Harrison, *et al.* 1993. Localization of the estrogen receptor locus (ESR) to chromosome 6q25.1 by FISH and a simple post-FISH banding technique. *Genomics* **17:** 263–265.
7. Sommer, S. & S.A. Fuga. 2001. Estrogen receptor and breast cancer. *Semin. Cancer Biol.* **11:** 339–352.
8. Rayter, Z. 1991. Steroid receptors in breast cancer. *Br. J. Surg.* **78:** 528–535.
9. de Jong, M.M., I.M. Nolte, G.J. te Meerman, *et al.* 2002. Genes other than BRCA1 and BRACA2 involved in breast cancer susceptibility. *J. Med. Genet.* **39:** 225–242.
10. Cai, Q., X. Shu, F. Jin, *et al.* 2003. Genetic polymorphisms in the estrogen receptor α gene and risk of breast cancer: result from the Shanghai Breast Cancer Study. *Cancer Epidemiol. Biomarkers Prev.* **12:** 853–859.
11. Newcomb, P.A., A.D. Trentham, K.M. Egan, *et al.* 2001. Fracture history and risk of breast and endometrial cancer. *Am. J. Epidemiol.* **153:** 1071–1078.
12. Yaich, L., W.D. Dupont, D.R. Cavener, *et al.* 1992. Analysis of the PvuII restriction fragment-length polymorphism and exon structure of the estrogen receptor gene in breast cancer and peripheral blood. *Cancer Res.* **52:** 77–83.
13. Zuppan, P., J.M. Hall, M.K. Lee, *et al.* 1991. Possible linkage of the estrogen receptor gene to breast cancer in a family with late-onset disease. *Am. J. Hum. Genet.* **48:** 1065–1068.
14. Hsiao, W.C., K.C. Young, S.L. Lin, *et al.* 2004. Estrogen receptor-α polymorphism in a Taiwanese clinical breast cancer population: a case-control study. *Breast Cancer Res.* **6:** R180–R186.
15. Colson, N., R.A. Lea, A. Rod, *et al.* 2006. No role for estrogen receptor I gene intron I PvuII and exon 4C325G polymorphisms in migraine susceptibility. *BMC Med. Genet.* **7:** 12–17.
16. Kang, D. 2003. Genetic polymorphism and cancer susceptibility of breast cancer in Korean women. *Rev. J. Biochem. Mol. Biol.* **36:** 28–34.
17. Roodi, N., L.R. Bailey, W.Y. Kao, *et al.* 1995. Estrogen receptor gene analysis in estrogen receptor-positive and receptor-negative primary breast cancer. *J. Natl. Cancer Inst.* **87:** 446–451.
18. Iwase, H., J.M. Greenman, D.M. Barnes, *et al.* 1996. Sequence variants of the estrogen receptor (ER) gene found in breast cancer patients with ER negative and progesterone receptor positive tumors. *Cancer Lett.* **108:** 179–184.
19. Vasconcelos, A., R. Medeiros, I. Veiga, *et al.* 2002. Analysis of estrogen receptor polymorphism in codon 325 by PCR-SSCP in breast cancer: association with lymph node metastasis. *Breast J.* **8:** 226–229.
20. Onay, V., L. Briollais, J.A. Knight, *et al.* 2006. SNP-SNP interactions in breast cancer susceptibility. *BMC Cancer* **6:** 114–129. 25
21. Southey, M.C., L.E. Batten, M.R. McCredie, *et al.* 1998. Estrogen receptor polymorphism at codon 325 and risk of breast cancer in women before age forty. *J. Natl. Cancer Inst.* **90:** 532–536.
22. Curran, J.E., R.A. Lea & S. Rutherford. 2001. Association of estrogen receptor and glucocorticoid receptor gene polymorphisms with sporadic breast cancer. *Int J. Cancer* **95:** 271–275.
23. Shearman, A.M., J.A. Cooper, P.J. Kotwinski, *et al.* 2005. Estrogen receptor alpha gene variation and the risk of stroke. *Stroke* **36:** 2281–2282.
24. Kang, H.J., S.W. Kim, H.J. Kim, *et al.* 2002. Polymorphisms in the estrogen receptor alpha gene and breast cancer risk. *Cancer Lett.* **178:** 175–180.
25. Wedre'n, S., L. Lovmar, K. Humphreys, *et al.* 2004. Oestrogen receptor α gene haplotype and postmenopausal breast cancer risk: a case control study. *Breast Cancer Res.* **6:** 437–449.
26. Coughlin, S.S. & M. Piper. 1999. Genetic polymorphism and breast cancer risk. *Cancer Epidemiol. Biomarker Prev.* **8:** 1023–1032.

27. Herynk, M.H & W.S. Fuqua. 2004. Estrogen mutation in human disease. *Endocrine Rev.* **6:** 869–898.

28. Larson, P.S., B.L. Schlechter, A. de las Morenas, *et al.* 2005. Allele imbalance, or loss of heterozygosity, in normal breast epithelium of sporadic breast cancer cases and BRCA1 gene mutation carriers is increased compared with reduction mamoplasty tissues. *J. Clin. Oncol.* **23:** 8613–8619.

29. Braakhuis, B.J., M.P. Tabor, J.A. Kummer, *et al.* 2003. A genetic explanation of Slaughter's concept of field cancerization: evidence and clinical implications. *Cancer Res.* **63:** 1727–1730.

30. Li, Z., D.H. Moore, Z.H. Meng, *et al.* 2002. Increased risk of local recurrence is associated with allelic loss in normal lobules of breast cancer patients. *Cancer Res.* **62:** 1000–1003.

31. Deng, G., Y. Lu, G. Zlotnikov, *et al.* 1996. Loss of heterozygosity in normal tissue adjacent of breast carcinomas. *Science* **274:** 2057–2059. 4

The Use of a Vacuum-assisted Biopsy Device (Mammotome) in the Early Detection of Breast Cancer in the United Arab Emirates

Issam Faour,[a] Suhail Al-Salam,[b] Hassan El-Terifi,[c] and Hakam El Taji[a]

[a]*Department of Surgery, and* [c]*Department of Pathology, Tawam Hospital, Al Ain, United Arab Emirates*

[b]*Department of Pathology, Faculty of Medicine and Health Sciences, UAE University, Al Ain, United Arab Emirates*

Stereotactic core needle biopsy has proven to be an accurate technique for evaluation of mammographically detected microcalcification. The development of the Mammotome biopsy system has led many medical centers to use this vacuum-assisted device for the sampling of microcalcifications in mammographically detected nonpalpable breast lesions. Ninety-six women underwent 101 stereotactic Mammotome core biopsies for mammographic calcifications over a 32-month period in the Department of Surgery at Tawam Hospital, the national referral oncology center in the UAE. The stereotactic procedure was performed by surgeons using the Mammotome biopsy system. Microcalcifications were evident on specimen radiographs and microscopic sections in 96% and 87% of the cases, respectively. Excisional biopsy was recommended for diagnoses of atypical ductal hyperplasia or carcinoma. Patients with benign diagnoses underwent mammographic follow-up. Eighty-one lesions were benign, 5 atypical ductal hyperplasias and 14 carcinomas were diagnosed (2 invasive lobular carcinoma, 4 invasive ductal carcinoma, and 8 intraductal carcinomas *in situ*: 1 comedo, 1 cribriform, 6 mixed cribriform and micropapillary). Surgical excision in four patients with atypia on Mammotome biopsy (one was lost to follow-up) showed atypical ductal hyperplasia. Surgical excision in seven patients diagnosed with intraductal carcinoma *in situ* (one patient lost to follow-up) showed intraductal carcinoma with no evidence of microinvasion. Similar diagnoses were made in all the invasive ductal and lobular carcinomas in both Mammotome and excisional biopsies. A diagnosis of atypia on Mammotome biopsy warranted excision of the atypical area, yet the underestimation rate for the presence of carcinoma remained low. The likelihood of an invasive component at excision was negligible for microcalcification diagnosed as intraductal carcinoma *in situ* on Mammotome biopsy. Mammotome biopsy proved to be an accurate technique for the sampling, diagnosis, and early detection of breast cancer.

Key words: breast; carcinoma; Mammotome

Introduction

Although nonpalpable breast lesions are detected with mammography, biopsy is necessary to make a diagnosis in most patients. Microcalcifications are frequent mammographic findings that account for approximately 50% of all biopsies of nonpalpable lesions.[1] Stereotactic core needle biopsy is a widely used technique for the diagnosis of nonpalpable breast lesions discovered on mammography.[2] Most studies published on the use of core needle biopsy for evaluation of mammary microcalcification

Address for correspondence: Dr. Suhail Al-Salam, MD, Department of Pathology, Faculty of Medicine and Health Sciences, United Arab Emirates University, Al Ain, UAE. Voice: +0097137672000 Ext-464; fax: +0097137671966. suhaila@uaeu.ac.ae

Ann. N.Y. Acad. Sci. 1138: 108–113 (2008). © 2008 New York Academy of Sciences.
doi: 10.1196/annals.1414.016

have utilized a stereotactic procedure with 14-gauge needles.[3–5] Stereotactic core needle biopsy with a prone position stereotactic mammography unit was used to obtain the tissue of nonpalpable lesions until the vacuum-assisted biopsy device (Mammotome) became available. The development of the Mammotome system, enabling eight core biopsies to be taken from one site, has been used to sample microcalcifications.[6,7] Subsequent studies have described improved sampling of mammary microcalcification compared with the traditional stereotactic method.[8,9]

The upright-type stereotactic mammography unit was not suitable for stereotactic core needle biopsy because it is difficult to keep the breast position strictly immobile. The vacuum-assisted biopsy device overcomes the shortcomings of the upright-type stereotactic mammography unit because a large volume of tissue could be obtained.[9] Breast carcinoma is the most common malignancy among females in the United Arab Emirates (UAE). Many efforts have been made to improve the rate of early detection of breast cancer. In this study we present the role of the vacuum-assisted biopsy device (Mammotome) in the early detection of breast cancer in the UAE and, to the best of our knowledge, this is the first study in the UAE.

Patients and Methods

One hundred and one stereotactic Mammotome core needle biopsies of indeterminate mammary microcalcification detected by routine mammography, without evidence of a mammographic density or mass, were obtained from 96 women with a mean age of 50 years (range 22–74). These were performed between January 2003 and August 2006 in Al Ain city at Tawam Hospital, a 600-bed tertiary care hospital and the National Oncology Referral center in the UAE. Five patients had microcalcifications in both breasts and bilateral biopsies were obtained. One patient had two distinct clusters of microcalcification biopsied

in the same breast. After obtaining informed consent from patients, surgeons performed the stereotactic procedure in the Radiology Department using the 11-gauge, directional, vacuum-assisted, Mammotome biopsy system (Johnson & Johnson, Ethicon Endo-surgery, Cincinnati, OH) mounted on a StereoGuide prone table (Lorad prone stereotactic breast biopsy system; Lorad Division Trex Medical Corp., Danbury, CT). The patient lay face down (prone) on this table. The patient's breast protruded through a hole in the table, lightly compressed and immobilized while a computer produced detailed images of the lesion. Local anesthetic was injected into the skin and deeper tissue of the breast. The probe was inserted through a small incision (5 mm) in the breast. After appropriate positioning of the probe in the area of concern a vacuum line drew the breast tissue into the sampling chamber of the device. The rotating cutting device was then advanced, and a tissue sample was captured, cut, and collected for examination. A mean of 10 (range 7–14) specimens were obtained. The specimens were radiographed for documentation of microcalcification, and those containing calcium were submitted for paraffin embedding in a container of 10% buffered formalin. In four cases the microcalcifications were not identified on tissue radiographs. In these patients the lesions were deeply seated near the chest wall, creating technical difficulties in obtaining biopsies. In these four cases excisional biopsies were recommended. The paraffin-embedded specimens were sectioned at 4 μm, leveled three times, and stained with hematoxylin and eosin. All specimens were accompanied by a data sheet that included information regarding menstrual status of the patient, past history of breast carcinoma, family history of breast carcinoma, and exogenous hormone intake. Sections of the specimens were evaluated for the presence of microcalcification, and, if necessary, additional levels were obtained. If calcification was not demonstrated on routine microscopic examination, polarization was performed. A radiopaque clip

TABLE 1. Distribution of Nonpalpable Lesions According to Site

Site of nonpalpable Lesions	Number of biopsies
Right breast	48
Left breast	48
Both left and right breasts	5

TABLE 2. Frequency of Microcalcifications in Different Procedures Performed on 101 Nonpalpable Breast Lesions

Procedure	Number
Mammographic calcifications	101
Tissue radiograph calcifications	97
Microscopic calcifications	87

TABLE 3. The Histologic Diagnosis of 101 Mammotome Biopsies

Histologic diagnosis	Number
Normal breast tissue	12
Nonproliferative fibrocystic disease	53
Proliferative fibrocystic disease	10
Fibroadenomatosis	1
Fibrosis	4
Fat necrosis	1
Radiation changes	1
Atypical ductal hyperplasia	5
Ductal carcinoma *in situ*	8
Invasive ductal carcinoma	4
Invasive lobular carcinoma	2
Total	101

TABLE 4. Comparison of the Diagnostic Accuracy of Mammotome Core Needle Biopsy and Excisional Biopsy of 17 Nonpalpable Breast Lesions

Type of procedure	ADH	DCIS	Invasive ductal carcinoma	Invasive lobular carcinoma
Mammotome core biopsy	4	7	4	2
Excisional biopsy	4	7	4	2

ADH: atypical ductal hyperplasia; DCIS: ductal carcinoma *in situ*.

was inserted into the biopsy site in patients at the time of biopsy when the entire cluster of microcalcification was removed. Excisional biopsy was recommended for all patients who had a diagnosis of atypical ductal hyperplasia (ADH) or carcinoma. Excisional biopsy specimens were inked for the assessment of margins and submitted for histologic evaluation. Patients with benign diagnoses were requested to undergo follow-up mammography 6 months later.

Results

One hundred and one Mammotome core needle biopsies were obtained (Table 1). Of the 101 biopsies that showed positive calcification on mammography, four specimen radiographs showed no evidence of calcification. Fourteen specimens (13%) showed no evidence of microcalcification on microscopic examination, and the diagnoses of all these cases were benign (Table 2).

Diagnoses were benign in 70, atypical in 5, carcinoma in 14, and normal breast tissue in 12 biopsies. Of the 70 benign biopsies, nonproliferative fibrocystic changes were identified in 53, proliferative fibrocystic changes in 10, fibroadenomatous lesions in 1, fibrosis

in 4, fat necrosis in 1, and radiation changes in 1. Five biopsies showed ADH. Of the 14 biopsies of carcinoma, 4 were invasive ductal carcinoma, 2 were invasive lobular carcinoma, and 8 were intraductal carcinoma *in situ*. Among the latter, a comedo type pattern was noted in one biopsy, a cribriform pattern in one biopsy, and a mixed cribriform and micropapillary pattern in six biopsies. (Table 3).

Two patients (2%) developed mild bruising, which resolved without treatment. Two other patients (2%) experienced mild hemorrhage after the biopsy, controlled by local application of pressure.

Excisional biopsy was performed in four patients with ADH and revealed fibrocystic change with atypical ductal epithelial hyperplasia but without any evidence of malignancy (Table 4). An appointment for excisional biopsy was made for the remaining patient who, unfortunately, defaulted. Seven of the eight patients diagnosed to have intraductal carcinoma *in situ* underwent surgical excision (Table 4). An appointment for excisional biopsy was made for the remaining patient but she also was lost to follow-up. In six of these patients, residual intraductal carcinoma *in situ* was present, while the remaining case showed no residual intraductal carcinoma *in situ* within the excisional specimen; however, ADH was noted. Four biopsies were diagnosed as invasive ductal carcinoma, which was followed by mastectomy and axillary clearance, a diagnosis compatible with the core needle biopsy. Another two biopsies were diagnosed as invasive lobular carcinoma, which was followed by mastectomy and axillary clearance, a diagnosis being compatible with the core needle biopsy.

Discussion

Vacuum-assisted stereotactic core needle biopsy has proved to be accurate in cases of mammary microcalcification.[10,11] The Mammotome system consists of a sterile probe and a nonsterile driver, which controls the probe. A vacuum pump pulls tissue from the probe and allows specimens to be removed without withdrawing the sterile probe between directional samplings.[12] With the standard core needle device, each core is obtained individually, and the needle must be reinserted between biopsies.

Microcalcification has been reported in specimen radiographs in 95–100% of biopsies performed with the vacuum-assisted device.[7] This contrasts with findings of microcalcification in 90.8% of biopsies performed by using the standard automated needle device.[8] In the current study, microcalcification was identified on a specimen radiograph in 96% of biopsies, and this yield is attributed to the greater volume of tissue obtained by Mammotome biopsy. Other studies have shown a five- to sixfold increase in tissue weights of specimens obtained with the 11-gauge Mammotome probe compared with those obtained with the automated 14-gauge Tru-cut system.[7] We found a lower rate of microcalcification in sections examined microscopically than in those obtained by specimen radiography. This is possibly explained by dissolution of the deposited calcium crystals during tissue processing, especially when they are fine and few, evident mainly in benign biopsies.

Mammograms obtained after Mammotome biopsy have shown air and hematoma, but these changes resolved quickly.[6] In a comparison study with mammograms obtained after stereotactic biopsy that used an automated gun, the mammograms after Mammotome biopsy more often show a decrease in the number of calcific deposits, air at the biopsy site, and complete removal of the lesion. These findings were attributed to the larger volume of tissue obtained by the vacuum-assisted device and the smaller size of the lesions sampled.[6] In the present study post-Mammotome mammography revealed absence of calcifications in 96% of our cases, which indicates complete removal of these lesions. In only four cases were we unable technically to remove the lesion completely and the post-Mammotome mammography showed residual microcalcification. This is attributable to finding that all these lesions were deep and near the chest wall and difficult to approach, especially if we take into consideration the prone position of the patients during biopsy taking. We recommended excisional biopsy of all four lesions.

Histologically, benign lesions predominated in our study and comprised 81% of the biopsies, while carcinoma and ADH comprised 14% and 5% of biopsies, respectively, findings in keeping with other reports.[5–9]

More accurate histologic diagnoses can be made when a larger volume of tissue is available for examination. A diagnosis of ADH on stereotactic core biopsy warrants surgical excision of the atypical area because over 50% of these lesions harbor carcinoma at the time of surgical excision. Interestingly, all the lesions that were diagnosed as ADH on Mammotome biopsy have had the diagnosis confirmed at the time of surgical excision, which indicates an early diagnosis for our patients.[13]

In one study, vacuum-assisted biopsy was shown to reduce the false negative rate for carcinoma to 18%.[8] This rate is higher than in the current study, where all the cases (available for follow-up) diagnosed with ADH, ductal carcinoma *in situ*, invasive ductal carcinoma, or invasive lobular carcinoma on Mammotome biopsy had the same diagnosis confirmed at surgical excision. None of our patients that were diagnosed to have ductal carcinoma *in situ* on Mammotome biopsy had any invasive component at surgical excision. This finding is superior to that reported with stereotactic core needle biopsy in other studies, where 16–31% of the biopsies reported to have ductal carcinoma *in situ* contained an invasive component at surgical excision.[14–17] We believe that the high accuracy rate in the histologic diagnosis of Mammotome core needle biopsy is related to the large volume of tissue obtained in each biopsy and the serial sectioning of each specimen on different levels. The reported complication rate for vacuum-assisted biopsy is similar to automated core biopsy.[7] Skin infection and pneumothorax have been reported.[7] Wong and colleagues reported moderate hemorrhage and severe bruising in 14% and 6.5% of their patients, respectively, after Mammotome stereotactic biopsies.[14] Weikel and colleagues reported postoperative deep hematoma in 3% of patients. In the current study, morbidity was low. Neither skin or chest-wall injuries, nor pain or intraoperative bleeding or infection were observed.[18] In the present study two patients (2%) developed mild bruising, which resolved without treatment. Two other patients (2%) had mild hemorrhage after the biopsy, and this was controlled by local application of pressure. Radiopaque clip placement was necessary in many patients after Mammotome biopsy

because complete removal of the mammographic abnormality is recommended in the presence of ADH or carcinoma. Complete removal of the mammographic calcification does not, however, ensure removal of the entire underlying lesion.[6] In six of eight biopsies diagnosed as intraductal carcinoma *in situ* in the current study, the entire cluster of microcalcifications were removed by Mammotome; however, residual intraductal carcinoma *in situ* was noted in excised specimens. We have also found that a diagnosis of carcinoma on Mammotome biopsy assists surgeons in the avoidance of unnecessary surgical procedures to achieve negative margins, thus facilitating breast conservation.[19] In conclusion, Mammotome biopsy proved to be a safe and accurate procedure for the investigation of mammographically detected microcalcification.

Conflicts of Interest

The authors declare no conflicts of interest.

References

1. Monsees, B.S. 1995. Evaluation of breast microcalcifications. *Radiol. Clin. N. Am.* **33:** 1109–1121.
2. Head, J.F., A.E. Haynes, M.C. Elliott, *et al.* 1996. Stereotaxic localization and core needle biopsy of nonpalpable breast lesions: two year follow up of a prospective study. *Am. Surg.* **62:** 1018–1023.
3. Elvecrog, E.L., M.C. Lechner & M.T. Nelson. 1993. Nonpalpable breast lesions: correlation of stereotaxic large-core needle biopsy and surgical biopsy results. *Radiology* **188:** 453–455.
4. Jackman, R.J., K.W. Nowels, M.J. Shepard, *et al.* 1994. Stereotactic large-core needle biopsy of 450 nonpalpable breast lesions with surgical correlation in lesions with cancer or atypical hyperplasia. *Radiology* **193:** 91–95.
5. Kettritz, U., K. Rotter I. Schreer, *et al.* 2004. Stereotactic vacuum-assisted breast biopsy in 2874 patients: a multicenter study. *Cancer* **100:** 245–251.
6. Liberman, L., L.E. Hann, D.D. Dershaw, *et al.* 1997. Mammographic findings after stereotactic 14-gauge vacuum biopsy. *Radiology* **203:** 343–347.
7. Meyer, J.E., D.N. Smith, S.C. Lester, *et al.* 1999. Large-core needle biopsy of nonpalpable breast lesions. *JAMA* **281:** 1638–1641.

8. Meyer, J.E., D.N. Smith, P.J. DiPiro, *et al.* 1997. Stereotactic breast biopsy of clustered microcalcifications with a directional, vacuum-assisted device. *Radiology* **204:** 575–576.

9. Cox, D., S. Bradley & D. England. 2006. The significance of mammotome core biopsy specimens without radiographically identifiable microcalcification and their influence on surgical management—a retrospective review with histological correlation. *Breast* **15:** 210–218.

10. Jackman, R., F. Burbank, S.H. Parker, *et al.* 1997. Atypical ductal hyperplasia diagnosed at stereotactic biopsy: improved reliability with 14-gauge, directional, vacuum assisted biopsy. *Radiology* **204:** 485–488.

11. Burbank, F. 1997. Stereotactic breast biopsy of atypical ductal hyperplasia and ductal carcinoma in situ lesions: improved accuracy with directional, vacuum-assisted biopsy. *Radiology* **203:** 673–677.

12. Parker, S.H. & A.J. Klaus. 1997. Performing a breast biopsy with a directional, vacuum-assisted biopsy instrument. *Radiographics* **17:** 1233–1252.

13. Liberman, L., M.A. Cohen, D.D. Dershaw, *et al.* 1995. Atypical ductal hyperplasia diagnosed at stereotaxic core biopsy of breast lesions: an indication for surgical biopsy. *AJR Am. J. Roentgenol.* **164:** 1111–1113.

14. Wong, T.T, P.S. Cheung, M.K. Ma, *et al.* 2005. Experience of stereotactic breast biopsy using the vacuum-assisted core needle biopsy device and the advanced breast biopsy instrumentation system in Hong Kong women. *Asian J. Surg.* **28:** 18–23.

15. Pijnappel, R.M., M. Van Den Donk, R. Holland, *et al.* 2004. Diagnostic accuracy for different strategies of image-guided breast intervention in cases of nonpalpable breast lesions. *Br. J. Cancer* **90:** 595–600.

16. Symmans, W.F., N. Weg, J. Gross, *et al.* 1999. A prospective comparison of stereotaxic fine-needle aspiration versus stereotaxic core needle biopsy for the diagnosis of mammographic abnormalities. *Cancer* **85:** 1119–1132.

17. Senn Bahls, E., V. Dupont Lampert, C. Oelschlegel, *et al.* 2006. Multitarget stereotactic core-needle breast biopsy (MSBB)—an effective and safe diagnostic intervention for non-palpable breast lesions: a large prospective single institution study. *Breast* **15:** 339–346.

18. Weikel, W., M. Hofmann, E. Steiner, *et al.* 2004. Stereotactic vacuum-assisted breast biopsy analysis of 166 cases. *Zentralbl. Gynakol.* **126:** 87–92.

19. Cangiarella, J., J. Gross, W.F. Symmans, *et al.* 2000. The incidence of positive margins with breast conserving therapy following mammotome biopsy for microcalcification. *J. Surg. Oncol.* **74:** 263–266.

An Immunohistochemistry Study of Tissue Bcl-2 Expression and Its Serum Levels in Breast Cancer Patients

Andalib Alireza, Shokohi Raheleh, Rezaei Abbass, Mokhtari Mojgan, Mohageri Mohamadreza, Mohageri Gholamreza, and Babazadeh Shadi

Departments of Immunology, Surgery, Pathology, and Oncology, Isfahan Medical School, Isfahan University of Medical Sciences, Isfahan, Iran

Variations in Bcl-2 expression have been reported in malignant tissues with various origins. In the case of breast cancer, the involvement of Bcl-2 overexpression in tumorigenicity and metastatic potential has been stated. However, association of tumor progression and loss of Bcl-2 in tumor cells is also being investigated. Augmentation of plasma levels of Bcl-2 was speculated in patients with metastatic breast cancer. The present study was designed to evaluate Bcl-2 protein expression in breast tumor paraffin-embedded fixed tissue and sought to investigate association with the Bcl-2 protein release in patient serum, as well as its relationship with clinicopathological features. Immunohistochemistry methods were applied to breast tumor sections from 35 surgically removed patient samples and 35 normal or benign tissue samples. The sera taken from both the patient and control groups were tested for soluble Bcl-2 (BMs244/3 Kit) using ELISA technique. Tumor type, grade, and size and patient menopause status and age were considered to analyze the association between these parameters. The analysis shows that 67.6% of the tumor sections were positive for Bcl-2 expression and 32.4% negative. Bcl-2 protein expression was positive in 57.1% of normal/benign section tumors. The Bcl-2 serum levels were 3.6 ± 1.1 ng/mL in the patient group and 3.23 ± 0.06 ng/mL in the control group. A weak correlation was found between Bcl-2 serum levels and tissue expression of the molecules ($r = 0.382$, $P = 0.049$). A negative association (but not statically significant) was obtained between Bcl-2 and low-grade stages ($r = -0.375$, $P = 0.08$). A positive and significant correlation was shown between Bcl-2 and menopause ($r = 0.523$, $P = 0.005$) and between age and serum Bcl-2 ($r = 0.488$, $P = 0.011$). Although a majority of the breast tumor tissue expresses Bcl-2, the mean Bcl-2 serum levels were not different between patient and control groups. The present data would lead us to use the Bcl-2 expression in tissue at the level of protein expression or would suggest the use of mRNA levels, but the use of serum levels would be very limited for clinical purposes.

Key words: breast cancer; Bcl-2 expression; immunohistochemistry

Introduction

The B cell lymphoma-2 (Bcl-2) proto-oncogene is normally expressed in the cells in a proliferation state, including hematopoietic

progenitor, breast, and ovarian cells.[1,2] Bcl-2 is physiologically expressed in ductal epithelia of normal breast.[3] In contrast, this protein is not expressed in some other tissues, including normal prostatic epithelium.[4] It is overexpressed in many cancers.[5] The Bcl-2 gene is implicated in a number of cancers, including melanoma and breast, prostate, and lung carcinomas.[6] It was recently proposed that Bcl-2 could inhibit cancer progression.[7] Alteration in protein

---

Address for correspondence: Andalib Alireza, Department of Immunology, Isfahan Medical School, Isfahan, Iran. Voice: +0913-313-4128; (Dept. office) 0311-7922431; fax (Med. School): +0311-6688597. andalib@med.mui.ac.ir

Ann. N.Y. Acad. Sci. 1138: 114–120 (2008). © 2008 New York Academy of Sciences.
doi: 10.1196/annals.1414.017

expression could help to evaluate the malignant tissue outcome, and it could also be used as a prognostic factor.

Tumor markers are used to evaluate cancer progression. During cancer development some molecular factors are altered in expression and/or production and can be measured in tumor tissue or, if the product released from tissue, in biological fluids, such as serum. Soluble tumor markers are detected in serum for clinical purposes, such as carcinoembryonic antigen in gastrointestinal cancer and alpha fetoprotein in hepatocellular carcinoma.[8]

Variations in Bcl-2 expression have been reported in various malignant tissues. For example, Alsabeh and colleagues showed that Bcl-2 was expressed in 79.3% of invasive breast carcinoma, whereas this protein was positive in only 5.6% and 8.3% of pulmonary and gastric carcinoma, respectively.[9] In contrast, Bargou and co-workers reported that Bcl-2 expression does not distinguish between normal breast epithelium and tumor tissue or breast cancer and nonmalignant epithelial cell lines.[6] In addition, others report that cancers overexpress Bcl-2.[3, 10, 11] However, it has been suggested that downregulation or loss of Bcl-2 expression may impair sustained tumor growth, which means the outcome of tumors could be evaluated by assessing Bcl-2 expression during tumor progression.[10] Bankfalvi and colleagues reported the worst prognosis for immunohistochemical Bcl-2-negative expression in breast carcinomas.[12] Barbareschi and colleagues showed an association between Bcl-2 expression and small tumor size, low tumor grade, and lack of p53 expression on breast cancer samples.[13]

In a breast cancer cell-line model, it has been shown that Bcl-2 overexpression enhances both tumorigenicity and metastatic potential.[14] Other research found no relationship between Bcl-2 and tumor size, differentiation status, type, or age at excision.[15] However, Leek and colleagues have shown that loss of Bcl-2 expression in breast cancer is associated with poor prognosis.[15] The intensity of Bcl-2 expression was considered in different samples. Alsabeh

and co-workers reported that breast cancer samples have more intense Bcl-2 staining than cancers with a different origin.[9]

Plasma levels of Bcl-2 have been investigated in patients with metastatic breast cancer by Gaballah and colleagues.[16] The mean level of Bcl-2 was 278.4 ± 383.2 U/L, compared with 64.4 ± 14.4 U/L ($P = 0.007$) for the control group. The research showed that levels of Bcl-2 were higher in patients less than 50 years old. In addition, other clinical factors, such as the site of metastatic disease and the number of metastatic sites, did not show statistically significant influences over Bcl-2 serum levels.[16] Thus Bcl-2 serum levels might be considered as a potential tumor marker, especially for breast cancer. Therefore, efforts have been made to evaluate the expression of tissue Bcl-2 and its serum levels in breast cancer samples, and our study focuses on the relationship between available clinicopathological factors and Bcl-2.

Materials and Methods

Patients

Patients with diagnosed breast cancer at Alzahra and Omid University Hospitals (2004–2005) were included. Serum of patients was obtained before surgery for evaluation of serum Bcl-2. Paraffin-embedded, fixed tissues were obtained from the Pathology Department. Bcl-2 was investigated in the normal mammary gland as well as in benign mammary dysplasia adjacent to breast cancer, as control samples. Samples were reviewed by two pathologists to ensure adequacy and that they were representative of the actual tumor. The medical records of the patients were reviewed to obtain relevant clinicopathological parameters including age, tumor size, tumor type, grade, stage of tumor, and treatment.

Immunohistochemistry

Immunostaining for Bcl-2 was performed on formalin-fixed, paraffin-embedded tissues based on an avidin-biotin-peroxidase complex technique. Sections were provided from formalin-fixed, paraffin-embedded tissues (3 μm thick). Sectioned tissues were deparaffined 1 h at 56°C and then by xylene (2 × 10 min) and rehydrated through descending strengths of alcohol (95%, 70%, 50%). Endogenous peroxidase activity was blocked by incubating specimens in 2% hydrogen peroxide in methanol for 5 min. The antigen retrieval step was performed by boiling sections for 15 min in 10 mmol/L citrate buffer at pH 6.0. The blocking step for nonspecific protein binding was performed with normal serum and bovine serum albumin. The slides were then incubated overnight at 4°C in a humidified chamber with a primary antibody (primary antibody used for detection of Bcl-2 was the DAKO (Denmark) antihuman Bcl-2 oncoprotein clone 124). The slides were rinsed with a tris buffer saline solution (TBS) for 9 min (3 × 3 min). The slides were incubated with the biotinylated secondary antibody for 30 min at room temperature. The slides were rinsed with TBS for 9 min (3 × 3 min). Then slides were incubated with avidin-biotin-horseradish peroxidase conjugate for 30 min. In this step, sections were stained with 0.04% diamino-benzidine tetrahydrochloride (Sigma, Germany) for 6 min and were counterstained with hematoxylin.

Counterstaining and Mounting of Sections

Counterstaining was carried out by light staining of slides with undistilled Lillie Mayer hematoxylin (Sigma) for 2 min. Slides were rinsed in TBS. Two fast dips in 0.6% acid-alcohol were carried out. Slides were washed for 30 s in water and blued in Scott solution (containing magnesium sulphate hydrated: 100 g; sodium hydrogen carbonate: 10 g; tap water 5000 mL; sodium azide: 5 g) for 10 s. A quick dip in tap water was carried out to remove excess salts from the Scott solution prior to dehydration and clearing. Dehydration involved 2 min in each of two 50%, 70%, 95%,

and 100% ethanol and cleared for 10 min in xylene. Slides were mounted using entelan.

Scoring of Immunostaining

Slides were evaluated by light microscope and scoring of immunostaining was detected. Scoring of immunostaining was as follows: The percentages of positively stained cells were segregated into the following groups: 0–4% into group N; 5–25%, weak 1+; 26–75%, moderate 2+; ≥75%, high 3+.

ELISA

The ELISA kit was provided from BenderMed Systems Company (Burlingame, CA) (Human Bcl-2 ELISA, No: BMS244/3). Briefly Bcl-2 molecules present in the serum samples were absorbed to the microwells, which were coated with anti-Bcl-2 monoclonal antibody. Then a biotin-conjugated monoclonal anti-Bcl-2 antibody was added that binds to Bcl-2 captured by the first antibody. Following incubation time, unbound biotin-conjugated anti-Bcl-2 was removed by washing, and then streptavidin-horseradish peroxidase was added to bind to the biotin-conjugated anti-Bcl-2. A colored product, the result of enzymatic reaction that terminated in appropriate time by acid and optical absorbance, was measured at 450 nm according to the manufacturer's recommendation.

Results

Subjects in this study included patients who had suffered from breast cancer ($n = 35$) and a control group ($n = 35$). The controls were persons who had benign breast masses and healthy persons. The clinicopathological features and results of the immunohistochemical stains of Bcl-2 are shown in Table 1. Type of breast cancer, size and grade of tumor, and menopausal status and age of patient were recorded. Tissue expression and serum

TABLE 1. Clinicopathological Features and Immunohistochemical Expression of Bcl-2

	Number of patients	Bcl-2 Positive	Bcl-2 Negative
Age			
<40 years	11	7	4
>40 years	24	17	7
Premenopause	25	16	9
Postmenopause	10	8	2
Tumor size			
>4 cm	14	10	4
>4 cm	21	14	7
Invasive ductal carcinoma	29	20	9
Infiltrating ductal carcinoma	3	3	-
Metastatic carcinoma	2	-	2
Medullary carcinoma	1	1	-

TABLE 2. Immunostaining of Bcl-2 Expression and Its Serum Level in Patients and the Control Group

Bcl-2 expression	Patients	Controls	P
Negative expression	32.4%	42.9%	
Weak expression	19.2%	31.4%	
Moderate expression	25.7%	14.3%	
Strong expression	22.8%	11.4%	
Overexpression*	48.5%	25.7%	0.03
Total positive	67.6%	57.1%	
Serum level (ng/mL)	3.6 ± 1.1	3.23 ± 0.7	0.57

*Bcl-2 overexpression was designated as the sum of moderate and strong expression.

Bcl-2 were evaluated. The age mean of patients and control groups were 46.9 ± 13.5 and 38.2 ± 16.0 years old, respectively. Twenty-nine patients were diagnosed with invasive ductal carcinoma, three with infiltrating ductal carcinoma, two with metastatic carcinoma, and one with medullary carcinoma. Twenty-one patients were categorized as grade I or II, 12 as grade III, and two as grade V disease. Mean tumor size was 4.8 ± 2.2 cm; 66.6% had a tumor larger than 4 cm. Bcl-2 cytoplasmic protein expression was negative in 11 of 35 (32.4%) tumors; 6 cases with weak staining (19.2%), 9 with moderate staining (25.7%), and 8 with strong staining (22.8%) were classified. For control tissue, Bcl-2 cytoplasmic protein expression was negative in 42.8%, 31.4% tissues had weak staining, 14.3% exhibited moderate staining, and 11.4% had strong staining.

The mean ± SD of serum Bcl-2 was 3.2 ± 0.7 ng/mL in the control group. The mean ± SD of serum Bcl-2 was 3.6 ± 1.1 ng/mL in patient groups. No significant statistically difference was found between patient and control groups ($P = 0.57$). A weak correlation was found between Bcl-2 serum levels and tissue expression of the molecules ($r = 0.382$, $P = 0.049$). A negative association (but not reaching statistical significance) was obtained between Bcl-2 and low-grade stages ($r = -0.375$, $P = 0.08$). Moreover, a positive and significant correlation was achieved between serum levels of Bcl-2 and menopausal status ($r = 0.523$, $P = 0.005$) and between age and serum Bcl-2 ($r = 0.488$, $P = 0.011$; Table 2). This yielded a comparison of Bcl-2 intensity of expression in tissues as well as mean Bcl-2 serum levels in both patients and the control group.

Discussion

In the present study, we have considered Bcl-2 expression in breast cancer tissues (Fig. 1), determined the levels of Bcl-2 in patient sera, and compared the relationship between serum levels, tissue expression, and several available clinicopathological features with a control group. Our data show that there is no difference in serum Bcl-2 levels between the patient and control groups. This result does not support a reported approximately fourfold increase for a metastatic breast cancer group compared with a control group.[16] To the best of our knowledge that report is the only study that observed augmentation in Bcl-2 serum levels in patients with breast cancer.

Our results show that 32.4% of our cases did not exhibit Bcl-2 cytoplasmic protein expression. In addition, 42.9% of the control tissues were also negative for the Bcl-2 expression.

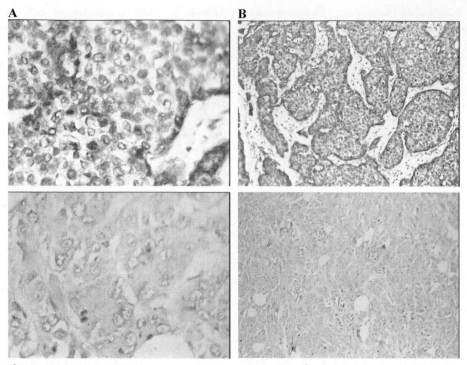

Figure 1. A representative immunostaining tumor tissue for Bcl-2 expression with intensity 3+ (**A**) and negative expression (**B**).

Coppola and colleagues reported that 46% of breast ductal carcinomas examined were negative for Bcl-2 expression.[2] Their work also showed that normal breast ductal cells were intensely Bcl-2 positive. In addition, Leek and co-workers reported 47.3% of breast cancer specimens were negative for Bcl-2 expression.[15] Provenzano and colleagues, however, reported 88% of metastatic breast carcinoma was negative for Bcl-2 expression, while only 26% of controls were negative.[17] Based on a literature survey,[18,19] normal Bcl-2 protein is usually synthesized in cells undergoing proliferation or in well-differentiated, noncycling cells (permanent cells). So, the trend in the literature suggests that losing Bcl-2 expression would be a feature of tumor progression, but our data do not consistently support this contention.

Coppola and colleagues[2] also concluded that low-grade breast tumors (I and II) were negative or exhibited decreased Bcl-2 expression when compared with the adjacent normal ducts. However, for high-grade carcinoma (III

and IV), intense Bcl-2 expression was observed in tumor cells. They stated that because of the small number of tumors studied statistical analysis would not be robust.[2] Moreover, in 1994, both Leek and co-workers and Haldar and colleagues indicated that Bcl-2 gene downregulation was evident both in pathological samples and *in vitro* in human breast carcinoma cell lines.[15,20]

In the present study, 65.7% of the tumor samples were positive for Bcl-2 expression with a majority of positive samples (73.8%) indicating moderate to strong molecule expression (Table 2). Analysis showed a weak negative correlation, not statistically significant, between low-grade stages and Bcl-2 expression ($r = -0.375$, $P = 0.08$). It may deserve additional investigation in a larger number of patients. The overexpression of Bcl-2 has been hypothesized as a phenomenon in tumor cells which may be important in the progression of breast carcinoma, with a significant association between Bcl-2 expression and high-grade breast tumors observed.[2] Bcl-2 overexpression in breast tumors has been considered favorable as a marker of progression in breast cancer patients.[21] In clinical practice the expression of Bcl-2 is used as an indicator of a favorable outcome following endocrine treatment in patients with limited disease[22-25] and as a predictor of treatment response in patients with advanced disease.[26] It has been speculated that Bcl-2 overexpression contributed, along with a low proliferation and weak or absent p53 expression, to the identification of the most favorable subsets.[24] Such findings provide further insight into the hypothesis that Bcl-2 expression should be viewed as a differentiation marker or a surrogate marker for other molecular or biological processes related to hormone sensitivity rather than a predictor of response to hormonal treatment.[21] As reports show, breast cancer may be stratified for Bcl-2 negative or positive expression with different intensity that investigators consider overexpression a factor for prediction of treatment response, but a consistent conclusion is still controversial.[21] Our results show a weak correlation between menopausal status and Bcl-2 expression, which would be related to patient hormonal status. The present work does not address the outcome of disease or treatment, but with these limited data we can conclude that Bcl-2 serum levels cannot be utilized as an evaluation marker for breast cancer and/or have no correlation with Bcl-2 tissue expression, although comments have been made for their tissue intensity expression. This is in agreement with other investigators who report that while there is a complex interaction between Bcl-2, tumor development, and clinical progression,[27] interpretation and validation[21] require further investigation to be conclusive.

Acknowledgments

This study was financially supported, in part, by the Research Council in Isfahan University of Medical Sciences with Grant No. 83171. The authors appreciate the kind technical cooperation of Mrs. Ostadi.

Conflicts of Interest

The authors declare no conflicts of interest.

Reference

1. Chan, W.Y., K.K. Cheung, J.O. Schorge, *et al.* 2000. Bcl-2 and p53 protein expression, apoptosis, and p53 mutation in human epithelial ovarian cancers. *Am. J. Pathol.* **156:** 409–417.
2. Coppola, D., E. Catalano & S.V. Nicosia. 1999. Significance of p53 and Bcl-2 protein expression in human breast ductal carcinoma. *Cancer Control* **6:** 181–187.
3. Binder, C., D. Marx, R. Overhoff, *et al.* 1995. Bcl-2 protein expression in breast cancer in relation to established prognostic factors and other clinicopathological variables. *Ann. Oncol.* **6:** 1005–1010.
4. Apakama, I., M.C. Robinson, N.M. Walter, *et al.* 1996. Bcl-2 overexpression combined with p53 protein accumulation correlates with hormone-refractory prostate cancer. *Br. J. Cancer* **74:** 1258–1262.
5. Arun, B., G. Kilic, C. Yen, *et al.* 2003. Correlation of bcl-2 and p53 expression in primary breast tumors and corresponding metastatic lymph nodes. *Cancer* **98:** 2554–2559.
6. Bargou, R.C., P.T. Daniel, M.Y. Mapara, *et al.* 1995. Expression of the bcl-2 gene family in normal and malignant breast tissue: low bax-alpha expression in tumor cells correlates with resistance towards apoptosis. *Int. J. Cancer* **60:** 854–859.
7. Bilalovic, N., S. Vranic, S. Hasanagic, *et al.* 2004. The bcl-2 protein: a prognostic indicator strongly related to ER and PR in breast cancer. *Bosn. J. Basic Med. Sci.* **4:** 5–12.
8. Lai, L.C., S.K. Cheong, K.L. Goh, *et al.* 2003. Clinical usefulness of tumour markers. *Malays. J. Pathol.* **25:** 83–105.
9. Alsabeh, R., C.S. Wilson, C.W. Ahn, *et al.* 1996. Expression of Bcl-2 by breast cancer: a possible diagnostic application. *Mod. Pathol.* **9:** 439–444.
10. Andersen, M.H., I.M. Svane, P. Kvistborg, *et al.* 2005. Immunogenicity of Bcl-2 in patients with cancer. *Blood* **105:** 728–734.
11. Biroccio, A., A. Candiloro, M. Mottolese, *et al.* 2000. Bcl-2 overexpression and hypoxia synergistically act to modulate vascular endothelial growth factor expression and in vivo angiogenesis in a breast carcinoma line. *FASEB J.* **14:** 652–660.
12. Bankfalvi, A., K. Tory, M. Kemper, *et al.* 2000. Clinical relevance of immunohistochemical expression of p53-targeted gene products mdm-2, p21 and Bcl-2 in breast carcinoma. *Pathol. Res. Pract.* **196:** 489–501.

13. Barbareschi, M., O. Caffo, S. Veronese, *et al.* 1996. Bcl-2 and p53 expression in node-negative breast carcinoma: a study with long-term follow-up. *Hum. Pathol.* **27:** 1149–1155.

14. Del Bufalo, D., A. Biroccio, C. Leonetti & G. Zupi. 1997. Bcl-2 overexpression enhances the metastatic potential of a human breast cancer line. *FASEB J.* **11:** 947–953.

15. Leek, R.D., L. Kaklamanis, F. Pezzella, *et al.* 1994. Bcl-2 in normal human breast and carcinoma, association with oestrogen receptor-positive, epidermal growth factor receptor-negative tumours and in situ cancer. *Br. J. Cancer* **69:** 135–139.

16. Gaballah, H.E., S.I. Abdel, W.N. Abdel & O.M. Mansour. 2001. Plasma Bcl-2 and nitric oxide: possible prognostic role in patients with metastatic breast cancer. *Med Oncol.* **18:** 171–178.

17. Provenzano, E., J.L. Hopper, G.G. Giles, *et al.* 2003. Biological markers that predict clinical recurrence in ductal carcinoma in situ of the breast. *Eur. J. Cancer* **39:** 622–630.

18. Hockenbery, D., G. Nunez, C. Milliman, *et al.* 1990. Bcl-2 is an inner mitochondrial membrane protein that blocks programmed cell death. *Nature* **348:** 334–336.

19. Nunez, G., L. London, D. Hockenbery, *et al.* 1990. Deregulated Bcl-2 gene expression selectively prolongs survival of growth factor-deprived hemopoietic cell lines. *J. Immunol.* **144:** 3602–3610.

20. Haldar, S., M. Negrini, M. Monne, *et al.* 1994. Down-regulation of Bcl-2 by p53 in breast cancer cells. *Cancer Res.* **54:** 2095–2097.

21. Daidone, M.G., A. Luisi, S. Veneroni, *et al.* 1999. Clinical studies of Bcl-2 and treatment benefit in breast cancer patients. *Endocr. Relat Cancer* **6:** 61–68.

22. Gasparini, G., M. Barbareschi, C. Doglioni, *et al.* 1995. Expression of Bcl-2 protein predicts efficacy of adjuvant treatments in operable node-positive breast cancer. *Clin. Cancer Res.* **1:** 189–198.

23. Kobayashi, S., H. Iwase, Y. Ito, *et al.* 1997. Clinical significance of Bcl-2 gene expression in human breast cancer tissues. *Breast Cancer Res. Treat.* **42:** 173–181.

24. Silvestrini, R., E. Benini, S. Veneroni, *et al.* 1996. P53 and Bcl-2 expression correlates with clinical outcome in a series of node-positive breast cancer patients. *J. Clin. Oncol.* **14:** 1604–1610.

25. Veronese, S., F.A. Mauri, O. Caffo, *et al.* 1998. Immunohistochemical expression in breast carcinoma: a study with long term follow-up. *Int. J. Cancer* **79:** 13–18.

26. Gee, J.M., J.F. Robertson, I.O. Ellis, *et al.* 1994. Immunocytochemical localization of Bcl-2 protein in human breast cancers and its relationship to a series of prognostic markers and response to endocrine therapy. *Int. J. Cancer* **59:** 619–628.

27. Yang, Q., T. Sakurai, G. Yoshimura, *et al.* 2003. Prognostic value of Bcl-2 in invasive breast cancer receiving chemotherapy and endocrine therapy. *Oncol. Rep.* **10:** 121–125.

Characterization of Breast Cancer Progression in the Rat

Wafa S. Al-Dhaheri,[a] Imam Hassouna,[b] Suhail Al-Salam,[c] and Sherif M. Karam[a]

Departments of [a]Anatomy and [c]Pathology, Faculty of Medicine & Health Sciences and [b]Department of Biology, Faculty of Science, UAE University, Al Ain, United Arab Emirates

The incidence of breast cancer is continuously increasing worldwide. This increasing trend is attributed partly to the fact that a considerable number of cases are related to environmental factors and partly to the little information available on the early changes that occur during mammary gland carcinogenesis. To characterize some of these early cellular changes, breast cancer was induced in female rats using a single intragastric dose of the environmental carcinogen 7,12-dimethylbenz[a]anthracene (DMBA; 80 mg/kg body weight). Mammary gland tissues of control and DMBA-treated rats were processed for routine histopathological examination and immunohistochemical analysis using an antibody specific for the proliferating cell nuclear antigen (PCNA). Microscopic examination of all mammary glands of DMBA-treated rats revealed a wide range of preneoplastic stages in addition to the well-characterized benign and malignant tumors that developed. The first stage was characterized by slightly dilated terminal ducts with accumulation of dead cells. This was designated the stage of cell death. Then, stages of hyperplasia, dysplasia, and carcinoma *in situ* followed. Immunohistochemical localization of PCNA in these preneoplastic lesions revealed an initial decrease followed by a gradual increase in the labeling index of PCNA. In conclusion, the DMBA-treated rats provide a useful model to dissect the early changes that occur during the multistep process of mammary gland carcinogenesis.

Key words: breast cancer; mammary gland; carcinogenesis; hyperplasia; cell death; PCNA

Introduction

Breast cancer is the most frequent type of cancer and the leading cause of cancer deaths in women worldwide.[1] In the United Arab Emirates (UAE), breast cancer is also the most common cancer among national females. According to UAE National Cancer Registry, 175 new breast cancer patients out of 538 female cancer cases (32.5%) were recorded from 1998 to 2002.

It is well known that the etiology of breast cancer is multifactorial and many risk factors contribute to its development including both endogenous and environmental estrogens, diet, lifestyle, geographic area of residence, and age at menarche or menopause.[2] However, in most cases there are no obvious factors predisposing to breast cancer, supporting the view that a variety of environmental carcinogens play a major role in the initiation of this disease.[3]

Experimental animal models are very useful for studying the events of mammary gland carcinogenesis. Chemically induced breast cancer in rats using the environmental carcinogen 7,12-dimethylbenz[a]anthracene (DMBA) is the most widely used model because tumors

Address for correspondence: Sherif M. Karam, Department of Anatomy, Faculty of Medicine & Health Sciences, UAE University, PO Box 17666, Al Ain, UAE. Voice: +971-3-7137493; fax: +971-3-7672033. skaram@uaeu.ac.ae

Ann. N.Y. Acad. Sci. 1138: 121–131 (2008). © 2008 New York Academy of Sciences.
doi: 10.1196/annals.1414.018

that develop in these rats closely mimic those of human breast cancer.[4]

DMBA is a synthetic, polycyclic aromatic hydrocarbon. Following its administration, the concentration of DMBA in the whole mammary gland is 110-fold higher than that obtained from collagenase-dissociated mammary epithelial cells. Therefore, it seems that the mammary fat pad serves as a reservoir for sustained release of the procarcinogen into the parenchymal tissues. This phenomenon explains the great susceptibility of the mammary epithelial cells to carcinogenesis by DMBA.[5]

It is well established that a single dose of DMBA results in a high yield of mammary tumors in rats at 50–56 days of age.[6] This optimal window of susceptibility to tumors is probably due to the active proliferation of the terminal ducts during this age.[7]

Even though much has been revealed concerning the pathogenesis of this disease, several questions remain to be answered. For example, the early preneoplastic events that occur during development of breast cancer are poorly understood. In the present study, we have used the DMBA rat model to characterize these preneoplastic stages. In addition, alteration in cell proliferation was studied and correlated with these early stages by detecting cells expressing the proliferating cell nuclear antigen (PCNA).

Materials and Methods

Animals

Female virgin Wistar rats (43–50 days old) were used in this study. Rats were supplied by the Animal House of the Faculty of Medicine and Health Sciences, UAE University. All rats were kept in standard conditions with light-dark regimen: 12–12 h and received food and water *ad libitum*.

To induce breast cancer, rats ($n = 21$) received a single intragastric dose of DMBA solution, 80 mg/kg body weight.[8] Control age- and weight-matched female rats ($n = 9$) received only vehicle, corn oil. All rats were examined weekly to detect any changes in general physical activity and body weight. In addition, the mammary glands were gently palpated to detect development of any abnormal mass. This protocol was approved by the Animal Ethics Committee of UAE University.

DMBA-treated and control rats were chosen randomly and killed by an overdose of anesthetic 25, 30, 35, or 40 weeks later. The mammary glands were dissected along with skin pelt and immediately immersed overnight (12–24 h) in Bouin's solution made of 70% picric acid, 10% formaldehyde, and 5% acetic acid.

Histopathological and Immunohistochemical Studies

Bouin-fixed mammary glands of each group of DMBA-treated rats and their controls were dehydrated and processed together for paraffin embedding. Some tissue sections of control and treated glands were processed for routine hematoxylin and eosin (H&E) staining to define the histopathological changes in the mammary glands and to classify tumors according to published criteria.[4]

For immunohistochemistry, 5-μm-thick tissue sections of control and DMBA-treated mammary glands showing different pathological conditions were mounted on the same slides, deparaffinized, hydrated, and then washed in phosphate buffered saline (PBS). To inhibit endogenous peroxidase activity, sections were incubated in 1% hydrogen peroxide for 30 min. To ensure equal conditions on all tissue sections to be probed, slides were drained off and areas around sections were wiped dry and circled with a thin film using PAP-pen (Dako, Glostrup, Denmark). Nonspecific binding was blocked by incubating sections in 1% bovine serum albumin containing 0.5% Tween-20 in PBS for 45 min. Then, sections were incubated with mouse monoclonal anti-PCNA antibody (clone 5A10, dilution 1:100;

Medical and Biological Laboratories Co., Nagoya, Japan) for overnight at 4°C. Then, sections were washed with PBS and incubated with biotinylated donkey-anti-mouse immunoglobulin (Ig) G (dilution 1:800; Jackson ImmunoResearch Laboratories Inc., West Grove, PA) for 30 min. Following PBS wash, sections were incubated in extravidin/peroxidase conjugate (dilution 1:1000, Sigma, St. Louis, MO) for 1 h. The antigen–antibody binding sites were revealed by incubating tissue sections with 3, 3′-diaminobenzidine tetrahydrochloride (DAB; Sigma) and counterstaining with periodic acid Schiff (PAS) technique.

To estimate the labeling index of PCNA immunostaining, for each mammary gland, images of at least three fields at ×640 magnification were randomly selected from two or more rats. The total number of PCNA-labeled cells per high-power field was counted. Data were expressed as mean ± standard error of the mean (SEM).

The intensity of PCNA immunolabeling of the cells was measured by using Scion Image Beta 4.02 software for Windows (http://www.scionimage.com/). Quantitative results of the optical density were reported in arbitrary units corresponding to DAB staining intensity, which was taken as an indication of the amount of PCNA in the sectioned cells. The measurements were presented as means of arbitrary units ± SEM.

The Student's *t*-test (SigmaPlot for Windows, version 9.0; Jandel Scientific, San Rafael, CA) was used to examine the differences in labeling intensity and labeling index in control and treated rats. $P < 0.05$ was considered statistically significant.

Results

Throughout this study, no changes were detected in the general activity and body weight of DMBA-treated rats as compared to control ones. However, all mammary glands of DMBA-treated rats were affected and exhibited a wide range of pathological changes.

Morphological Features of the Mammary Glands in DMBA-treated Rats

Gross observation and gentle palpation of the mammary glands of control and DMBA-treated rats revealed the development of some subcutaneous nodular masses in about 29% of the rats. These masses were of variable sizes, and the covering skin appeared normal. They were provisionally considered to be tumors (Fig. 1A). They developed in different topographical locations of the mammary glands; some were observed in the cervical region, others in the thoracic and abdomino-inguinal regions. Nevertheless, these tumors were more frequent in the cervical region than in other regions (Table 1).

To confirm the nature of these tumors and to detect the early microscopic changes that occur during development of breast cancer, H&E stained tissue sections of all the mammary glands of control and DMBA-treated rats were examined, including those that did not show any masses and appeared like control ones.

The mammary glands of control rats showed the normal ductal epithelial lining surrounding narrow lumen and external discontinuous layer of myoepithelial cells. The latter were supported by some fibrous connective tissue, which was surrounded by massive amount of adipocytes (Fig. 1B).

Microscopic examination of all mammary glands of rats treated with DMBA revealed various degrees of morphological changes which were usually a combination of more than one abnormal pattern. Most DMBA-treated mammary glands had moderately dilated ducts with groups of small cells in their lumens (Fig. 1C). These free luminal cells had eosinophilic cytoplasm and small hyperchromatic nuclei. These cells were considered to be dead. In some other ducts, a sign of increased secretory activity was evident with the accumulation of homogeneous secretory material in their lumens. Therefore, these mammary glands seemed to have unbalanced cell dynamics and enhanced secretory activity. All DMBA-treated rats had such

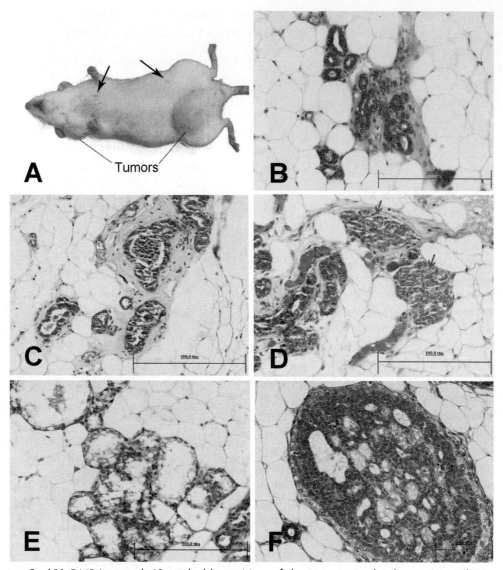

Figure 1. (A) DMBA-treated 42-week-old rat. Most of the mammary glands appear to have normal size and shape (*arrows*). Note that two tumors developed in cervical and abdomino-inguinal regions. **(B–F)** Mammary glands of a control rat **(B)** and DMBA-treated rats that did not develop any palpable mass or tumor, similar to the upper ones in (A), as they appear in paraffin sections stained with H&E. **(B)** Control mammary gland showing normal small ducts surrounded by a small amount of fibrous connective tissue and much adipose tissue. **(C)** Stage of cell death in the mammary gland showing early sign of morphological change. Notice the moderate dilatation of the ducts and presence of dead cells in their lumens. Two ducts in the lower third of the micrograph show some secretory material in their lumens. **(D)** Typical hyperplasia with an increased cellularity and number of terminal small ducts (*arrows*). **(E)** Dysplastic mammary gland showing dilated ducts and decreased amount of connective tissue. **(F)** *In situ* cribriform carcinoma exhibiting a localized area of dilated ducts partially filled with tumor cells. Note the numerous peripheral mitotic figures. Magnification: ×400.

changes in some of their mammary glands. Of the total number of DMBA-treated mammary glands examined ($n = 78$), 46% showed altered cellular dynamics (Table 2).

The second type of lesion observed in the mammary glands of DMBA-treated rats was characterized by an increase in the cell number, which led to an apparent increase in the density

TABLE 1. Summary of Tumors Developed in DMBA-treated Rats

	Age groups of rats			
	32 weeks	37 weeks	42 weeks	47 weeks
No. of rats	6	5	5	5
Rats with tumor	1	1	3	1
Tumor location	Cervical	*In situ*	Cervical, thoracic, and abdomino-inguinal	Cervical
Weight of tumor (g)	15	No mass (*in situ*)	No mass in 2 rats (*in situ*)—3.2; 13.8; 3; 3.1	3
Type of tumor	Ductal solid and cribriform carcinoma *In situ* cribriform carcinoma	*In situ* cribriform carcinoma	Lactating adenoma Ductal solid and cribriform carcinoma Papillary carcinoma *In situ* cribriform carcinoma	Squamous cell papilloma

TABLE 2. Numbers of Mammary Glands Showing Preneoplastic and Neoplastic Lesions following DMBA Administration into Rats (total number of DMBA-treated mammary glands examined = 78)

Mammary gland lesions	Number
Stage of cell death	36 (46%)
Hyperplasia	-
Dysplasia	1 (1.2%)
Stage of cell death + hyperplasia	21 (27%)
Stage of cell death + dysplasia	4 (5%)
Stage of cell death + hyperplasia + dysplasia	8 (10%)
In situ carcinoma + stage of cell death + hyperplasia + dysplasia	1 (1.2%)
In situ carcinoma + stage of cell death + hyperplasia	1 (1.2%)
Tumors	6 (8%)

of the cells forming the terminal ducts (Fig. 1D). Mammary glands with these changes were referred to as hyperplastic. However, those also showing lesions with altered cell dynamics, as described in the previous paragraph, were referred to as mammary glands in the stage of cell death.

Hyperplastic mammary glands also showed some small ducts with signs of cell death or other preneoplastic lesions. These mammary glands with mixed lesions represented about 39% of all DMBA-treated mammary glands examined (Table 2).

The third kind of lesion observed was characterized by increased number of epithelial duct cells, which was manifested with an increase in the number of small ducts, and many of them showed an apparent increase in the secretory activity and accumulation of secretory material. In the epithelial cells of these ducts, many of the nucleoli became prominent. Mammary glands with these features were referred to as dysplastic (Fig. 1E). Dysplastic mammary glands were developed in about 17% of all examined DMBA-treated mammary glands. A few of these glands (1.2%) showed only signs of dysplasia. The others were mixed with signs of cell death and hyperplasia (Table 2).

Two of the DMBA-treated rats (9.5%) developed large microscopic lesions made of dilated ducts which were mostly filled with cells. The nuclei of these cells were variable in density and were frequently seen in mitosis. There were some spaces in between the cells that formed secondary lumens. This lesion was typical of the cribriform type of carcinoma *in situ* (Fig. 1F). It was estimated that 2.4% of DMBA-treated mammary glands showed *in situ* cribriform carcinoma. These mammary glands also showed

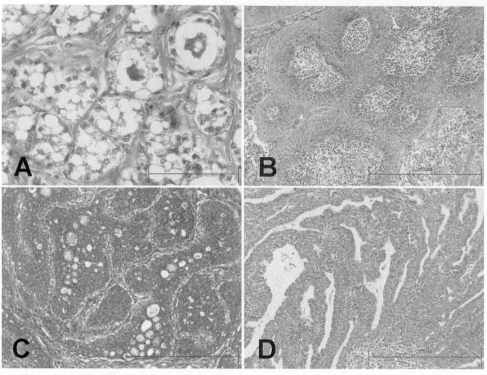

Figure 2. Benign **(A, B)** and malignant **(C, D)** tumors as they appear in DMBA-treated rats. **(A)** Lactating adenoma showing numerous round profiles; some contain secretory material. **(B)** Squamous cell papilloma showing multiple layers of epithelial cells (*arrows*). **(C)** Invasive cribriform carcinoma with solid sheets of cells interrupted by secondary lumens. **(D)** Papillary carcinoma characterized by the epithelial papillary growth with scanty connective tissue. Magnification: A = ×640; B–D = ×200.

signs of cell death, hyperplasia, and dysplasia (Table 2).

Advanced palpable pathological lesions were developed in five rats and showed various histopathological features. These lesions were either benign or malignant. Benign lesions were developed in rats sacrificed at 42 and 47 weeks of age, with incidence of 14% of the total number of tumors (Table 2). The first type, lactating adenoma, was characterized by numerous round profiles. Lumens of these alveolar structures had a serrated appearance due to decapitation or supranuclear vacuolization of the lining epithelium. The size of these alveoli may increase due to accumulation of secreted material inside the lumens (Fig. 2A). The other benign lesion, squamous cell papilloma (Fig. 2B), was developed in the 47-week-old rat. Ductal structures were maintained with multilayered epithelial cells surrounding the lu-

men, which was full of dead cells. The presence of keratin and a decrease in the amount of connective tissue were typical features of this tumor.

In the DMBA-treated rats, malignant lesions were more frequent (19%) than benign lesions and developed in one of the 32-week-old-rats and two of the 42-week-old rats. The first type of malignant lesions observed was typical of invasive cribriform carcinoma. It was characterized by solid sheets of neoplastic epithelial cells that were interrupted by round or irregularly shaped secondary lumens of variable sizes (Fig. 2C). Individual neoplastic cells were moderately pleomorphic.

The second malignant tumor observed was invasive papillary carcinoma. It was characterized by numerous papillary projections with a thinner fibrovascular core. Papillae were lined by columnar cells that were continuous with a

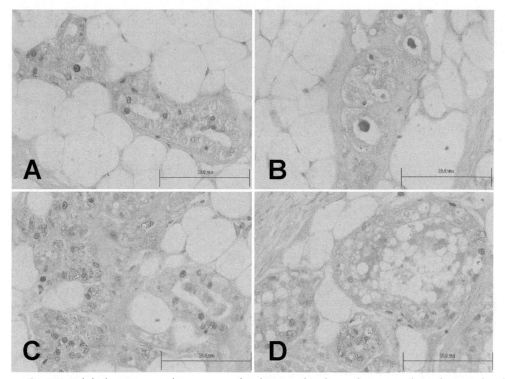

Figure 3. PCNA labeling in control mammary gland **(A)** and in the early preneoplastic lesions developed in DMBA-treated rats **(B–D)**. **(A)** PCNA-labeled nuclei appear brownish in some epithelial duct cells of control mammary gland. **(B)** Stage of "cell death" lesion showing a few PCNA-labeled cells. Notice increased secretory activity of the cells with accumulation PAS-stained material in the lumen. **(C)** Severe hyperplasia showing an increased number of PCNA-labeled cells. **(D)** Dysplastic mammary gland showing dilated ducts with an increased number of PCNA-labeled cells and accumulation of secretory material in their lumen. Magnification: ×640.

multilayered and pleomorphic epithelium. Mitotic figures were frequently observed in this tumor. Nucleoli appeared prominent and often multiple (Fig. 2D).

Immunohistochemical Localization of PCNA

Immunolocalization of PCNA in the mammary glands of control rats revealed the presence of proliferating cells in some small terminal ducts (Fig. 3A). In addition, PCNA-labeled nuclei of myoepithelial cells in these control rats were occasionally observed. The number of PCNA-labeled cells was counted per high-power field in the mammary glands of all control and DMBA-treated rats examined. The PCNA labeling index was then calculated and averaged. Comparing the labeling indices in

different preneoplastic and neoplastic lesions developed in the mammary glands after treatment with DMBA revealed an increase in the number of PCNA-labeled cells starting from hyperplasia, followed by dysplasia (Fig. 3C and D, respectively), and progressing to malignant lesions. However, during the stage of cell death, the PCNA-labeling index was lower than that of control mammary glands (Fig. 3B; Table 3).

In mammary glands with palpable benign and malignant tumors, the PCNA-labeling indices were higher than those in the control and other nonpalpable lesions. The PCNA labeling was highest in the case of cribriform carcinoma (Table 3).

When PCNA immunolabeling was examined in various mammary gland tissues of rats treated with DMBA and compared with labeling in tissues of control rats, some variation in

TABLE 3. PCNA-labeling Indices (means ± SEM) Estimated in Normal Tissues of Control Rats as well as in Various Preneoplastic and Neoplastic Lesions Developed in Rats Treated with DMBA

Tissues	Labeling index
Control	12.3 ± 4.1
Stage of cell death	2.3 ± 0.3
Hyperplasia	12.7 ± 4.2
Dysplasia	42.7 ± 13.9
In situ cribriform	64.5 ± 27.6
Lactating adenoma	25.3 ± 6.9
Squamous cell papilloma	121.3 ± 20.3
Papillary carcinoma	120.0 ± 5.3
Cribriform carcinoma	179.7 ± 15.1

the labeling intensities was observed. These tissue sections were processed, cut, mounted, and immunoprobed together. Measurements using the Scion computer program revealed no significant difference in PCNA labeling intensity in the lesions developed in DMBA-treated rats when compared with those of control rats.

Discussion

In the present study, the early morphological preneoplastic changes that occur during development of breast cancer have been characterized in female Wister rats treated with DMBA.

The Sequence of Events That Occur during Development of Preneoplastic Lesions in DMBA-treated Rats

A series of microscopic changes have been observed in the mammary glands of DMBA-treated rats. These changes are taken to be representative of the multistep process that occurs before development of breast cancer.

In the past, Beckmann and colleagues[9] described the first two stages of breast cancer development in humans as hyperplasia and carcinoma *in situ*. When breast cancer was induced in Sprague Dawley rats with 1-methyl-1-nitrosourea, hyperplasia was also the first histopathological change observed.[10] Even though these hyperplastic ducts of mammary glands are poorly studied, their presence has

become a valuable indicator of malignant progression in both humans and rats.[11,12]

In the DMBA-treated rats examined in this study, some mammary glands developed hyperplasia in association with other preneoplastic lesions (42.4% of all mammary glands examined in DMBA-treated rats). In a few mammary glands (2.4%), carcinoma *in situ* was also observed.

The majority of DMBA-treated mammary glands (93.4%) examined in the present study developed another form of histopathological change. These glands exhibited moderately dilated terminal ducts characterized by numerous dead cells extruded into their lumens. This morphological change was observed either alone (46% of all DMBA-treated mammary glands examined) or in association with other preneoplastic lesions (47.4%). It is generally believed that when a cell dies, it releases some factors that stimulate neighboring postmitotic cells to re-enter the cell cycle. It was reported earlier that in lymphoid and vascular epithelial tissues, apoptosis precedes and leads to hyperplasia.[13,14] Thus, the stage of cell death described in this study has been considered to occur earlier than hyperplasia, and is taken to be the first stage in the multistep process of breast cancer development in the DMBA-treated Wister rats.

Dysplasia of the mammary glands is the third preneoplastic lesion detected in the DMBA-treated rats. Dysplasia appeared either alone (1.2%) or, more commonly (18.2%), in association with other preneoplastic lesions. Similar features of this lesion were also described by Xie and co-workers when breast cancer was induced in rats with a combination of 17β-estradiol and testosterone.[15]

It has been reported earlier that preneoplastic changes of the mammary gland include intraductal noninfiltrating carcinoma, or carcinoma *in situ*.[16] In the present study, 9.5% of the rats treated with DMBA developed intraductal noninfiltrating carcinoma *in situ*. When all the DMBA-treated mammary gland are considered, it is estimated that carcinoma *in situ* occurs in only 2.4% of them. It occurs in association with other preneoplastic lesions. It has already been shown that DMBA treatment alters the normal process of mammary gland differentiation of terminal ducts to alveoli and lobules, producing instead the sequence of terminal ducts → intraductal proliferation → carcinoma *in situ* → invasive carcinoma.[17] Extensive studies on the unique features of *in situ* carcinoma reveal its significance in predicting the aggressiveness of breast cancer.[18,19]

Tumors Developed in the Mammary Glands of DMBA-treated Wistar Rats Are Mostly Malignant

In this study, the incidence of mammary tumors induced in Wistar rats using DMBA was 29%. In contrast, Bojkova and colleagues. found that administration of 20 mg of DMBA in Wistar:Han rats resulted in about 8% tumor incidence.[20] Repeated DMBA administration (3 doses of 10 mg/rat) increased the incidence to 85%. These differences in rat susceptibility could, possibly, be due to the age when the carcinogen was administered. The incidence reached the highest rate between postnatal days 40–46, when cells of the terminal ducts have maximal proliferative activity. The physiological changes through seasons may also play a substantial role in determining the susceptibility to carcinogenesis.[21] All rats used in the present study received DMBA at almost the same age and during the same season.

The vast majority of tumors observed in DMBA-treated rats in the present study were carcinomas. This is consistent with previous studies using DMBA or 1-methyl-1-nitrosourea as a carcinogenic agent.[8,22,23]

The most highly malignant tumors in the rat have some common features with infiltrating ductal carcinoma of the human.[24] In this study, two different forms of carcinoma were observed: cribriform and papillary; the former was observed more commonly. However, Russo and Russo reported that invasive papillary carcinoma is the most typical and frequent DMBA-induced tumor.[4]

Two other forms of tumors were also observed in the present study and classified as "benign." They include: 1) lactating adenoma, which was previously identified and well characterized,[4,23] and 2) squamous cell papilloma, which was identified in the present study in DMBA-treated rats for the first time. Based on the features described in the results section, it is hypothesized that the origin of squamous cell papilloma is probably the lactiferous or large ducts, which are close to the nipple.

While benign tumors of the mammary glands that occur in the rats closely resemble those of humans, they are observed more frequently in humans than in rats treated with 1-methy-l-nitrosourea.[10,24] However, Liska and colleagues were not able to detect any benign tumors by using similar carcinogen in rats.[22] In the present study, benign tumors are observed less frequently than malignant lesions. It is postulated that the less differentiated terminal ducts develop invasive cancer lesions when attacked by DMBA, while benign lesions, such as adenomas, arise from the more differentiated large ducts.[24] If this is the case, then the reason for developing more carcinomas than benign lesions could simply be due to the structural organization of the tree-like branching duct system of the mammary gland, in which the small terminal ducts are much more numerous than the big ones.

An Initial Decrease followed by a Gradual Increase in Cell Proliferation Characterizes Breast Cancer Development in DMBA-treated Rats

PCNA has been described as an important predictive and prognostic factor which is used widely as a marker for cell proliferation in the clinical assessment of various tumors including breast cancer.[25] In the present study, PCNA labeling has also been used to correlate the rate of cell proliferation with each of the various preneoplastic and neoplastic changes observed in DMBA-treated rats.

The nuclear expression of PCNA in the mammary glands of control rats shows that cell proliferation is mainly found in the small terminal ducts. This finding confirms previously published data.[26] The occasional presence of PCNA-labeled myoepithelial cells indicates that these differentiated cells maintain some capacity for mitosis.

In DMBA-treated rats, progression toward breast cancer is found to be associated with an increase in the number of PCNA-labeled cells starting at the stage of hyperplasia (Table 3). This observation correlates with those of Funakoshi and colleagues, who studied canine mammary gland tumors.[27] However, unexpectedly, there was a reduction in PCNA labeling during the initial stage of "cell death." This might be related to the deregulation phenomena of neoplastic progression.[28]

In an attempt to evaluate the correlation between breast cancer progression and the intensity of PCNA labeling, quantitative measurements were carried out using the Scion image program. It is generally noticed that the intensity of staining gradually increases with progression toward breast cancer. Similarly, Mo and co-workers reported that the expression of PCNA was significantly related to progression of nasopharyngeal tumor in humans.[29] However, Surowiak and colleagues used another proliferation marker, Ki-67, and found it useful in correlating its labeling intensity with the grading of ductal breast cancer.[30]

In conclusion, a series of histopathological changes were characterized in the mammary glands of Wister rats treated with a single intragastric dose of DMBA. These changes included poorly characterized preneoplastic changes in addition to the previously well-characterized neoplastic changes. The former appeared to be representative of the early multistep events of mammary gland carcinogenesis. The present study suggests that alteration of cellular dynamics and enhanced cell death were the first preneoplastic events observed. These were followed by hyperplastic and dysplastic changes leading to carcinoma *in situ*. Malignant lesions appeared in two forms—cribriform and papillary carcinomas—and were more common than benign tumors: lactating adenoma and squamous papilloma. These morphological changes were associated with alteration in the expression of PCNA protein. An initial downregulation followed by upregulation of PCNA follows the sequence of the morphological changes. It is very likely that the observations reported in the present study are applicable to humans because: 1) the overall organization of the epithelial duct cells of rat mammary glands are comparable to those of the human, 2) DMBA is a well-known environmental factor that may contribute to the etiology of breast cancer in humans, and 3) most of the neoplastic changes observed in the mammary glands of DMBA-treated rats are similar to those reported in humans. Therefore, one of the important challenges now is to know whether this very early stage of pre-hyperplastic cell death also occurs in humans. Next, gene-profiling technology could be used to identify some genes involved and use them as early markers for screening of high-risk women susceptible to develop breast cancer.

Acknowledgments

This study is funded in part by the Faculty of Graduate studies UAEU to W.S.A. and by a grant from Terry fox Funds for Cancer Research to S.M.K.

Conflicts of Interest

The authors declare no conflicts of interest.

References

1. Smymiotis, V., T. Theodosopoulos, A. Marinis, *et al.* 2005. Metastatic disease in the breast from nonmammary neoplasms. *Eur. J. Gynaecol. Oncol.* **26:** 547–550.
2. Martin, A. & B.L. Weber. 2000. Genetic and hormonal risk factors in breast cancer. *J. Natl. Cancer Inst.* **92:** 1126–1135.
3. Steinetz, B.G., T. Gordon, S. Lasano, *et al.* 2006. The parity-related protection against breast cancer is compromised by cigarette smoke during rat pregnancy: observations on tumorigenesis and

immunological defenses of the neonate. *Carcinogenesis* **27:** 1146–1152.

4. Russo, J. & I.H. Russo. 2000. Atlas and histologic classification of Tumors of rat mammary gland. *J. Mamm. Gland Biol. Neoplasia* **5:** 187–200.

5. Menon, R., J. Bartley, S. Som & M.R. Banerjee. 1987. Metabolism of 7, 12-Dimethylbenz[a]anthracene by mouse mammary cells in serum-free organ culture medium. *Eur. J. Cancer Clin. Oncol.* **23:** 395–400.

6. Sinha, D.K., J.E. Pazik & T.L. Dao. 1983. Progression of rat mammary development with age and its relationship to carcinogenesis by a chemical carcinogen. *Int. J. Cancer* **31:** 321–327.

7. Ariazi, J.L., J.D. Haag, M.J. Lindstrom & M.N. Gould. 2005. Mammary glands of sexually immature rats are more susceptible than those of mature rats to the carcinogenic, lethal, and mutagenic effects of N-Nitroso-N-Methylurea. *Mol. Carcinogenesis* **43:** 155–164.

8. Russo, I.H. & J. Russo. 1996. Mammary gland neoplasia in long-term rodent studies. *Environ. Health Prospect.* **104:** 938–967.

9. Beckmann, M.W., D. Niederacher, H.G. Schnurch, *et al.* 1997. Multistep carcinogenesis of breast cancer and tumour heterogeneity. *J. Mol. Med.* **75:** 429–439.

10. Singh, M., J.N. McGinley & H.J. Thompson. 2000. A comparison of the histopathology of premalignant and malignant mammary gland lesions induced in sexually immature rats with those occurring in the human. *Lab. Investig.* **50:** 221–231.

11. Lee, S., S.K. Mohsin, S. Mao, *et al.* 2006. Hormones, receptors, and growth in hyperplastic enlarged lobular units: early potential precursors of breast cancer. *Breast Cancer Res.* **8:** R6.

12. Weroha, S.J., S.A. Li, O. Tawfik & J.J. Li. 2006. Overexpression of cyclins D1 and D3 during estrogen-induced breast oncogenesis in female ACI rats. *Carcinogenesis* **27:** 491–498.

13. Volkmann, A., R. Doffinger, U. Ruther & B.A. Kyewski. 1996. Insertional mutagenesis affecting programmed cell death leads to thymic hyperplasia and altered thymopoiesis. *J. Immunol.* **156:** 136–145.

14. Izumi, Y., S. Kim, M. Yoshiyama, *et al.* 2003. Activation of apoptosis signal-regulating kinase 1 in injured artery and its critical role in neointimal hyperplasia. *Circulation* **108:** 2812–2818.

15. Xie, B., S.W. Tsao & Y.C. Wong. 1999. Induction of high incidence of mammary tumour in female Nobel rats with a combination of 17β-oestradiol and testosterone. *Carcinogenesis* **20:** 1069–1078.

16. Komitowski, D., B. Sass & W. Laub. 1982. Rat mammary tumor classification: notes on comparative aspects. *J. Natl. Cancer Inst.* **68:** 147–156.

17. Russo, J., L.K. Tay & I.H. Russo. 1982. Differentiation of the mammary gland and susceptibility to carcinogesis. *Breast Cancer Res. Treat.* **2:** 5–73.

18. Lennington, W.J., R.A. Jensen, L.W. Dalton & D.L. Page. 1994. Ductal carcinoma in situ of the breast. *Cancer* **73:** 118–24.

19. Rehman, S., J. Crow & P.A. Revell. 2000. Bax protein expression in DCIS of the breast in relation to invasive ductal carcinoma and other molecular markers. *Pathol Oncol. Res.* **6:** 256–263.

20. Bojkova, B., I. Ahlers, P. Kubatka, *et al.* 2000. Repeated administration of carcinogen in critical development periods increases susceptibility of female Wistar:Han rats to mammary carcinogenesis induction. *Neoplasma* **47:** 230–233.

21. Kubatka, P., E. Ahlersova, I. Ahlers, *et al.* 2002. Variability of mammary carcinogenesis induction in female Sprague-Dawley and Wistar:Han rats: the effect of season and age. *Physiol. Res.* **51:** 633–640.

22. Liska, J., S. Galbavy, D. Macejova, *et al.* 2000. Histopathology of mammary tumours in female rats treated with 1-methyl-1-nitrosourea. *Endocrine Regul.* **34:** 91–96.

23. Costa, I., M. Solanas & E. Escrich. 2002. Histopathologic characterization of mammary neoplastic lesions induced with 7, 12-dimethylbenz[a]anthracene in the rat. *Arch. Pathol. Lab. Med.* **126:** 915–927.

24. Russo, J., B.A. Gusterson, A.E. Rogers, *et al.* 1990. Biology of disease: comparative study of human and rat mammary tumorigenesis. *Lab. Investig.* **62:** 244–278.

25. Wu, K., Z. Weng, Q. Tao, *et al.* 2003. Stage-specific expression of breast cancer-specific genc γ-Synuclein. *Cancer Epidemiol. Biochem. Prev.* **12:** 920–925.

26. Qiu, C., L. Shan, M. Yu & E.G. Snyderwine. 2005. Steroid hormone receptor expression and proliferation in rat mammary gland carcinoma induced by 2-amino-1-phenylimidazo[4, 5-*b*-]pyridine. *Carcinogenesis* **26:** 763 769.

27. Funakoshi, Y., H. Nakayama, K. Uetsuka, *et al.* 2000. Cellular proliferative and telomerasc activity in canine mammary gland tumors. *Vet. Pathol.* **37:** 177–183.

28. Hoshino, T. 1992. Cell kinetics of glial tumours. *Revue Neurologigue* **148:** 396–401.

29. Mo, H.Y., C.Q. Zhang, K.T. Feng, *et al.* 2004. Expression of P53 and PCNA in nasopharyngeal carcinoma and their relation with clinical stage, VCA/IgA, EA/IgA, radiation sensibility, and prognosis. *Aizheng Chinese J. Cancer* **23**(11 Suppl): 1551–1554.

30. Surowiak, P., M. Pudelko, A. Maciejczyk, *et al.* 2005. The relationship of the expression of proliferation—related antigens Ki67 and PCNA in the cells of ductal breast cancer with the differentiation grade. *Ginekologia Polska* **76:** 9–14.

Targeted Intra-operative Radiotherapy—TARGIT for Early Breast Cancer

Can We Spare the Patient Daily Journeys to the Radiotherapist?

Michael Baum[a] and Jayant S. Vaidya[b]

[a]University College London, The Portland Hospital, London, United Kingdom

[b]Department of Surgery and Molecular Oncology, Ninewells Hospital and Medical School, University of Dundee, Scotland, United Kingdom

Breast conservation by wide local excision for early breast cancer is now considered safe and should be considered default therapy wherever possible. Unfortunately, this requires access to costly radiotherapy centers. Many women in the developing world or for that matter in wealthy countries with large land masses and small populations do not have access to radiotherapy and are therefore denied the option of breast-conserving surgery. Whole-breast radiation by external beam after tumorectomy is predicated on the belief that latent foci of subclinical cancer outside the index quadrant are responsible for local recurrence. We do not think this is the case, as over 90% of these recurrences occur in the index quadrant. In this paper we describe a novel system for intra-operative radiotherapy using a mobile unit that should, in theory, be able to replace 6 weeks of external beam from a linear accelerator. The technique, TARGIT, is currently undergoing a multinational clinical trial in comparison with conventional external beam. If we can prove at least equivalence in outcome, then breast-conserving surgery might become available to all women in the developing world and to those living long distances from the nearest radiotherapy center.

Key words: early breast cancer; intra-operative radiotherapy; technology for developing world

Introduction

We would like to begin this paper with an anecdote. One of us (MB) frequently looks after patients with breast cancer from the UAE. They come to London for diagnostic work-up and surgery and return home for postoperative radiotherapy and adjuvant systemic therapy. One woman, who lives in Dubai, had to make the daily trek by car, one and a half hours each way, to Al Ain for her radiotherapy. This involved 42 return journeys. On one occasion her driver fell asleep and they were involved in a serious crash. The injuries she received have to be considered as serious adverse events related to postoperative radiotherapy.

It is of course a pity that a wealthy city like Dubai with over 2 million inhabitants, does not support a radiotherapy unit, but this pattern is repeated every day around the world in equally wealthy countries with large rural areas and difficult access to the nearest major city. Furthermore, in the poorest countries in the world, women with early breast cancer cannot be offered breast-conserving surgery

Address for correspondence: Prof. Michael Baum, University College London, Portland Hospital, 212-214 Great Portland Street, London W1W 5QN, UK. michael@mbaum.freeserve.co.uk because of inadequate provision of radiotherapy units. Assuming there never will be a golden age when all women in the world suffering with breast cancer have easy access to postoperative radiotherapy, we need some original thinking "outside the box" to offer a solution. If the woman cannot get to the radiotherapy unit, then the radiotherapy unit must come to the woman.

In this paper, we wish to describe the rationale and the technique that may answer the problem with a simple mobile radiotherapy unit that can provide a one-shot intra-operative treatment targeting the area around the primary tumor, that in theory might be equivalent or even better than 5–7 weeks of conventional external beam treatment.

Rationale—Logical

The rationale for targeting the area around the primary tumor comes from clinical correlation of whole organ analysis of mastectomy specimens. It has been well demonstrated that the female breast frequently harbors more than one tumor and these are found if one looks hard enough. This has been demonstrated in autopsy studies (e.g., undiagnosed cancer present in 20% of women with a median age of 39[1]) as well as in mastectomy specimens.[2] However, this widespread three-dimensional distribution does not correspond to the location of recurrences after breast-conserving surgery,[3,4] which occurs most commonly (in about 90% of cases) in the area around the scar of primary excision (that is, in the index quadrant). Hence it follows that radiotherapy after surgical excision should be targeted to the area around the primary tumor—the tumor bed.

Rationale—Biological

The conventional standard radiotherapy is very successful and reduces the rate of local recurrence by two-thirds, but conversely, it fails in one-third of cases. This could be because of intrinsic resistance or due to the radiotherapy dose "geographically" missing the target tissues and "temporally" missing the window of optimal opportunity. It is interesting that the proportional reduction of the risk does not change with increasing size of excision. Hence just excising the cancer with a larger margin will not eliminate the risk. This raises the question as to whether the trauma of surgery itself may contribute to the risk. The wound fluid after surgery is found to stimulate cancer cell growth, motility, and invasiveness, and we have found that targeted intra-operative radiotherapy impairs the stimulatory effect of surgery.[5] As it is delivered immediately after surgery, targeted intra-operative radiotherapy may avoid both the geographical and temporal missing of the target.

Rationale—Mathematical Model

We have devised a mathematical model[6,7] that simulates breast cancer growth, recurrence, and response to radiotherapy. In this model we have introduced the cells that have suffered a loss of heterozygosity in the tumor suppression genes. These cells would have been derived from the same ductal tree and would surround the area of the primary tumor. They would be morphologically normal and would withstand the usual fractionated (low) doses of radiotherapy, but would not able to tolerate the high dose delivered in the single shot of intra-operative radiotherapy. Our model predicts that the single well-directed dose may be superior to conventional radiotherapy.

The New Approach

In 1998 we pioneered the approach of *targ*eted *i*ntra-operative radio*t*herapy (TARGIT).[8–10] With our technique, using the Intrabeam™ system (Carl Zeiss Meditec, Jena, Germany), a single fraction of 20 Gy is delivered to the surface of the tumor bed using a spherical applicator, from within the breast. The surgeon "wraps" (or conforms) the pliable tumor bed around the applicator (something we discovered while testing out our initial applicator designs), ensuring close apposition of the target tissue to the radiotherapy source. The technique[11] needs to be meticulous but is relatively straightforward, and over 1000 patients have been treated worldwide.

Although the approach of concentrating on the tumor bed is not new, modern technology has allowed it to be used with relative ease in a routine operating theater and with a potential for significant economic savings. The latest analysis of our large phase II study using Intrabeam in place of a conventional boost, has given us the courage of our convictions to go ahead and test the approach in a large multicenter randomized clinical trial.[11] Several other investigators have also started testing the same approach: the ELIOT trial in Milan, the NSABP-B32 trial in the United States, and the GEC-ESTRO, RAPID, and IMPORT trials in Europe and the United Kingdom.

The Randomized Trials

After successful completion of a pilot study,[9] we launched the TARGIT (Alone) trial in March 2000. In this trial, we are selecting women who are older than 45 years and who do not face a high risk of developing recurrent or multiple cancers in the breast. In fact, these women form the majority of breast cancer patients. The randomly allocated treatment that follows wide excision of the cancer (lumpectomy) is either targeted intra-operative radiotherapy or the usual 4- to 7-week course of external beam radiotherapy. The initial slow uptake of the trial has now accelerated as confidence with this approach has grown, and currently 21 centers on three continents contribute to a steep recruitment curve. The aim of the trial is modest—to investigate if the two treatments are equivalent. But if proven, the prize is great—women could then avoid the 30–40 visits to the radiotherapy center and still conserve their breast. If it turns out to be superior then that will be an added bonus.

For women outside the criteria for entry to the trial who may need "prophylactic" radiotherapy to the whole breast in addition, the intra-operative dose to the tumor bed could be the better way of giving the usual tumor bed boost for the reasons already stated. In our series of 302 cancers, we found a very low recurrence rate,[12] and this has prompted us to launch a second trial, TARGIT-B, to assess if it yields superior results to an external beam boost. The prize if this trial is successful would be a significant reduction in local recurrence, which may translate into a definite, albeit small, survival benefit.

Conflicts of Interest

Michael Baum declares a consultancy arrangement with Karl Zeiss that pays 1,000 euros a month. Jayant S. Vaidya's salary was partly funded by a research grant from Photoelectron Corporation (PeC), the initial manufacturer of Intrabeam from October 1996 to September 1999.

References

1. Nielsen, M., J.L. Thomsen, S. Primdahl, *et al.* 1987. Breast cancer and atypia among young and middle-aged women: a study of 110 medicolegal autopsies. *Br J. Cancer* **56:** 814–819.
2. Holland, R., S.H. Veling, M. Mravunac & J.H. Hendriks. 1985. Histologic multifocality of Tis, T.1-2 breast carcinomas. Implications for clinical trials of breast-conserving surgery. *Cancer* **56:** 979–990.
3. Vaidya, J.S., J.J. Vyas, I. Mittra & R.F. Chinoy. 1995. Multicentricity and its influence on conservative breast cancer treatment strategy. *Hongkong International Cancer Congress: Abstract* 44.4.
4. Baum, M., J.S. Vaidya & I. Mittra. 1997. Multicentricity and recurrence of breast cancer [letter; comment]. *Lancet* **349:** 208.

5. Massarut, S., G. Baldassare, B. Belleti, *et al.* 2006. Intraoperative radiotherapy impairs breast cancer cell motility induced by surgical wound fluid. *J. Clin. Oncol.* **24:** 10611.

6. Enderling, H., A.R. Anderson, M.A. Chaplain, *et al.* 2006. Mathematical modelling of radiotherapy strategies for early breast cancer. *J. Theor. Biol.* **241:** 158–171.

7. Enderling, H., A.R.A. Anderson, M.A.J. Chaplain & J.S. Vaidya. 2006. A mathematical model of breast cancer development, local treatment and recurrence. *J. Theor. Biol.* **246:** 245–259.

8. Vaidya, J.S. 2002. A novel approach for local treatment of early breast cancer. PhD Thesis, University of London. http://www.targit.org.uk/ (accessed Aug. 15, 2008).

9. Vaidya, J.S., M. Baum, J.S. Tobias, *et al.* 2001. Targeted intra-operative radiotherapy (Targit): an innovative method of treatment for early breast cancer. *Ann. Oncol.* **12:** 1075–1080.

10. Vaidya, J.S., M. Baum, J.S. Tobias, *et al.* 2002. The novel technique of delivering targeted intraoperative radiotherapy (Targit) for early breast cancer. *Eur. J. Surg. Oncol.* **28:** 447–454.

11. Vaidya, J.S., M. Baum, J.S. Tobias & J. Houghton. 1999. Targeted Intraoperative Radiotherapy (TARGIT)—trial protocol. *Lancet*: http://www.thelancet.com/journals/lancet/misc/protocol/99 PRT-47 (accessed Aug. 15, 2008).

12. Vaidya, J.S., M. Baum, J.S. Tobias, *et al.* 2006. Targeted intraoperative radiotherapy (TARGIT) yields very low recurrence rates when given as a boost. *Int. J. Rad. Oncol. Biol. Phys.* **66:** 1335–1338.

The Potential of PARP Inhibitors in Genetic Breast and Ovarian Cancers

Yvette Drew and Hilary Calvert

Northern Institute for Cancer Research, Newcastle University, Newcastle-upon-Tyne, United Kingdom

The abundant nuclear enzyme poly(ADP-ribose) polymerase-1 (PARP-1), represents an important novel target in cancer therapy. PARP-1 is essential to the repair of DNA single-strand breaks via the base excision repair pathway. Inhibitors of PARP-1 have been shown to enhance the cytotoxic effects of ionizing radiation and DNA damaging chemotherapy agents, such as the methylating agents and topoisomerase I inhibitors. There are currently at least five PARP inhibitors in clinical trial development. Recent *in vitro* and *in vivo* evidence suggests that PARP inhibitors could be used not only as chemo/radiotherapy sensitizers, but as *single* agents to selectively kill cancers defective in DNA repair, specifically cancers with mutations in the breast cancer associated (BRCA) 1 and 2 genes. This theory of selectively exploiting cells defective in one DNA repair pathway by inhibiting another is a major breakthrough in the treatment of cancer. BRCA1/2 mutations are responsible for the majority of genetic breast/ovarian cancers, known as the hereditary breast ovarian cancer syndrome. This review summarizes the preclinical and clinical evidence for the potential of PARP inhibitors in genetic breast and ovarian cancers.

Key words: breast cancer; ovarian cancer; BRCA1 gene; BRCA2 gene; cancer genetics; poly(ADP-ribose) polymerase-1 (PARP-1); PARP inhibitors

Introduction

Breast cancer is the most common malignancy in women; one in eight women will be diagnosed during their lifetime.[1] Ovarian cancer is less common, affecting one in 70 women, but this must be balanced against its poorer 5-year survival rate of 44.7%, compared to 88.5% observed in patients with breast cancer.[1] A positive family history is reported in between 10–20% of patients, and individuals with an affected first-degree relative have a two- to threefold increased risk of developing the cancers over the general population.[2–4] Between 5–10% of all breast and ovarian cancer cases are associated with a known inherited genetic mutation. Inheriting a mutation in either BRCA genes, known as the hereditary breast ovarian cancer syndrome (HBOCS), is associated with a high lifetime risk of cancer.[5,6] Mutations in other genes have been linked to an increased lifetime risk of breast and/or ovarian cancer. They include CHEK2 (1100delC mutation),[7] the tumor-suppressor gene p53,[8] PTEN,[9] the ataxia telangiectasia mutated gene (ATM),[10] STK11,[11] the Fanconi anemia genes FANCD2 and FANCJ,[12] and the DNA mismatch repair genes[13] (Table 1).

Hereditary Breast Ovarian Cancer Syndrome

Inheriting a mutation in either the BRCA1 or the BRCA2 gene, renders the individual at high lifetime risk of developing cancer.[6] Breast and ovarian cancer are the most commonly

Address for correspondence: Dr Yvette Drew, Specialist Registrar in Medical Oncology and Clinical Research Fellow, MBBS (Newcastle), MRCP (London), Northern Institute for Cancer Research, Paul O'Gorman Building, Newcastle University, Newcastle-upon-Tyne, UK NE2 4HH. Yvette.drew@ncl.ac.uk

Ann. N.Y. Acad. Sci. 1138: 136–145 (2008). © 2008 New York Academy of Sciences.
doi: 10.1196/annals.1414.020

TABLE 1. Gene Mutations Linked to Increased Lifetime Risk of Breast and/or Ovarian Cancer

Gene	Associated syndrome	Chromosome site	Cancer phenotype	Reference
BRCA1	HBOC	17q21	Breast Ovary	6
BRCA2/FANCD1	HBOC	13q12	Breast Ovary	6
ATM	Ataxia-telangiectasia	11q22–23	Breast	10
CHEK2 (1100delC mutation)		22q12	Breast	7
p53	Li fraumeni	17p13.1	Breast	8
PTEN	Cowden's	10q22–23	Breast	9
MMR genes	HNPCC/Lynch syndrome II		Ovary Breast	13
STK11	Peutz-jeghers	19p13.3	Breast Ovary	11
Other FA genes:FANCJ, FANCD2	Fanconi anemia		Breast	12

observed, but an increased risk of other cancers has also been documented, including prostate, pancreatic, fallopian tube, and primary peritoneal carcinoma.[14,15]

The lifetime risk of breast cancer in female BRCA1 mutation carriers has been reported to be as high as 84% and between 60–80% in BRCA2 mutation carriers.[2,5] In men breast cancer is rare accounting for <1% of all cancers, but in BRCA2 and BRCA1 mutations carriers, the lifetime risk was recently estimated to be 80–100-fold and 58-fold times that of the general male population, respectively.[13,16]

The lifetime risk of ovarian cancer for BRCA1 and BRCA2 mutation carriers is estimated at 40–50% and 10–20%, respectively.[17] The frequency of BRCA1/2 mutations in the general population is reported to be between 0.1–0.8%.[18] Carriers of the mutations are not limited to a particular population, but specific groups with high prevalence have been identified, such as women of Ashkenazi Jewish descent.[19] The autosomal dominant mode of genetic transmission means that *both* the male and female children of a carrier have a 50% chance of inheriting the mutation in their germline. One defective BRCA1 or BRCA2 copy is enough to predispose to cancer, but loss of the second allele is consistently found in cancer cells confirming the classic Knudson two-hit hypothesis for tumor suppressor genes.[20]

BRCA1/2 Genes

The BRCA1/2 tumor suppressor genes were identified by positional cloning in 1994 and 1995, respectively.[21,22] The BRCA1 gene, located on chromosome 17q21, has a variety of proposed functions including DNA damage signaling response and repair, transcriptional regulation, cell cycle control, and ubiquitylation.[23]

BRCA1 forms part of a large complex known as the BRCA1-associated genome surveillance complex (BASC), which acts as a sensor for DNA damage. BRCA1 is phosphorylated following recognition of DNA double-strand breaks (DSBs) and plays a major role in DSB repair by homologous recombination (HR).[24] HR is a complex, error-free pathway that repairs DSBs that occur in late S and G2 phase of the cell cycle. HR also has a key role in repairing DSBs that arise as a result of replication fork stalling following an unrepaired single-strand break (SSB).[25]

The BRCA2 gene, later confirmed to also be the Fanconi anemia gene FANCD1, is located on chromosome 13q12.[26] Its main function is in HR-mediated DSB repair, in particular through its direct interaction with the eukaryotic homolog of the prokaryotic RecA protein (RAD51). The binding of BRCA2 to RAD51, is thought to be essential for HR to take place. Recent work suggests that BRCA2 not only brings RAD51 to the site of DNA damage but also has a role in regulating its DNA-binding activity, holding it in an inactive state when it is not needed.[27] BRCA2 may also have a role as a regulator of cell cycle progression, in particular at the mitotic checkpoint.[28]

Current Treatment of BRCA1/2-associated Cancers

Over the past 10 years the management of those identified as BRCA1/2 mutation carriers has focused on cancer prevention through prophylactic surgery and hormone therapy and early cancer detection through screening.[29]

Prophylactic oophorectomy (PO) reduces the risk of ovarian cancer by about 90%. Prophylactic bilateral mastectomy (PM) can reduce the risk of breast cancer by about 90%.[29] PO has also been shown to halve the risk of death from breast cancer, presumably through the anti-estrogen effect of a surgical menopause.

Despite these interventions, some BRCA1/2 carriers will develop cancer and many will already have cancer at the time their mutation status is diagnosed. The current treatment of patients with a BRCA-associated cancer is identical to that given to patients with the sporadic form of the same cancer. However, there is mounting evidence to suggest they should, in respect of systemic therapies, be treated differently. Several preclinical studies have shown BRCA1/2-deficient cell lines are more sensitive than BRCA1/2 wild-type controls to agents that cause DNA damage through DSBs or DNA cross-links, such as the platinums.[30] This sensitivity is not seen with the taxanes, which act on microtubules.[31] This is currently being investigated in BRCA1/2 mutation–associated metastatic breast cancer in a Cancer Research UK–sponsored randomized phase II clinical trial, randomizing patients to either carboplatin or the taxane–docetaxel.[32]

More recently, a potential novel strategy for treating these inherited cancers has emerged using inhibitors that target the nuclear enzyme poly(ADP-ribose) polymerase 1 (PARP-1).

PARP-1 and Its Functions

The PARP super-family was first identified over 40 years ago,[33] and to date, 17 members have been identified.[34] PARP-1 and PARP-2 are the only members known to be activated by DNA damage, and PARP-1, the best characterized, is the focus of this review.

PARP-1, 113 kDa nuclear enzyme, consists of six domains, A–F, and is illustrated in Figure 1. PARP-1 is expressed in all nucleated human cells except neutrophils[35] and is reported to be overexpressed in certain tumor types.[36] PARP-1 plays a crucial role in the repair of DNA SSBs via the base excision repair (BER) pathway.[34] PARP-1 binds with high affinity via its zinc finger DNA-binding domains to the site of SSBs (Fig. 2). Once bound it catalyzes the synthesis of the successive transfer of ADP-ribose units from the substrate nicotinamide adenine dinucleotide (NAD^+) to a variety of acceptor proteins, including PARP-1 itself, to produce linear and/or branched polymers of poly(ADP-ribose) (PAR). This poly(ADP-ribosyl)ation creates a negatively charged target at the SSB, which recruits the enzymes required to form the BER multiprotein complex. This complex is made up of XRCC1 (X-ray repair cross-complementing 1), DNA ligase III, and the DNA polymerase pol β. Following ADP-ribosylation, PARP-1 has reduced affinity for DNA and is released, opening up the chromatin and allowing access to the damaged site to the other repair complex proteins. The subsequent degradation of the PAR polymers is performed by poly(ADP-ribose) glycohydrolase (PARG).

The role of PARP-1 is not limited to SSB repair. It is also stimulated by DSBs and although

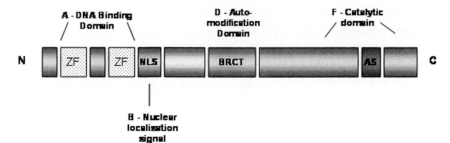

Figure 1. The structure of PARP-1: N terminal consists of a DNA-binding domain containing two zinc finger (ZF) motifs that are specific for DNA SSBs. Domain B contains a nuclear localization signal (NLS) domain and a caspase-3 cleavage site. Domain D is the automodification zone and contains a BRCA1 C terminus (BRCT) motif for interactions with BRCT on other BER proteins. Domain F, found at the C-terminal, is the catalytic domain and contains the active site (AS). To date the functions of domains C and E are not known.

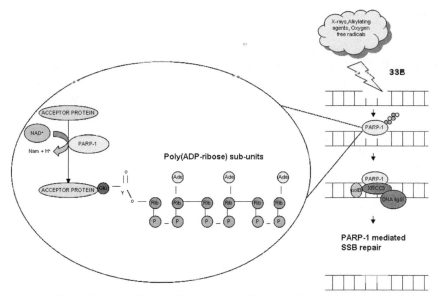

Figure 2. The role of PARP in SSB repair: Following DNA damage poly(ADP-ribose) polymerase (PARP), specifically PARP-1 and PARP-2, is activated and binds to the exposed SSB. Once bound it catalyzes the successive transfer of ADP-ribose units from the substrate NAD$^+$ (nicotinamide adenine dinucleotide) to a variety of acceptor nuclear proteins. The reaction is initiated by the formation of an ester bond between the amino acid receptor (Glu, Asp, COOH Lys). This produces linear and/or branched polymers of poly(ADP-ribose) (PAR). This "poly(ADP-ribosyl)ation" creates a negatively charged target at the SSB, which recruits the enzymes required for successful long or short patch base excision repair (BER) forming the BER multiprotein complex, which consists of XRCC1 (X-ray repair cross-complementing 1), DNA ligase III, and the DNA polymerase pol β (shown).

no *direct* role in the nonhomologous end joining (NHEJ) or HR pathways has been shown, roles in the DSB repair response and regulation have been proposed. Increased sister chromatid exchange and spontaneous RAD51 formation have been demonstrated in PARP-1$^{-/-}$ knockout mice, PARP-deficient cells lines, and after PARP inhibition in normal cells, suggesting an upregulation of the HR repair pathway.[37]

Activation of ATM, which is required for DSB repair, has also been observed following PARP inhibition.[38]

PARP-1 has also been shown to regulate gene transcription, mediate p53-regulated apoptosis, and initiate necrotic cell death in response to extensive DNA damage, such as that occurring after myocardial infarction, stroke, and septic shock.[39]

The Development of PARP Inhibitors

Over 20 years ago the first inhibitor of PARP, 3-aminobenzamide (3-AB), was identified following the observation that nicotinamide and 5-methylnicotinamide competed with NAD^+ as a PARP substrate.[40] 3-AB causes 96% PARP inhibition but requires millimolar intracellular concentrations to achieve this. Furthermore, it lacks specificity as it is also known to inhibit *de novo* purine synthesis.[41] Such shortcomings led to the development of more potent and more specific inhibitors, which inhibit PARP by the same mechanism: competitive inhibition of NAD^+. In the preclinical setting, inhibitors of PARP-1 have been shown to enhance the cytotoxic effects of ionizing radiation and DNA-damaging chemotherapy agents, such as monofunctional alkylating agents and topoisomerase I inhibitors.[42]

At the time of writing there are at least five PARP inhibitors in anticancer clinical trial development[43–46] (Table 2).

AG014699, an intravenous, potent, selective inhibitor of PARP-1, was the first PARP inhibitor to enter anticancer clinical trials. A phase I trial of AG014699 in combination with the oral alkylating agent temozolomide in patients with advanced cancers was completed in 2005.[43] No adverse effects were observed with AG014699 alone at any dose level. The recommended PARP inhibitory dose ($12 \, mg/m^2$) in combination with temozolomide ($200 \, mg/m^2$) was taken forward into a phase II trial in patients with metastatic melanoma. The results of this trial, published in abstract form only, report 7/40 partial responses (18%) and prolonged (>6 months) disease stabilization in 40% of patients.[44] AG014699 was shown to potentiate the myelosuppressive effects of temozolomide, but again, *no* specific toxic effects of single-agent AG014699 were observed.

Recent *in vitro* and *in vivo* evidence suggests that PARP inhibitors could be used not only as chemo/radiotherapy sensitizers, but as *single* agents to selectively kill cancers defective in DNA repair, specifically cancers with mutations in the BRCA genes.[47,48]

Increased Sensitivity of BRCA1/2 Mutated Cells to PARP Inhibitors

In 2005, two paired papers were published in *Nature* demonstrating the sensitivity of BRCA1- and BRCA2-deficient cell lines to different PARP inhibitors. The first paper, by Bryant and colleagues, used the PARP inhibitors NU1025 and AG14361, both forerunners to AG014699.[47] They demonstrated reduced survival of V-C8 (BRCA2-deficient) cell lines after continuous exposure to NU1025 or 24 hours exposure to AG14361. In mouse xenograft models, three out of five V-C8 tumors responded to a 5-day dosing of AG14361, with one mouse showing complete remission and no sign of tumor at autopsy. In V-C8 cell lines, after exposure to NU1025, an increase in γH2AX foci (representing DSB formation) was seen but not in RAD51 (indicating HR). They concluded that BRCA2-deficient cells were sensitive to PARP inhibition and that *monotherapy* with a DNA-repair inhibitor could selectively kill cancer cells. In the sister *Nature* paper, Farmer and colleagues demonstrated sensitivity of *both* BRCA1- and BRCA2-deficient cell lines to the specific inhibition of PARP-1 by two small-molecule PARP-1 inhibitors—KU0058684 and KU0058948.[48] They demonstrated that 24 hours exposure to the PARP inhibitor resulted in permanent G2/M cell-cycle arrest or apoptosis. The similar findings from two independent groups using different BRCA-deficient models and different chemical classes of PARP inhibitors suggest that this effect is definitely related to PARP

TABLE 2. PARP Inhibitors in Cancer Clinical Trial Development, 2007

Agent	Company	Route of administration	Clinical status	Ref (if published)
AG014699	Pfizer	Intravenous (i.v)	Phase I in combination with oral temozolomide in advanced solid malignancies—complete	43
			Phase II in combination with oral temozolomide in metastatic melanoma—complete	44
			Phase II as single agent in known BRCA1/2 mutation carriers with advanced breast/ovarian cancer—ongoing	
KU0059436/ AZD2281	AstraZeneca/ KuDOS	oral	Phase I as single agent in advanced solid malignancies including known BRCA patients—ongoing	45
			Phase II x2 as single agent in known BRCA1/2 mutation carriers with advanced breast and ovarian cancer—planned	
ABT-888	Abbott Laboratories	oral	Phase 0 as single agent in advanced solid tumors and hematological malignancies—ongoing	46
BSI-201	Bipar	intravenous	Phase I as single agent in advanced solid malignancies—ongoing	
INO-1001	Genentech/Inotek	intravenous	Phase Ib in combination with oral temozolomide in patients with newly diagnosed or recurrent stage III/IV melanoma—ongoing	
GPI 21016	MGI Pharma	oral	Phase I—planned	

inhibition. Farmer and colleagues also reported (data unpublished) a threefold increase in sensitivity over the DNA-damaging agent cisplatin for BRCA1/2-deficient cells.

First Clinical Evidence that BRCA1/2-Mutated Cancers May Be Sensitive to PARP Inhibitors

The first clinical evidence that BRCA-mutated cancers may be sensitive to PARP inhibitor monotherapy was presented at the 2007 American Society of Clinical Oncology meeting. Yap and co-workers presented preliminary data for the phase I trial of the oral, small-molecule PARP inhibitor, AZD2281

(previously known as KU-0059436).[45] In an enriched phase I population for BRCA mutation carriers, partial responses either radiological or by reduction in tumor markers were seen in 4 out of 10 evaluable ovarian cancer patients with confirmed BRCA1 mutations. Data for the BRCA mutation–associated breast cancers were too immature and therefore not presented.

Why Might PARP Inhibitors *Selectively* Kill BRCA1/2-Mutated Cancers?

Inhibition of PARP-1 leads to failure of SSB repair, which when encountered by a DNA replication fork will result in a DSB.[49] In

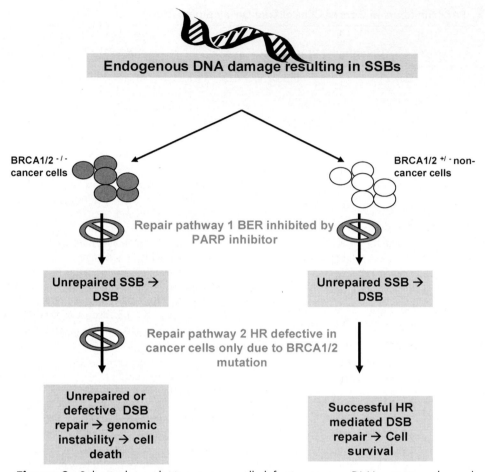

Figure 3. Selectively exploiting cancer cell defective in one DNA repair pathway by inhibiting another.

normal cells this DSB would be repaired by the error-free mechanism HR with no deleterious effect seen. However in cells in which HR is defective, such as the BRCA-mutated cells, repair is dependent on the upregulated more error-prone NHEJ pathway resulting in chromosome aberrations and loss of viability. In BRCA1/2-deficient cancers it is believed that only the cancer cells are homozygous for the mutation and that normal cells retain HR function via the sole functioning allele. Therefore, inhibition of BER by PARP inhibitors may be selectively lethal to cancer cells (Fig. 3). This hypothesis will be tested in forthcoming phase II clinical trials, which will treat proven BRCA1/2 mutation carriers suffering from advanced ovarian or breast cancer with PARP inhibitor monotherapy. The Pfizer compound

AG014699 will be tested in a combined phase II trial for patients with breast or ovarian cancer, whereas AZD2281 will be tested in separate trials for each cancer.

If the trials are positive, they will raise many more questions, such as whether PARP inhibitors can act as chemopreventative treatment in BRCA1/2 mutation carriers and whether there is a wider role for single-agent PARP inhibitors in sporadic cancers.

The Potential of PARP Inhibitors in Sporadic Breast/Ovarian Cancers

As previously stated, inherited genetic mutations account for only 5–10% of all breast/ovarian cancers. However, loss of BRCA1/2 function is not exclusive to inheriting a mutation in the BRCA1 or 2 genes. Epigenetic gene inactivation is a well-recognized mechanism by which the function of tumor suppressor genes can be silenced in the absence of mutation.[50] The most studied epigenetic event is the aberrant methylation of CpG islands found on gene promoters, which results in loss of transcription. Interestingly, aberrant methylation of the BRCA1 promoter is reported in 11–14% of sporadic breast cancers[51] and in up to 31% of ovarian cancers.[52] In addition, overexpression of the novel gene EMSY, which represses BRCA2 resulting in loss of function, has been observed in 13% of sporadic breast cancers and 17% of high-grade sporadic ovarian cancers.[53] Cancers with genetic or epigenetic defects in *other* components of the HR pathway, such as the Fanconi anemia genes, may confer sensitivity to PARP inhibitors. We know that Fanconi Anaemia Complementation Group F gene (FANCF) methylation occurs in many sporadic cancers including ovarian cancer.[54] If biomarkers could be developed to easily identify these "BRCA-like" sporadic tumors, the role of PARP inhibitors could be extended beyond the niche of genetic breast/ovarian malignancies. To date few such biomarkers exist and their development is the focus of much research.

Conclusions

PARP-1 represents an important novel target in cancer therapy. The PARP inhibitor AG014699 has successfully completed phase I and II clinical trials in combination with temozolomide, with no specific study-drug toxicity reported. Preclinical evidence and preliminary phase I data suggest that PARP inhibitors can be used not only as chemo/radiotherapy sensitizers but as single agents to selectively kill cancers defective in DNA repair. To be able to target cancer cells by selectively exploiting cells defective in one DNA repair pathway by inhibiting another represents a major potential breakthrough in the treatment of cancer. It may

mean efficacy without toxicity, the ultimate goal of any cancer therapy. We await the results of these ongoing clinical trials.

Conflicts of Interest

The authors declare no conflicts of interest.

References

1. Ries, L.A.G. *et al.* (Eds.). 2007. SEER Cancer Statistics Review, 1975–2004, National Cancer Institute, Bethesda, MD. http://seer.cancer.gov/csr/1975–2004/ (accessed May 25, 2007).
2. Malone, K., J.R. Daling, J.D. Thompson, *et al.* 1998. BRCA1 mutations and breast cancer in the general population: analyses in women before age 35 years and in women before age 45 years with first-degree family history. *JAMA* **279:** 922–929.
3. Kerlikowske, K., J.S. Brown & D.G. Grady. 1992. Should women with familial ovarian cancer undergo prophylactic oophorectomy? *Obstet. Gynecol.* **80:** 700–707.
4. Pharoah, P., N.E. Day, S. Duffy, *et al.* 1997. Family history and the risk of breast cancer: a systematic review and meta-analysis. *Int. J. Cancer* **71:** 800–809.
5. Stratton, J., S.A. Gayther, P. Russell, *et al.* 1997. Contribution of BRCA1 mutations to ovarian cancer. *N. Engl. J. Med.* **336:** 1125–1130.
6. Venkitaraman, A.R. 2002. Cancer susceptibility and the functions of BRCA1 and BRCA2. *Cell* **108:** 171–182.
7. The CHEK2 Breast Cancer Case-Control Consortium. 2004. CHEK2*1100delC and susceptibility to breast cancer: a collaborative analysis involving 10,860 breast cancer cases and 9,065 controls from 10 studies. *Am. J. Hum. Genet.* **74:** 1175–1182.
8. Malkin, D., F.P. Li, L.C. Strong, *et al.* 1990. Germ line p53 mutations in a familial syndrome of breast cancer, sarcomas and other neoplasms. *Science* **250:** 1233–1238.
9. Lynch, E.D., E.A. Ostermeyer, M.K. Lee, *et al.* 1997. Inherited mutations in PTEN that are associated with Breast Cancer, Cowden disease, and Juvenile Polyposis. *Am. J. Hum. Genet.* **61:** 1254–1260.
10. Renwick, A., D. Thompson, S. Seal, *et al.* 2006. ATM mutations that cause ataxia-telangiectasia are breast cancer susceptibility alleles. *Nat. Genet.* **38:** 873–875.
11. Giardiello, F.M., J.D. Brensinger, A.C. Tersmette, *et al.* 2000. Very high risk of cancer in familial Peutz-Jeghers syndrome. *Gastroenterology* **119:** 1447–1453.
12. Barroso, E., R.L. Milne, L.P. Fernandez, *et al.* 2006. FANCD2 associated with sporadic breast cancer risk. *Carcinogenesis* **27:** 1930–1937.

13. Aarnio, M., J. Mecklin, L.A. Aaltonen, *et al.* 1995. Lifetime risk of different cancers in hereditary non-polyposis colorectal cancer (HNPCC) syndrome. *Int. J. Cancer* **64:** 430–433.

14. Brose, M.S., T.R. Rebbeck, K.A. Calzone, *et al.* 2002. Cancer risk estimates for BRCA1 mutation carriers identified in a risk evaluation program. *J. Natl. Cancer Inst.* **94:** 1365–1372.

15. The Breast Cancer Linkage Consortium. 1999. Cancer risks in BRCA2 mutation carriers. *J. Natl. Cancer Inst.* **91:** 1310–1316.

16. Liede, A., B.Y. Karlan, S.A. Narod, *et al.* 2004. Cancer risks for male carriers of germline mutations in BRCA1 or BRCA2: A review of the literature. *J. Clin. Oncol.* **22:** 735–742.

17. Ford, D., D.F. Easton, D.T. Bishop, *et al.* 1994. Risks of Cancer in BRCA1-Mutation Carriers. *Lancet* **343:** 692–695.

18. Risch, H.A., J.R. Mclaughlin, D.E.C. Cole, *et al.* 2006. Population BRCA1 and BRCA2 mutation frequencies and cancer penetrances: a kin-cohort study in Ontario, Canada. *J. Natl. Cancer Inst.* **98:** 1694–1706.

19. Levy-Lahad, E., R. Catane, S. Eisenberg, *et al.* 1997. Founder BRCA1 and BRCA2 mutations in Ashkenazi Jews in Israel: frequency and differential penetrance in ovarian cancer and in breast-ovarian cancer families. *Am. J. Hum. Genet.* **60:** 1059–1067.

20. Knudson, A.G. 1971. Mutation and Cancer—Statistical Study of Retinoblastoma. *Proc. Natl. Acad. Sci. USA* **68:** 820–823.

21. Miki, Y., J. Swensen, D. Shattuck-Eidens, *et al.* 1994. A strong candidate for the breast and ovarian cancer susceptibility gene BRCA1. *Science* **266:** 66–71.

22. Wooster, R., G. Bignell, J. Lancaster, *et al.* 1995. Identification of the breast cancer susceptibility gene BRCA2. *Nature* **378:** 789–792.

23. Gudmundsdottir, K. & A. Ashworth. 2006. The roles of BRCA1 and BRCA2 and associated proteins in the maintenance of genomic stability. *Oncogene* **25:** 5864–5874.

24. Zhong, Q., C.F. Chen, S. Li, *et al.* 1999. Association of BRCA1 with the hRad50-hMre11-p95 complex and the DNA damage response. *Science* **285:** 747–750.

25. O'Driscoll, M. & P.A. Jeggo. 2006. The role of double-strand break repair—insights from human genetics. *Nat. Rev. Genet.* **7:** 45–54.

26. Stewart, G. & S.J. Elledge. 2002. The two faces of BRCA2, a FANCtastic discovery. *Mol. Cell.* **10:** 2–4.

27. Davies, A.A., J.-Y. Masson, M.J. Mcllwraith, *et al.* 2001. Role of BRCA2 in control of the RAD51 recombination and DNA repair protein. *Mol. Cell.* **7:** 273–282.

28. Marmorstein, L.Y., A.V. Kinev, G.K.T. Chan, *et al.* 2001. A human BRCA2 complex containing a structural DNA binding component influences cell cycle progression. *Cell* **104:** 247–257.

29. Domchek, S.M. & B.L. Weber. 2006. Clinical management of BRCA1 and BRCA2 mutation carriers. *Oncogene* **25:** 5825–5831.

30. Bhattacharyya, A., U.S. Ear, B.H. Koller, *et al.* 2000. The breast cancer susceptibility gene BRCA1 is required for subnuclear assembly of Rad51 and survival following treatment with the DNA cross-linking agent cisplatin. *J. Biol. Chem.* **275:** 23899–23903.

31. Tassone, P., P. Tagliaferri, A. Perricelli, *et al.* 2003. BRCA I expression modulates chemosensitivity of BRCA I-defective HCC1937 human breast cancer cells. *Br. J. Cancer* **88:** 1285–1291.

32. The BRCA Trial. Breakthrough breast cancer. Clinical trials. www.breakthroughresearch.org.uk (accessed July 21, 2008).

33. Chambon, P., J.D. Weill & P. Mandel. 1963. Nicotinamide mononucleotide activation of a new DNA-dependent polyadenylic acid synthesizing nuclear enzyme. *Biochem. Biopys. Res. Commun.* **11:** 39–43.

34. Schreiber, V., F. Dantzer, J.C. Ame, *et al.* 2006. Poly(ADP-ribose): novel functions for an old molecule. *Nat. Rev. Mol. Cell Biol.* **7:** 517–528.

35. Oei, S.L., H. Herzog, M. Hirschkauffmann, *et al.* 1994. Transcriptional regulation and autoregulation of the Human Gene for ADP-Ribosyltransferase. *Mol. Cell. Biochem.* **138:** 99–104.

36. Alderson, T. 1990. New targets for cancer chemotherapy: Poly(ADP- ribosylation) processing and Polyisoprene metabolism. *Biol. Rev.* **65:** 623–641.

37. Schultz, N., E. Lopez, N. Saleh-Gohari, *et al.* 2003. Poly(ADP-ribose) polymerase (PARP-1) has a controlling role in homologous recombination. *Nucleic Acids Res.* **31:** 4959–4964.

38. Bryant, H.E. & T. Helleday. 2006. Inhibition of poly(ADP-ribose) polymerase activates ATM which is required for subsequent homologous recombination repair. *Nucleic Acids Res.* **34:** 1685–1691.

39. Kim, M.Y., T. Zhang, L. Kraus, *et al.* 2005. Poly(ADP-ribosyl)ation by PARP-1: 'PAR-laying' NAD (+) into a nuclear signal. *Genes Dev.* **19:** 1951–1967.

40. Purnell, M.R. & W.J.D. Whish. 1980. Novel inhibitors of Poly(ADP-ribose) synthetase. *Biochem. J.* **185:** 775–777.

41. Milam, K.M. & J.E. Cleaver. 1984. Inhibitors of poly(adenosine diphosphate ribose) synthesis-effect on other metabolic processes. *Science* **223:** 589–591.

42. Calabrese, C.R., R. Almassay, S. Barton, *et al.* 2004. Anticancer chemosensitization and radiosensitization by the novel poly(ADP-ribose) polymerase-1 inhibitor AG14361. *J. Natl. Cancer Inst.* **96:** 56–67.

43. Plummer, R., M. Middleton, M.R. Wilson, *et al.* 2005. First in human phase I trial of the PARP inhibitor AG-014699 with Temozolomide (TMZ) in patients (pts) with advanced solid tumours. *Proc. Am. Soc. Clin. Oncol.* Abstract: 3065.

44. Plummer, R., P. Lorigan, J. Evans, *et al.* 2006. First and final report of a phase II study of the poly(ADP-ribose) polymerase (PARP) inhibitor, AG014699, in combination with Temozolomide (TMZ) in patients with metastatic malignant melanoma (MM). *Proc. Am. Soc. Clin. Oncol.* Abstract: 8013.

45. Yap, T.A., D.S. Boss, P.C. Fong, *et al.* 2007. First in human phase 1 pharmacokinetic and pharmacodynamic study of KU-0059436 (Ku), a small molecule inhibitor of Poly(ADP-ribose) polymerase (PARP) in cancer patients including BRCA1/2 mutation carriers. *Proc. Am. Soc. Clin. Oncol.* Abstract: 3529.

46. Kummar, S., R. Kinders, M. Gutierrez, *et al.* 2007. Inhibition of poly (ADP-ribose) polymerase (PARP) by ABT-888 in patients with advanced malignancies: results of a phase 0 trial. *J. Clin. Oncol.*, ASCO Annual Meeting Proceedings Part I. Vol 25, No. 18S (June 20 Supplement): 3518.

47. Bryant, H.E., N. Schultz, H.D. Thomas, *et al.* 2005. Specific killing of BRCA2-deficient tumours with inhibitors of poly(ADP-ribose) polymerase. *Nature* **434:** 913–917.

48. Farmer, H., N. McCabe, C.J. Lord, *et al.* 2005. Targeting the DNA repair defect in BRCA mutant cells as a therapeutic strategy. *Nature* **434:** 917–921.

49. Hoeijmakers, J.H.J. 2001. Genome maintenance mechanisms for preventing cancer. *Nature* **411:** 366–374.

50. Jones, P.A. & S.B. Baylin. 2002. The fundamental role of epigenetic events in cancer. *Nat. Rev. Genet.* **3:** 415–428.

51. Esteller, M., J.M. Silva, G. Dominguez, *et al.* 2000. Promoter hypermethylation and BRCA1 inactivation in sporadic breast and ovarian tumors. *J. Natl. Cancer Inst.* **92:** 564–569.

52. Baldwin, R.L., E. Nemeth, H. Tran, *et al.* 2000. BRCA1 promoter region hypermethylation in ovarian carcinoma: a population-based study. *Cancer Res.* **60:** 5329–5333.

53. Hughes-Davies, L., D. Huntsman, M. Ruas, *et al.* 2003. EMSY links the BRCA2 pathway to sporadic breast and ovarian cancer. *Cell* **115:** 523–535.

54. Kennedy, R.D. & A.D. D'Andrea. 2006. DNA repair pathways in clinical practice: lessons from pediatric cancer susceptibility syndromes. *J. Clin. Oncol.* **24:** 3799–3808.

Validation of the European Organization for Research and Treatment of Cancer Quality of Life Questionnaires for Arabic-speaking Populations

Manal A. Awad,[a] Srdjan Denic,[b] and Hakam El Taji[c]

[a] University of Sharjah, Sharjah, United Arab Emirates

[b] United Arab Emirates University, Al Ain, United Arab Emirates

[c] Tawam Hospital, Al Ain, United Arab Emirates

Information about quality of life in patients with cancer in Arab populations in 21 countries is inadequate. The objective of this study was to assess the psychometric properties of the Arabic version of the European Organization for Research and Treatment of Cancer (EORTC) general quality of life questionnaire (QLQ-C30) and of the breast cancer–specific questionnaire (QLQ-BR23) in Arab breast cancer patients. The questionnaires were administered to 87 breast cancer patients 3 months after surgery. The mean age of patients was 48.6 years (SD: 9.9), 76% were married, all had staged disease (I, 9%; II, 46%; III, 44%; IV, 1%). The percentage of patients who underwent mastectomy and lumpectomy were 49% and 51%, respectively. Questionnaire reliability was assessed using Cronbach's alpha coefficient, in which the values were all >0.7, with the exception of cognitive function and pain in the QLQ-C30 (Cronbach's alpha 0.67 and 0.51, respectively) and breast symptoms in the QLQ-BR23 (Cronbach's alpha 0.50). The questionnaires' validity was confirmed using "known group comparisons," which showed that the QLQ-C30 discriminated between mastectomy and lumpectomy patients on the emotional and cognitive function scales ($P < 0.001$) and QLQ-BR23 discriminated as well on the function scales and for systemic side effects ($P < 0.001$). For the most part, QLQ-C30 and QLQ-BR23 distinguished clearly between subgroups of patients differing in their Hospital Anxiety and Depression Scale. In summary, the Arabic versions of the EORTC QLQ-C30 and QLQ-BR23 are reliable and valid tools for assessment of quality of life in Arab patients with cancer.

Key words: breast cancer; quality of life; European Organization for Research and Treatment of Cancer (EORTC); QLQ-BR23; Hospital Anxiety and Depression Scale (HADS)

Introduction

Breast cancer diagnosis and treatment are often associated with psychological distress and reduced quality of life (QoL).[1–3] Studies of the QoL of cancer patients can identify subgroups of patients at the greatest risk of psychological morbidity, who could benefit from interventions designed to assist them in coping with the disease and its treatment.[3,4] In Arabic-speaking countries, which comprise 300 million people in 21 countries, QoL of patients with cancer is inadequately studied. The European Organization for Research and Treatment of Cancer (EORTC) has developed several questionnaires to assess QoL. Among these are a 30-item general QoL questionnaire for all cancer patients (QLQ-C30)[5] and disease-specific questionnaires, including one for breast cancer (QLQ-BR23).[2] The English-language

Address for correspondence: Manal Awad, PhD, College of Dentistry, University of Sharjah, UAE. Voice: +971-6-5057306. awad@sharjah.ac.ae versions of these questionnaires were successfully tested[2,5] and translated into several languages.[1,6-9] The QLQ-C30 and QLQ-BR23 questionnaires were previously translated into Arabic but were not efficiently validated for use in Arabic-speaking patients.

Studies have shown that patient-based outcomes could be affected by cultural experiences and ethnic backgrounds.[10,11] An individual's perception and evaluation of symptoms, psychological well-being, and social functioning are likely to be affected by culture, beliefs, and values. For example, perceptions of illness in Western societies tend to be organized around dimensions of severity and contagion. In Eastern cultures, such as India and China, illness perception also includes spiritual and psychological dimensions.[11] Arab women share a unique set of cultural norms and beliefs. Therefore, assessment of QoL in breast cancer patients after treatment, may reveal findings that will ultimately require different approaches for assistance in coping with their condition. For these reasons, an important first step is to evaluate the psychometric properties of QoL questionnaires for future use in Arab populations. Although the QLQ-C30 questionnaire was previously tested among Moroccan cancer patients in the Netherlands,[6] 50% of these patients did not speak the standard Arabic language. Therefore, the main objective of the present study is to assess the validity and reliability of the standard Arabic version of the general (QLQ-C30) and breast-specific (QLQ-BR23) questionnaires in an Arab breast cancer population.

Patients and Methods

From September 2005 to December 2006, 87 women of Arabic origin who had a confirmed diagnosis of breast cancer and attended the Breast Cancer Clinic at Tawam Hospital, Al Ain, United Arab Emirates, were recruited in the study. The hospital is the principal oncology center in the country, with an estimated 85% catchment of all patients with cancer nationally. Patients suffering from any serious psychiatric disorder, such as psychosis, untreated major depression, and severe personality disorder, were excluded. Data were collected from patients 3 months after surgical treatment. The study protocol was approved by the Research and Ethics Committee at the University of Sharjah and the Ethics Committee at Tawam Hospital.

Data Collection

Data on tissue diagnosis, cancer stage, and treatment were obtained from the Tumor Registry located in the hospital. Cancer staging criteria were as per the fifth edition of the American Joint Committee on Cancer. All interviews were conducted by a single female Arab nurse, trained in oncology patient care, in the outpatient department of the hospital.

Health Related Quality of Life Questionnaires

The Arabic version of the QLQ-C30 was developed and translated by the EORTC.[5] This questionnaire assesses general QoL using five functional scales (physical, role, cognitive, emotional, and social), three symptom scales (fatigue, pain, and nausea and vomiting), and a single global health status/QoL scale. In addition, the questionnaire contains five symptom scales that are commonly reported by cancer patients (dyspnea, loss of appetite, insomnia, constipation, and diarrhea) and the perceived financial impact of the disease scale. The Arabic version of the QLQ-BR23 comprises two functional scales (body image and sexuality), three symptom scales (arm symptoms, breast symptoms, and systemic therapy side effects), a single item that measures sexual enjoyment, and another that assesses future perspective.[2] Due to cultural considerations, only married women were asked about sexual function. The scoring algorithm recommended by the EORTC[12] was used to analyze participants' responses to the QLQ-C30 and QLQ-BR23 questionnaires. In summary, the algorithm creates an average from component item responses and then transforms this to a value on a 0–100 scale. For the functional and global QoL scales, a higher score corresponds to better function and QoL. For symptom scales, a higher score corresponds to more frequent and/or a more intense symptoms.

Hospital Anxiety and Depression Scale (HADS)

The HADS is a 14-item scale designed to detect anxiety and depression, independent of somatic symptoms.[13] The reliability and validity of the Arabic version of the HADS questionnaire has been previously tested.[14] It has two, 7-item subscales measuring depression and anxiety. Each item is assessed on a 4-point response scale (from 0, representing absence of symptoms, to 3, representing maximum symptomatology) with possible scores for each subscale ranging from 0 to 21. Higher scores indicate higher levels of anxiety and depression.

Statistical Analysis

Reliability

The internal consistency of the Arabic versions of both QLQ-C30 and QLQ-BR23 questionnaires was assessed for the multi-item questionnaire scales using Cronbach's alpha coefficients. Internal consistency of a magnitude of 0.70 or greater was sought.

Multitrait Scaling

Multitrait scaling analysis was used to examine the extent to which items of the questionnaire could be combined into the hypothesized multi-item scales. This technique is based on item–scale correlations. Evidence of item-convergent validity was defined as a correlation of ≥0.40 between an item and its own scale.

Validity

Two approaches were used to evaluate the validity of the QLQ-C30 and QLQ-BR23. The first approach involved clinical validity of the QLQ-C30 and QLQ-BR23 using "known group comparisons," which evaluate the extent to which the questionnaires are able to discriminate between clinical subgroups of patients. The clinical parameter used to form mutually exclusive patient subgroups was the type of previous surgery (mastectomy versus lumpectomy). Scores of each QoL scale were analyzed separately according to the type of treatment received, using the independent *t*-test. In the second approach, patients were categorized into three HADS scores according to their responses. The HADS scores are grouped into categories as 0–7 (normal), 8–10 (borderline anxious depressed), and 11–20 (probable case anxiety/depression).[13] Univariate analysis of variance (ANOVA) was performed to compare QLQ-C30 and QLQ-BR23 scores with these three groups in order to establish known groups (discriminate) validity. It is expected that patients with better HADS status would also report better QoL. To compensate for multiple testing, $P < 0.001$ was considered significant.

Results

The demographic and clinical characteristics of the 87 patients are shown in Table 1. The mean age was 48.6 (SD = 9.9) years, and most patients were married (76%). The majority of patients were diagnosed with stage 2 or 3 cancer (90%). In addition, a similar percentage of patients underwent mastectomy and lumpectomy (49% and 51%, respectively). Patients found the questionnaires acceptable and easy to understand.

Reliability

The internal consistency of multi-item scales (Cronbach's alpha coefficient) for both

TABLE 1. Sociodemographic and Clinical Characteristics of Patients

Characteristics	$N = 87$
Age, years, mean (SD)	48.6 (9.9)
Education:	
University degree complete/incomplete	52
Marital Status	
Married(%)	76
Stage of Cancer(%)	
Stage 1	9
Stage 2	46
Stage 3	44
Stage 4	1
Treatment (%)	
Mastectomy	49
Lumpectomy	51
Chemotherapy	89
Radiotherapy	86

TABLE 2. Descriptive Statistics and Scale Reliability of the QLQ-C30

Scale	Number of items	Mean (SD)	Cronbach's alpha value
Functional scales			
Physical	5	73.8 (22.6)	0.76
Role	2	82.5 (27.6)	0.84
Cognitive	4	74.0 (30.7)	0.67
Emotional	2	65.8 (32.8)	0.87
Social	2	85.1 (26.0)	0.79
Symptoms scales			
Fatigue	3	35.8 (30.5)	0.84
Nausea and vomiting	2	21.8 (33.4)	0.86
Pain	2	85.0 (26.9)	0.50
Dyspnea	1	21.1 (30.1)	
Sleep disturbance	1	44.7 (42.7)	
Appetite loss	1	31.8 (39.3)	
Constipation	1	25.20 (37.9)	
Diarrhea	1	11.24 (27.8)	
Financial impact	1	10.47 (26.7)	
Global quality of life	2	74.6 (18.0)	0.86

QLQ-C30 and QLQ-BR23 are shown in Tables 2 and 3. Reliability of six of eight multi-item scales in QLQ-C30 was high (Cronbach's alpha >0.7); less reliable were cognitive and pain scales (Cronbach's alpha of 0.67 and 0.50, respectively). In the QLQ-BR23 questionnaire, four of five multi-item scales were reliable; less reliable was the breast symptoms scale (Cronbach's alpha 0.51).

The correlations between the items in multi-item scales are shown in Table 4. The correlation coefficient exceeded the 0.40 criterion for the item-convergent validity of role functioning, cognitive functioning, social functioning, and fatigue (QLQ-C30). For the QLQ-BR23, the item–scale correlations exceeded the 0.40 criterion for body image, sexual functioning, systemic side effects, and arm symptoms.

Clinical Validity

Known Group Comparisons

Patients who underwent mastectomy reported significantly lower levels of emotional and cognitive functions, as well as worse nausea and vomiting symptoms, than patients who had undergone lumpectomy ($P < 0.01$). In addi-

TABLE 3. Descriptive Statistics and Scale Reliability of the QLQ-BR23

Scale	Number of items	Mean (SD)	Cronbach's alpha value
Functional scales			
Body image	4	69.4 (26.5)	0.75
Sexual functioning	2	62.6 (28.7)	0.84
Sexual enjoyment	1	59.0 (31.8)	
Future perspective	1	47.3 (39.4)	
Symptoms scales			
Systemic side effects	7	38.4 (22.6)	0.72
Breast symptoms	4	21.4 (18.5)	0.51
Arm symptoms	3	32.0 (31.1)	0.78
Upset by hair loss	1	63.2 (13.5)	

tion, mastectomy patients reported significantly more side effects of treatment and arm symptoms ($P < 0.01$) (Table 5).

In general, patients who were more anxious and depressed (had higher HADS scores) were less functional and more symptomatic (in QLQ-C30 and QLQ-BR23 questionnaires) (Tables 6 and 7). Subgroup differences in the anxiety scores were observed in the symptom scales of both the QLQ-C30 (fatigue, pain, dyspnea, and loss of appetite) and

TABLE 4. Item-convergent Validity of the QLQ-C30 and QLQ-BR23

	Item–scale correlations
QLQ C30	
Functional scales	
Physical	0.31–0.72
Role	0.83
Cognitive	0.68
Emotional	0.60–0.87
Social	0.67
Symptoms scales	
Fatigue	0.64–0.79
Pain	0.32
Nausea and vomiting	0.77
QLQ-BR23	
Functional scales	
Body image	0.22–0.77
Sexual	0.72
Symptoms scales	
Systemic therapy	0.30–0.55
Breast symptoms	0.13–0.40
Arm symptoms	0.50–0.62

TABLE 5. QLQ-C30 and QLQ-BR23 Scores according to Treatment Received*

	Lumpectomy mean (SD)	Mastectomy mean (SD)
QLQ-C30		
Global quality of life	74.4 (18.2)	75.0 (17.2)
Functional scales		
Physical	74.8 (23.4)	72.3 (19.7)
Role	89.2 (24.2)	75.4 (17.9)
Emotional	77.9 (27.3)	57.5 (34.2)*
Cognitive	84.6 (22.5)	65.0 (34.8)*
Social function	87.5 (24.7)	83.3 (25.6)
Symptom scales/items		
Fatigue	28.8 (28.3)	41.9 (32.1)
Nausea and vomiting	15.8 (31.3)	25.4 (34.6)*
Pain	22.2 (28.4)	31.6 (32.4)
Insomnia	39.2 (42.6)	52.5 (42.6)
Dyspnea	18.3 (27.2)	24.2 (32.0)
Loss of appetite	25.8 (38.1)	35.0 (39.9)
Constipation	23.1 (36.0)	24.2 (38.5)
Finance	09.4 (26.4)	11.7 (28.8)
Diarrhea	08.3 (23.6)	15.8 (32.9)
QLQ-BR23		
Functional scales		
Body image	77.5 (26.7)	66.7 (23.4)
Sexual functioning	55.2 (22.4)	61.3 (48.5)
Sexual enjoyment	60.6 (31.9)	59.7 (34.2)
Future perspective	55.8 (40.9)	40.8 (36.6)
Symptom scales/items		
Systemic side effects	30.9 (21.8)	44.0 (20.8)*
Breast symptoms	23.6 (17.7)	19.9 (18.3)
Arm symptoms	25.8 (28.6)	39.2 (32.2)
Upset by hair loss	57.9 (45.0)	65.7 (42.2)

*$P < 0.01$ for difference between treatments, based on independent t-test.

QLQ-BR23 (systemic side effects and arm symptoms) ($P < 0.001$). The depression scores of the HADS yield significant differences for the emotional, cognitive, and social function scales as well as fatigue and nausea in the QLQ-C30. Furthermore, lower levels of body image were significantly associated with higher levels of depression ($P < 0.001$).

Discussion

The EORTC QoL questionnaires (QLQ-C30 and QLQ-BR23) have been extensively used in clinical studies in Western populations.[2,4,5,15] We tested these instruments' psychometric characteristics in Arab women with breast cancer, and found them to be valid and reliable tools for QoL assessments.

In this study, interviews were conducted by one female interviewer, an Arabic-speaking oncology nurse. This facilitated the interviewing process and increased patient comfort. We found that the questions related to sexual function were acceptable to participants in this study. A similar observation was made in validation of the QLQ-BR23 questionnaire in Iranian women, who are expected in general to share many cultural characteristics with Arab patients.[1] This observation suggests that, among sexually active Arab patients with breast cancer, sexual counseling could be feasible. This is especially important because Arab patients with breast cancer in this and other studies[16,17] are relatively younger than Western patients.[5,18,19]

The mean time required for conducting the interviews was 15 min, the same time reported in studies from other countries.[1,7]

TABLE 6. Summary of ANOVA of the QLQ-C30 Functional and Symptom Scores by HADS Status

	HADS anxiety scores		
Scales	0–7 (n = 64) mean (SD)	8–10 (n = 15) mean (SD)	11–20 (n = 8) mean (SD)
Functional scales			
Physical	77.8 (21.6)	66.7 (19.2)	54.2 (25.6)*
Role	86.9 (22.7)	74.4 (36.1)	62.5 (12.8)
Emotional	74.87 (27.3)	45.6 (31.5)	65.8 (32.8)*
Cognitive	80.5 (26.5)	57.8 (33.3)	50.0 (40.8)
Social	77.8 (21.6)	66.7 (19.2)	54.2 (25.6)*
Symptom scales			
Fatigue	27.9 (24.7)	53.3 (36.2)	65.3 (32.2)*
Nausea and vomiting	15.1 (29.1)	38.9 (37.1)	43.8 (41.7)*
Pain	19.4 (25.3)	41.11 (27.4)	58.3 (42.8)*
Dyspnea	13.5 (25.0)	35.6 (32.0)	54.2 (35.3)*
Insomnia	36.5 (41.9)	71.1 (35.3)	58.3 (42.8)
Appetite loss	21.8 (33.7)	55.6 (39.1)	66.6 (47.2)*
Constipation	22.2 (36.9)	31.1 (38.2)	37.5 (45.2)
Diarrhea	06.3 (12.3)	35.6 (40.8)	4. 2 (11.8)
Financial difficulties	05.0 (20.3)	24.4 (36.7)	20.83 (39.6)

	HADS depression scores		
	0 7 (n = 61) mean (SD)	8–10 (n = 18) mean (SD)	11–20 (n = 8) mean (SD)
Functional scales			
Physical	76.8 (23.2)	70.4 (19.8)	56.2 (16.7)
Role	88.0 (22.8)	72.2 (34.8)	64.6 (32.7)
Emotional	77.7 (24.9)	39.4 (34.5)	34.4 (28.7)*
Cognitive	83.3 (24.7)	54.6 (34.2)	42.9 (28.6)*
Social	93.9 (18.0)	71.3 (26.7)	47.9 (32.7)*
Symptoms scales			
Fatigue	26.9 (25.1)	54.3 (36.5)	61.1 (20.6)*
Nausea and vomiting	15.6 (30.6)	32.4 (32.6)	45.8 (42.5)
Pain	20.3 (26.6)	33.3 (29.5)	62.5 (29.2)*
Dyspnea	13.7 (24.6)	35.2 (33.3)	45.8 (39.6)*
Insomnia	35.6 (42.6)	64.8 (37.0)	66.7 (35.6)
Appetite loss	21.8 (34.8)	50.0 (40.0)	66.7 (39.8)*
Constipation	21.7 (36.3)	38.88 (44.6)	20.8 (30.5)
Diarrhea	7.2 (22.9)	13.8 (33.5)	37.5 (37.5)
Financial difficulties	6.1 (20.8)	20.4 (34.56)	20.83 (39.6)

*$P < 0.001$ for ANOVA among three groups.

Overall, the reliability and validity of the QLQ-C30 and QLQ-BR23 are satisfactory. In general, the internal reliability of both scales was high. This is confirmed by the Cronbach's alpha values that exceeded 0.70 for all scales except those for pain (0.50) and cognitive func- tion (0.68). The latter finding is similar to that in a recent validation of the QLQ-C30 among Moroccan cancer patients.[12] The highest value of Cronbach's alpha for the QLQ-BR23 was found for sexual functioning (alpha: 0.84), a finding previously reported among

TABLE 7. Summary of ANOVA of the QLQ-BR23 Functional and Symptom Scores by HADS Status

	HADS anxiety scores		
Scales	0–7 (n = 64) mean (SD)	8–10 (n = 15) mean (SD)	11–20 (n = 8) mean (SD)
Functional scales			
Body image	73.1 (26.7)	59.8 (23.5)	69.5 (26.6)
Sexual function	59.9 (29.9)	68.5 (26.9)	71.4 (23.0)
Sexual enjoyment	56.6 (32.8)	66.7 (29.8)	73.3 (27.9)
Future perspective	56.1 (39.2)	26.7 (25.8)	16.7 (35.6)
Symptoms scales			
Systemic side effects	31.0 (18.4)	59.8 (19.2)	59.5 (23.2)*
Breast symptoms	18.5 (17.1)	26.7 (18.7)	34.3 (23.3)
Arm symptoms	23.9 (27.1)	58.5 (25.7)	50.0 (34.6)*
Upset by hair loss	59.8 (44.9)	76.9 (34.4)	66.7 (47.1)
	HADS depression scores		
	0–7 (n = 61) mean (SD)	8–10 (n = 18) mean (SD)	11–20 (n = 8) mean (SD)
Functional scales			
Body image	78.0 (22.8)	52.9 (23.3)	41.7 (25.5)*
Sexual function	59.5 (29.7)	71.7 (26.1)	69.4 (24.5)
Sexual enjoyment	56.6 (32.8)	66.7 (33.3)	75.0 (16.7)
Future perspective	56.3 (40.6)	27.5 (29.4)	20.8 (17.3)*
Symptoms scales			
Systemic side effects	32.4 (20.7)	46.1 (18.2)	66.1 (20.3)*
Breast symptoms	16.9 (14.9)	26.9 (22.1)	42.7 (18.1)*
Arm symptoms	21.7 (25.2)	51.9 (30.3)	69.4 (20.4)*
Upset by hair loss	56.2 (45.7)	83.3 (32.2)	70.8 (37.5)

*$P < 0.001$ for ANOVA among groups.

Iranian and Western women.[1,2] This suggests that sex-related determinants of QoL are perceived similarly by patients with different cultural backgrounds.

The validity of the Arabic version of the QLQ-C30 was evident by its ability to discriminate between subgroups of patients known to differ in clinical status. The role function subscale, which measures the effect of the disease on the ability to carry out job and home duties, discriminated well between lumpectomy and mastectomy patients. This finding is consistent with previous studies in Western patients with breast cancer.[4,20]

Overall QoL of Arab women who underwent mastectomy was not different from those who received lumpectomy. These findings are in agreement with those reported among Australian patients with breast cancer.[18] This indicates that patients' perceptions extend beyond the negative physical and functional impact of cancer to the individuals' perceptions of their general well-being.

Previous QoL studies in breast cancer reported that body image, after treatment, was more negatively affected by more extensive surgery, and morbidity was higher after mastectomy.[1] However, in this study, the body-image scale ratings were the same for patients who had mastectomy and those who underwent lumpectomy. Nonetheless, high levels of depression were, as expected, associated with significantly lower ratings of body image. The latter finding provides additional evidence that the QLQ-BR23 questionnaire is able to discriminate between subgroups of patients according to their performance on the HADS scale.

A limitation of the study is that the EORTC general QoL questionnaire QLQ-C30 was tested only in patients with breast cancer. This questionnaire is applicable to all cancer patients, and we are planning to conduct additional testing on a larger group of Arab patients with different types of malignancies.

In summary, the Arabic versions of the QLQ-C30 and QLQ-BR23 questionnaires have acceptable reliability and validity, which are comparable to those reported in other languages.[1,7,8] This will permit their use among Arabic-speaking patients and allow identification of subgroups of patients most in need of emotional support. In addition, both questionnaires could be used in clinical trials that evaluate the impact of specific interventions on the QoL of Arab patients with breast cancer.

Acknowledgments

The authors wish to thank the EORTC Study Group on Quality of Life for providing the Arabic translation of the QLQ-C30 and QLQ-BR23. Special thanks to Ms. Reema Khalil for conducting the interviews. We are also grateful for the financial support received from Sheikh Hamdan Bin Rashed Al Maktoum Awards for Medical Sciences and University of Sharjah Grant Office.

Conflicts of Interest

The authors declare no conflicts of interest.

References

1. Montazeri, A., I. Harirchi, M. Vahdani, *et al.* 2000. The EORTC breast cancer-specific quality of life questionnaire (EORTC QLQ-BR23): translation and validation study of the Iranian version. *Qual. Life Res.* **9:** 177–184.

2. Sprangers, M.A., M. Groendvold, J.I. Arraras, *et al.* 1996. The European Organization for Research and Treatment of Cancer cancer specific quality-of-life questionnaire module: first results from a three country field study. *J. Clin. Oncol.* **14:** 2756–2768.

3. Goodwin, P.J., M. Ennis, L.J. Bordeleau, *et al.* 2004. Health-related quality of life and psychological status in breast cancer prognosis: analysis of multiple variables. *J. Clin. Oncol.* **22:** 4184–4192.

4. Coates, A., F. Porzosolt & D. Osoba. 1997. Quality of life in oncology practice: prognostic value of EORTC QLQ-C30 scores in patients with advanced malignancy. *Eur. J. Cancer* **33:** 1025–1030.

5. Aaronson, N.K., S. Ahmedzai, B. Bergman, *et al.* 1993. The European Organization for Research and Treatment of Cancer QLQ-C30: a quality of life instrument for use in international clinical trials in oncology. *J. Natl. Cancer Inst.* **85:** 365–376.

6. Hoopman, R., M.J. Muller, C.B. Terwee, *et al.* 2006. Translation and validation of the EORTC QLQ-C30 for use among Turkish and Moroccan ethnic minority cancer patients in the Netherlands. *Eur. J. Cancer* **42:** 1839–1847.

7. Kyriaki, M., T. Eleni, P. Efi, *et al.* 2001. The EORTC Core Quality of Life questionnaire (QLQ-C30, version 3.0) in terminally ill cancer patients under palliative care: validity and reliability in a Hellenic sample. *Int. J. Cancer* **94:** 135–139.

8. Chie, W.C., K.J. Chang, C.S. Huang, *et al.* 2003. Quality of life of breast cancer patients in Taiwan: validation of the Taiwan Chinese version of the EORTC QLQ-C30 and EORTC-BR23. *Psychooncology* **12:** 729–735.

9. Zhao, H. & K. Kanda. 2000. Translation and validation of the standard Chinese version of the EORTC QLQ-C30. *Qual. Life Res.* **9:** 129–137.

10. Bates, M.S., L. Rankin-Hill & M. Sanchez-Ayendez. 1997. The effects of the culture context of health care on treatment of and response to chronic pain and illness. *Soc. Sci. Med.* **45:** 1433–1447.

11. Taleghani, F., Z. Parsa & A.N. Nasrabadi. 2006. Coping with breast cancer in newly diagnosed Iranian women. *J. Adv. Nurs.* **54:** 265–272.

12. Fayer, P., N. Aaronson, S. Bordal, *et al.* 1995. EORTC-C30 scoring manual. Brussels: EORTC Study Group on Quality of Life.

13. Zigmond, A.S. & R.P. Snaith. 1983. The hospital anxiety and depression scale. *Acta Psychiatr. Scand.* **67:** 361–370.

14. El-Rufai, O.E.F. & G. Absood. 1987. Validity study of the Hospital Anxiety and Depression Scale among a group of Saudi patients. *Br. J. Psych.* **151:** 687–688.

15. Curran, D., J.P. van Dongen, N.K. Aaronson, *et al.* 1998. Quality of life of early stage breast cancer patients treated with radical mastectomy or breast-conserving procedures: results of EORTC Trial 10801. The European Organization for Research and Treatment of cancer (EORTC), Breast Cancer Co-operative Group (BCCG). *Eur. J. Cancer* **34:** 307–314.

16. Nissan, A., R.M. Spira, T. Hamburger, *et al.* 2004. Clinical profile of breast cancer in Arab and Jewish women in the Jerusalem area. *Am. J. Surg.* **188:** 62–67.

17. Ibrahim, E.M., F.A. al-Mulhim, A. Al-Amir, *et al.* 1998. Breast cancer in the eastern province of Saudi Arabia. *Med. Oncol.* **15:** 241–247.

18. King, M.T., P. Kenny, J. Shiell, *et al.* 2000. Quality of life three months and one year after first treatment for early stage breast cancer: influence of treatment and patient satisfaction. *Qual. Life Res.* **9:** 789–800.

19. Efficace, F., L. Biganzoli, M. Piccart, *et al.* 2004. Baseline health-related quality-of-life data as prognostic factors in a phase III multicentre study of women with metastatic breast cancer. *Eur. J. Cancer* **40:** 1021–1030.

20. Bottomely, A., P. Therasse, P. Piccart, *et al.* 2005. Health-related quality of life in survivors of locally advanced breast cancer: an international randomised controlled phase III trial. *Lancet Oncol.* **6:** 287–294.

Laparoscopy in Gastrointestinal Malignancies

Fawaz Chikh Torab,[a] **Bernard Bokobza,**[b] **and Frank Branicki**[a]

[a]*Department of Surgery, Faculty of Medicine & Health Sciences, UAE University, Al Ain, United Arab Emirates*

[b]*Hospital Group of Le Havre, Le Havre, France*

This paper presents an update of the role of minimally invasive surgery (MIS) in gastrointestinal malignancy. A review of indications, surgical technique, and radicality of laparoscopy in the field of gastrointestinal cancer surgery is discussed. The feasibility and safety of laparoscopic procedures are compared with established and implemented standards in the diagnosis and treatment of oncological disorders. It is important to appreciate that only the "access" is different with all its attendant advantages. The use of laparoscopy in tumor staging and palliative and curative resection is evaluated on review of the literature, and special indications for a laparoscopic approach in gastrointestinal malignancy in different organs are discussed. In conclusion, MIS is safe and feasible, with many short-term advantages; long-term results should be further assessed in randomized controlled studies. Until the outcomes of such studies are available MIS for malignant disease should be performed by experienced surgeons in specialized centers.

Key words: gastrointestinal tract; malignancy; laparoscopy

Introduction

Endoscopic surgery has now been accepted in general and subspecialty surgical interventions, and this is regarded as a milestone in surgical practice. However, the new videoendoscopic surgical methods still require critical appraisal, especially in surgical oncology. This is attributable mainly to a lack of long-term survival data and to the technical difficulties encountered at operation, such as lymph node dissection. For these reasons, minimally invasive cancer surgery has largely been performed only in specialized centers by surgeons with sufficient experience in the field. The efficacy of various procedures is still being evaluated in the context of multicenter studies. With the development of modern instruments, such as high-resolution cameras, projection of the procedure on a monitor, and use of computer-controlled (robotic) devices, endoscopic surgery is regarded as so-called high-tech medicine. This kind of surgery has become more popular with patients as information relating to these new developments finds its way into the public domain.

Despite the above-mentioned advantages of minimally invasive surgical procedures, there are particular indications and limitations. In this article we highlight some examples of the implementation of minimally invasive surgery (MIS) in the field of gastrointestinal oncology.

Tumor Staging

If preoperative oncological assessment in patients with suspected abdominal malignancy is not able to identify metastatic disease, the use of laparoscopy will often help to correctly stage the disease and to prevent unnecessary laparotomy in these patients. Staging laparoscopy

Address for correspondence: Dr. Fawaz Chikh Torab, Department of Surgery, Faculty of Medicine and Health Sciences, UAE University, P. O. Box 17666, Al Ain, UAE. Voice: +00971-3-7137578; fax: +00971-3-7672067. ftorab@uaeu.ac.ae

Ann. N.Y. Acad. Sci. 1138: 155–161 (2008). © 2008 New York Academy of Sciences.
doi: 10.1196/annals.1414.022

prevented a nontherapeutic laparotomy in 10% of patients submitted to operation for potentially curative partial hepatectomy and in 33% of patients scheduled for pump placement only.[1] Preventing unnecessary laparotomy with laparoscopy was associated with decreased hospital stay and early administration of systemic chemotherapy.[1] In pancreatic cancer, stratification of patients into those with locally advanced disease alone and those with metastatic disease is imperative for accurate evaluation of treatment outcomes. Shoup and colleagues showed that neither primary tumor size nor location influenced the incidence of metastatic disease.[2] Laparoscopy identified metastatic disease not seen on preoperative imaging in 37% of patients. Staging investigations precluded resection in one-third of patients with esophagogastric carcinoma, the greatest yield being for laparoscopy in gastric carcinoma.[3]

The limitation of laparoscopy in oncology is that it can fail, even with the addition of laparoscopic ultrasound (LUS), to identify metastatic disease. Following computed tomography, 15% of patients with metastatic colorectal carcinoma were found to have unresectable disease. Laparoscopy had identified only half of this group. Laparoscopy was of no greater value in staging synchronous compared with metachronous metastases.[4] In a retrospectively analyzed study,[5] the efficacy of diagnostic laparoscopy (DL) combined with LUS for liver malignancies was assessed in the light of improved imaging and revised criteria for resection. DL combined with LUS was, in this study, an adequate staging modality for primary liver malignancies, but of lower efficacy for colorectal liver metastasis because of more liberal resection criteria, a high failure rate due to adhesions from previous surgery, and better preoperative imaging. Tumor location will also affect the efficacy of DL. All of the staging failures in patients with gastroesophageal junction carcinomas were related to posterior tumor extension into the lesser sac.[3] The surgeon's experience plays a major role in such circumstances. A detailed examination of the whole abdominal cavity (peritoneum, omentum, colon, bowel, and liver) is recommended. Even during laparoscopic cholecystectomy, abdominal malignancies can be missed.[6]

Palliative Surgery

For unresectable tumors, laparoscopy can provide accurate staging of the disease along with the opportunity, at the same time, to perform a palliative procedure, thus avoiding laparotomy. A laparoscopic approach can be used safely and effectively to perform palliative gastrojejunostomy for advanced recurrent gastric cancer after Billroth I resection, or for unresectable pancreatic cancer.[7,8]

Laparoscopy has gained acceptance in the field of palliative care without the need for controlled studies.[9] Obvious examples of palliative resections are distal gastrectomy in the presence of liver metastasis, left colon resection to avoid obstructive symptoms, and rectal resection to control hemorrhage at anastomotic or other sites.

MIS was used to facilitate other palliative treatment modalities, such as radiofrequency thermal ablation for liver metastasis. In 2003, success was reported with laparoscopic radiofrequency ablation as an alternative to major hepatic resection in patients with a solitary hepatic gastrinoma[10] and with liver metastasis from colorectal cancer.[11] The laparoscopic approach is also used to safely place a hepatic artery infusion pump as a novel treatment option for patients with colorectal liver metastases.[12]

Laparoscopic gastric and biliary bypass and bilateral thoracoscopic splanchnicotomy have been combined to provide safe and effective minimally invasive palliation of incurable pancreatic cancer.[13] Gastrostomy is another example of the use of laparoscopy in palliative treatment for unresectable cancer of the head of the pancreas.[14]

Curative Resection

The application of a minimally invasive approach in the field of cancer surgery raised several outstanding questions regarding indications, surgical technique, the timing of conversion, radicality, oncological quality, value, advantages and disadvantages, and port-site metastasis, as well as the training of surgeons. In principle, established and implemented standards in the diagnosis, treatment, and postoperative management of tumors should not be neglected in the implementation of MIS. It is evident that it is only "access" that is different, with all its advantages, but this must not be pursued at the expense of principles of oncological treatment.

Thus, one of the important issues raised with the use of laparoscopic surgery in oncology is the need to maintain internationally accepted oncological standards and quality control. In colon cancer, the prognosis of T3N0 tumors is dependent on the number of lymph nodes examined. This was concluded from a prospective study of 35,787 patients with T3N0 colon cancer who were surgically treated and reported between 1985 to 1991.[15] In this study, the 5-year relative survival rate for T3N0M0 colon cancer varied from 64% if one or two lymph nodes were examined to 86% if >25 lymph nodes were retrieved. A minimum of 13 lymph nodes should be examined to label a T3 colon cancer as node negative. The question is whether the laparoscopic approach will yield enough lymph nodes at resection to provide sufficient prognostic information.

The second issue is to evaluate the oncological value of laparoscopic approach. In a prospective observational, multicenter study of 500 operations, of which 231 (46%) were performed for cancer, significant differences were noted between participating centers in relation to the number of lymph nodes resected.[16] The mean number of lymph nodes harvested was 13 (11.5–14.6) with 2.2 (0.9–3.4) positive lymph nodes harvested. The mean distal resection margin was 39 (33–45) mm, and in eight of these resections there was a positive margin. The conclusion of the study was that the oncological results of laparoscopic colorectal procedures for cancer were similar to those obtained at laparotomy, but these differ among centers and depend on surgical experience.

Many advantages of laparoscopic surgery have been proven in numerous studies. The extent of lymphadenectomy after laparoscopic distal gastrectomy for gastric cancer is sufficient for adequate TNM classification; however, the number of lymph nodes harvested by the open approach was reported to be significantly higher.[17] In a multi-institutional study comparing laparoscopic colectomy and open surgery for cancer, the rates of recurrent cancer at 3 years were similar (16% versus 18%, respectively, $P = 0.32$). This study suggested that the laparoscopic approach is an acceptable alternative to open surgery for colon cancer.[18] When using a laparoscopic approach for colorectal surgery, the blood loss measured by estimated losses, fall in hemoglobin level, and transfusion requirements is significantly less than for matched open colectomy (OC) cases.[19] Laparoscopy-assisted colectomy (LAC) has been shown to be superior to OC for treatment of colon cancer in terms of morbidity, hospital stay, tumor recurrence, and cancer-related survival.[20]

One of the prerequisites for the use of laparoscopic approach for resection of malignant disease is the need for precise preoperative tumor staging using multiple modalities, including total colonoscopy, ultrasound, and CT scanning. Many developments to improve the accuracy of intraoperative staging, such as of intraoperative ultrasound during laparoscopic surgery, have been introduced. The possibility of conversion to open operation is another disadvantage of the laparoscopic approach. This rate varies between 5 and 20% depending on the bulk of the tumor, presence of carcinosis, difficulty in dissection, and the occasional difficulty encountered in localization of the tumor. The same problems are responsible for longer duration of operative procedures.

Incisional scar recurrence after curative resection has been a cause for concern. The known rate after laparotomy varies between 0.9 and 3.3%.[21,22] In a literature review of 20 studies performed between 1993 and 2000 in 3436 patients, the mean rate of port-site metastasis was 1.8% (range 0–21%). Three prospective randomized studies showed 0% port-site metastasis on follow-up at 17–21 months.[23–25] It is important to consider these findings carefully. The first studies regarding port metastasis were reported in the early 1990s, when experience with laparoscopy was very limited. The highest rates of port-site metastasis were reported after resection of Dukes B or C lesions, with only a few patients having Dukes A tumors. Higher rates were reported in multicenter studies when compared with a rate of <1% in single-center reports. This led to postulation that the rate of port-site metastasis is reduced with increasing experience. The suggested mechanisms for tumor implantation in the port site are tumor cell spillage by surgical manipulation, contamination of instruments, changes in the peritoneal surface due to carbon dioxide and increased intraperitoneal pressure, CO_2-induced immune modulation and stimulation of cell growth, a chimney effect with gas leakage/ischemia, and necrosis at port sites.

Results of Laparoscopic Surgery in Different Tumor Sites

Esophagus

The advantage of using laparoscopy in the transhiatal approach for subtotal esophagectomy is that the dissection clearly visualizes the azygos vein.[26] A thoracoscopic or a thoracoscopic-assisted approach is very useful in achieving tumor mobilization and retrieval of lymph nodes.[27,28] Thoracoscopy can also be performed in the prone position.[26]

Stomach

The laparoscopic approach is used mainly for subtotal gastrectomy. Laparoscopy-assisted subtotal gastrectomy and D2 lymph node dissection is safe and effective in terms of morbidity and meets oncological principles.[29] Laparoscopy-assisted distal gastrectomy has been found to be superior to conventional open distal gastrectomy for early gastric cancer in relation to estimated blood loss, acute-phase systemic response, and the rate of postoperative complications.[30,31] Comparing obese and nonobese patients with early gastric cancer who underwent laparoscopic gastrectomy, there was no significant difference in regards to hospital stay and postoperative morbidity.[32]

Liver

Laparoscopy has recently been introduced for use in hepatic surgery. It can be performed safely and efficaciously and appears to provide several distinct advantages over traditional open hepatic operations. There is still a need to develop the technique to better control hemorrhage and avoid bile leakage.[33] Hand-assisted laparoscopic partial hepatectomy has been shown to be safe and feasible for primary liver cancer when performed in selected patients.[34] Small tumors located in the left-lateral segment are the most appropriate for the laparoscopic approach. This highly advanced laparoscopic surgery requires experience and the availability of technologies for safe dissection of liver parenchyma.[35] In a study comparing 30 laparoscopic liver resections (LLR) with 30 open liver resections (OLR), minor LLR of anterior segments has shown the same rates of morbidity and mortality as OLR. However, the laparoscopic approach reduces blood loss and postoperative hospital stay.[36]

Pancreas

A laparoscopic approach has been employed for a growing number of pancreatic procedures since the early 1990s. These have been performed for a variety of lesions including chronic pancreatitis, pancreatic trauma, congenital hyperinsulinism, and pancreatic tumors.

A combination of laparoscopic pancreatic resection and an *en bloc* lymph node dissection has also been performed for invasive carcinoma. The long-term results after laparoscopic resection for invasive pancreatic cancer, however, are still not well documented. Based on retrospective analyses of collective series and case reports, the advantages of laparoscopic distal pancreatectomy are reduced postoperative pain, shorter hospital stay, a quicker return to normal activity, and better cosmesis. Laparoscopic proximal pancreatectomy is technically feasible, however, laparoscopic reconstruction is not yet generally accepted, and its performance is limited to the personal experiences of a small number of laparoscopic surgeons.[37,38] In a series of 27 patients with malignant pancreatic disease, resection with no macroscopic residual disease and clear resection margins (R0) was achieved in 90% of patients with ductal adenocarcinoma and in all of those with other malignant tumors. The median survival for patients with ductal adenocarcinoma was 14 months. This series demonstrated that laparoscopic pancreatic resection is feasible and safe and that it is suitable for lesions with a benign appearance as well as malignant neoplasms of the pancreas.[39]

Colon and Rectum

All kinds of colorectal resections are feasible laparoscopically. In a retrospective case-controlled study of right hemicolectomy for malignant disease comparing the laparoscopic approach with an age-matched and stage-matched series of patients who underwent open surgery, overall survival was not compromised after laparoscopic resection, with the advantage of a shorter period of postoperative ileus and decreased analgesic requirements.[40] A randomized study comparing the efficacy of LAC and OC for the treatment of nonmetastatic colon cancer has shown that LAC is superior to OC for the treatment of colon cancer in terms of morbidity, hospital stay, tumor recurrence, and cancer-related survival.[20] However, survival rates at 2 and 5 years were lower for patients in the converted group compared to patients with LAC.[41] Laparoscopic left colectomy was safely performed in obese patients without compounding technical difficulties or causing an adverse impact on postoperative outcomes.[42] In the case of acute colonic obstruction due to colorectal cancer, the use of endoscopic colonic stent insertion can effectively relieve obstruction, allowing safe elective surgery. The use of stents does not preclude a laparoscopic approach.[43,44] In a review of 48 studies comparing laparoscopic mesorectal excision (LTME) with open mesorectal excision, there was evidence that LTME results in less blood loss, a quicker return to normal diet, less pain, less narcotic usage, and a lesser immune response. LTME was associated with longer operative time and higher costs. No results relating to quality of life were reported.[45]

As mentioned above, laparoscopic colectomy for malignant disease is technically feasible, but the most important question still concerns long-term outcome. In a retrospective, multicenter study conducted in Japan to evaluate preliminary long-term results of laparoscopic surgery for colorectal cancer, of 1495 patients with colon cancer, cancer recurred in 61 (4.1%) of 1367 curatively treated patients with colon cancer (median follow-up period, 32 months; range, 6–125 months). The 5-year survival rate for patients with colon cancer was 96.7% for stage I, 94.8% for stage II, and 79.6% for stage III disease. Of 541 patients with rectal cancer, cancer recurred in 30 (5.6%) of 476 curatively treated patients with rectal cancer (median follow-up period, 25 months; range 6–102 months). The 5-year survival rate for patients with rectal cancer was 95.2% for stage I, 85.2% for stage II, and 80.8% for stage III disease. These findings indicate that laparoscopic surgery for colorectal cancer yields an oncological outcome as good as that reported for conventional open surgery in the Japanese Registry for all disease stages.[46]

Conclusion

Minimally invasive surgeons, who have enough experience in laparoscopy, have endeavored to perform laparoscopically a whole range of abdominal procedures for gastrointestinal malignancy, even in pediatric patients and pregnant women, including the most complicated procedures, such as a pancreatectomy or liver resection. It is doubtful whether all of these procedures are performed in the patients' best interests or rather just to satisfy surgical prowess—that every operation can be done using an MIS approach. In this paper, we have reviewed fields wherein results achieved by MIS are more rewarding or challenging, many difficulties being as yet unsolved in the field of surgical gastrointestinal oncology. Thus, it is essential that MIS oncological procedures be conducted within the confines of prospective randomized trials in centers that possess particular expertise in these techniques.

Conflicts of Interest

The authors declare no conflicts of interest.

References

1. Grobmyer, S.R., Y. Fong, M. D'Angelica, *et al.* 2004. Diagnostic laparoscopy prior to planned hepatic resection for colorectal metastases. *Arch. Surg.* **139:** 1326–1330.
2. Shoup, M., C. Winston, M.F. Brennan, *et al.* 2004. Is there a role for staging laparoscopy in patients with locally advanced, unresectable pancreatic adenocarcinoma? *J. Gastrointest. Surg.* **8:** 1068–1071.
3. Clements, D.M., D.J. Bowrey & T.J. Havard. 2004. The role of staging investigations for oesophagogastric carcinoma. *Eur. J. Surg. Oncol.* **30:** 309–312.
4. Koea, J., M. Rodgers, P. Thompson, *et al.* 2004. Laparoscopy in the management of colorectal cancer metastatic to the liver. *ANZ. J. Surg.* **74:** 1056–1059.
5. de Castro, S.M., E.H. Tilleman, O.R. Busch, *et al.* 2004. Diagnostic laparoscopy for primary and secondary liver malignancies: impact of improved imaging and changed criteria for resection. *Ann. Surg. Oncol.* **11:** 522–529.
6. Wysocki, A., W. Lejman & A. Bobrzynski. 2001. Abdominal malignancies missed during laparoscopic cholecystectomy. *Surg. Endosc.* **15:** 959–961.
7. Cogliandolo, A., G. Scarmozzino, R.R. Pidoto, *et al.* 2004. Laparoscopic palliative gastrojejunostomy for advanced recurrent gastric cancer after Billroth I resection. *J. Laparoendosc. Adv. Surg. Tech. A* **14:** 43–46.
8. Croce, E., S. Olmi, M. Azzola, *et al.* 1999. Surgical palliation in pancreatic head carcinoma and gastric cancer: the role of laparoscopy. *Hepatogastroenterology* **46:** 2606–2611.
9. Bruch, H.P., O. Schwandner & R. Keller. 2003. [Limitations of laparoscopic visceral surgery in oncology]. *Chirurg* **74:** 290–300.
10. Deol, Z.K., E. Frezza, S. DeJong & J. Pickleman. 2003. Solitary hepatic gastrinoma treated with laparoscopic radiofrequency ablation. *JSLS* **7:** 285–289.
11. Croce, E., S. Olmi, A. Bertolini, *et al.* 2003. Laparoscopic liver resection with radiofrequency. *Hepatogastroenterology* **50:** 2088–2092.
12. Cheng, J., D. Hong, G. Zhu, *et al.* 2004. Laparoscopic placement of hepatic artery infusion pumps: technical considerations and early results. *Ann. Surg. Oncol.* **11:** 589–597.
13. Ali, A.S. & B.J. Ammori. 2003. Concomitant laparoscopic gastric and biliary bypass and bilateral thoracoscopic splanchnotomy: the full package of minimally invasive palliation for pancreatic cancer. *Surg. Endosc.* **17:** 2028–2031.
14. Pelton, J.J. 1998. Routine diagnostic laparoscopy is unnecessary in staging tumors of the pancreatic head. *South. Med. J.* **91:** 182–186.
15. Swanson, R.S., C.C. Compton, A.K. Stewart & K.I. Bland. 2003. The prognosis of T3N0 colon cancer is dependent on the number of lymph nodes examined. *Ann. Surg. Oncol.* **10:** 65–71.
16. Kockerling, F., M.A. Reymond, C. Schneider, *et al.* 1998. Prospective multicenter study of the quality of oncologic resections in patients undergoing laparoscopic colorectal surgery for cancer. The Laparoscopic Colorectal Surgery Study Group. *Dis. Colon Rectum* **41:** 963–970.
17. Miura, S., Y. Kodera, M. Fujiwara, *et al.* 2004. Laparoscopy-assisted distal gastrectomy with systemic lymph node dissection: a critical reappraisal from the viewpoint of lymph node retrieval. *J. Am. Coll. Surg.* **198:** 933–938.
18. Clinical Outcomes of Surgical Therapy Study Group. 2004. A comparison of laparoscopically assisted and open colectomy for colon cancer. *N. Engl. J. Med.* **350:** 2050–2059.
19. Kiran, R.P., C.P. Delaney, A.J. Senagore, *et al.* 2004. Operative blood loss and use of blood products after

laparoscopic and conventional open colorectal operations. *Arch. Surg.* **139:** 39–42.

20. Lacy, A.M., J.C. Garcia-Valdecasas, S. Delgado, *et al.* 2002. Laparoscopy-assisted colectomy versus open colectomy for treatment of non-metastatic colon cancer: a randomised trial. *Lancet* **359:** 2224–2229.

21. Hughes, E.S., F.T. McDermott, A.L. Polglase & W.R. Johnson. 1983. Tumor recurrence in the abdominal wall scar tissue after large-bowel cancer surgery. *Dis. Colon Rectum* **26:** 571–572.

22. Reilly, W.T., H. Nelson, G. Schroeder, *et al.* 1996. Wound recurrence following conventional treatment of colorectal cancer. A rare but perhaps underestimated problem. *Dis. Colon Rectum* **39:** 200–207.

23. Lacy, A.M., S. Delgado, J.C. Garcia-Valdecasas, *et al.* 1998. Port site metastases and recurrence after laparoscopic colectomy. A randomized trial. *Surg. Endosc.* **12:** 1039–1042.

24. Milsom, J.W., B. Bohm, K.A. Hammerhofer, *et al.* 1998. A prospective, randomized trial comparing laparoscopic versus conventional techniques in colorectal cancer surgery: a preliminary report. *J. Am. Coll. Surg.* **187:** 46–54.

25. Stage, J.G., S. Schulze, P. Moller, *et al.* 1997. Prospective randomized study of laparoscopic versus open colonic resection for adenocarcinoma. *Br. J. Surg.* **84:** 391–396.

26. Costi, R., J. Himpens, B. Essola, *et al.* 2004. Totally laparoscopic esophago-gastrectomy. *Acta Biomed.* **75:** 188–191.

27. Bonavina, L., D. Bona, P.R. Binyom & A. Peracchia. 2004. A laparoscopy-assisted surgical approach to esophageal carcinoma. *J. Surg. Res.* **117:** 52–57.

28. Luketich, J.D., M. Alvelo-Rivera, P.O. Buenaventura, *et al.* 2003. Minimally invasive esophagectomy: outcomes in 222 patients. *Ann. Surg.* **238:** 486–494.

29. Han, H.S., Y.W. Kim, N.J. Yi & G.D. Fleischer. 2003. Laparoscopy-assisted D2 subtotal gastrectomy in early gastric cancer. *Surg. Laparosc. Endosc. Percutan. Tech.* **13:** 361–365.

30. Huscher, C.G., A. Mingoli, G. Sgarzini, *et al.* 2005. Laparoscopic versus open subtotal gastrectomy for distal gastric cancer: five-year results of a randomized prospective trial. *Ann. Surg.* **241:** 232–237.

31. Migoh, S., K. Hasuda, K. Nakashima & H. Anai. 2003. The benefit of laparoscopy-assisted distal gastrectomy compared with conventional open distal gastrectomy: a case-matched control study. *Hepatogastroenterology* **50:** 2251–2254.

32. Yasuda, K., M. Inomata, N. Shiraishi, *et al.* 2004. Laparoscopy-assisted distal gastrectomy for early gastric cancer in obese and nonobese patients. *Surg. Endosc.* **18:** 1253–1256.

33. Buell, J.F., M.J. Thomas, T.C. Doty, *et al.* 2004. An initial experience and evolution of laparoscopic hepatic resectional surgery. *Surgery* **136:** 804–811.

34. Su, S.Y., L. Fei & Z.J. Zhen. 2004. [Hand-assisted laparoscopic partial hepatectomy in the treatment of primary liver cancer]. *Di Yi. Jun. Yi. Da. Xue. Xue. Bao.* **24:** 1084–1086.

35. Gagner, M., T. Rogula & D. Selzer. 2004. Laparoscopic liver resection: benefits and controversies. *Surg. Clin. North Am.* **84:** 451–462.

36. Morino, M., I. Morra, E. Rosso, *et al.* 2003. Laparoscopic vs open hepatic resection: a comparative study. *Surg. Endosc.* **17:** 1914–1918.

37. Gagner, M. & A. Pomp. 1997. Laparoscopic pancreatic resection: Is it worthwhile? *J. Gastrointest. Surg.* **1:** 20–25.

38. Takaori, K. & N. Tanigawa. 2007. Laparoscopic pancreatic resection: the past, present, and future. *Surg. Today* **37:** 535–545.

39. Fernandez-Cruz, L., R. Cosa, L. Blanco, *et al.* 2007. Curative laparoscopic resection for pancreatic neoplasms: a critical analysis from a single institution. *J. Gastrointest. Surg.* **11:** 1607–1622.

40. Baker, R.P., L.V. Titu, J.E. Hartley, *et al.* 2004. A case-control study of laparoscopic right hemicolectomy vs. open right hemicolectomy. *Dis. Colon Rectum* **47:** 1675–1679.

41. Leroy, J., P. Ananian, F. Rubino, *et al.* 2005. The impact of obesity on technical feasibility and postoperative outcomes of laparoscopic left colectomy. *Ann. Surg.* **241:** 69–76.

42. Moloo, H., J. Mamazza, E.C. Poulin, *et al.* 2004. Laparoscopic resections for colorectal cancer: does conversion survival? *Surg. Endosc.* **18:** 732–735.

43. Balague, C., E.M. Targarona, S. Sainz, *et al.* 2004. Minimally invasive treatment for obstructive tumors of the left colon: endoluminal self-expanding metal stent and laparoscopic colectomy. Preliminary results. *Dig. Surg.* **21:** 282–286.

44. Stipa, F., B. Bascone, A. Cimitan, *et al.* 2006. [Endoscopic-laparoscopic treatment of neoplastic occlusion of the left colon]. *Chir. Ital.* **58:** 197–201.

45. Breukink, S., J. Pierie & T. Wiggers. 2006. Laparoscopic versus open total mesorectal excision for rectal cancer. *Cochrane Database Syst. Rev.* CD005200.

46. Kitano, S., M. Kitajima, F. Konishi, *et al.* 2006. A multicenter study on laparoscopic surgery for colorectal cancer in Japan. *Surg. Endosc.* **20:** 1348–1352.

Cellular Origin of Gastric Cancer

Sherif M. Karam

Department of Anatomy, Faculty of Medicine and Health Sciences, UAE University, Al Ain, United Arab Emirates

Gastric cancer is the second leading cause of cancer deaths worldwide. Although the link between *Helicobacter pylori* infection and gastric cancer is well established, little is known about the early development and detection of this malignant disease. Cancer is the disease of epithelia and recently, it has been suggested that some cancers originate in adult stem cells. Advances have been made in identifying the gastric epithelial stem cells and their immediate descendents, which act as progenitors giving rise to mucus-, acid-, pepsinogen-, and hormone-secreting cell lineages. Analyses of some genetically manipulated animal models in which the proliferation and differentiation program of the gastric stem/progenitor cells was altered by different approaches have provided some clues to the cellular origin of gastric cancer. Despite the challenges and the similarity between gastric epithelial progenitors and their differentiation program in mice and humans, it remains to be determined whether observations made in genetically engineered mice are also applicable to humans.

Key words: stomach; stem cell; gastric carcinogenesis; cell differentiation; cell dynamics; radioautography

Introduction

The majority of cancers are derived from epithelia. It is estimated that about 92% of all human cancers arise from the covering or lining epithelial tissues in various locations, such as the skin, lung, uterine cervix, breast, prostate, colon, and stomach.[1] To understand the pathogenesis of cancer in these organs, one has to first study the biological and dynamic features of their epithelia, and then to trace the early changes that occur during development of preneoplastic and neoplastic lesions.

In the stomach, the epithelial lining produces acid, pepsinogen, mucus, peptides, and hormones. These products are secreted by different cell types which are organized to form numerous epithelial units. Each unit is made of a short pit continuous with a long tubular gland. The pit contains mucus-secreting pit cells and the gland is divisible into three regions according to the predominance of three main types of cells. Immature progenitor cells predominate in the isthmus region, mucus-secreting neck cells in the neck region, and pepsinogen-secreting zymogenic (chief) cells in the base region. Both the acid-secreting parietal (oxyntic) cells and the enteroendocrine cells are scattered in the three gland regions and, in mice, these cells are also found in the pits.[2]

More than 50 years ago, Stevens and Leblond[3] proposed that the mucus-secreting pit cells of the stomach undergo normal physiological renewal. The evidence was based on: 1) the presence of mitotic figures at the bottom of the pits, 2) the increasing amount of periodic acid Schiff-stained mucus toward the luminal surface, and 3) the presence of some degenerated cells on the luminal surface. Some years later, with the advent of 3H-thymidine radioautography, additional evidence was added. The migration, with time, of 3H-thymidine-labeled pit cells toward the luminal surface

Address for correspondence: Sherif M. Karam, Department of Anatomy, Faculty of Medicine and Health Sciences, UAE University, P. O. Box: 17666, Al Ain, UAE. Voice: +00971-3-7137-493; fax: +00971-3-7672-033. skaram@uaeu.ac.ae

Ann. N.Y. Acad. Sci. 1138: 162–168 (2008). © 2008 New York Academy of Sciences.
doi: 10.1196/annals.1414.023

was documented.[4] Finally, combining detailed electron microscopic analysis with radioautographic studies following different modalities of 3H-thymidine administration has made it possible to demonstrate the continuous renewal not only of pit cells, but of all cell types of the gastric gland and to define their cellular origin.[5]

Stem Cell Identification

In renewing epithelia, stem cells are generally defined by their morphological and functional features. Morphologically, they are undifferentiated and exhibit embryonic cell-like features as described above. Functionally, they are highly proliferative and capable of replacing other mature cells of the epithelium while maintaining their own population.[6]

It was Plenk[7] who first reported that some cells in the gastric glands are capable of mitosis. This observation was confirmed by Stevens and Leblond[3] and then demonstrated with 3H-thymidine radioautography by various investigators.[4,5,8–10] The identity of these cells was unknown, and no information was available regarding their dynamics, differentiation, and role in the renewal of the other epithelial cell types.

Electron microscopy combined with 3H-thymidine radioautography has revealed that these highly proliferative cells in the mouse oxyntic glands include three different types: granule-free, prepit, and preneck cells.[5] While granule-free cells have no secretory granules, prepit and preneck cells have a few membrane-bound secretion granules, which appear similar to but smaller than those of pit and neck cells, respectively.[5]

Detailed ultrastructural analysis of the three proliferative cell types has shown not only that the nucleus-to-cytoplasm ratios are high in these cells, but also that the surface areas of their nucleoli are large (2.0–2.5 μm^2) and the mitochondrial diameters are small, 300–375 nm, relative to those of mature cell types.[5]

Examination of the Golgi region of the granule-free cells in tissues fixed in mixed aldehyde solution and tannic acid and postfixed in osmium tetroxide partially reduced with potassium ferrocyanide has revealed that these cells include three different subtypes. Two of these subtypes are characterized by the presence of a few small prosecretory vesicles next to the trans face of the Golgi apparatus. These vesicles indicate that the Golgi apparatus is starting to show some secretory activity to produce secretion granules. The prosecretory vesicles contain secretion material that appears similar to that in prosecretory vesicles of prepit or preneck cells. In prepit cells, the contents of such vesicles appear uniform but at various stages of condensation. In preneck cells the prosecretory granules have pale peripheral contents against darker background. In the third subtype of granule-free cells, the Golgi apparatus is very primitive and its trans face lacks any prosecretory vesicles, indicating that this subtype is not involved in the production of secretory granules. Therefore, this third subtype of granule-free cells is named the "undifferentiated granule-free cell."[5]

In addition to their primitive Golgi, the undifferentiated granule-free cell is characterized by a high nucleus-to-cytoplasm ratio. The large nucleus contains much diffuse chromatin and large reticulated nucleoli. While the scanty cytoplasm includes many free ribosomes, there are only a few small mitochondria and cisternae of rough endoplasmic reticulum. Thus, the ultrastructural features of undifferentiated granule-free cells appear similar to those of primitive undifferentiated embryonic cells.[11] In addition, 30 min 3H-thymidine labeling has indicated that granule-free cells are the most proliferative, labeling index 32.4%. This proliferative activity ensures the production of other cells and their own maintenance. In brief, granule-free cells are the least differentiated and most proliferative and, hence, fulfill the morphological and functional features of a stem cell.[5] While no molecular markers are yet available to label and identify specifically the gastric epithelial stem cells, these combined ultrastructural and dynamic features described above can be used to pinpoint them.

Analysis of the entire length of the oxyntic glands at different levels has revealed that these three types of epithelial progenitors are all found in the isthmus region. While granule-free cells can be seen at any level of the isthmus, prepit cells are found next to the isthmus–pit border and preneck cells, next to the isthmus–neck border.[5]

Stem Cell Proliferation Dynamics

In addition to the 30-min labeling of granule-free cells with 3H-thymidine, two more experiments were used to study their proliferation dynamics.[5] In the first experiment, a small single dose of 3H-thymidine, 1 μCi/gm body weight, was injected into mice which were then sacrificed at 3, 6 or, 12 h or 1, 2, 4, or 8 days (pulse–chase experiment). Following radioautography, estimation of the 3H-thymidine labeling indices of granule-free cells at each of these time intervals revealed an initial increase in labeling index from 33.3% at 3 h to 51% at 6 h. Then, the labeling indices deceased dramatically from 46% at 12 h to 22% and 8% at 1 and 2 days. Finally, 3H-thymidine-labeled granule-free cells almost disappear by 4 days. Therefore, granule-free cells turn over very rapidly.

The overall turnover time of granule-free cells was estimated from the second experiment, in which a very small dose of 3H-thymidine, 0.1 μCi/gm body weight/day was continuously infused into mice subcutaneously for 1, 2, 3, or 4 days (cumulative labeling experiment). Estimation of the 3H-thymidine labeling indices of granule-free cells after these different time intervals and analysis of their increasing slope with time have confirmed their rapid renewal. The overall turnover time of granule-free cells averages 2.6 days.[5]

Stem Cell Hierarchies

Three immediate descendants of the undifferentiated granule-free cell have been identified: prepit, preneck, and preparietal cell progenitors. The latter is identified in a transgenic animal model expressing the H,K-ATPase beta subunit-simian virus 40 large T antigen fusion gene.[12] These immediate progenitors are responsible for the production of the three main gastric epithelial cell lineages: pit, zymogenic, and parietal.

In the mouse stomach, morphological and radioautographic evidence indicates that the undifferentiated granule-free stem cell also gives rise to pre-enteroendocrine and precaveolated cells, which in turn give rise to enteroendocrine and caveolated cell lineages.[5]

Regulation of Stem Cell Dynamics

Several lines of evidence suggest that parietal cells are the source of some factors that are necessary for maintaining normal proliferation and differentiation of the gastric epithelial stem cells: 1) parietal cells complete their differentiation and maturation within the stem cell (isthmus) region[13]; 2) block of parietal cell differentiation in transgenic mice leads to an increase in stem cell proliferation and alteration in their commitment program[14,15]; 3) inhibition of parietal cells' secretory activity induces not only an enhancement of their degeneration but also an increase in the number of mitotic progenitor cells[16,17]; 4) ablation of parietal cells in transgenic mice is associated with an amplification of progenitor cell populations and alteration of their commitment and/or differentiation program[15,18]; and finally, 5) Mills and Gordon have applied the powerful tools of laser capture microdissection and gene profiling to parietal cell population to reveal the expression of five genes that could be candidates for stem cell regulation—insulin-like growth factor binding protein-2, growth hormone binding protein, parathyroid hormone-like peptide, vascular endothelial growth factor-B, and CD-36.[19]

Gastrin has long been known to be involved in growth of the gastric mucosa.[20] It is also known that hypergastrinemia is associated with hypertrophy of the gastric mucosa and gastrin deficiency leads to atrophic gastric mucosa. Nakajima and colleagues[21] have found that gastrin enhances cell proliferation by induction of its own receptors in gastric progenitor cells. When gastrin synthesis was deficient in mice, there was an alteration in stem cell proliferation followed by a sequence of pathologic changes ending in gastric adenocarcinoma.[22]

Glucocorticoids are also known to influence both cell proliferation and differentiation in the gastric glands.[23–25] While a short-term treatment with glucocorticoids decreases cell proliferation, its chronic administration for 2 months induces a highly significant increase in cell proliferation.[23]

Trefoil factor 1 (or pS2) has recently been shown to play a role in the commitment program of gastric stem cell hierarchies. Detailed immunohistochemical and electron microscopic analysis of the gastric mucosa of pS2 knockout mice has suggested that the lack of pS2 alters the subpopulation of prepit cells which originally committed to differentiate into parietal cells. This subpopulation of prepit cells was redirected into pit cell–differentiation pathway, and a deficiency in parietal cell production developed without any effect on cell proliferation but an enhancement in pit cell production.[26]

Vitamin A is also an important factor that appears to be involved in the regulation of progenitor cells in the gastric glands. Recently, the expression of some retinoid and/or retinoic acid receptors was demonstrated in the gastric progenitor cells of various species including mice, rabbits, and humans.[27] Also, retinoic acid administration has been found to enhance both proliferation of gastric epithelial progenitors and differentiation of pit and zymogenic cell lineages in mice.[28] Furthermore, in developing rabbits, retinol has been shown to enhance the differentiation of gastric parietal cells.[29]

Lymphoid cells have long been recognized as a feature of the gastrointestinal mucosa.[30,31] Therefore, in addition to the intestinal lymphoid nodules (Peyer's patches), some lymphoid cells are also scattered in the epithelial lining of the gastric glands and in the connective tissue of the lamina propria around them. These cells are mainly T cells and also include some macrophages, which have been reported earlier to be involved in the turnover of the cells that migrate toward the bottom of the gastric glands.[13] Intraepithelial lymphoid cells secrete a variety of cytokines that may be important in regulation of epithelial cell renewal. Since many intraepithelial lymphocytes have been observed in the vicinity of the isthmal progenitor cells of the gastric glands (S.M. Karam, unpublished observation), it is possible that these lymphoid cells are involved in the regulation the self-renewal of gastric progenitor cells and/or their commitment to differentiation.

Stem Cell Origin of Gastric Cancer

A fundamental problem in cancer research is the identification of each cancer's cellular origin. These cells are capable of initiating and sustaining neoplasia in the gastric mucosa. Nowell[32] proposed that cancer is monoclonal and originates from a single gastric stem cell as a result of several genetic alterations.

Recently, Houghton and colleagues,[33] have demonstrated that *Helicobacter pylori* infection, in mice, drives mesenchymal bone marrow stem cells into the gastric epithelium where they subsequently develop into gastric cancer. Therefore, the role of gastric epithelial tissue-specific stem/progenitor cells in the origin of cancer was questioned. The answer may come from another study in transgenic mice expressing the regulatory elements of H,K-ATPase beta subunit/DT 176 fusion gene.[15] When the stomachs of these mice were infected with *Helicobacter pylori*, the bacteria grew in the achlorohydric environment of the stomach and attached to amplified epithelial progenitors expressing glycan-specific *H pylori* adhesins.[34] The bacteria then invaded the cytoplasm of these cells and formed small communities which were possible to visualize at different stages of their development.[35]

A lineage progenitor has typically been thought to be committed to the production of a mature cell type that performs a specific function. Thus, a preparietal cell gives rise to a parietal cell, not an enteroendocrine cell.[13] A recent analysis of a transgenic mouse model of gastric cancer has provided some evidence for more plasticity for progenitor cell commitment and differentiation than previously considered possible. In these mice, the transcriptional regulatory elements of the H,K-ATPase beta-subunit gene were used to deliver the product of simian virus 40 large T antigen gene to preparietal cells. This forced expression of an oncoprotein in preparietal cells, induced their proliferation from day 1 of postnatal life,[12] and led to a massive (50- to 70-fold) expansion in their population by 1–2 months of age.[14]

When these mice became 3–6 months old, preparietal cell hyperplasia became associated with progressive mucosal thickening and glandular cyst formation. Areas of dysplasia were also developed. They were characterized by nuclear heterogeneity, loss of polarity, and stratification of glandular epithelial cells. In 10-month-old transgenic mice, areas with typical features of carcinoma *in situ* developed. These areas were characterized by complete loss of glandular architecture. Invasive epithelial cells formed loose trabeculae or ribbons. The cells had large nuclear-to-cytoplasmic ratio and much condensed heterochromatin. By 1 year of age, invasive gastric cancer developed with local and distal (hepatic) metastases.[36]

Immunohistochemical characterization of the gastric epithelial cells that form the invasive carcinoma revealed a surprising result. The transition from preparietal cell hyperplasia to neoplasia is marked by increased expression of neuroendocrine cell markers and loss of preparietal cell marker (H,K-ATPase). Therefore sites of focal neoplasia are characterized by expression of chromogranin A and dopa decarboxylase, and loss of H,K-ATPase. So, it seemed as if preparietal cells had switched their phenotype from H,K-ATPase synthesizing cells to enteroendocrine-type synthesizing chromogranin A and dopa decarboxylase. Electron microscopic examination of these focal neoplastic areas demonstrated the transdifferentiation of preparietal cells into enteroendocrine cells.[36] These findings may provide a possible explanation for the cellular origin of neuroendocrine cancer in the stomach, which appears to be more common than generally thought.[37]

Stem Cell Molecular Fingerprint

There are still many key questions to be answered regarding the biological features of gastric stem cells. What are the mechanisms that regulate the fundamental decision of a stem cell to either self-renew or to commit to differentiate into one lineage or another? The first step toward answering this question is to determine genes differentially expressed in gastric stem cells. It was Gordon and co-workers in St. Louis[38] who first revealed the molecular properties of gastric epithelial stem cells. They used the diphtheria toxin transgenic mouse model in which parietal cells were ablated and hence, enriched populations of gastric stem cells became available.[15] They also used embryonic day–18 mouse stomach, which is rich in the gastric stem cells.[12] Using navigated laser capture, groups of stem cells were microdissected and processed for gene profiling and compared with genes expressed in normal mouse stomach. A total of 147 genes differentially expressed in transgenic and embryonic stomachs are considered to form the molecular signature of gastric stem cells.

Many of these genes provided some insights into the regulation of stem cell proliferation and differentiation. Some genes appear to be growth regulators. In addition to PCNA, they include: Akt, beta-catenin, N-myc down-regulated 1 (NDRG1), bHLH antagonist Id2, cdk4, RPA3, RPA1, and Rad51. The expression of both IGF1, IGF1-R at high levels in microdissected gastric stem cells indicated a role for IGF pathway in regulating stem cell functions. Lactoferrin is also a feature of stem cells; it binds to IGHBP3 to increase bioavailability of IGF.[38]

Several genes involved in protein turnover and mRNA processing are also enriched in microdissected gastric stem cells. These include N-terminal asparagine amidase, X-chromosome ubiquitin-activating enzyme, ubiquitin-conjugating enzymes (Ubc6 and Ubc10), small ubiquitin-related modifier proteins (SUMO1 and SUMO2), three proteosomal subunits (Pas1, regulatory subunit S10, and Psmb3), and Mago-m.[38] This molecular signature of gastric stem cells would hopefully provide the means to differentiate between normal, preneoplastic, and neoplastic gastric stem cells.

Conclusion

In this perspective we have attempted to address the fundamental properties of gastric stem cells, to describe the extent to which they have been identified in mice, to describe their dynamics in normal stomach, and to analyze the effects of some factors that are found to control their proliferation and differentiation program. This has therefore provided the starting point for better understanding of gastric epithelial cell biology.

Acknowledgments

The author's recent research summarized in this review is funded by Terry Fox Funds for Cancer Research and the Research Administration of the Faculty of Medicine and Health Sciences, UAE University. This review is dedicated to the memory of Dr. C.P. Leblond, who has inspired the author throughout the years on the subject of stem cells.

Conflicts of Interest

The author declares no conflicts of interest.

References

1. Tu, S.M., S.H. Lin & C.J. Logothetis. 2002. Stem-cell origin of metastasis and heterogeneity in solid tumours. *Lancet Oncol.* **3:** 508–513.
2. Karam, S.M. & C.P. Leblond. 1992. Identifying and counting epithelial cell types in the "corpus" of the mouse stomach. *Anat. Rec.* **232:** 231–246.
3. Stevens, C.E. & C.P. Leblond. 1953. Renewal of the mucous cells in the gastric mucosa of the rat. *Anat. Rec.* **115:** 231–245.
4. Messier, B. & C.P. Leblond. 1960. Cell proliferation and migration as revealed by radioautography after injection of thymidine-H3 into male rats and mice. *Am. J. Anat.* **106:** 247–285.
5. Karam, S.M. & C.P. Leblond. 1993. Dynamics of epithelial cells in the corpus of the mouse stomach. I. Identification of proliferative cell types and pinpointing of the stem cell. *Anat. Rec.* **236:** 259–279.
6. Leblond, C.P. 1981. The life history of cells in renewing systems. *Am. J. Anat.* **160:** 114–158.
7. Plenk, H. 1932. Der Magen. In *Handbuch der Mikroskopischenm Anatomie des Menschen.* Vol. 5, Part 2. W. Von Mollendorff, Ed.: 1–234. Springer-Verlag. Berlin.
8. Hunt, T.E. & E.A. Hunt. 1962. Radioautographic study of proliferation in the stomach of the rat using thymidine-H3 and compound 48/80. *Anat. Rec.* **142:** 505–517.
9. Willems, G., P. Galand, Y. Vansteenkiste & P. Zeitoun. 1972. Cell population kinetics of zymogen and parietal cells in the stomach of mice. *Z. Zellforsch. Mikrosk. Anat.* **134:** 505–518.
10. Kataoka, K., A. Kantani-Matsumoto & Y. Takeoka. 1989. Epithelial cell proliferation and differentiation in the gastric mucosa: comparisons between histogenetic and cell renewal processes. *Prog. Clin. Biol. Res.* **295:** 309–316.
11. Mizuno, T. & A. Ishizuya. 1982. Electron microscopic study of in vitro differentiation of the small intestinal endoderm in young bird embryo in presence or absence of mesenchyme. *C. R. Seances Soc. Biol. Fil.* **176:** 580–584.
12. Karam, S.M., Q. Li & J.I. Gordon. 1997. Gastric epithelial morphogenesis in normal and transgenic mice. *Am. J. Physiol.* **272**(5 Pt 1): G1209–1220.

13. Karam, S.M. 1993. Dynamics of epithelial cells in the corpus of the mouse stomach. IV. Bidirectional migration of parietal cells ending in their gradual degeneration and loss. *Anat. Rec.* **236:** 314–332.

14. Li, Q., S.M. Karam & J.I. Gordon. 1995. Simian virus 40 T antigen-induced amplification of pre-parietal cells in transgenic mice. Effects on other gastric epithelial cell lineages and evidence for a p53-independent apoptotic mechanism that operates in a committed progenitor. *J. Biol. Chem.* **270:** 15777–15788.

15. Li, Q., S.M. Karam & J.I. Gordon. 1996. Diphtheria toxin-mediated ablation of parietal cells in the stomach of transgenic mice. *J. Biol. Chem.* **271:** 3671–3676.

16. Karam, S.M. & J.G. Forte. 1994. Inhibiting gastric H(+)-K(+)-ATPase activity by omeprazole promotes degeneration and production of parietal cells. *Am. J. Physiol.* **266**(4 Pt 1): G745–G758.

17. Karam, S.M. & G. Alexander. 2001. Blocking of histamine H2 receptors enhances parietal cell degeneration in the mouse stomach. *Histol. Histopathol.* **16:** 469–480.

18. Canfield, V., A.B. West, J.R. Goldenring & R. Levenson. 1996. Genetic ablation of parietal cells in transgenic mice: a new model for analyzing cell lineage relationships in the gastric mucosa. *Proc. Natl. Acad. Sci. USA* **93:** 2431–2435.

19. Mills, J.C. & J.I. Gordon. 2001. A molecular profile of the mouse gastric parietal cell with and without exposure to Helicobacter pylori. *Proc. Natl. Acad. Sci. USA* **98:** 13687–13692.

20. Johnson, L.R. 1988. Regulation of gastrointestinal mucosal growth. *Physiol. Rev.* **68:** 456–502.

21. Nakajima, T., Y. Konda, Y. Izumi, *et al.* 2002. Gastrin stimulates the growth of gastric pit cell precursors by inducing its own receptors. *Am. J. Physiol. Gastrointest. Liver Physiol.* **282:** G359–66.

22. Zavros, Y., K.A. Eaton, W. Kang, *et al.* 2005. Chronic gastritis in the hypochlorhydric gastrin-deficient mouse progresses to adenocarcinoma. *Oncogene* **24:** 2354–2366.

23. Gunin, A.G. & D.V. Nikolaev. 2000. Two-month glucocorticoid treatment increases proliferation in the stomach and large intestine of rats. *Digestion* **61:** 151–156.

24. Tseng, C.C., K.L. Schmidt & L.R. Johnson. 1987. Hormonal effects on development of the secretory apparatus of parietal cells. *Am. J. Physiol.* **253**(3 Pt 1): G284–289.

25. Tseng, C.C., K.L. Schmidt & L.R. Johnson. 1987. Hormonal effects on development of the secretory apparatus of chief cells. *Am. J. Physiol.* **253**(3 Pt 1): G274–283.

26. Karam, S.M., C. Tomasetto & M.C. Rio. 2004. Trefoil factor 1 is required for the commitment programme of mouse oxyntic epithelial progenitors. *Gut* **53:** 1408–1415.

27. Karam, S.M., W.M. Hassan & R. John. 2005. Expression of retinoid receptors in multiple cell lineages in the gastric mucosae of mice and humans. *J. Gastroenterol. Hepatol.* **20:** 1892–1899.

28. Karam, S.M., R. John, D.H. Alpers & A.S. Ponery. 2005. Retinoic acid stimulates the dynamics of mouse gastric epithelial progenitors. *Stem Cells* **23:** 433–441.

29. Karam, S.M., H.R. Ansari, W.S. Al-Dhaheri & G. Alexander. 2004. Retinol enhances differentiation of the gastric parietal cell lineage in developing rabbits. *Cell Physiol. Biochem.* **14:** 333–342.

30. Nakagawa, K., K. Higuchi, T. Arakawa, *et al.* 2000. Phenotypical and morphological analyses of intraepithelial and lamina propria lymphocytes in normal and regenerating gastric mucosa of rats in comparison with those in intestinal mucosa. *Arch. Histol. Cytol.* **63:** 159–167.

31. Foss, H.D., A. Schmitt-Graff, S. Daum, *et al.* 1999. Origin of primary gastric T-cell lymphomas from intraepithelial T-lymphocytes: report of two cases. *Histopathology* **34:** 9–15.

32. Nowell, P.C. 1976. The clonal evolution of tumor cell populations. *Science* **194:** 23–28.

33. Houghton, J., C. Stoicov, S. Nomura, *et al.* 2004. Gastric cancer originating from bone marrow-derived cells. *Science* **306:** 1568–1571.

34. Syder, A.J., J.L. Guruge, Q. Li, *et al.* 1999. Helicobacter pylori attaches to NeuAc alpha 2,3Gal beta 1,4 glycoconjugates produced in the stomach of transgenic mice lacking parietal cells. *Mol Cell.* **3:** 263–274.

35. Oh, J.D., S.M. Karam & J.I. Gordon. 2005. Intracellular Helicobacter pylori in gastric epithelial progenitors. *Proc. Natl. Acad. Sci. USA* **102:** 5186–5191.

36. Syder, A.J., S.M. Karam, J.C. Mills, *et al.* 2004. A transgenic mouse model of metastatic carcinoma involving transdifferentiation of a gastric epithelial lineage progenitor to a neuroendocrine phenotype. *Proc. Natl. Acad. Sci. USA* **101:** 4471–4476.

37. Modlin, I.M., M. Kidd, I. Latich, *et al.* 2005. Current status of gastrointestinal carcinoids. *Gastroenterology* **128:** 1717–1751.

38. Mills, J.C., N. Andersson, C.V. Hong, *et al.* 2002. Molecular characterization of mouse gastric epithelial progenitor cells. *Proc. Natl. Acad. Sci. USA* **99:** 14819–14824.

Surgical Treatment of Pancreatic Cancer

Martin Loos,[a] **Jörg Kleeff,**[a] **Helmut Friess,**[a]
and Markus W. Büchler[b]

[a]*Department of Surgery, Technische Universität München, Munich, Germany*

[b]*Department of General Surgery, University of Heidelberg, Heidelberg, Germany*

Pancreatic cancer is an aggressive disease with an overall 5-year survival rate of less than 5%. Up to date, surgical resection represents the basis of treatment for localized pancreatic cancer and remains the only chance for cure. Due to continuous improvements in surgical techniques and perioperative care, pancreatic resections have evolved into safe surgical procedures with low mortality and acceptable morbidity rates for experienced surgeons in high-volume centers. Recently, more aggressive approaches including extended lymphadenectomy, vascular resection, surgery for metastastic or recurrent disease, and multimodal regimens have been suggested to improve long-term outcome. This article provides an overview on current standard procedures and summarizes new strategies in the surgical treatment of pancreatic cancer.

Key words: **pancreas; cancer; pancreatectomy**

Introduction

Pancreatic ductal adenocarcinoma (PDAC) is one of the most fatal human malignancies. At present, PDAC is the fourth leading cause of cancer-related deaths in the Western world.[1] Due to its aggressive growth behavior, with early local spread into the surrounding tissues mostly along neural sheets, early metastasis, and resistance to radiation and most systemic therapies, the prognosis remains poor, with an overall 5-year survival rate of only 1–4%.[1] Surgical treatment still represents the only chance for cure.[2] Recent large series report a 5-year survival rate in the range of 15–25% following surgical resection.[3–6]

Although pancreatic surgery is considered one of the most technically demanding and challenging surgical disciplines, steady improvement in surgical techniques and advances in perioperative supportive care, based on a

modern interdisciplinary approach that includes anesthesiology, oncology, radiology, and nursing, have reduced the mortality rates to less than 5% in high-volume centers.[3,7–12] However, only a minority of patients (10–20%) present with resectable disease at the time of diagnosis.[13]

Pancreaticoduodenectomy (PD) is the standard procedure in pancreatic surgery, because most PDACs arise in the head of the pancreas. For many years, the classical PD, which was first described by Kausch and Whipple, was the procedure of choice.[14,15] However, recent studies have demonstrated that pylorus-preserving PD (PPPD) is equally effective for the treatment of PDAC, with comparable perioperative morbidity and long-term outcome.[16–22] Other surgical procedures include distal pancreatectomy, for tumors located in the pancreatic body or tail, as well as total pancreatectomy and segmental resection for rare indications.[9,23–24]

Despite constant progress in pancreatic surgery, new approaches are needed to improve the outcome of patients with PDAC. Rather disappointing results come from several trials that could not confirm better survival

Address for correspondence: Markus W. Büchler, MD, Department of General Surgery, University of Heidelberg, Im Neuenheimer Feld 110, 69120 Heidelberg, Germany. Voice: +49 6221 56 6202; fax: +49 6221 56 6903. markus.buechler@med.uni-heidelberg.de rates with more extensive radical surgery, including vascular resections and extended lymphadenectomy.[25–30] In contrast, multimodal approaches with adjuvant chemotherapy have shown promising results. The ESPAC-1 and the CONKO-001 trials demonstrated that adjuvant chemotherapy improves survival after radical pancreatic cancer surgery.[31] Even better results were achieved by the Virginia Mason approach, demonstrating 5-year survival of 55% in pancreatic cancer patients who received adjuvant chemo-radio-immunotherapy along with surgery.[32] Unfortunately, there was no control arm in this trial. Still controversial is the role of surgery for metastatic or recurrent pancreatic cancer, as well as the role of adjuvant chemoradiation and neoadjuvant therapy in the multimodal treatment concept.[33–36]

Resection for Tumors of the Head of the Pancreas

Classical Kausch–Whipple Procedure

For many years, the classical Kausch–Whipple procedure was the surgical procedure of choice for tumors located in the head of the pancreas.[37] It consists of the resection of the pancreatic head and duodenum along with a distal gastrectomy, cholecystectomy, removal of the common bile duct and proximal jejunum, and *enbloc* resection of regional lymph nodes.

After performance of a midline or roof-top incision to enter the abdominal cavity, a thorough examination of the peritoneal lining and the liver is mandatory in order to exclude generalized disease. A Kocher maneuver is then performed to assess the retroperitoneum for evidence of invasion. Furthermore, the relationship of the tumor to the superior mesenteric artery (SMA) is evaluated to confirm resectability. Subsequently, the superior mesenteric vein (SMV) is identified and traced to the inferior margin of the pancreas. In order to mobilize the posterior aspect of the pancreas, a tunnel is then carefully created between the neck of the pancreas and the SMV–portal vein

(PV) trunk. This step is accompanied by the exposure of the PV at the superior margin of the pancreas. For preparation of the *enbloc* removal of the specimen, the gallbladder and the common bile duct are removed. The hepatic artery is then identified and traced proximally towards the common hepatic artery to identify the gastroduodenal artery (GDA). It is essential to clearly identify the GDA before dividing the vessel. The pancreas can then be transected at its neck, ventral to the SMV–PV trunk. The specimen is finally removed, along with an *enbloc* removal of the distal stomach and duodenum.

Pylorus-preserving Pancreaticoduodenectomy

This procedure, first introduced by Watson in 1942, did not become popular until Traverso and Longmire reintroduced it in 1978.[38,39] Although the procedure was originally described for the treatment of periampullary tumors, PPPD is now performed by many surgeons for cancer of the pancreatic head. The rationale behind preservation of the stomach is to improve gastrointestinal function. To retain a functioning pylorus, the entire stomach and 2 cm of the first part of the duodenum are preserved along with their neurovascular supply. Following the division of the right gastric and right gastroepiploic arteries, the duodenum is skeletonized distal to the pylorus. The duodenal bulb is then transected with a stapling device.

There has been controversy over whether PPPD is a sufficiently radical treatment for pancreatic cancer with respect to tumor outgrowth to the pylorus and spread to lymph nodes along the greater and lesser curvatures of the stomach.[40,41] In addition, previous studies reported a higher incidence of delayed gastric emptying following PPPD.[42–44] In the meantime, a number of randomized controlled trials and a meta-analysis have demonstrated that both perioperative morbidity and long-term outcome are equal with the pylorus-preserving and the classical Whipple approach.[17,19,20,22,28,45]

Therefore, both the classical Kausch–Whipple procedure and the pylorus-preserving procedure are the recommended operations for patients with resectable pancreatic and peri-ampullary tumors.[46]

Pancreatic Anastomosis

Pancreatic leak represents the major cause of procedure-related morbidity and mortality in pancreatic surgery.[47] Different techniques for performing a safe pancreatic anastomosis have been described in the literature. Although the technique of pancreatico-enteric anastomosis has been highly standardized in individual centers, there is still no consensus as to how to perform a safe pancreatic anastomosis.[48] Several prognostic factors have been identified for pancreatic anastomosis failure, including the pancreatic tissue texture (soft versus hard), the surgical technique (traumatic versus meticulous), the extent of resection (multivisceral versus standard), and the extent of dilatation of the pancreatic duct.[49–52] According to the literature, the pancreatic leakage rate ranges from 0 to >10% in centers with experience in pancreatic surgery.[7,53,54]

The two most common pancreatic anastomosis techniques are pancreaticojejunostomy (PJ) and pancreaticogastrostomy (PG). The PJ can be performed by invaginating the transected pancreas into the jejunum. Another possibility is the duct-to-mucosa technique, anastomosing the pancreatic duct directly to the jejunum. Separate duct-to-mucosa adaptation helps to keep the duct orifice open, allowing the unobstructed flow of pancreatic juice through the anastomosis. Using the end-to-side anastomosis, the jejunal opening can be adapted specifically to the requirements of the pancreatic remnant. Another technique often used is to anastomose the pancreatic remnant to the stomach. Observational clinical studies reported the superiority of PG over PJ, showing a reduced rate of pancreatic leak and mortality.[55] In contrast, randomized controlled trials and a recent meta-analysis could not confirm

the advantage of a particular technique, suggesting equal results for PG and PJ.[56–59]

As a third option, the pancreatic duct can be occluded by sutures, glue, or biologic material.[55] This practice, however, has been associated with higher fistula rates and an increased risk of exocrine and endocrine pancreatic insufficiency.[60] Fibrin glue, whether used for temporary ductal occlusion or sealing of the pancreatico-enteric anastomosis, has been shown to be ineffective in preventing intra-abdominal complications in controlled trials.[60–62] As a result, ductal occlusion has largely been abandoned.

Based on current data, there is no evidence in favor of one particular technique. As long as the three basic requirements of a safe anastomosis are met—namely, a tension-free adaptation, well-perfused tissues, and no distal obstruction—any pancreatico-enteric anastomotic technique can result in good outcome.

Resection for Tumors of the Body/Tail of the Pancreas

Distal Pancreatectomy

Distal pancreatectomy represents the surgical procedure of choice for tumors arising in the body or tail of the pancreas.[63] This operation entails the removal of that portion of the pancreas extending to the left of the midline.[24] In contrast to PD, the duodenum and distal bile duct are not resected. The pancreas is usually divided to the left of the SMV–PV trunk; the exact line of transection, however, is dependent on the location of the tumor. The conventional method for preventing leakage of pancreatic juice from the cut surface is ligation of the main pancreatic duct and additional suturing of the stump to approximate the anterior and posterior capsule.[9] With the advent of surgical stapling devices, a new tool became available for sealing the pancreatic stump, joining the harmonic scalpel, fibrin glue, and prolamine injection.

Adjuvant Chemotherapy

Probably the most progress in pancreatic cancer treatment has been achieved during the past decade using multimodal approaches. Several randomized controlled trials on the role of adjuvant chemotherapy in pancreatic cancer have been published, including an early study by Bakkevold and colleagues.[102] This study demonstrated a significant increase in median survival time to 23 months in patients receiving adjuvant chemotherapy along with surgical resection, in comparison to 11 months in the control group. However, the study included not only patients suffering from pancreatic cancer, but also periampullary cancer patients. A significant survival benefit was not seen when only patients with pancreatic cancer were analyzed. Although it may be difficult to draw final conclusions from this underpowered study, which included only 61 PDAC patients, there was a tendency toward prolonged overall and recurrence-free survival with adjuvant chemotherapy.

Similarly, a study by Takada and co-workers also contained both periampullary and pancreatic malignancies, but each tumor entity was analyzed separately.[103] In total, 508 patients were included in this trial, of which 158 patients with pancreatic cancer were analyzed. In contrast to the Bakkevold study, patients receiving adjuvant chemotherapy had a poorer outcome, with a 5-year survival rate of 11.5% compared to 18% in the control group. However, this difference did not reach statistical significance.

ESPAC-1, the first trial of the European study group for pancreatic cancer, demonstrated for the first time in an international trial that adjuvant chemotherapy improves survival in patients after radical pancreatic cancer surgery.[31] Patients were included and randomized into one of four arms: chemotherapy, chemoradiation, neither, or both. 5-Fluorouracil (5-FU)/folinic acid (FA) was used as chemotherapy, and chemoradiation comprised 20 Gy beam radiation plus a bolus of 5-FU intravenously. The final result of the study revealed a median survival of 20.1 months among the 147 patients who received chemotherapy in comparison to 15.5 months among 142 the patients who did not receive chemotherapy.[31] Although some concerns regarding standardized pathological examination and the adherence to the treatment protocols have been raised, the study demonstrated that chemotherapy confers a survival benefit.

A recent meta-analysis by Stocken and colleagues that analyzed five randomized controlled trials on adjuvant treatment of pancreatic cancer was generally consistent with what has been shown by the ESPAC-1 trial, revealing a combined median survival of 19 months with chemotherapy and 13.5 months without chemotherapy.[104]

Oettle and co-workers conducted the most recent randomized controlled clinical trial.[105] Patients underwent curative-intended resection for pancreatic cancer. After R0 or R1 resection, patients were randomized into an adjuvant chemotherapy arm (gemcitabine) and an observation arm; 179 patients in the gemcitabine group and 175 patients in the control group met the eligibility criteria and constituted the intent-to-treat population for the primary endpoint analysis. The median disease-free survival in the gemcitabine group was 13.4 months, versus 6.9 months in the control group. The 5-year survival rate with adjuvant gemcitabine treatment reached 23% versus 12% without treatment.[105] Overall, the existing data show a clear benefit for postoperative adjuvant chemotherapy (5-FU or gemcitabine). Further information on the optimal adjuvant chemotherapy regimen in pancreatic cancer will soon be available, as other ongoing randomized trials will be completed soon. The ESPAC-3 study, which compares the adjuvant chemotherapy regimen 5-FU/FA with gemcitabine, represents one of the largest trials assessing adjuvant chemotherapy in pancreatic disease. Up to date, more than 1300 patients have been recruited.

Adjuvant Chemoradiation

Early studies on the effect of adjuvant therapy with 5-FU in combination with radiation demonstrated a favorable effect in advanced pancreatic cancer. However, most of the studies analyzed the effect of chemoradiation in a nonrandomized fashion. A randomized controlled trial carried out by the Gastrointestinal Tumor Study Group in 1985 compared postoperative adjuvant combined therapy in resected pancreatic cancer patients with no adjuvant therapy.[106] Due to a significant survival benefit, with a median survival of 20 months in the treatment group versus 11 months in the control group, the study had to be discontinued prematurely.[106] In contrast, the multicenter randomized trial by Klinkenbijl and colleagues concluded that adjuvant chemoradiation was a well-tolerated treatment regimen but was not superior to surgery alone.[107]

A recent meta-analysis pointed toward a survival benefit for adjuvant chemoradiation.[108] However, in addition to four randomized controlled trials,[31,107,109,110] one prospective study was included in this analysis, and the significant effect was not seen when only trials after 1997 were analyzed.[108] Thus, the data of this meta-analysis do not point to a convincing effect of chemoradiation in the adjuvant setting.

In the meta-analysis of adjuvant treatment by Stocken and colleagues,[104] no survival differences were seen with chemoradiation. Nonetheless, a subgroup analysis showed that chemoradiation was more effective than chemotherapy alone in patients with positive resection margins. However, there is increasing evidence that negative resection margins depend not only on the surgeons' technique but also to a large extent on the definition used and the experience of the pathologists. A recent analysis reports R1 resection rates of as high as 85% for pancreatic cancer.[111]

Adjuvant chemoradiation can therefore not be recommended as a standard treatment for resectable pancreatic cancer. Further randomized controlled trials should be conducted in the future to determine the value of chemoradiation (for margin-positive patients, for example).

Recently, a promising but nonrandomized study using adjuvant chemoradiation together with interferon-alpha was published by Picozzi and co-workers, showing 2-year and 5-year survival rates of 64% and 55%, respectively.[32] Thus, several randomized controlled trials have been initiated to confirm these data on a larger scale in a randomized fashion. In one of these studies (the CapRI study), interferon-alpha, cisplatin, radiation, and 5-FU are being compared to 5-FU alone (ESPAC-1 chemotherapy arm).[112]

Surgery for Metastasized or Recurrent Pancreatic Cancer

Distant metastasis is generally considered to be a contraindication for surgery. However, the majority of PDAC patients have distant metastases.[13] We analyzed 29 patients who were selected for resection in the presence of liver or distant lymph node metastases.[113] The overall in-hospital morbidity and mortality of R0/R1 pancreatic resection for M1 disease was 24.1% and 0%, in comparison to 32.4% and 4.2% for M0 disease ($n = 287$). The median survival in patients with metastatic interaortocaval lymph nodes was 27 months, compared with 11.4 months for those with liver metastases and 12.9 months for patients with peritoneal metastases.[113] Hence, pancreatic resection with M1 disease is feasible, with acceptable safety in highly selected patients. However, resection of liver and peritoneal metastases cannot be generally recommended until randomized controlled trials have been carried out.

Recurrence of PDAC occurs in up to 80% of patients within 2 years following curative resection. A recent analysis of 30 patients who underwent resection for recurrent pancreatic cancer showed a tendency toward an increase in median survival in patients undergoing additional resection. However, resection for recurrent pancreatic cancer does not appear to change the natural course of the disease in most patients.[114]

Conclusion

Pancreatic surgery has clearly progressed in recent decades. In high-volume centers, surgery for pancreatic cancer is safe, with morbidity and mortality rates that are not different from those of major surgery for other gastrointestinal cancers. Five-year survival rates after pancreatic resection for PDAC have increased to 15–25%. However, the overall prognosis of PDAC has barely changed over the years. Therefore, new approaches, including multimodal therapies, are being established in order to improve outcome in PDAC. Adjuvant chemotherapy (5-FU or gemcitabine) but not adjuvant chemoradiation has been shown to improve the prognosis in resectable pancreatic cancer. Isolated PV involvement does not generally represent a contraindication for resection. In contrast, extended radical lymphadenectomy did not prove to be of benefit. Hence, standard lymphadenectomy and postoperative chemotherapy have been established as the standard of care for resectable pancreatic cancer. Surgery for M1 and recurrent disease remains questionable, although recent data seem promising.

Conflicts of Interest

The authors declare no conflicts of interest.

References

1. Jemal, A. *et al.* 2007. Cancer statistics 2007. *CA Cancer J. Clin.* **57:** 43–66.
2. Ozawa, F. *et al.* 2001. Treatment of pancreatic cancer: the role of surgery. *Dig. Dis.* **19:** 47–56.
3. Cameron, J.L. *et al.* 2006. One thousand consecutive pancreaticoduodenectomies. *Ann. Surg.* **244:** 10–15.
4. Richter, A. *et al.* 2003. Long-term results of partial pancreaticoduodenectomy for ductal adenocarcinoma of the pancreatic head. *World J. Surg.* **27:** 324–329.
5. Carpelan-Holmstrom, M. *et al.* 2005. Does anyone survive pancreatic ductal adenocarcinoma? A nationwide study re-evaluating the data of the Finnish Cancer Registry. *Gut* **54:** 385–387.
6. Wagner, M. *et al.* 2004. Curative resection is the single most important factor determining outcome in patients with pancreatic adenocarcinoma. *Br. J. Surg.* **91:** 586–594.
7. Yeo, C.J. *et al.* 1997. Six hundred fifty consecutive pancreaticoduodenectomies in the 1990s: pathology, complications, and outcomes. *Ann. Surg.* **226:** 248–257.
8. Buchler, M.W. *et al.* 2003. Changes in morbidity after pancreatic resection: toward the end of completion pancreatectomy. *Arch. Surg.* **138:** 1310–1314.
9. Fernandez-del Castillo, C. *et al.* 1995. Standards for pancreatic resection in the 1990s. *Arch. Surg.* **130:** 295–299.
10. Neoptolemos, J.P. *et al.* 1997. Low mortality following resection for pancreatic and periampullary tumors in 1026 patients: UK survey of specialist pancreatic units. UK Pancreatic Cancer Group. *Br. J. Surg.* **84:** 1370–1376.
11. Birkmeyer, J.D. *et al.* 2002. Hospital volume and surgical mortality in the United States. *N. Engl. J. Med.* **346:** 1128–1137.
12. Begg, C.B. *et al.* 1998. Impact of hospital volume on operative mortality for major cancer surgery. *JAMA* **280:** 1747–1751.
13. Sener, S.F. *et al.* 1999. Pancreatic cancer: a report of treatment and survival trends for 100,313 patients diagnosed from 1985–1995, using the national cancer database. *J. Am. Coll. Surg.* **189:** 1–7.
14. Kausch, W. *et al.* 1912. Das Karzinoma der Papilla duodeni und seine radikale Entfernung. *Beitr. Klin. Chir.* **78:** 439–486.
15. Whipple, A.O. *et al.* 1935. Treatment of carcinoma of the ampulla of Vater. *Ann. Surg.* **102:** 763–768.
16. Seiler, C.A. *et al.* 2000. Randomized prospective trial of pylorus-preserving vs. classical duodenopancreatectomy (Whipple Procedure): Initial clinical results. *J. Gastrointest. Surg.* **4:** 443–452.
17. Seiler, C.A. *et al.* 2005. Randomized clinical trial of pylorus-preserving duodenopancreatectomy versus classical Whipple resection—long term results. *Br. J. Surg.* **92:** 547–556.
18. Lin, P.W. *et al.* 1999. Prospective randomized comparison between pylorus-preserving and standard pancreaticoduodenectomy. *Br. J. Surg.* **86:** 603–607.
19. Lin, P.W. *et al.* 2005. Pancreaticoduodenectomy for pancreatic head cancer: PPPD versus Whipple procedure. *Hepatogastroenterology* **52:** 1601–1604.
20. Tran, K.T. *et al.* 2004. Pylorus preserving pancreaticoduodenectomy versus standard Whipple procedure: a prospective, randomized, multicenter analysis of 170 patients with pancreatic and periampullary tumors. *Ann. Surg.* **240:** 738–745.

21. Wenger, F.A. *et al.* 1999. [Gastrointestinal quality of life after duodenopancreatectomy in pancreatic carcinoma. Preliminary results of a prospective randomized study: pancreatoduodenectomy or pylorus-preserving pancreatoduodenectomy]. *Chirurg* **70:** 1454–1459. German.

22. Diener, M.K. *et al.* 2007. A systematic review and meta-analysis of pylorus-preserving versus classical pancreaticoduodenectomy for surgical treatment of periampullary and pancreatic carcinoma. *Ann. Surg.* **245:** 187–200.

23. Pedrazzoli, S. *et al.* 1999. A surgical and pathological based classification of resective treatment of pancreatic cancer. *Dig. Surg.* **16:** 337–345.

24. Lillemoe, K.D. *et al.* 1999. Distal pancreatectomy: indications and outcomes in 235 patients. *Ann. Surg.* **229:** 693–700.

25. Henne-Bruns, D. *et al.* 2000. Surgery for ductal adenocarcinoma of the pancreatic head: staging, complications, and survival after regional versus extended lymphadenectomy. *World J. Surg.* **24:** 595–601.

26. Gazzaniga, G.M. *et al.* 2001. D1 versus D2 pancreatoduodenectomy in surgical therapy of pancreatic head cancer. *Hepatogastroenterology* **48:** 1471–1478.

27. Farnell, M.B. *et al.* 2005. A prospective randomized trial comparing standard pancreatoduodenectomy with pancreatoduodenectomy with extended lymphadenectomy in resectable pancreatic head adenocarcinoma. *Surgery* **138:** 618–630.

28. Yeo, C.J. *et al.* 2002. Pancreaticoduodenectomy with or without extended distal gastrectomy and extended retroperitoneal lymphadenectomy for periampullary adenocarcinoma, part 2: randomized controlled trial evaluating survival, morbidity, and mortality. *Ann. Surg.* **236:** 355–368.

29. Pedrazzoli, S. *et al.* 1998. Standard versus extended lymphadenectomy associated with pancreatoduodenectomy in the surgical treatment of adenocarcinoma of the head of the pancreas: a multicenter, prospective, randomized study. Lymphadenectomy Study Group. *Ann. Surg.* **228:** 508–517.

30. Nimura, Y. *et al.* 2004. Regional versus extended lymph node dissection in radical pancreaticoduodenectomy for pancreatic cancer: a multicenter, randomized controlled trial. *HPB* **6**(Suppl. 1): S2.

31. Neoptolemos, J.P. *et al.* 2004. A randomized trial of chemoradiotherapy and chemotherapy after resection of pancreatic cancer. *N. Engl. J. Med.* **350:** 1200–1210.

32. Picozzi, V.J. *et al.* 2003. Interferon-based adjuvant chemoradiation therapy after pancreaticoduodenectomy for pancreatic adenocarcinoma. *Am. J. Surg.* **185:** 476–480.

33. Czito, B.G. *et al.* 2006. Increased toxicity with gefitinib, capecitabine, and radiation therapy in pancreatic and rectal cancer: phase I trial results. *J. Clin. Oncol.* **24:** 656–662.

34. Mornex, F. *et al.* 2006. Feasibility of preoperative combined radiation therapy and chemotherapy with 5-fluorouracil and cisplatin in potentially resectable pancreatic adenocarcinoma: the French SFRO-FFCD 97–04 Phase II trial. *Int. J. Radiat. Oncol. Biol. Phys.* **65:** 1471–1478.

35. Krempien, R. *et al.* 2005. Randomized phase II study evaluating EGFR targeting therapy with cetuximab in combination with radiotherapy and chemotherapy for patients with locally advanced pancreatic cancer—PARC: study protocol. *BMC Cancer* **5:** 131.

36. Kastl, S. *et al.* 2000. Neoadjuvant radiochemotherapy in advanced primarily non-resectable carcinomas of the pancreas. *Eur. J. Surg. Oncol.* **26:** 578–582.

37. Bramhall, S.R. *et al.* 1995. Treatment and survival in 13560 patients with pancreatic cancer, and incidence of the disease, in the West Midlands: an epidemiological study. *Br. J. Surg.* **82:** 111–115.

38. Watson, K.. 1944. Carcinoma of the ampulla of Vater. Successful radical resection. *Br. J. Surg.* **31:** 368.

39. Traverso, L.W. & W. P. Longmire Jr. 1978. Preservation of the pylorus in the pancreaticoduodenectomy. *Surg. Gynecol. Obstet.* **146:** 959–962.

40. Friess, H. *et al.* 1999. The impact of different types of surgery in pancreatic cancer. *Eur. J. Surg. Oncol.* **25:** 124–131.

41. Grace, P.A. *et al.* 1990. Pylorus-preserving pancreatoduodenectomy: an overview. *Br. J. Surg.* **77:** 968–974.

42. Warshaw, A.L. *et al.* 1985. Delayed gastric emptying after pylorus-preserving pancreaticoduodenectomy. *Surg. Gynecol. Obstet.* **160:** 1–4.

43. Roder, J.D. *et al.* 1992. Pylorus-preserving versus standard pancreatico-duodenectomy: an analysis of 110 pancreatic and periampullary carcinomas. *Br. J. Surg.* **79:** 152–155.

44. Park, Y.C. *et al.* 2003. Factors influencing delayed gastric emptying after pylorus-preserving pancreatoduodenectomy. *J. Am. Coll. Surg.* **196:** 859–865.

45. Poon, T.P. *et al.* 2001. Opinions and commentary on treating pancreatic cancer. *Surg. Clin. North Am.* **81:** 625–636.

46. American Gastroenterological Association. 1999. Medical Position Statement: epidemiology, diagnosis, and treatment of pancreatic ductal adenocarcinoma. *Gastroenterology* **117:** 163–1484.

47. Berberat, P.O. *et al.* 1999. Prevention and treatment of complications in pancreatic cancer surgery. *Dig. Surg.* **16:** 327–336.

48. Z'graggen, K. *et al.* 2002. How to do a safe pancreatic anastomosis. *J. Hepatobiliary Pancreat. Surg.* **9:** 733–737.

49. van Berge Henegouwen, M.I. *et al.* 1997. Incidence, risk factors, and treatment of pancreatic leakage after pancreaticoduodenectomy: drainage versus resection of the pancreatic remnant. *J. Am. Coll. Surg.* **185:** 18–24.

50. Muscari, F. *et al.* 2006. Risk factors for mortality and intra-abdominal complications after pancreatoduodenectomy: multivariate analysis in 300 patients. *Surgery* **139:** 591–598.

51. Bartoli, F.G. *et al.* 1991. Pancreatic fistula and relative mortality in malignant disease after pancreaticoduodenectomy. Review and statistical meta-analysis regarding 15 years of literature. *Anticancer Res.* **11:** 1831–1848.

52. Lin, J.W. *et al.* 2004. Risk factors and outcomes in postpancreaticoduodenectomy pancreaticocutaneous fistula. *J. Gastrointest. Surg.* **8:** 951–959.

53. Schafer, M. *et al.* 2002. Evidence-based pancreatic head resection for pancreatic cancer and chronic pancreatitis. *Ann. Surg.* **236:** 137–148.

54. Kazanijan, K.K. *et al.* 2005. Management of pancreatic fistulas after pancreaticoduodenectomy: results in 437 consecutive patients. *Arch. Surg.* **140:** 849–854.

55. Zenilman, M.E.. 2000. Use of pancreaticogastrostomy for pancreatic reconstruction after pancreaticoduodenectomy. *J. Clin. Gastroenterol.* **31:** 11–18.

56. Bassi, C. *et al.* 2005. Reconstruction by pancreaticojejunostomy versus pancreaticogastrostomy following pancreatectomy: results of a comparative study. *Ann. Surg.* **242:** 767–771.

57. Duffas, J.P. *et al.* 2005. A controlled randomized multicenter trial of pancreatogastrostomy or pancreatojejunostomy after pancreatoduodenectomy. *Am. J. Surg.* **189:** 720–729.

58. Yeo, C.J. *et al.* 1995. A prospective randomized trial of pancreaticogastrostomy versus pancreaticojejunostomy after pancreaticoduodenectomy. *Ann. Surg.* **222:** 580–588.

59. Wente, M.N. *et al.* 2007. Pancreaticojejunostomy versus pancreaticogastrostomy: a systematic review and meta-analysis. *Am. J. Surg.* **193:** 171–183.

60. Tran, K. *et al.* 2002. Occlusion of the pancreatic duct versus pancreaticojejunostomy: a prospective randomized trial. *Ann. Surg.* **236:** 422–428.

61. D'Andrea, A.A. *et al.* 1994. Human fibrin sealant in pancreatic surgery: is it useful in preventing fistula? A prospective randomized study. *Ital. J. Gastroenterol.* **26:** 283–286.

62. Suc, B. *et al.* 2003. Temporary fibrin glue occlusion of the main pancreatic duct in the prevention of intra-abdominal complications after pancreatic resection. *Ann. Surg.* **237:** 57–65.

63. Pedrazzoli, S. *et al.* 2002. Role of surgery in the treatment of bilio-pancreatic cancer: the European experience. *Semin. Oncol.* **29**(6, Suppl. 20): S23–S30.

64. Sheehan, M.K. *et al.* 2002. Distal pancreatectomy: does the method of closure influence fistula formation? *The Am. Surgeon* **68:** 264–268.

65. Aldridge, M.C. *et al.* 1991. Distal pancreatectomy with and without splenectomy. *Br. J. Surg.* **78:** 976–979.

66. Kleeff, J. *et al.* 2007. Distal pancreatectomy: risk factors for surgical failure in 302 consecutive cases. *Ann. Surg.* **245:** 573–582.

67. Shoup, M. *et al.* 2002. The value of splenic preservation with distal pancreatectomy. *Arch. Surg.* **137:** 164–168.

68. Richardson, D.Q. *et al.* 1989. Distal pancreatectomy with and without splenectomy. *Am. Surg.* **55:** 21–25.

69. Warshaw, A.L. *et al.* 1988. Conservation of the spleen with distal pancreatectomy. *Arch. Surg.* **123:** 550–553.

70. Schwarz, R.E. *et al.* 1999. The impact of splenectomy on outcomes after resection of pancreatic adenocarcinoma. *J. Am. Coll. Surg.* **188:** 516–521.

71. Fabre, J.M. *et al.* 1996. Surgery for left-sided pancreatic cancer. *Br. J. Surg.* **83:** 1065–1070.

72. Johnson, C.D. *et al.* 1993. Resection for adenocarcinoma of the body and tail of the pancreas. *Br. J. Surg.* **80:** 1177–1179.

73. Brennan, M.F. *et al.* 1996. Management of adenocarcinoma of the body and tail of the pancreas. *Ann. Surg.* **223:** 506–512.

74. Sohn, T.A. *et al.* 2000. Resected adenocarcinoma of the pancreas—616 patients: results, outcomes, and prognostic indicators. *J. Gastrointest. Surg.* **4:** 567.

75. Fortner, J.G. 1973. Regional resection and pancreatic carcinoma. *Surgery* **73:** 799–800.

76. Fortner, J.G. *et al.* 1984. Regional pancreatectomy for cancer of the pancreas, ampulla, and other related sites. Tumor staging and results. *Ann. Surg.* **199:** 418–425.

77. Pedrazzoli, S. *et al.* 1999. A surgical and pathological based classification of resective treatment of pancreatic cancer. Summary of an international workshop on surgical procedures in pancreatic cancer. *Dig. Surg.* **16:** 337–345.

78. Ishikawa, O. *et al.* 1988. Practical usefulness of lymphatic and connective tissue clearance for the carcinoma of the pancreatic head. *Ann. Surg.* **208:** 215–220.

79. Manabe, T. *et al.* 1989. Radical pancreatectomy for ductal cell carcinoma of the head of the pancreas. *Cancer* **64:** 1132–1137.

80. Kayahara, M. *et al.* 1993. An evaluation of radical resection for pancreatic cancer based on the mode of recurrence as determined by autopsy and diagnostic imaging. *Cancer* **72:** 2118–2123.

81. Nagai, H. 1987. [An anatomical and pathological study of autopsy material on the metastasis of pancreatic cancer to para-aortic lymph nodes]. *Nippon Geka Gakkai Zasshi* **88:** 308–317.

82. Nagakawa, T. *et al.* 1989. The spread and prognosis of carcinoma in the region of the pancreatic head. *Jpn. J. Surg.* **19:** 510–518.

83. Ozaki, H. *et al.* 1983. Lymph node dissection in radical resection for carcinoma of the head of the pancreas and periampullary region. *Jpn. J. Clin. Oncol.* **13:** 371–377.

84. Ishikawa, O. *et al.* 1992. Preoperative indications for extended pancreatectomy for locally advanced pancreatic cancer involving the portal vein. *Ann. Surg.* **215:** 231–236.

85. Ishikawa, O. *et al.* 1984. [Clinico-pathological study on the appropriate range of pancreatic head cancer]. *Nippon Geka Gakkai Zasshi* **85:** 363–369.

86. Kawarada, Y. *et al.* 1999. Modified standard pancreaticoduodenectomy for the treatment of pancreatic head cancer. *Digestion* **60**(Suppl. 1): S120–S125.

87. Goldberg, M. *et al.* 1987. Wide local excision as an alternative treatment for periampullary carcinoma. *Am. J. Gastroenterol.* **82:** 1169–1171.

88. Miyazaki, I.. 1989. [Significance of extensive surgery in pancreatic cancer]. *Gan To Kagaku Ryoho* **16**(4 Pt 2–1): 1064–1069.

89. Miyazai, I. *et al.* 1992. [Extensive radical surgery for carcinomas of the head of the pancreas]. *Gan To Kagaku Ryoho* **19:** 2333–2337.

90. Nagakawa, T. *et al.* 1996. Results of extensive surgery for pancreatic carcinoma. *Cancer* **77:** 640–645.

91. Sindelar, W.F. 1989. Clinical experience with regional pancreatectomy for adenocarcinoma of the pancreas. *Arch. Surg.* **124:** 127–132.

92. Imaizumi, T. *et al.* 1998. Extended radical Whipple resection for cancer of the pancreatic head: operative procedures and results. *Dig. Surg.* **15:** 299–307.

93. Riall, T.S. *et al.* 2005. Pancreaticoduodenectomy with or without distal gastrectomy and extended retroperitoneal lymphadenectomy for periampullary adenocarcinoma—part 3: update on 5-year survival. *J. Gastrointest. Surg.* **9:** 1191–1204.

94. Michalski, C.W. *et al.* 2007. Systematic review and meta-analysis of standard and extended lymphadenectomy in pancreaticoduodenectomy for pancreatic cancer. **94:** 265–273.

95. Fuhrman, G.M. *et al.* 1996. Rationale for en bloc vein resection in the treatment of pancreatic adenocarcinoma adherent to the superior mesenteric-portal vein confluence. *Ann. Surg.* **223:** 154–162.

96. Harrison, L.E. *et al.* 1996. Isolated portal vein involvement in pancreatic adenocarcinoma: a contraindication to resection? *Ann. Surg.* **224:** 342–349.

97. Leach, S.D. *et al.* 1998. Survival following pancreaticoduodenectomy with resection of superior mesenteric-portal vein confluence for adenocarcinoma of the pancreatic head. *Br. J. Surg.* **85:** 611–617.

98. Hartel, M. *et al.* 2002. Benefit of venous resection for ductal adenocarcinoma of the pancreatic head. *Eur. J. Surg.* **168:** 707–712.

99. Evans, D.B.. 2005. Preoperative chemoradiation for pancreatic cancer. *Semin. Oncol.* **32**(6, Suppl. 9): S25–S29.

100. Pipas, J.M. *et al.* 2005. Docetaxel/Gemcitabine followed by gemcitabine and external beam radiotherapy in patients with pancreatic adenocarcinoma. *Ann. Surg. Oncol.* **12:** 995–1004.

101. Kleeff, J. *et al.* 2007. Neoadjuvant therapy for pancreatic cancer. *Br. J. Surg.* **94:** 261–262.

102. Bakkevold, K.E. *et al.* 1993. Adjuvant combination chemotherapy (AMF) following radical resection of carcinoma of the pancreas and papilla of Vater—results of a controlled, prospective, randomized multicenter study. *Eur. J. Cancer* **29A:** 698–703.

103. Takada, T. *et al.* 2002. Is postoperative adjuvant chemotherapy useful for gallbladder carcinoma? A phase III multicenter prospective randomized controlled trial in patients with resected pancreaticobiliary carcinoma. *Cancer* **95:** 1685–1695.

104. Stocken, D.D. *et al.* 2005. Meta-analysis of randomized adjuvant therapy trials for pancreatic cancer. *Br. J. Cancer* **92:** 1372–1381.

105. Oettle, H. *et al.* 2007. Adjuvant chemotherapy with gemcitabine versus observation in patients undergoing curative-intent resection of pancreatic cancer. A randomized controlled trial. *JAMA* **297:** 267–277.

106. Kalser, M.H. *et al.* 1985. Pancreatic cancer. Adjuvant combined radiation and chemotherapy following curative resection. *Arch. Surg.* **120:** 899–903.

107. Klinkenbijl, J.H. *et al.* 1999. Adjuvant radiotherapy and 5-fluorouracil after curative resection of cancer of the pancreas and periampullary region: phase III trial of the EORTC gastrointestinal tract cancer cooperative group. *Ann. Surg.* **230:** 776–782.

108. Khanna, A. *et al.* 2006. Is adjuvant 5-FU-based chemoradiotherapy for resectable pancreatic adenocarcinoma beneficial? A meta-analysis of an unanswered question. *J. Gastrointest. Surg.* **10:** 689–697.

109. The Gastrointestinal Tumor Study Group. 1979. A multi-institutional comparative trial of radiation therapy alone and in combination with 5-fluorouracil for locally unresectable pancreatic carcinoma. *Ann. Surg.* **189:** 205–208.

110. Yeo, C.J. *et al.* 1997. Pancreaticoduodenectomy for pancreatic adenocarcinoma: postoperative adjuvant chemoradiation improves survival. A prospective, single-institution experience. *Ann. Surg.* **225:** 621–633.

111. Verbeke, C.S. *et al.* 2006. Redefining the R1 resection in pancreatic cancer. *Br. J. Surg.* **93:** 1232–1237.

112. Knaebel, H.P. *et al.* 2005. Phase III trial of postoperative cisplatin, interferon alpha-2b, and 5-FU combined with external radiation treatment versus 5-FU alone for patients with resected pancreatic adenocarcinoma—CapRI: study protocol. *BMC Cancer* **5:** 37.

113. Shrikhande, S.V. *et al.* 2007. Pancreatic resection for M1 pancreatic ductal adenocarcinoma. *Ann. Surg.* **14:** 118–127.

114. Kleeff, J. *et al.* 2007. Surgery for recurrent pancreatic ductal adenocarcinoma. *Ann. Surg.* **245:** 566–572.

Review of the Apoptosis Pathways in Pancreatic Cancer and the Anti-apoptotic Effects of the Novel Sea Cucumber Compound, Frondoside A

X. Li,[a,e] A. B. Roginsky,[a] X.-Z. Ding,[a] C. Woodward,[b] P. Collin,[b] R. A. Newman,[c] R. H. Bell, Jr.,[a] and T. E. Adrian[a,d]

[a]Department of Surgery and Robert H. Lurie Comprehensive Cancer Center, Northwestern University Feinberg School of Medicine, Chicago, Illinois, USA

[b]Coastside Research, Stonington, Maine, USA

[c]Department of Experimental Therapeutics, The University of Texas MD Anderson Cancer Center, Houston, Texas, USA

[d]Department of Physiology, Faculty of Medicine and Health Sciences, UAE University, Al Ain, United Arab Emirates

[e]Current Address: Department of Hematology, Chinese Wujing General Hospital, Beijing, China

Pancreatic cancer cells are resistant to the growth-inhibitory and apoptosis-inducing effects of conventional chemotherapeutic agents. There are multiple genetic and epigenetic events during the process of carcinogenesis that enable the cancer cells to avoid normal growth constraints and apoptosis. Investigation of the mechanisms involved has led to multiple strategies that encourage cell death and apoptosis to occur. The pathways involved are summarized in this review, together with some recently developed strategies to promote cell death in this cancer and with a particular focus on the frondoside A, a novel triterpenoid glycoside isolated from the Atlantic sea cucumber, *Cucumaria frondosa*. Frondoside A inhibited proliferation of AsPC-1 human pancreatic cancer cells in a concentration- and time-dependent manner, as measured by ^{3}H-thymidine incorporation and cell counting. In concert with inhibition of cell growth, frondoside A induced significant morphological changes consistent with apoptosis. Propidium iodide DNA staining showed an increase of sub-G0/G1 cell population of apoptotic cells induced by frondoside A. Frondoside A–induced apoptosis was confirmed by annexin V binding and TUNEL assay. Furthermore, western blotting showed a decrease in expression of Bcl-2 and Mcl-1, an increase in Bax expression, activation of caspases 3, 7, and 9, and an increase in the expression of the cyclin-dependent kinase inhibitor, p21. These findings show that frondoside A induced apoptosis in human pancreatic cancer cells through the mitochondrial pathway and activation of the caspase cascade. Finally, a very low concentration of frondoside A (10 μg/kg/day) inhibited growth of AsPC-1 xenografts in athymic mice. In conclusion, new chemotherapeutic agents are desperately needed for pancreatic cancer because of the poor responsiveness to currently available treatment options. Frondoside A has potent growth inhibitory effects on human pancreatic cancer cells, and the inhibition of proliferation is accompanied by marked

Address for correspondence: Thomas E. Adrian, Ph.D., F.R.C.Path., Department of Physiology, Faculty of Medicine and Health Sciences, United Arab Emirates University, P.O. Box 17666, Al Ain, UAE. Voice: +971 3 7137551; fax: +971 3 7671966. tadrian@uaeu.ac.ae

Ann. N.Y. Acad. Sci. 1138: 181–198 (2008). © 2008 New York Academy of Sciences.
doi: 10.1196/annals.1414.025

apoptosis. Frondoside A may be valuable for the treatment or chemoprevention of this devastating disease.

Key words: frondoside A; pancreatic cancer; apoptosis pathways

Introduction

Pancreatic Cancer and its Resistance to Chemotherapy

Pancreatic adenocarcinoma is a devastating disease with a median survival of less than 6 months after diagnosis, which is the worst survival outcome of any human cancer.[1] Symptoms occur late in the development of pancreatic malignancy and conventional chemotherapy has little impact on the outcome.[2] Less than 20% of patients are candidates for potentially curative resection, and the vast majority of even this preselected group of patients eventually succumbs to metastatic disease.[2,3] It is claimed that 20% 5-year survival after surgery is responsible for an overall 5-year survival of 2–4%. However, even this low figure has been disputed recently.[3,4] Clearly, new therapeutic strategies are necessary to improve this dismal situation.

Chemotherapy and radiation therapy provide only limited palliation, without a meaningful improvement in survival in patients with nonresectable disease.[2,5] The reasons for this are hard to define and evidence suggests that they are complex.[6,7] Meaningful studies on the mechanisms of resistance to therapy can only be performed once a highly effective drug has been found, and at present that appears to be a distant hope. Resistance to chemotherapeutic drugs is partly due to the intrinsic properties of the cancer cells, such as their ability to overcome normal cellular growth constraints and to resist apoptosis, and partly due to resistance acquired from therapy, such as the upregulation of multidrug resistance proteins, which are pumps that lower intracellular drug concentrations. In the case of pancreatic cancers, a host of genetic and epigenetic changes enable

avoidance of normal growth constraints.[6,8,9] These include upregulation and activation of growth pathways and loss of function of tumor-suppressor proteins. These pathways provide a number of potential targets for inhibition of pancreatic cancer cell growth and induction of apoptosis. With application of therapies targeted to these pathways, we can hopefully improve on the dismal outcome of this disease in the future.

The Apoptosis Pathways in Pancreatic Cancer

Programmed cell death, known as apoptosis, plays a pivotal role in cellular homeostasis. Abnormal cells are eliminated by apoptosis, but cancer cells develop mechanisms to prevent this process just as they manage to avoid cellular growth constraints.[10,11] There are two pathways through which apoptosis can be triggered. The first involves death receptors belonging to the tumor necrosis factor (TNF) super family. The second is triggered by environmental stresses or drugs that result in permeabilization of the mitochondrial outer membrane and release of apoptotic factors into the cytoplasm.[10,11] Apoptosis is mediated by activation of a cascade of serine proteases, called caspases. There are initiator caspases (caspases 8 and 9) that trigger the cascade and effector or executioner caspases (caspases 3, 6, 7, and others) that are responsible for cleavage of substrates that directly or indirectly lead to cell death. In contrast to necrosis, cellular contents remain membrane bound and subsequently undergo phagocytosis in apoptosis, thus preventing inflammation. In some cells, activation of caspase-8 through the death receptors is sufficient to directly activate the central effector caspase, caspase-3, and to trigger apoptosis directly.[10,11] In other cells, the mitochondrial pathway has to be involved in the apoptotic process. In pancreatic cancer cells, regardless of whether apoptosis is triggered by death receptors or by the stress or drug-activated mechanism, the mitochondrial pathway is always involved.[10,11]

The death receptor pathway, involves binding of TNF, the Fas ligand, or the TNF-related apoptosis-inducing ligand (TRAIL) to their respective specific receptors, which share a common internal region called the death domain. Ligand binding causes receptor trimerization and recruitment of Fas-associated death domain protein (FADD) and caspase-8 to form the death-inducing signaling complex (DISC), then caspase-8 is activated by cleavage.[12] In pancreatic cancer cells the signal-enhancing effect of mitochondria is needed and the Bcl-2 family member, BID, mediates the activation of mitochondria in response to death receptor activation. BID is cleaved by caspase-8 to tBID, which becomes integrated into the mitochondrial membrane and induces release of cytochrome c and other apoptogenic factors. In the cytoplasm, cytochrome c forms a complex with apoptotic protease-activating factor (Apaf-1), ATP, and caspase-9, called the apoptosome. Caspase-9 is another initiator caspase. It is activated by cleavage at the apoptosome and in turn activates the executioner caspases, caspase-3, -6, and -7. These executioner caspases then cleave substrates that result in DNA fragmentation, cleavage of cytoskeletal proteins, and cell death. Most studies have shown that while the Fas ligand and receptor are produced in pancreatic cancer cells, they are resistant to apoptosis through this pathway. This may be due to nonfunctional receptors or to changes in the downstream pathway, with upregulation of Bcl-x_L or other family members.[12] The secreted Fas ligand may be important in evasion of the immune response to the tumor. Similarly, resistance to TRAIL is not related to lack of receptors, but rather to upregulation of anti-apoptosis proteins, such as Bcl-x_L, XIAP, and FLIP$_S$.[13,14] Inhibition of produc-

tion of these proteins sensitizes the cells to the apoptosis-inducing effects of TRAIL.[13,14]

Key factors in the cell's balance of apoptosis or survival are the Bcl-2 family of apoptosis regulators. This is a large family of at least 16 members including anti-apoptotic proteins (such as Bcl-2, Mcl-1, Bcl-x_L) and pro-apoptotic proteins (such as Bax, Bak, and Bad). These regulators interact with other proteins through a helical region, called the Bcl homology domain. This interaction is important for regulation of apoptosis. The pro-apoptotic Bcl proteins activate permeabilization of the mitochondrial membrane, either by forming tetrameric channels themselves or by interaction with the mitochondrial permeability pore complex, allowing cytochrome c to pass into the cytoplasm. The anti-apoptotic members of the family prevent cytochrome c release, and it is probably the balance between these effectors that determines whether apoptosis will proceed or not. Bcl-x exists in two molecular forms, a long form (Bcl-x_L) that is anti-apoptotic and a short form (Bcl-x_S) that is pro-apoptotic. There is some evidence in pancreatic cancer cells that Bcl-x_L is more important than Bcl-2 in protecting against apoptosis triggered by the Fas ligand or TRAIL.[15] Bcl-x_L is constitutively over-expressed in pancreatic cancer cells. However, Bcl-2 itself and Mcl-1 appear to be important in resistance to drug-induced apoptosis.[16,17] Like Bcl-2, Bcl-x_L prevents cytochrome c release, but it also binds to Apaf-1 and thereby prevents association of caspase-9 with Apaf-1 and activation of this caspase.[18] Bcl-x_L or other family members might be useful targets for pancreatic cancer therapy, and certainly knockout of Bcl-x_L function results in an increase in apoptosis and sensitivity to gemcitabine, the cytotoxic agent that is the mainstay of therapy in pancreatic cancer.[19,20] Similarly, over-expression of Bax increases the sensitivity of pancreatic cancer cells to drug-induced apoptosis.[21] Expression of another family member, Bak, and apoptosis occur in the areas of inflammation surrounding the cancer, but not in the cancer cells themselves. This may actually promote tumor growth. There is considerable effort aimed at restoring the function of the pro-apoptotic Bcl-2 family members in the tumor cells using peptide mimetics and drugs that mimic the function of these proteins.[22]

The complex control of apoptosis also involves a series of caspase inhibitors. One class of these is the FADD-like ICE inhibitory proteins (FLIPs). Long ($FLIP_L$) and short ($FLIP_S$) forms of FLIP have been characterized.[20] $FLIP_L$, which is a homologue of caspase-8 but lacks the amino acids necessary for caspase activity, competes with caspase-8 for binding to FADD at the DISC, preventing activation of the caspase.[23] $FLIP_L$ is over-expressed in pancreatic cancer cells that are resistant to Fas-mediated apoptosis, and thus a potential target for therapy.[12] Indeed, peroxisome proliferator-activated receptor γ (PPARγ) agonists sensitize tumor cells to apoptosis by decreasing FLIP expression.[24] FLIP is also involved in activation of nuclear factor κB (NFκB) by recruiting adaptor proteins, such as TRAF, which in turn activates expression of several genes involved in tumor growth and progression.[25,26]

Another group of caspase inhibitors is the inhibitor of apoptosis (IAP) family, including cIAP, XIAP, and survivin.[27] These proteins contain a region called the baculoviral IAP repeat domain, through which they bind to caspases. The cellular function of the IAPs is not clear, but their expression is increased in cancer cells resistant to Fas and TRAIL-induced apoptosis. Forced expression of cIAP1, cIAP2, and XIAP suppresses apoptosis.[27] Survivin is a member of the IAP family, but has a unique structure that discriminates it from the other family members.[27] It is expressed in the G2/M phase of the cell cycle in a regulated manner. Survivin binds and inhibits both caspase-3 and caspase-7, which are the major executioner caspases.[28] It is not expressed in normal differentiated cells from any organ in adults, but is highly expressed in a wide range of cancers, including pancreatic cancer. Survivin expression steadily increases through the developmental stages of pancreatic intraepithelial neoplasias (PanINs),

which are the precursor lesions of pancreatic cancer.[29] Since survivin is such a potent caspase inhibitor, its over-expression in cancer is implicated in the resistance to different apoptotic stimuli, including chemotherapy. It may be a major reason for the resistance of pancreatic cancer to therapeutic agents. Several studies have shown that knockdown of survivin or XIAP expression using small inhibitory RNA (siRNA) can induce apoptosis in a number of different cancer cell types, including pancreatic cancer, and increase sensitivity to gemcitabine and 5-fluorouracil.[30–32] That is why these proteins are of such interest as targets in cancer therapy and also for chemoprevention.

The function of IAPs is inhibited by a protein called second mitochondria-derived activator of caspase (SMAC), which is also known as direct AIP binding protein with low pI (DIABLO).[33] The precursor form of SMAC is localized to mitochondria and it is released into the cytosol by cellular stress.[30] Its release, like that of cytochrome c, is suppressed by Bcl-2.[33] Upregulation of SMAC/DIABLO or its function may be valuable in pancreatic cancer therapy. A small fragment of the N-terminal sequence of SMAC/DIABLO coupled to a carrier peptide is able to enhance the antiproliferative effect, and apoptosis induction stimulated by wide range of antineoplastic agents.[34]

Procaspase-3 expression is increased in pancreatic cancer and levels are related to the invasiveness of the cancer cells.[35] Attempts to increase its expression would, therefore be futile. Recently, it came to light that the dormancy of the proenzyme is maintained by a regulatory "safety catch," which prevents accidental apoptosis.[36] The safety catch comprises a triplet of aspartic acid residues contained within the proenzyme itself that blocks access to the Ile-Glu-Thr-Asp (IETD) proteolytic activation site. It appears that the safety catch becomes disabled under the low cellular pH conditions that accompany apoptosis, enabling activation of this executioner caspase by caspase-9 or autoactivation.[36] This safety catch clearly represents an important drug target, since procaspase-3 is upregulated in pancreatic cancer and its activation results in apoptosis. These observations triggered the search for a small molecule that would directly activate this executioner caspase and bypass the upstream apoptosis regulatory pathways. A screen of more than 20,000 diverse small molecules revealed four compounds that could increase hydrolysis of a peptidic caspase-3 substrate.[37] One compound in particular showed a strong dose-dependent effect on procaspase-3 activation. This compound, named procaspase activating compound 1 (PAC-1) induces apoptosis in a wide range of cell lines and retarded growth of tumors in three different mouse models of cancer.[37] PAC-1 is active when administered orally.[37] Hopefully, PAC-1 or a similar compound can be developed as an anticancer agent.

The Growth Pathways in Pancreatic Cancer

Genetic mutations in oncogenes and tumor suppressor genes leads to upregulation of growth factors, their receptors, and downstream signaling pathways in pancreatic cancer. These tumors are largely independent of extrinsic growth factors, rendering them a distinct growth advantage. Removal of autocrine growth factor support triggers apoptosis, and many targeted therapy strategies are focused on these pathways. Important targets include the phosphoinositol 3-kinase (PI3K) and protein kinase B (AKT) pathway, the epidermal growth factor (EGF)-receptor-mediated pathway, the NFκB pathway, the p53 tumor suppressor gene, and the lipoxygenase and cyclooxygenase pathways.

The PI3K/AKT pathway is activated by growth factor receptors, such as the EGF and insulin-like growth factor 1 receptors. This pathway is important for cellular survival as well as growth. Activation of AKT induces upregulation of anti-apoptotic Bcl family members, as well as p27[KIP1] and NFκB.[38,39] AKT also phosphorylates and thereby inactivates the pro-apoptotic Bcl family member, Bad, as well

as caspase-9.[40,41] The activity of PI3K is inhibited by a protein called PTEN. In pancreatic cancer cells, PI3K, AKT, growth factors, and their receptors are over-expressed, while expression of PTEN is often suppressed. Because of the survival advantage that this pathway renders, it provides an important target for sensitizing cells to apoptosis. Wortmannin, a potent PI3K inhibitor blocks proliferation, induces apoptosis, and enhances the effects of gemcitabine in pancreatic cancer cells.[42,43] Other PI3K inhibitors are currently under investigation for cancer therapy.

The EGF receptor is over-expressed in the majority of pancreatic cancer cells and several of the ligands for this receptor are also upregulated, including EGF itself, transforming growth factor α, amphiregulin, and heparin-binding EGF.[44] High-affinity binding of these ligands to the receptor triggers a growth-stimulatory signaling cascade that involves *K-ras*, which is mutated and constitutively active in about 95% of pancreatic cancers. This pathway is, therefore, extremely important for growth and survival of this cancer, and several therapeutic strategies targeting the pathway are being pursued. These include various strategies to normalize the function of *K-ras*. Previous studies have shown that protein kinase C (PKC) activation by tumor-promoting phorbol esters causes a paradoxical inhibition of pancreatic cancer cell proliferation.[45] A recent study showed that phosphorylation of the *K-ras* oncogene on S181 results in translocation from the plasma membrane to intracellular membranes, including the outer mitochondrial membrane, where it interacts with Bcl-x$_L$ to promote apoptosis.[46] The PKC partial agonist bryostatin-1 inhibited the growth *in vitro* and *in vivo* of cells transformed with oncogenic *K-ras* in a S181-dependent mechanism. These findings provide a direct link between PKC activation and apoptosis and provide a possible explanation for PKC activation–mediated growth inhibition. Furthermore, since *K-ras* is mutated in almost all pancreatic cancers, these findings suggest that bryostatin may be effective in the treatment of these tumors.[46] Another important approach to targeting the EGF growth pathway is the use of EGF receptor tyrosine kinase inhibitors, the first of which (erlotinib) has been FDA approved for treating the disease.[47,48] However, it is now clear that a small subset of patients with EGF receptor mutations are the ones that respond well to the effects of these agents.[49] Other approaches to targeting this pathway include chimeric or humanized monoclonal antibodies that target the EGF receptor, such as cetuximab and matuzumab,[50,51] as well as inhibitors of the extracellular regulated kinases.[52] Another member of the EGF receptor family, ErbB2, also known as Her-2/neu has also been targeted with a monoclonal antibody marketed as Herceptin.[53]

NFκB is a transcription factor involved in diverse cellular activities including inflammation and the immune response. NFκB induces transcription of multiple target genes, including Bcl-x_L, cIAPs, and FLIPs.[54] Normally, NFκB is kept in an inactive state in the cytoplasm by another protein called IκBα. Cytokines, growth factors, and cellular stress activate NFκB by degradation of IκBα, whereupon it is translocated to the nucleus to increase expression of several anti-apoptotic genes listed above. NFκB appears to be constitutively activated in pancreatic cancer cells and is certainly activated by several chemotherapeutic agents, indicating that this transcription factor contributes to resistance to apoptosis in this cancer.[27] Inhibitors of NFκB, such as genestein, gliotoxin, and sulfaslazine, sensitize pancreatic cancer cells to chemotherapeutic drugs with an increase in apoptosis.[55,56] Such agents are likely to be valuable in enhancing the effect of chemotherapeutic drugs in pancreatic cancer.

In normal cells, the p53 protein inhibits growth by triggering cell-cycle arrest and apoptosis. It acts directly, by binding and inactivating Bcl-2 and Bcl-x_L, and indirectly, by increasing the expression of pro-apoptotic Bcl family members, such as Bax, Bid, and Bim.[56] The p53 tumor-suppressor gene is inactivated in more than 60% of pancreatic cancers, giving the cells a growth advantage.[9] Forced expression of wild-type p53 suppresses growth of pancreatic cancer cells and sensitizes them to apoptosis. Thus an important therapeutic approach for pancreatic cancer is to normalize p53 function.[57]

Lipoxygenases (particularly 5-LOX, 12-LOX) and cyclooxygenases (COX-2), which are key enzymes of arachidonic acid metabolism, play a major role in development and progression of pancreatic cancers.[17,58,59] These enzymes are not expressed in normal ductal cells, but are expressed pancreatic cancers as well as in the precursor, PanIN lesions.[60,61] LOX and COX metabolites stimulate growth of pancreatic cancer cells, while inhibitors of these enzymes block growth both *in vitro* and *in vivo*.[17,58,59,62–65] The LOX enzymes are upregulated in response to growth factor stimulation, while inhibitors of these enzymes block growth factor-induced growth and MAP kinase activation, indicating interaction of these pathways. COX and LOX inhibitors and receptor antagonists for the downstream metabolite, leukotriene B4, induce apoptosis *in vitro* and *in vivo* and enhance the effectiveness of gemcitabine against these cancer cells.[1,59,64,65] These pathways are clearly valuable targets for pancreatic cancer therapy and chemoprevention.

Novel Agents Recently Shown to Inhibit Pancreatic Cancer Growth with Apoptosis

There are many naturally occurring substances that have been recently shown to potently inhibit growth of pancreatic cancer cells with induction of apoptosis. These include genistein, a flavonoid from soy beans[56]; resveratrol, a phytoalexin found in high concentrations in grape skins and red wine[66]; apigenin, a flavonoid found in herbs, such as parsley, thyme, and peppermint[67]; gingerol, a major phenolic compound in root ginger[68]; frondoside A, a triterpine glycoside from the skin of the edible Atlantic sea cucumber; and sansalvamide,

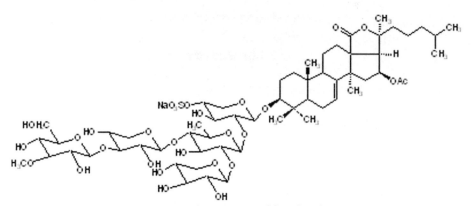

Figure 1. The structure of frondoside A.

a small cyclic depsipeptide from a marine fungus.[69] All of these compounds appear to have low toxicity and may be developed into therapeutic agents themselves or as adjuncts to conventional chemotherapeutic drugs.

Frondoside A

Sea cucumbers (phylum: *Echinodermata*, class: *Holothuroidea*) are consumed, especially in Asian cultures. They also have been employed for various medicinal purposes for hundreds of years. Sea cucumber toxins or holotoxins have been isolated in crystalline form and shown to contain a mixture of saponins.[70–72] Some glycosylated triterpenoid saponins have been shown to possess anticancer activity.[73–78] Frondoside A is a bioactive triterpenoid saponin isolated from the edible Atlantic sea cucumber, *Cucumaria frondosa*. To illustrate the effects of a novel agent on growth and apoptosis, we investigated the effects of frondoside A on growth and apoptosis of human pancreatic cells (AsPC-1) *in vivo* and *in vitro*.

Materials and Methods

Reagents

Frondoside A was diluted to the appropriate concentrations in serum-free medium for the experiments. The structure of frondoside

A is shown in Figure 1, and the purity and molecular mass of the compound are shown in Figure 2. This analysis was carried out by Dr. Thomas McCloud at the National Cancer Institute, Natural Products Branch (Frederick, MD). The enhanced chemiluminescence system was obtained from Santa Cruz Biotechnology, Inc. (Santa Cruz, CA). The mouse monoclonal antibodies against Bax, Bcl-2, Mcl-1, P21[wafl], and P27[kip1] and the rabbit polyclonal antibodies against caspase-3, caspase-7, and caspase-9 were purchased from Santa Cruz Biotechnology, Inc. Unless otherwise stated, all other chemicals were purchased from Sigma Chemicals (St. Louis, MO).

Cell Culture

The poorly differentiated human pancreatic cancer line, AsPC-1, was purchased from the American Type Culture Collection (Manassas, VA). Cells were cultured in minimal essential medium supplemented with penicillin G (100 U/mL), streptomycin (100 U/mL), and 10% fetal bovine serum at 37°C in humidified air with 5% CO_2. Cells were harvested by incubation in trypsin-EDTA solution for 10–15 mins. Then cells were centrifuged at 300 g for 5 min and cell pellets were suspended in fresh culture medium prior to seeding into culture flasks or plates.

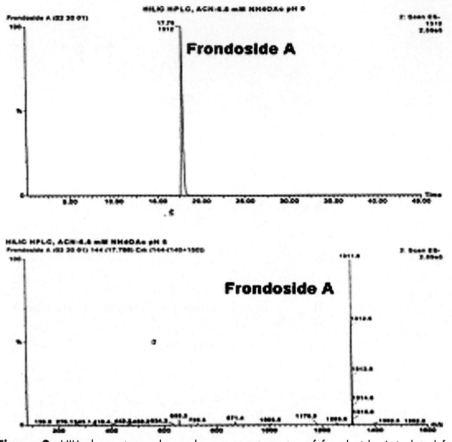

Figure 2. HILI chromatography and mass spectrometry of frondoside A isolated from *Cucumaria frondosa*. *Top Panel*: HILI chromatography showing purity of frondoside A. The column was eluted with acetonitrile with 5.5 mM ammonium acetate, pH 5.0. *Bottom Panel*: Tandem electrospray mass spectrometry of frondoside A showing a molecular mass (mass of charge ratio) of 1312. Note that a single Na+ ion is lost in this analysis, thus the true molecular weight is 1334. This analysis was carried out by Dr. Thomas McCloud at the National Cancer Institute, Natural Products Branch (Frederick, MD).

Morphological Studies

The photomicrographs of cell morphological changes were taken with a Kodak DC 120 digital zoom camera (Eastman Kodak Company, Rochester, NY) under an inverted microscope ($\times$400) following treatment with or without 4 μg/mL frondoside A for different time periods from 24 to 72 h.

Cell Proliferation Assay

Cell growth was analyzed by the ^{3}H-methyl thymidine incorporation and cell counting. Following treatment of pancreatic cancer cells with a series of concentrations of frondoside A from 1 μg/mL to 16 μg/mL, cellular DNA synthesis was assayed by adding ^{3}H-methyl thymidine 0.5 μCi/well. After 2 h incubation, the cells were washed twice with phosphate-buffered saline (PBS), precipitated with 10% TCA for 2 h, and solubilized from each well with 0.5 mL of 0.4 N NaOH. Incorporation of ^{3}H-methyl thymidine into DNA was measured by adding scintillation liquid, and counting in a scintillation counter (LKB BackBeta, Wallac, Turku, Finland). For cell counting, cells were seeded in 12-well plates and cultured with serum-free medium for 24 h prior to frondoside A treatment and then switched to serum-free medium with or without 4 μg/mL frondoside A for the respective treatment time points (24, 48, and 72 h). The cells were removed from the plate by trypsinization to produce a single cell suspension for cell counting. The cells were counted using Z1-Coulter Counter (Luton, UK).

Annexin V assay

Cells grown on coverslips were treated with or without 4 μg/mL frondoside A, in serum-free media, for 4 h. The cells were then rinsed with PBS and 500 μL of assay buffer once. Then, 200 μL of assay buffer, 4 μL of annexin-V fluorescein isothiocyanate (FITC), and 20 μL of propidium iodide were added to each coverslip. The coverslips were then incubated at room temperature for 15 min in the dark and washed once with PBS. Cells were finally viewed under fluorescence microscope using a dual filter set for FITC and rhodamine, and pictures were taken using a Kodak DC 120 digital zoom camera.

Terminal Deoxynucleotidyl Transferase-mediated Deoxyuridine Triphosphate Nick-end Labeling (TUNEL) Assay

The assay was carried out for terminal incorporation of fluorescein 12-dUTP by terminal deoxynucleotidyl transferase into fragmented DNA in cancer cells (TUNEL assay kits, Promega, Madison, WI). Cells were cultured to 50–60% confluence in T75 flasks in serum-free conditions for 24 h and then in the presence or absence of 4 μg/mL frondoside A for 72 h. Cells were then trypsinized and fixed in 1% methanol-free formaldehyde-PBS for 15 min. At the end of treatment, cells were then harvested with trypsin-EDTA solution to produce a single cell suspension. Cells were then pelleted by centrifugation and washed twice with PBS. The cell pellets were then suspended in 0.5 mL PBS and fixed in ice-cold 70% ethanol at 4°C. Fixed cells were

centrifuged at 300 *g* for 10 min and pellets were washed with PBS. After resuspension with 1 mL PBS, cells were incubated with 10 μL of RNase I (10 mg/mL) and 100 μL of propidium iodide (400 μg/mL; Sigma) and shaken for 1 h at 37°C in the dark. Samples were analyzed by flow cytometry. Laser flow cytometry was used to quantify the green fluorescence of fluorescein-12-dUTP incorporated against the red fluorescence of propidium iodide.

Western Blotting

Cells were seeded into flasks and cultured to 50–60% confluence for 24 h. Cells were then placed in serum-free medium in the presence or absence of 4 μg/mL frondoside A for periods of 0, 24, 48, and 72 h. Proteins were extracted from attached and floating cells in lysis buffer containing 4% SDS. Protein concentrations were determined using the bicinchoninic acid assay with bovine serum antigen as standard. Western blotting was carried out. In brief, equal amounts protein in the cell lysates were separated on 15% SDS-PAGE and the proteins then transferred onto nitrocellulose membranes. After blocking nonspecific sites with dried milk, membranes were incubated with the appropriate dilution of primary antibody. Membranes were then incubated with a horseradish peroxidase conjugated secondary antibody. Proteins were detected using an enhanced chemiluminescence detection system.

Animal Study

Athymic mice (BALB/c nu/nu, 5-week-old females) were purchased from Charles River Laboratories (Wilmington, MA). Mice were acclimatized to the animal facility for 1 week prior to receiving xenografts. Xenografts of 3 million AsPC-1 cells were injected into the flanks of mice, once visible tumors were evidenced, 4–5 days after injection, the animals were divided equally into two groups (six animals/group) and treated with frondoside A (10 μg/kg/day) or control vehicle (100 μL PBS) by intraperitoneal injection. Animal weight and tumor size were recorded every 3 days. The formula used for tumor volume: volume = (length) × (width) × (length + width/2) × 0.526.[79] After 4 weeks of treatment, the animals were euthanized and the tumors were carefully dissected and tumors weighed.

Statistical Analysis

Thymidine incorporation data was analyzed by ANOVA with Dunnett's multiple comparison post-test, for significance between individual groups. The time-course experiments measuring cell number and the *in vivo* studies of xenografts in athymic mice were analyzed by two-way ANOVA with treatment and time as the independent variables. Analysis was performed with the Prism software package (GraphPad, San Diego, CA). Data are expressed as mean ± SEM. All other data shown are representative of at least three different experiments.

Results

Effect of Frondoside A on Thymidine Incorporation in Pancreatic Cancer Cells

Frondoside A caused marked inhibition of thymidine incorporation in AsPC-1 cells in a concentration-dependent manner at concentrations ranging from 1 μg/mL to 16 μg/mL (ANOVA: $F(5,30) = 55.6$, $P < 0.0001$; Fig. 3). Cytotoxicity was seen only following treatment with frondoside A concentrations higher than 16 μg/mL, which caused cell necrosis (data not shown).

Effect of Frondoside A on Pancreatic Cancer Cell Proliferation Measured by Cell Counting

Frondoside A significantly inhibited proliferation of pancreatic cancer cells in a time-dependent manner, as measured by cell num-

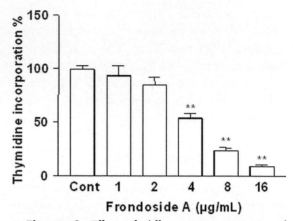

Figure 3. Effect of different concentrations of frondoside A on proliferation of AsPC-1 human pancreatic cancer cells, measured by ^{3}H-methyl thymidine incorporation. Data are expressed as percent of untreated control with mean ± SEM of three separate experiments. ANOVA: $F(5,30) = 55.6$, $P < 0.0001$, **$P < 0.01$ compared to control.

ber in AsPC-1 cells (two-way ANOVA, drug effect: $F(1,40) = 45.9$, $P < 0.0001$; time effect: $F(3,40) = 28.3$, $P < 0.0001$; interaction $F(3,40) = 13.6$, $P < 0.0001$, Fig. 4). During the first 24 h, no obvious effect was seen compared to control. At 48 and 72 h, frondoside A resulted in a marked and progressive decrease in cell number compared to control.

Apoptosis of Pancreatic Cancer Cells Induced by Frondoside A

Within 24 h, 4 μg/mL frondoside A caused the marked morphological changes characteristic of apoptosis, including shrinkage of cytoplasm, membrane blebbing, nuclear condensation, and loss of adhesion (Fig. 5). To further characterize the apoptosis observed, the early apoptotic changes in the cellular membrane were investigated by annexin V binding assay, and late changes by analysis of DNA fragmentation was carried out using the TUNEL assay. Annexin V binding was observed in response to 4 μg/mL frondoside A treatment within 3 h (Fig. 6). TUNEL staining of pancreatic cancer cells was markedly increased by 4 μg/mL frondoside A treatment at

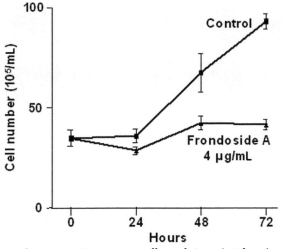

Figure 4. Time-course effect of 4 μg/mL frondoside A on cell number of AsPC-1 human pancreatic cancer cells. Data represent means ± SEM of three separate experiments. Two-way ANOVA, drug effect: $F(1,40) = 45.9$, $P < 0.0001$; time effect: $F(3,40) = 28.3$, $P < 0.0001$; interaction $F(3,40) = 13.6$, $P < 0.0001$.

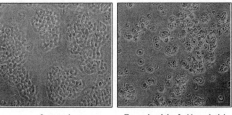
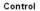

Figure 5. Frondoside A-induced morphological changes in AsPC-1 cells. Cells were treated with 4 μg/mL frondoside A and photomicrographs were taken at 72 h. Frondoside A induced shrinkage of cytoplasm, membrane blebbing, and nuclear condensation. Results are representative of three separate experiments.

72 h (control 2.4%, frondoside A 36.1%, $P < 0.001$).

Effect of Frondoside A on Activation of Caspase 3, 7, and 9 Proteins

The expression and activation of caspases 3, 7, and 9 by cleavage were observed by western blotting. In response to frondoside A, procaspase-3 was cleaved into products of lower molecular weight, including bands of 17 and

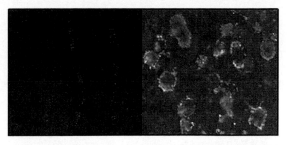

Figure 6. Western blot showing the effect of 4 μg/mL frondoside A on annexin V binding in AsPC-1 pancreatic cancer cells. There is no detectable fluorescence in control cells but marked fluorescence in cells treated with 4 μg/mL frondoside A. The results are representative of three different experiments.

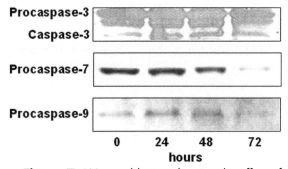

Figure 7. Western blotting showing the effect of 4 μg/mL frondoside A on caspases 3, 7, 9 in AsPC-1 cells. Procaspases 3, 7, 9 were identified using specific antibodies. The *top panel* shows increased cleavage of procapsase-3 into active fragments over time. The *other panels* show a reduction in content of procaspases 7 and 9 over time. The results are representative of three separate experiments.

11 kDa, indicating activation (Fig. 7). Only the uncleaved 32 kDa procaspase-3 was seen in untreated controls. Activation of caspases 7 and 9 was confirmed by a reduction in the amounts of the respective procaspase forms, as the antibodies do not recognize the active fragments (Fig. 7). Activation of caspases 3, 7, and 9 was induced in a time-dependent manner, coincident with the induction of apoptosis.

Effect of Frondoside A on Expression of Bax, Bcl-2, and Mcl-1 Proteins

Treatment with frondoside A decreased expression of the anti-apoptotic proteins, Bcl-2

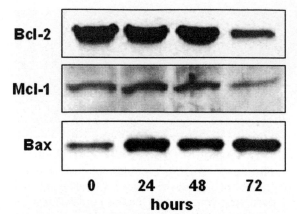

Figure 8. Western blot showing the effect of 4 μg/mL frondoside A on the Bcl-2, Mcl-1, and Bax proteins in AsPC-1 cells. The results are representative of three separate experiments.

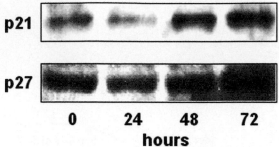

Figure 9. Western blot showing the effect of 4 μg/mL frondoside A on the cyclin-dependent kinase inhibitors, p21 and p27, in AsPC-1 cells. The results are representative of three separate experiments.

and Mcl-1 in a time-dependent manner (Fig. 8). In contrast, concentrations of the pro-apoptotic protein Bax increased (Fig. 8).

Effect of Frondoside A on Expression of p21 and p27

In response to frondoside A, expression of the cyclin-dependent kinase inhibitor, $p21^{wafl}$ was markedly increased in a time-dependent manner, while expression of $p27^{kip1}$ was not changed (Fig. 9).

Effect of Frondoside A on Pancreatic Cancer Growth *in vivo*

The growth inhibitory effect of frondoside A was confirmed in an *in vivo* study. Frondoside A (10 μg/kg/day) markedly inhibited the growth of subcutaneously transplanted AsPC-1 cells in athymic mice after 4 weeks of treatment, as measured by both tumor volume and tumor weight (two-way ANOVA, drug effect: $F(1,148) = 7.9$, $P < 0.0001$; time effect: $F(8,40) = 56.3$, $P < 0.0001$; interaction $F(8) = 4.6$, $P < 0.0027$, Fig. 10). No toxicity of was seen with frondoside A through the treatment period, and there was no significant difference between the body weights of control and treated animals.

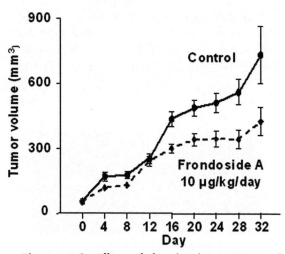

Figure 10. Effect of frondoside A (10 μg/kg/day) on growth of AsPC-1 human pancreatic cancer xenografts in athymic mice. Frondoside A substantially reduced growth of the subcutaneous tumors, particularly through the last 2 weeks of treatment. Two-way ANOVA, drug effect: $F(1,148) = 7.9$, $P < 0.0001$; time effect: $F(8,40) = 56.3$, $P < 0.0001$; interaction $F(8) = 4.6$, $P < 0.0027$.

Discussion

Sea cucumbers are important components of traditional Chinese medicine and some health-food supplements sold in the United States. Active compounds isolated from these echinoderms have interesting biological properties and potential clinical use. One group of active compounds is glycosylated triterpenoid saponins, some of which have been shown to have anticancer activity.[73–78] One such compound is Frondoside A, which is derived from the Atlantic sea cucumber, *Cucumaria frondosa,* a species that is very abundant on the North Atlantic coast of America. The effects of this agent on proliferation and apoptosis of cancer cells have not previously been reported. We investigated the effects of frondoside A in pancreatic cancer, which is a major cause of cancer death in the Western world.

In preliminary experiments, we tested a series of concentrations of frondoside A ranging from 1 μg/mL to 32 μg/mL. The results showed that concentrations higher than 16 μg/mL frondoside A caused immediate necrosis of cells, indicating a cytotoxic effect. Therefore, concentrations between 1 μg/mL and 16 μg/mL frondoside A were used for subsequent experiments on induction of apoptosis in pancreatic cancer cells, to avoid cytotoxicity. At low concentrations, frondoside A inhibited growth and induced apoptosis in a concentration-dependent manner in AsPC-1 cells. Because 4 μg/mL frondoside A reduced incorporation of ^{3}H-methyl thymidine into DNA by approximately 50% within 24 h, we tested the effect of this concentration on cell number over a prolonged time period from 24 to 72 h. The results showed profound inhibition of growth that is time-dependent. The cyclin-dependent kinase inhibitor, p21^{wafl} mediates cellular responses to DNA damaging agents.[80] The present studies revealed a marked time-dependent increase in expression of p21^{wafl} in response to frondoside A, while expression of P27^{kip1} protein was not changed. These results suggest that the p21^{wafl} protein might play a role in the growth inhibition of pancreatic cancer cells, induced by frondoside A.

The inhibitory effect of frondoside A on pancreatic cancer cell growth was confirmed in the athymic mouse xenograft model. A very low concentration of frondoside A caused a substantial inhibition of tumor growth throughout the period of study. Dose–response experiments were not carried out because of the limited availability of the compound.

Morphological changes are characteristic features of cells undergoing apoptosis and these are readily observed microscopically. Specific apoptotic morphological changes were identified following frondoside A treatment within 48 h, and the proportion of apoptotic cells increased with the time of treatment. To confirm the effect of frondoside A on apoptosis in pancreatic cancer cells, annexin V staining and TUNEL assay were carried out. During early apoptosis, phosphatidylserine, a phospholipid usually located on the inner surface of the plasma membrane, translocates to the outer plasma membrane.[10] Annexin V preferentially binds to negatively charged phosphatidylserine. By conjugating fluorescein to annexin V, it can be used to identify early apoptosis by flow cytometry or fluorescence microscopy. Annexin V binds to early apoptotic cells, but they do not exhibit intracellular staining with propidium iodide. As the cells progress through apoptosis, the integrity of the plasma membrane is lost, allowing propidium iodide to penetrate and label the cells with a strong yellow-red fluorescence. The results showed strong annexin V staining in AsPC-1 cell after frondoside A treatment for 3 h, but no staining in control untreated cells. In the late stages of apoptosis, genomic DNA is cleaved in fragments due to activation of endonucleases. The TUNEL assay identifies these DNA fragments in apoptotic cells by use of a fluorescent indicator that attaches to the ends of DNA fragments. The TUNEL assay results confirmed marked apoptosis in frondoside A–treated pancreatic cancer cells.

The ability to induce apoptosis of cancer cells is an attractive feature of anticancer agents.[81] Because the caspase cascade plays an important role in the apoptotic program of cells,[82–84] we analyzed caspases 3, 7, and 9 by western blotting. All three caspases were activated by frondoside A. Sequence alignment of caspases 3, 7, and 9 reveals the structural basis of their functions. The executioner caspases 3 and 7 share 54% sequence homology and the backbone structures are nearly identical.[85] These effector caspases are activated by the initiator, caspase-9 through proteolytic cleavage at specific internal Asp residues. In turn, caspases 3 and 7 are responsible for initiating the apoptotic program.[82–84] The Bcl-2 protein family is broadly classified into two categories, according to their role in apoptosis, as anti-apoptotic members, such as Bcl-2, Mcl-1, and Bcl-x_L and pro-apoptotic members, such as Bax, Bad, Bak, and Bag. These proteins indirectly regulate the activation of the caspase cascade.[86,87] It is believed that the ratio of anti-apoptotic proteins and pro-apoptotic proteins, which can form homodimers or interact with each other to form heterodimers, determines whether or not cells will undergo apoptosis.[86,87] The increase of Bax and the decrease of Bcl-2 and Mcl-1 concentrations indicate that the balance has changed in favor of apoptosis. When considered together, the results indicate that the mitochondrial pathway to caspase cascade activation plays an important role in frondoside A–induced apoptosis.

The ability to induce apoptosis in cancer cells, without affecting healthy cells, as well as minimizing side effects, are major goals for the development of new anticancer agents. The results from the present study indicate that frondoside A inhibits cell proliferation, coincident with an increase in p21 expression, and induces apoptosis in pancreatic cancer cells via the mitochondrial pathway of caspase cascade activation. Low concentrations of frondoside A caused a marked decrease in tumor growth in a mouse xenograft model using a highly malignant, poorly differentiated human pancreatic cancer cell line. In summary, these findings indicate frondoside A has potent antiproliferative effects on human pancreatic cancer cells with induction of apoptosis.

Conclusions

The complex pathways involved in apoptosis are controlled by a variety of pro- and anti-apoptotic factors, the balance of which ensures tissue homeostasis. Activation or downregulation of pro- and anti-apoptotic genes can influence cancer cell viability and sensitivity to chemotherapy or radiotherapy, tumor development, and progression. There are a number of potential targets for inducing and enhancing apoptosis in this disease, including enhancing or mimicking the effects of pro-apoptotic Bcl family members; blocking the effects of caspase inhibitors; upregulating SMAC/DIABLO function; inhibition of the PI3K/AKT pathway; blocking growth factor (such as EGF) pathways; inhibiting NFκB; normalizing p53 function; and inhibiting 5-LOX, 12-LOX, and/or COX-2 activity or blocking the downstream pathways for their metabolites. Such therapeutic strategies, perhaps in combination, may help to improve outcomes in pancreatic cancer. Pancreatic cancer cells are relatively resistant to conventional therapeutics and so discovery of novel agents that can induce apoptosis in these cells is important for the future therapy of pancreatic cancer. Frondoside A is one such agent that may be valuable in the treatment of the devastating disease and is worthy of further investigation.

Acknowledgments

The authors are grateful for the chromatographic analysis and mass spectrometry of frondoside A carried out by Dr. Thomas McCloud at the National Cancer Institute, Natural Products Branch (Frederick, MD). The work was supported by a grant from the National Cancer Institute RAPID program, the Maine Technology Institute, and the Michael Rolfe Foundation for Pancreatic Cancer Research. Patent Pending. There are no commercial affiliations, licensing agreements, or other potential conflicts of interest.

Conflicts of Interest

The authors declare no conflicts of interest.

References

1. Jema, A., R. Siegel, E. Ward, *et al.* 2006. Cancer statistics, 2006. *CA. Cancer J. Clin.* **56:** 106–130.

2. Cardenes, H.R., E.G. Chiorean, J.J. DeWitt, *et al.* 2006. Locally advanced pancreatic cancer: current therapeutic approach. *Ocologist* **11:** 612–623.

3. Cameron, J.L., H.A. Pitt & C.J. Yeo. 1993. One hundred and forty-five consecutive pancreaticoduodenectomies without mortality. *Ann. Surg.* **217:** 430–438.

4. Carpelan-Holmström, M., S. Nordling, E. Pukkala, *et al.* 2005. Does anyone survive pancreatic ductal adenocarcinoma? A nationwide study re-evaluating the data of the Finnish Cancer Registry. *Pancreas* **54:** 385–387.

5. Serafini, F.M. & A.S. Rosemurgy. 2000. New direction in systemic therapy of pancreatic cancer. *Cancer Control* **7:** 437–444.

6. Giovannetti, E., V. Mey, S. Nannizzi, *et al.* 2006. Pharmacogenetics of anticancer drug sensitivity in pancreatic cancer. *Mol. Cancer Ther.* **6:** 1387–1395.

7. Nakano, Y., S. Tanno, K. Koizumi, *et al.* 2007. Gemcitabine chemoresistance and molecular markers associated with gemcitabine transport and metabolism in human pancreatic cancer cells. *Br. J. Cancer* **96:** 457–463.

8. Talar-Wojnarowska, R. & E. Malecka-Panas. 2006. Molecular pathogenesis of pancreatic adenocarcinoma: potential clinical implications. *Med. Sci. Monit.* **2:** 186–193.

9. Schneider, G. & R.M. Schmid. 2003. Genetic alterations in pancreatic carcinoma. *Mol. Cancer* **2:** 15.

10. Okada, H. & T.W. Mak. 2004. Pathways of apoptotic and non-apoptotic death in tumor cells. *Nature Rev. Cancer* **4:** 592–603.

11. Ghobrial, I.M., T.E. Witzig & A.A. Adjei. 2005. Targeting apoptosis pathways in cancer therapy. *CA Cancer J. Clin.* **55:** 178–194.

12. Elnemr, A., T. Ohta, A. Yachie, *et al.* 2001. Human pancreatic cancer cells disable function of Fas receptors at several levels in Fas signal transduction pathway. *Int. J. Oncol.* **2:** 311–316.

13. Matsuzaki, H., B.M. Schmied, A. Ulrich, *et al.* 2001. Combination of tumor necrosis factor-related apoptosis-inducing ligand (TRAIL) and actinomycin D induces apoptosis even in TRAIL-resistant human pancreatic cancer cells. *Clin. Cancer Res.* **2:** 407–414.

14. Vogler, M., K. Durr, M. Jovanovic, *et al.* 2007. Regulation of TRAIL-induced apoptosis by XIAP in pancreatic cancer cells. *Oncogene* **26:** 248–257.

15. Hinz, S., A. Trauzold, L. Boenicke, *et al.* 2000. Bcl-x$_L$ protects pancreatic adenocarcinoma cells against CD95- and TRAIL-receptor-mediated apoptosis. *Oncogene* **19:** 5477–5486.

16. Li, X., X. Ding & T.E. Adrian. 2003. Arsenic trioxide induces apoptosis in pancreatic cancer cells via changes in cell cycle, caspase activation, and GADD expression. *Pancreas* **27:** 174–179.

17. Tong, W.G., X.Z. Ding, R.C. Witt & T.E. Adrian. 2002. Lipoxygenase inhibitors attenuate growth of human pancreatic cancer xenografts and induce apoptosis through the mitochondrial pathway. *Mol. Cancer Ther.* **1:** 929–935.

18. Hu, Y., M.A. Benedict, D. Wu, *et al.* 1998. Bcl-x$_L$ interacts with Apaf-1 and inhibits Apaf-1-dependent caspase-9 activation. *Proc. Natl. Acad. Sci. U.S.A.* **95:** 4386–4391.

19. Xu, Z., H. Friess, M. Solioz, *et al.* 2001. Bcl-x$_L$ antisense oligonucleotides induce apoptosis and increase sensitivity of pancreatic cancer cells to gemcitabine. *Int. J. Cancer* **94:** 268–274.

20. Shi, X., S. Liu, J. Kleeff, *et al.* 2002. Acquired resistance of pancreatic cancer cells towards 5-fluorouracil and gemcitabine is associated with altered expression of apoptosis-regulating genes. *Oncology* **62:** 354–362.

21. Xu, Z.W., H. Friess, M.W. Büchler & M. Solioz. 2002. Overexpression of Bax sensitizes human pancreatic cancer cells to apoptosis induced by chemotherapeutic agents. *Cancer Chemother. Pharmacol.* **49:** 504–510.

22. Baell, J.B. & D.C. Huang. 2002. Prospects for targeting the Bcl-2 family of proteins to develop novel cytotoxic drugs. *Biochem. Pharmacol.* **64:** 851–863.

23. Krueger, A., S. Baumann, P.H. Krammer & S. Kirchoff. 2001. FLICE-inhibitory proteins: Regulators of death receptor-mediated apoptosis. *Mol. Cell Biol.* **21:** 8247–8254.

24. Kim, Y., N. Suh, M. Sporn & J.C. Reed. 2002. An inducible pathway for degradation of FLIP protein sensitizes tumor cells to TRAIL-induced apoptosis. *J. Biol. Chem.* **277:** 22320–22329.

25. Kataoka, T., R.C. Budd, N. Holler, *et al.* 2000. The caspase-8 inhibitor FLIP promotes activation of NFκB and Erk signaling pathways. *Curr. Biol.* **10:** 640–648.

26. Bharti, A.C. & B.B. Aggarwal. 2002. Nuclear factor-κ-B and cancer: Its role in prevention and therapy. *Biochem. Pharmacol.* **64:** 883–888.

27. Deveraux, Q.L. & J.C. Reed. 1999. IAP family proteins-suppressors of apoptosis. *Genes Dev.* **13:** 239–252.

28. Tamm, I., Y. Wang, E. Sausville, *et al.* 1998. IAP-family protein survivin inhibits caspase activity and apoptosis induced by Fas (CD95), Bax, caspases, and anticancer drugs. *Cancer Res.* **58:** 5315–5320.

29. Bhanot, U., R. Heydrich, P. Moller & C. Hasel. 2006. Survivin expression in pancreatic intraepithelial neoplasia (PanIN): steady increase along the

developmental stages of pancreatic ductal adenocarcinoma. *Am. J. Surg. Pathol.* **30:** 754–759.

30. Shrikhande, S.V., J. Kleeff, H. Kayed, *et al.* 2006. Silencing of X-linked inhibitor of apoptosis (XIAP) decreases gemcitabine resistance in pancreatic cancer cells. *Anticancer Res.* **26:** 3265–3273.

31. Li, Y., Z. Jian, K. Xia, *et al.* 2006. XIAP is related to the chemoresistance and inhibited its expression by RNA interference sensitize pancreatic carcinoma cells to chemotherapeutics. *Pancreas* **32:** 288–296.

32. Guan, H.T., X.H. Xue, Z.J. Dai, *et al.* 2006. Downregulation of survivin expression by small interfering RNA induces pancreatic cancer cell apoptosis and enhances its radiosensitivity. *World J. Gastroenterol.* **12:** 2901–2907.

33. Verhagan, A.M., P.G. Ekert, M. Pakusch, *et al.* 2000. Identification of DIABLO, a mammalian protein that promotes apoptosis by binding to and antagonizing IAP proteins. *Cell* **102:** 43–53.

34. Arnt, C.R., M.V. Chiorean, M.P. Heldebrant, *et al.* 2002. Synthetic Smac/DIABLO peptides enhance the effects of chemotherapeutic agents by binding XIAP and cIAP in situ. *J. Biol. Chem.* **277:** 44236–44243.

35. Satoh, K., K. Kaneko, M. Hirota, *et al.* 2000. The pattern of CPP32/caspase-3 expression reflects the biological behavior of the human pancreatic duct cell tumors. *Pancreas* **21:** 532–537.

36. Roy, S., C.I. Bayly, Y. Gareau, *et al.* 2001. Maintenance of caspase-3 proenzyme dormancy by an intrinsic "safety catch" regulatory tripeptide. *Proc. Natl. Acad. Sci. U.S.A.* **98:** 6132–6137.

37. Putt, K.S., G.W. Chen, J.M. Pearson, *et al.* 2006. Small-molecule activation of procaspase-3 to caspase-3 as a personalized anticancer strategy. *Nature Chem. Biol.* **2:** 543–550.

38. Graff, J.R., B.W. Konicek, A.M. McNulty, *et al.* 2000. Increased AKT activity contributes to prostate cancer progression by dramatically accelerating prostate tumor growth and diminishing p27^{KIP1} expression. *J. Biol. Chem.* **275:** 24500–24505.

39. Jones, R.G., M. Parsons, M. Bonnard, *et al.* 2000. Protein kinase B regulates T lymphocyte survival, nuclear factor κB activation and Bcl-x$_L$ levels in vivo. *J. Exp. Med.* **191:** 1721–1734.

40. Gilmore, A.P., A.J. Valentjin, P. Wang, *et al.* 2002. Activation of BAD by therapeutic inhibition of epidermal growth factor receptor and transactivation by insulin-like growth factor receptor. *J. Biol. Chem.* **277:** 27643–27650.

41. Kermer, P., R. Ankerhold, N. Klocker, *et al.* 2000. Caspase-9: Involvement in secondary death of axotomized rat retinal ganglion cells in vivo. *Brain Res. Mol. Brain Res.* **85:** 144–150.

42. Ng, S.S.W., M.S. Tsao, S. Chow & D.W. Hedley. 2000.

Inhibition of phophatidylinositide 3-kinase enhances gemcitabine-induced apoptosis in human pancreatic cancer cells. *Cancer Res.* **60:** 5451–5455.

43. Ng, S.S., M.S. Tsau, T. Nicklee & D.W. Hedley. 2001. Wortmannin inhibits pkb/akt phosphorylation and promotes gemcitabine antitumor activity in orthotopic human pancreatic cancer xenografts in immunodeficient mice. *Clin. Cancer Res.* **7:** 3269–3275.

44. Korc, M., B. Chandraseker, Y. Yamanaka, *et al.* 1992. Overexpression of the epidermal growth factor receptor in human pancreatic cancer is associated with comcomitant increases in the level of epidermal growth factor and transforming growth factor alpha. *J. Clin. Invest.* **90:** 1352–1360.

45. Salabat, M.R., X.Z. Ding, J.B. Flesche, *et al.* 2006. On the mechanisms of 12-otetradecanoylphorbol-13-acetate -induced growth arrest in pancreatic cancer cells. *Pancreas* **33:** 148–155.

46. Bivona, T.G., S.E. Quatela, B.O. Bodemann, *et al.* 2006. PKC regulates a farnesyl-electrostatic switch on K-Ras that promotes its association with Bcl-XL on mitochondria and induces apoptosis. *Mol. Cell* **21:** 481–493.

47. Moore, M.J., D. Goldstein, J. Hamm, *et al.* 2005. Erlotinib improves survival when added to gemcitabine in patients with advanced pancreatic cancer. A phase III trial of the National Cancer Institute of Canada Clinical Trials Group (NCIC-CTG). *J. Clin. Oncology* **23**(Suppl.): 1.

48. Tang, P.A., M.S. Tsao & M.J. Moore. 2006. A review of erlotinib and its clinical use. *Expert. Opin. Pharmacother.* **7:** 177–193.

49. Kwak, E.L., J. Jankowski, S.P. Thayer, *et al.* 2006. Epidermal growth factor receptor kinase domain mutations in esophageal and pancreatic adenocarcinomas. *Clin. Cancer Res.* **12:** 4283–4287.

50. Xiong, H.Q., A. Rosenberg, A. LoBuglio, *et al.* 2004. Cetuximab, a monoclonal antibody targeting the epidermal growth factor receptor, in combination with gemcitabine for advanced pancreatic cancer: a multicenter phase II trial. *J. Clin. Oncol.* **22:** 2610–2616.

51. Graeven, U., B. Kremer, T. Sudhoff, *et al.* 2006. Phase I study of the humanized anti-EGFR monoclonal antibody matuzumab (EMD 72000) combined with gemcitabine in advanced pancreatic cancer. *Br. J. Cancer* **94:** 1293–1299.

52. Messersmith, W.A., M. Hidalgo, M. Carducci & S.G. Eckhardt. 2006. Novel targets in solid tumors: MEK inhibitors. *Clin. Adv. Hematol. Oncol.* **4:** 831–836.

53. Safran, H., D. Iannitti, R. Ramanathan, *et al.* 2004. Herceptin and gemcitabine for metastatic pancreatic cancers that overexpress Her-2/neu. *Cancer Invest.* **22:** 706–712.

54. Karin, M. & A. Lin. 2002. NF-κB at the crossroads of life and death. *Nature Immunol.* **3:** 221–222.

55. Arlt, A., J. Vorndamm, M. Breitenbroich, *et al.* 2001. Inhibition of NF-κB sensitizes human pancreatic carcinoma cells to apoptosis induced by etoposide (VP16) or doxorubicin. *Oncogene* **20:** 859–868.

56. Li, Y., F. Ahmed, S. Ali, *et al.* 2005. Inactivation of nuclear factor κB by soy isoflavone genestein contributes to increased apoptosis induced by chemotherapeutic agents in human cancer cells. *Cancer Res.* **65:** 6934–6942.

57. Ghaneh, P., W. Greenhalf, M. Humphreys, *et al.* 2001. Adenovirus-mediated transfer of p53 and p16 (INK4a) results in pancreatic cancer regression in vitro and in vivo. *Gene Ther.* **8:** 199–208.

58. Ding, X.Z., C.A. Kuszynski, T.H. El-Metwally & T.E. Adrian. 1999. Lipoxygenase inhibitors induce apoptosis, morphological changes and carbonic anhydrase expression in pancreatic cancer cells. *Biochem. Biophys. Res. Comm.* **266:** 392–399.

59. Ding, X.Z., W.G. Tong & T.E. Adrian. 2000. Blockade of cyclooxygenase-2 inhibits proliferation and induces apoptosis in human pancreatic cancer cells. *Anticancer Res.* **20:** 2625–2631.

60. Hennig, R., X.Z. Ding, W.G. Tong, *et al.* 2002. 5-Lipoxygenase and leukotriene B(4) receptor are expressed in human pancreatic cancers but not in pancreatic ducts in normal tissue. *Am. J. Pathol.* **161:** 421–428.

61. Hennig, R., P. Grippo, X.Z. Ding, *et al.* 2005. 5-Lipoxygenase, a marker for early pancreatic intraepithelial neoplastic lesions. *Cancer Res.* **65:** 6011–6016.

62. Ding, X.Z., W.G. Tong & T.E. Adrian. 2001. 12-lipoxygenase metabolite 12(S)-HETE stimulates human pancreatic cancer cell proliferation via protein tyrosine phosphorylation and ERK activation. *Int. J. Cancer* **94:** 630–636.

63. Ding, X.Z., W.G. Tong & T.E. Adrian. 2003. Multiple signal pathways are involved in the mitogenic effect of 5(S)-HETE in human pancreatic cancer. *Oncology* **65:** 285–294.

64. Tong, W.G., X.Z. Ding & T.E. Adrian. 2002. Leukotriene B4 receptor antagonist LY293111 inhibits proliferation and induces apoptosis in human pancreatic cancer cells. *Clin. Cancer Res.* **8:** 3232–3242.

65. Hennig, R., J. Ventura, R. Segersvard, *et al.* 2005. LY293111 improves efficacy of gemcitabine therapy on pancreatic cancer in a fluorescent orthotopic model in athymic mice. *Neoplasia* **7:** 417–425.

66. Ding, X.Z. & T.E. Adrian. 2002. Resveratrol inhibits proliferation and induces apoptosis in human pancreatic cancer cells. *Pancreas* **25:** e71–e76.

67. Ujiki, M.B., X.Z. Ding, M.R. Salabat, *et al.* 2006. Apigenin inhibits pancreatic cancer cell proliferation through G2/M cell cycle arrest. *Mol. Cancer* **5:** 76.

68. Park, Y.J., J. Wen, S. Bang, *et al.* 2005. [6]-Gingerol induces cell cycle arrest and cell death of mutant p53-expressing pancreatic cancer cells. *Yonsei Med. J.* **47:** 688–697.

69. Ujiki, M.B., B. Milam, X.Z. Ding, *et al.* 2006. A novel peptide sansalvamide analogue inhibits pancreatic cancer cell growth through G0/G1 cell-cycle arrest. *Biochem. Biophys. Res. Commun.* **340:** 1224–1228.

70. Elyakov, G.B., T.A. Kuznetsova, *et al.* 1969. A chemical investigation of the trepeng (Stychopus japonicus Selenka): the structure of triterpenoid aglycones obtained from trepeng glycosides. *Tetrahedron Lett.* **15:** 1151–1154.

71. Maltsev, I.I., V.A. Stonik, A.I. Kalinovsky & G.B. Elyakov. 1984. Triterpene glycosides from sea cucumber Stichopus japonicus Selenka. *Comp. Biochem. Physiol. B.* **78:** 421–426.

72. Halstead, B.W. 1969. Marine biotoxins: a new source of medicinals. *Lloydia* **32:** 484–488.

73. Kashiwada, Y., T. Fujioka, K. Mihashi, *et al.* 1997. Antitumor agents.180. Chemical studies and cytotoxic evaluation of cumingianosides and cumindyoside A, antileukemic triterpene glucosides with a 14, 18-cycloapotirucallane skeleton. *J. Nat. Prod.* **60:** 1105–1114.

74. Friess, S.L., F.G. Standaert, E.R. Whitcomb, *et al.* 1960. Some pharmacologic properties of holothurin A a glycosidic mixture from the sea cucumber. *Ann. N. Y. Acad. Sci.* **17:** 893–901.

75. Pettit, G.R., C.L. Herald & D.L. Herald. 1976. Antineoplastic agents XLV: sea cucumber cytotoxic saponins. *J. Pharm. Sci.* **65:** 1558–1559.

76. Friess, S.L., F.G. Standaert, E.R. Whitcomb, *et al.* 1959. Some pharmacologic properties of holothurin, an active neurotoxin from the sea cucumber. *J. Pharm. Exp. Ther.* **126:** 323–329.

77. Kuznetsova, T.A., M.M. Anisimov, A.M. Popov, *et al.* 1982. A comparative study in vitro of physiological activity of triterpene glycosides of marine invertebrates of echinoderm type. *Comp. Biochem. Physiol. C.* **73:** 41–43.

78. Zou, Z.R., Y.H. Yi, H.M. Wu, *et al.* 2003. Intercedensides A-C, three new cytotoxic triterpene glycosides from the sea cucumber Mensamaria intercedens Lampert. *J. Nat. Prod.* **66:** 1055–1060.

79. Naito, K., N. Kanbayashi, S. Nakajima, *et al.* 1994. Inhibition of growth of human tumor cells in nude mice by a metalloproteinase inhibitor. *Int. J. Cancer* **58:** 730–735.

80. Waldman, T., K.W. Kinzler & B. Vogelstein. 1995. p21 is necessary for the p53-mediated G1 arrest in human cancer cells. *Cancer Res.* **55:** 5187–5190.

81. Houghton, J.A. 1999. Apoptosis and drug response. *Curr. Opin. Oncol.* **11:** 475–481.

82. Thornberry, N.A. & Y. Lazebnik. 1998. Caspase: enemies within. *Science* **281:** 1312–1316.

83. Mancini, M., D.W. Nicholson, S. Roy, *et al.* 1998. The caspase-3 precursor has a cytosolic and mitochondrial distribution: implications for apoptotic signaling. *J. Cell Biol.* **140:** 1485–1495.

84. Kothakota, S., T. Azuma, C. Reinhard, *et al.* 1997. Caspase-3 generated fragment of gelsolin: effector of morphological change in apoptosis. *Science* **278:** 294–298.

85. Chai, J., E. Shiozaki, S.M. Srinivasula, *et al.* 2001. Structure basis of caspase-7 inhibition by XIAP. *Cell* **104:** 769–780.

86. Boucher, M.J., J. Morisset, P.H. Vachon, *et al.* 2000. MEK/ERK signaling pathway regulates the expression of Bcl-2, Bcl-X(L), and Mcl-1 and promotes survival of human pancreatic cancer cells. *J. Cell. Biochem.* **79:** 355–369.

87. Harris, M.H. & C.B. Thompson. 2000. The role of the Bcl-2 family in the regulation of outer mitochondrial membrane permeability. *Cell Death Differ.* **7:** 1182–1191.

Profile of Patients with Colorectal Cancer at a Tertiary Care Cancer Hospital in Pakistan

Natasha Anwar,[a] **Farhana Badar,**[b] **and Muhammad Aasim Yusuf**[c]

[a]*Basic Sciences Research,* [b]*Cancer Registry and Clinical Data Management, Abdul Hafeez Cancer Research Wing, and* [c]*Internal Medicine Department, Shaukat Khanum Memorial Cancer Hospital and Research Centre, Lahore, Punjab, Pakistan*

The following study describes the basic demography of colorectal cancer patients and characteristics of the disease seen at a regional tertiary care cancer hospital. The study highlights the influence of gender and age on the occurrence of this malignancy in patients in Pakistan. In general, this population shares many epidemiological features of developing countries for colorectal carcinoma. These include a younger age at presentation (mean age of patients was 46.5 years), subsite distribution (72.5% had left-sided tumors), and delayed presentation of the disease in an advanced stage. We stress the significance of public awareness regarding colorectal cancer to improve the outcome.

Key words: epidemiology; colorectal cancer; developing country; Pakistan; younger age presentation

Introduction

Colorectal cancer (CRC) is one of the most common forms of gastrointestinal cancer in the world today, with an incidence of 20.1 and 14.6 per 100,000 per year for men and women, respectively.[1] In recent years it has been noted that CRC is no longer a disease of only developed or more economically viable countries, with approximately 36% of new cases of CRC in the year 2000 occurring outside industrialized countries.[2]

Shaukat Khanum Memorial Cancer Hospital and Research Centre (SKMCH & RC) is the only tertiary care cancer facility in Pakistan. The hospital is located in the Northeastern city of Lahore, which has an estimated population of 10 million and is the second-largest city in the country. The hospital was established in 1994 and registers over 3000 new cancer patients every year; almost 70% of these patients are treated free of cost, according to international protocols and guidelines.

CRC appears to be an uncommon cancer in Pakistan; data from the only population-based epidemiology study conducted in Pakistan indicates an age standardized rate of 5.9 per 100,000 per year in men and 5.0 per 100,000 in women, making CRC the seventh most frequent cancer in men and the ninth most frequent in women.[3]

The aims of our study were to investigate the basic demography of CRC patients and characteristics of CRC diagnosed at our institution and to determine the influence of gender and age on the occurrence of CRC in this group of patients.

Patients and Methods

A total of 591 medical records were reviewed of CRC patients registered at the SKMCH &

Address for correspondence: Dr. Natasha Anwar, Research Scientist, Basic Sciences Research, Abdul Hafeez Cancer Research Wing, Shaukat Khanum Memorial Cancer Hospital & Research Centre 7A, Block R3, Johar Town, Lahore, Punjab 54000, Pakistan. Voice: +92425945100 ext. 2350. natasha@skm.org.pk

Ann. N.Y. Acad. Sci. 1138: 199–203 (2008). © 2008 New York Academy of Sciences.
doi: 10.1196/annals.1414.026

RC in Lahore, Pakistan. The registration period was between January 1995 and December 2004. The patients under study were adults (>18 years), whose disease could be evaluated by a standardized staging evaluation method using the American Joint Committee on Cancer (AJCC) 2002 staging system.[4] One hundred eighty patients whose disease stage could not be determined due to incomplete work-up and/or failure to return after one or two visits were not included in this study; neither were 22 patients under 18 years of age. Information was collected on gender, presenting age, site/subsite, histology, stage, grade, colonoscopy findings, final patient status, and survival. Judgment criteria used for survival was overall survival, which was measured from the date of diagnosis to the date of death, regardless of cause. Patients who had not died at the time of analysis were censored at the most recent date they were known to be alive. Survival was estimated using the Kaplan-Meier method. Results were generated using the Statistical Package for Social Sciences software, version 10 (SPSS Inc., Chicago, IL).

Results

Of the 591 patients, 388 (65.7%) were male compared to 203 female. More than 50% of the individuals were under 50 years of age. Mean age at presentation was 46.5 years (SD 15.2, range 19–107). Figure 1 is a histogram depicting age distribution of the patients. Family history of cancer was positive in 74 (12.5%), negative in 401 (67.9%), and not recorded in 116 (19.6%). More than half the patients (312, 53%) presented with rectal bleeding, either alone or in combination with other symptoms. Two hundred forty five (41%) presented with altered bowel habits, tenesmus, and obstructive bowel symptoms, whereas in 34 records (5.8%) there was no mention of precise presenting symptoms. Left-sided tumors were found in 428 patients (72.5%); these included 336 originating in the rectum. Right-sided cancers were reported in 122 (20.7%), while 24 (4.1%) pa-

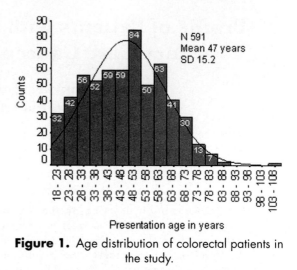

Figure 1. Age distribution of colorectal patients in the study.

tients were found to have tumors in the transverse colon. The subsite was not specified in 17 (2.9%) records. The commonest histologic subtype was adenocarcinoma, diagnosed in 547 patients (92.5%). Squamous cell carcinoma was seen in five cases (0.84%), and carcinoid tumor in one patient. Thirty-eight patients (6.4%), had carcinoma, not otherwise specified. Histologic grades were as follows: moderately differentiated 267 (45.2%), well differentiated 70 (11.8%), poorly differentiated 68 (11.5%), and undetermined grade 186 (31.5%). The staging classification revealed that, at presentation, 36 patients (6.1%) were in stage I, 145 (24.5%) in stage II, 170 (28.8%) in stage III, and 240 (40.6%) in stage IV of the disease. Table 1 and Figure 2 show differences in presenting age stratified by disease stage.

A total of three hundred eighty-one patients underwent colonoscopy at the hospital. Of these, 271 had a single tumor, 6 had multiple tumors, 24 had a solitary tumor with associated colonic polyps, and 2 had multiple polyposis syndromes.

When the study ended, 152 patients (25.7%) were alive and 164 (27.7%) were known to have died; 76 patients who had not completed their work-up did not get any treatment at the hospital and 199 (33%) were lost to follow-up. The overall median survival was 54 months. The median survival times for stages I–IV were

TABLE 1. Details of Age at Presentation according to Disease Stage

Stage	N	Mean Age (y)	Std. Deviation	Minimum	Maximum
I	36	48.81	17.62	21	85
II	145	48.94	14.45	20	82
III	170	43.82	14.74	19	75
IV	240	46.77	15.38	19	107
Total	591	46.58	15.21	19	107

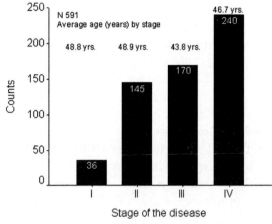

Figure 2. Proportional distribution of cases by disease stage and average age at presentation within each stage.

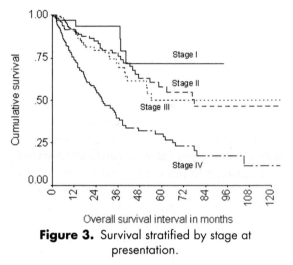

Figure 3. Survival stratified by stage at presentation.

90+, 77, 54, and 27 months, respectively. The 5-year cumulative probability of survival was 72% for stage I, 57% for stage II, 50% for stage III, and 30% for stage IV. Figure 3 depicts survival curves stratified by stage.

Discussion

CRC is the sixth commonest tumor treated at our tertiary care cancer hospital. A review of the data collected between January 1995 and December 2004 revealed both similarities and differences when compared to data from studies in more developed countries. The male-to-female preponderance in our study was 1.9:1 for the group as a whole, higher than that reported in a large study from the United States, which showed that males had a higher incidence of both colon and rectal cancers compared to women, but that this was more marked for rectal cancers, 1.2:1.0 and 1.7:1.0, respec-

tively.[3] Three hundred thirty-six patients in our cohort were recorded as having rectal cancer during the review period, of whom 220 were males and 116 were females (1.9:1); there was thus no difference in the male-to-female ratio between colon and rectal cancer at our institution.

The mean age at presentation of CRC in our study population was calculated to be 46.5 years, which is considerably lower than the age of presentation seen in the West, and almost a full decade lower than that reported in a study of 200 patients attending a major referral center in Iran.[5] This is despite the fact that Pakistan has a demographically similar population to that of Iran, with 39.1% versus 43.4% < 15 years of age, 56% versus 53% between 15–64 years of age, and 4.3% versus 3.5% over 65 years of age.[6] A characteristic feature of CRC in the developed world is that 90% of cases occur in those over 70 years of age. By contrast, 50% of the patients at our center were found to be less than 50 years of age. A small study from Pakistan, which assessed 85 resected specimens from patients with CRC, reported sex distributions and mean age at presentation similar to those seen in our study.[7]

It has been suggested that the age distribution of CRC seen in developing countries is a reflection of the fact that the mean age of the population is lower. The authors of a study from Iran reported the incidence and age distribution of CRC in five provinces of Iran and concluded that the lower mean age of presentation of CRC in Iran, and possibly in neighboring countries, was related to the lower mean age of the population, as well as to a lower incidence of CRC in older individuals in those countries.[8] Two other studies from Iran have shown a sharp increase in the incidence of CRC seen at the two major referral centers in that country over the last 30 years. There was no difference in the mean age at the time of diagnosis for men or women.[9,10]

Delayed presentation was a major problem for our patients: more than 69% presented in stage III or IV. Others from the region have reported similar problems with delayed diagnosis.[11] This may be due to a number of factors, including poverty, lack of access to healthcare, a reliance on traditional healers in the first instance, and a tendency for poorly trained primary-care physicians to assume all rectal bleeding to be due to hemorrhoids and to provide (inappropriate) treatment accordingly.

Additionally, delayed treatment decisions by the patient also contributed to late-stage presentation. It was noted that most of the rectal cancer cases had already seen three or four physicians prior to their arrival at SKMCH & RC. These patients had been recommended abdominoperineal resection (APR) as part of their treatment. There is a great reluctance among our patient population to accept a permanent colostomy, and it is thus common for us to see patients in whom APR has been recommended by two or three other physicians before they come to us and finally accept that this will be necessary. This leads to considerable delay

in provision of treatment and to upstaging of the disease.

The paucity of published data from Pakistan may also help to explain why physicians are unaware of the lower mean age of presentation of CRC in our country and are therefore less likely to consider it a possible diagnosis when confronted with a young patient presenting with altered bowel habit or rectal bleeding.

In keeping with other studies from our region, the majority of patients presented with left-sided tumors and with adenocarcinoma.[12] Overall, a family history had been sought in over 80% of cases and was found to be present in 12.5%. Familial adenomatous polyposis syndrome and hereditary nonpolyposis CRC are hereditary forms of CRC. There have been no genetic studies conducted on CRC in Pakistan. Therefore, detailed molecular characterization of CRC is required in order to ascertain any genetic component or susceptibility of this disease in our patients.

We report an overall median survival of 53.6 months in our patient group. The 5-year cumulative probability of survival was 72% for stage I, 57% for stage II, 50% for stage III, and 30% for stage IV. Results from a study in the United States showed similar survival rates, where stage I was 66–78%, stage II was between 55 and 62%, and survival in stage III was 31–42%.[13]

In conclusion, we have found a high incidence of CRC in patients presenting to our institution. The mean age at presentation is lower than that reported within our region, and much lower than that seen worldwide. Patients tend to present at an advanced stage, but this patient population is similar to others in having a preponderance of left-sided disease and adenocarcinoma as the most frequent histologic diagnosis.

There is clearly a need to educate the public as well as physicians about CRC. We are currently undertaking a prospective study to investigate environmental and genetic factors associated with the development of CRC in our population.

Conflicts of Interest

The authors declare no conflicts of interest.

References

1. Ferlay, J., F. Bray, P. Pisani, *et al.* 2000. Cancer Incidence, Mortality and Prevalence Worldwide, Version 1.0. IARC CancerBase No. 5. Lyon: IARC, 2001 http://www-dep.iarc.fr/globocan/globocan. htm (accessed April 2007).
2. Boyle, P. & M.E. Leon. 2002. Epidemiology of colorectal cancer. *Br. Med. Bull.* **64:** 1–25.
3. Bhurgri, Y. 2001. Epidemiology of Cancers in Karachi (1995–1999). Chapter 2. Incidence Data Karachi South 1995–1999; 23–39.
4. Greene, F.L., D.L. Page, I.D. Fleming, *et al.* (Eds.) 2002. *AJCC Cancer Staging Manual*, 6th ed. Springer-Verlag. New York.
5. Matanoski, G., X.G. Tao, L. Almon, *et al.* 2006. Demographics and tumor characteristics of colorectal cancers in the United States, 1998–2001. *Cancer* 1:**107**(5 Suppl): 1112–1120.
6. Pahlavan, P.S. & R. Kanthan. 2006. The epidemiology and clinical findings of colorectal cancer in Iran. *J. Gastrointestin. Liver Dis.* **15:** 15–19.
7. Ahmad, Z., R. Idrees, R. Ahmed, *et al.* 2005. Colorectal carcinoma, extent and spread in our population. Resection specimens give valuable information. *J. Pak. Med. Assoc.* **55:** 483–485.
8. Ansari, R., M. Mahdavinia, A. Sadjadi, *et al.* 2006. Incidence and age distribution of colorectal cancer in Iran: results of a population-based cancer registry. *Cancer Lett.* **240:** 143–147.
9. Yazdizadeh, B., A.M. Jarrahi, H. Mortazavi, *et al.* 2005. Time trends in the occurrence of major GI cancers in Iran. *Asian Pac. J. Cancer Prev.* **6:** 130–134.
10. Hosseini, S.V., A. Izadpanah & H. Yarmohammadi. 2004. Epidemiological changes in colorectal cancer in Shiraz, Iran: 1980–2000. *ANZ J. Surg.* **74:** 547–549.
11. Deo, S.V., N.K. Shukla, G. Srinivas, *et al.* 2001. Colorectal cancers—experience at a regional cancer centre in India. *Trop. Gastroenterol.* **22:** 83–86.
12. Ayyub, M.I., A.O. Al-Radi, A.M. Khazeindar, *et al.* 2002. Clinicopathological trends in colorectal cancer in a tertiary care hospital. *Saudi Med. J.* **23:** 160–163.
13. Jessup, J.M., A.K. Stewart & H.R. Menck. 1998. The National Cancer Data Base report on patterns of care for adenocarcinoma of the rectum, 1985–95. *Cancer* **83:** 2408.

The Transforming Functions of PI3-kinase-γ Are Linked to Disruption of Intercellular Adhesion and Promotion of Cancer Cell Invasion

Samir Attoub,[a,b] **Olivier De Wever,**[c] **Eric Bruyneel,**[c] **Marc Mareel,**[c] **and Christian Gespach**[a]

[a]*INSERM U 673, Molecular and Clinical Oncology of Solid Tumors, University Pierre et Marie Curie Paris VI, Hospital Saint-Antoine, Paris, France*

[b]*Department of Pharmacology & Therapeutics, Faculty of Medicine and Health Sciences, UAE University, Al Ain, United Arab Emirates*

[c]*Laboratory of Experimental Cancerology, University Hospital, Gent, Belgium*

The involvement of phosphoinositide 3-kinases class IA (PI3K-α and -β) in cancer cell proliferation, survival, motility, and invasiveness is now well established. However, the possible contribution of the class IB PI3Kγ in cancer cell transformation remains to be explored. In this study, we have stably transfected the PI3Kγ-deficient human colon cancer cell line HCT8/S11 with expression vectors encoding either wild-type PI3Kγ, its plasma membrane targeted form CAAX-PI3Kγ, or the PI3Kγ lipid and protein kinase-dead mutant (CAAX-K832R). We provide evidence that the constitutively active CAAX-PI3Kγ variant induced collagen type I invasion in HCT8/S11 cells through disruption of cell–cell adhesion, with no apparent impact on cell proliferation and motility. The proinvasive activity of CAAX-PI3K-γ was abolished by pharmacological inhibitors targeting PI3-K activities (wortmannin), Rho-GTPases, and the Rho-Rho kinase axis (C3T exoenzyme and Y27632, respectively). Conversely, the wild-type PI3Kγ and its double mutant CAAX-K832R were ineffective on cancer cell invasion measured under control or stimulated conditions operated with the proinvasive agents leptin and intestinal trefoil factor. Taken together, our data indicate that PI3Kγ exerts transforming functions via several mechanisms in human colon epithelial cancer cells, including alterations of homotypic cell–cell adhesion and induction of collagen type I invasion through canonical proinvasive pathways.

Key words: leptin; trefoil peptides; Rho-GTPases; MAPK; cell proliferation; motility

Introduction

Phosphoinositide 3-kinases (PI3Ks) belong to a large family of enzymes, grouped in three classes, I, II, and III, based on their sequence and substrate preference for PI, PIP, PI(3,4)P2, or PI(3,5)P2.[1] Class I of PI3K is subdivided into two families. Class IA are heterodimers composed of a regulatory p85 and a catalytic p110 subunit (α, β, or δ), and are ubiquitously expressed in mammalian cells. The catalytic subunits p110α, p110β, and p110δ catalyze the phosphorylation of phosphoinositides at position 3 of the inositol ring.[1] These dual lipid–protein kinases are activated by extracellular cytokines and receptor kinase signals induced by insulin, insulin-like growth factor, epidermal growth factor, platelet derived growth factor, scatter factor/hepatocyte growth factor, leptin,

Address for correspondence: Dr. Samir Attoub, Department of Pharmacology, Faculty of Medicine and Health Sciences, UAE University, P.O. Box 17666, Al Ain, UAE. Voice: +9713-7137-219; fax: +9713-767-2033. samir.attoub@uaeu.ac.ae

Ann. N.Y. Acad. Sci. 1138: 204–213 (2008). © 2008 New York Academy of Sciences.
doi: 10.1196/annals.1414.027

and stem cell factor.[2,3] In addition, PI3Kα is activated by intracellular nonreceptor tyrosine kinases, such as the src family kinases, and by the transforming small GTPases Rac1 and Ras.[4,5] Inositol lipids phosphorylated by PI3K act as second messengers for several downstream targets, including the serine–threonine kinase Akt, the ribosomal S6 kinase pp70^{S6K}, and glycogen synthase kinase-3.[6,7] The activation of receptor tyrosine kinases by growth and survival factors increases the activity of PI3K.[8] Class IA PI3Ks are also a frequent target of mutational activation. Mutation in the *PIK3CA* gene, which encodes the p110α catalytic subunit of PI3K, has been reported in several human cancers, namely glioblastoma and colorectal, gastric, breast, and lung cancers. The acquisition of PIK3CA mutations may be an important event in progression toward more aggressive and invasive phenotypes.[9] In this context, increased PI3Kα activity has been identified in 86% of colorectal cancers.[10] Insulin and some growth factors preferentially signal through p110β, but there is also evidence for the elevation of p110β (PIK3CB) expression and activity in colon and bladder tumors.[11] All these PI3K mutations identified in human cancer are oncogenic. Consequently this activation of PI3-kinases class IA is a crucial step in tumor cell proliferation, differentiation, survival, cytoskeleton rearrangement, motility, invasion, and angiogenesis.[12] The class IB (PI3Kγ) in contrast is mainly activated by G-protein coupled receptors (GPCR) via the heterotrimeric GαGβγ complex through direct association of the p110γ regulatory subunit p101 and the Gβγ dimer at the plasma membrane.[13,14] In contrast with the other members of the PI3K family, PI3Kγ is not activated by receptor tyrosine kinases, according to our knowledge. In addition to its lipid kinase activity, PI3Kγ exhibits intrinsic protein kinase activity with unknown functional and biological significance. Two major oncogenic pathways emerge from PI3Kγ, the lipid kinase–phosphoinositides cascade linked to Akt, ribosomal protein S6 kinase, Jun N-terminal kinase

activation,[15,16] and the PI3Kγ protein kinase cascade linked to Mitogen-Activated Protein Kinase (MAPK)/Stress-Activated Protein Kinase activation and Janus-Activated Kinase 2 signals.[17,18] Both the lipid and protein kinase activities of PI3Kγ are sensitive to the PI3K inhibitors wortmannin and LY294002.[19]

Increased levels of PI3K products have been observed in colorectal and breast cancers.[10,20] A screening study also demonstrated that high levels of PI3K activity are associated with the proliferation and anti-apoptotic signaling in small-cell lung cancer.[21] In addition, PI3Kγ-deficient mice displayed an impaired T cell proliferation phenotype. However, the possible contribution of PI3Kγ in neoplastic transformation is, until now, largely unknown. We have presented new evidence that ectopic expression of PI3Kγ promoted survival and pro-invasive responses in human colon cancer cells HCT8/S11.[22] Subsequent studies reported that both p110γ and its interacting adaptor p101 implicate the PI3Kγ signaling system as a putative oncogenic pathway.[23] It is now well accepted that PI3Kγ is expressed in hematopoietic cells (normal neutrophils and leukemia K-562 and U-937 cells), endothelial cells, and cardiac myocytes, and plays a crucial role in macrophage motility.[13,24] Lipid products of PI3Kγ accumulate at the leading edge of migrating neutrophils and activate Rho GTPases and actin polymerization.[25] Accordingly, PI3Kγ mediates actin rearrangement at the leading edge of fibroblasts activated by chemokines via the downstream small GTPase Rac.[26]

In this work we investigated the impact of PI3Kγ on cellular adhesion, motility, proliferation, and invasion in human colon cancer cells that are deficient for the expression of PI3Kγ. We have demonstrated that the human colon cancer cell lines HCT8/S11, HT29, HCT116, and LoVo do not express p110γ[22] (and unpublished results). Immunoblotting experiments revealed that colorectal SW-480 cells lack the catalytic PI3K p110γ and p110α isoforms, but express the heterodimeric isoform p85/p110β.[27] Other studies indicate that p110γ transcripts are absent in DLD-1, LoVo, and SW-480 colon cancer cells and are detected at very low levels in Colo205 and HCT-15 cells.[28] Thus, we focused the present study on the transforming potential of PI3Kγ using the human colon cancer cell line HCT8/S11.

Materials and Methods

Cell Culture and Reagents

Human colorectal cancer cell line HCT8/S11 was maintained in Roswell Park Memorial Institute medium 1640 (RPMI) (Invitrogen, Cergy Pontoise, France) supplemented with 10% fetal bovine serum (FBS) (Roche Molecular Biochemicals, Meylan, France). Recombinant human leptin was from R&D Systems Europe Ltd. (Oxon, UK). Human trefoil factor TFF3 was produced in yeast and purified as described. The p42/44 MAPK inhibitor PD98059 and the PI3-kinase inhibitor wortmannin were from Calbiochem (Meudon, France). *Clostridium botulinum* exoenzyme C3 transferase (C3T), which ADP-ribosylates and inactivates the Rho-like small GTPases, was a gift from Dr. Gilles Flatau (INSERM U627, Nice, France). The ROCK inhibitor Y27632 was kindly provided by Yoshitomi Pharmaceutical Industries Ltd (Osaka, Japan).

Expression Vectors and Cell Transfection

The expression vectors pEGFP.C1/p110γ-CAAX and pEGFP.C1/p110γ-K832R-CAAX were a gift from Dr. Reinhard Weitzker (Institute of Molecular Cell Biology, University of Jena, Germany). The p110γ-CAAX variant encodes a constitutively active, membrane-targeted PI3Kγ. The lipid and protein kinase-inactive mutant p110γ-K832R was prepared by a point mutation (Lys-832 to Arg) in the DNA sequence encoding the predicted domain required for ATP binding. The expression vector pcDNA3 encoding the wild-type (wt) form of PI3Kγ (p110γ-wt) was a gift from Prof. Matthias Wymann (Institute of Biochemistry and Genetics, University of Basel, Switzerland). HCT8/S11 cells were plated for 24 h on 60-mm-diameter dishes and stably transfected by lipofection (LipofectAMINE Reagent Plus, Invitrogen), according to the manufacturer's instructions. Cells were transfected with 4 μg of the expression vectors pcDNA3/p110γ-wt, pEGFP.C1/p110γ-CA-AX, or pEGFP.C1/p110γ-K832R-CAAX carrying the neomycin resistance gene. The next day, cultures were split into two 100-mm-diameter dishes and selected for 10 days in the culture medium supplemented with 400 μg/mL of G418. Resistant colonies were ring-cloned as individual clones or pooled. Expression of the transgene was determined by western blotting.

Wound Healing Migration and Cell Proliferation Assays

Cells were grown in six-well tissue culture dishes until confluence. Cultures were incubated for 10 min with Moscona buffer. A scrape was made through the confluent monolayer with a plastic pipette tip of 1 mm diameter. Afterwards, Moscona buffer was removed, and the dishes were washed twice and incubated at 37°C in fresh RPMI containing 10% FBS. Cell viability was checked by the trypan blue exclusion test. At the underside of each dish, a mark was made at six arbitrary places where the width of the wound was measured with an inverted microscope (objective × 4). Migration was expressed as the average ± SEM of the difference between the measurements at time zero and the time points 2 h, 5 h, and 8 h. Parental and stably transfected PI3Kγ-HCT8/S11 cells were plated at the density of 2×10^5 cells into 60-mm dishes supplemented with 10% FBS. After 24, 48, 72, and 96 h, the cells were trypsinized, collected in 1 mL of medium, and counted using a Coulter Counter (Northwell, England).

Aggregation and Collagen Invasion Assays

The fast aggregation assay was performed as described.[29] Briefly, single-cell suspensions were prepared using an E-cadherin saving procedure. Cells were incubated in an isotonic buffer containing 1.25 mM Ca^{2+} under gyratory shaking for 30 min at 37°C. Particle diameters were measured in a particle size counter (LS 200; Beckman Coulter, Miami, FL) at the start (t_0) and after 30-min incubation (t_{30}), and plotted against percentage volume distribution. For invasion of collagen gels by HCT8/S11 cells, six-well tissue culture dishes were filled with 1.35 mL of neutralized type I collagen (Upstate Biotechnology, Lake Placid, NY) and incubated overnight at 37°C to allow gelling. Cells were harvested using Moscona buffer and trypsin/EDTA, and seeded on top of the collagen gels. Cultures were incubated for 24 h at 37°C, in the presence or absence of the indicated agents. The depth of cell migration inside the gels was measured using an inverted microscope. Invasive and superficial cells were counted in 12 fields of 0.157 mm^2. The invasion index corresponds to the ratio of the number of cells invading the gel over the total number of cells counted in each field.

Statistical Analysis

Data are means ± SEM for the number of experiments indicated. The statistical significance between experimental values was assessed by the unpaired Student's *t*-test and $P < 0.05$ was considered to be statistically significant.

Results

Disruption of Cellular Adhesion by Constitutively Active CAAX-PI3Kγ in HCT8/S11 Human Colon Cancer Cells

Given that PI3Kγ is abundantly expressed in hematopoietic cells, but not in normal and transformed human colon epithelial cells, including the human colon cancer cell line HCT8/S11[22] (and unpublished results), we have established an heterologous model of HCT8/S11 cells expressing either wt PI3Kγ, the membrane-targeted CAAX-PI3Kγ variant, or the K832R-PI3Kγ mutant deficient in both lipid and protein kinase activities. Positive clones and pools of stably transfected HCT8/S11 cell populations were then selected according to neomycin resistance, and validated for the expression of the PI3Kγ transgenes by western blots (not shown) and further functional characterization (see below).

The acquisition of a motile phenotype during tumor cell invasion is often associated with alterations in intercellular adhesion between epithelial cells. Using the fast aggregation assay, which determines the size of the cluster particles formed by HCT8/S11 cells, we showed that a rapid formation of HCT8/S11 aggregates, as shown in Figure 1A. A similar aggregation profile was observed following stable expression of the wt or the K832R-PI3Kγ lipid and protein kinase–dead mutant in HCT8/S11 cells. In contrast, cell–cell adhesion was remarkably disrupted in the CAAX-PI3Kγ HCT8/S11 cell line expressing the constitutively activated form of the enzyme (Fig. 1A). The mechanism for this effect may involve molecular interactions between CAAX-PI3Kγ and homotypic cellular adhesion mechanisms between epithelial cells, such as the E-cadherin/β-catenin system. One can postulate that the membrane-targeted PI3Kγ-CAAX is recruited to the plasma membrane at the vicinity of cell–cell junctions by the E-cadherin/p120/β-catenin-containing scaffolds in HCT8/S11 epithelial cells. This scenario was recently demonstrated for class IA PI3 kinase in the context of the E-cadherin adhesive functions in keratinocytes.[30] Taken together with these reports, our data suggest that the ectopic expression of PI3Kγ-CAAX counteracts epithelial cell–cell contacts via a negative contribution to E-cadherin-mediated cellular adhesion. Next,

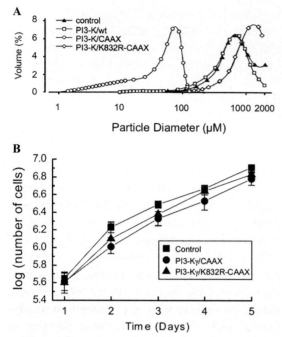

Figure 1. Impact of wt-PI3Kγ and its constitutively activated or kinase-dead mutants on cellular adhesion and proliferation in HCT8/S11 cells. **(A)** Disruption of cellular aggregation by membrane-targeted, constitutively activated CAAX-PI3Kγ. Human cancer cells HCT8/S11 (control), HCT8/S11-PI3Kγ-wt, HCT8/S11-CAAX-PI3Kγ, and HCT8/S11-CAAX-K832R were allowed to aggregate in a gyratory shaker. Cell aggregation was measured by particle size counting. **(B)** Effects of CAAX-PI3Kγ and its kinase-dead mutant K832R on cellular proliferation. HCT8/S11, HCT8/S11-CAAX-PI3Kγ, and HCT8/S11-CAAX-K832R cells were seeded in 60 mm Petri dishes (200,000 cells/dish). Parental and PI3Kγ -stably transfected cells were counted daily for 5 days. The data are means ± SEM of three independent experiments.

we tested whether alterations of cell–cell adhesion in HCT8/S11-PI3Kγ-CAAX cells affected their proliferation potential *in vitro*. Thus, HCT8/S11, HCT8/S11-PI3Kγ-CAAX, and HCT8/S11-PI3Kγ-K832R-CAAX cells were seeded into plates (2×10^5 cells/well) in 10% FBS. All the cell lines had similar growth rates (Fig. 1B), indicating that ectopic expression of the membrane-bound PI3Kγ is not a mitogenic signal for HCT8/S11 cells cultured in the presence of serum. In support of our findings, PI3Kγ-deficient mice did not show any

alterations in heart size, indicating that this kinase is not involved in growth control under developmental situations.

Impact of PI3Kγ on Cellular Migration and the Invasive Potential in HCT8/S11 Cells

Cellular motility is a crucial feature of several physiological and pathological processes, including embryogenesis, wound healing, immune functions, and angiogenesis. The acquisition of a motile phenotype by cancer cells, leading to local invasion in growing tumors, is the hallmark of the cancerous transformation. First, we assessed whether the membrane-targeted form of PI3Kγ stimulated intestinal epithelial cell migration, utilizing a classic *in vitro* wound-healing model. Experiments performed on subconfluent cell cultures showed that PI3Kγ-CAAX was ineffective to regulate significantly the motility of HCT8/S11 cells ($P = 0.071$) within 8 h after wounding (Fig. 2A). Recent data indicate that constitutively active PI3Kγ is associated with a reduced chemotactic response and directional movement in leukocytes.[31] In contrast, PI3Kγ expression and activity are linked to increased cell survival and tumorigenesis in fibroblasts[23] and were essential features for cellular motility induced by autotaxin in human melanoma cells.[32]

Next, we assessed the impact of PI3Kγ on the invasive potential of HCT8/S11 cells. As shown in Figure 2B, parental cells, as well as HCT8/S11 cells stably transfected with the wt and K832R-CAAX forms of PI3Kγ, were not spontaneously invasive in collagen gels. Interestingly, stable expression of PI3Kγ-CAAX in HCT8/S11 cells induced a remarkable invasive response in collagen type I gels. We have also observed that the pro-invasive activity of leptin and intestinal trefoil factor TFF3[33] was not potentiated by the ectopic expression of wt-PI3Kγ in HCT8/S11 cells, suggesting that human cancer cells are not equipped with the signal transduction adaptors involved in the activation of the PI3K-γ subtype under basal or stimulated conditions (Fig. 3A). In contrast, we

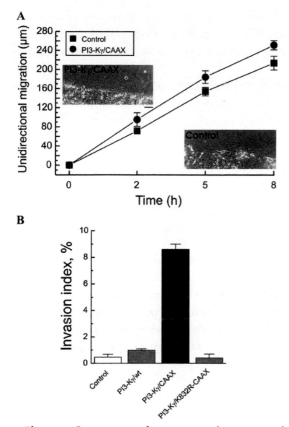

Figure 2. Impact of constitutively activated CAAX- PI3Kγ on cellular motility and invasion in HCT8/S11 cells. **(A)** Wounds were introduced in confluent monolayers of parental HCT8/S11 cells (control) and their counterparts stably transfected by CAAX-PI3Kγ. Cells were then cultured at 37°C for 2, 5, and 8 h. The mean distance that cells traveled from the edge of the scraped area was measured in a blinded fashion, using an inverted microscope (4 × magnifications, insets). Values shown are means ± SEM of three independent experiments, each performed in triplicate. **(B)** Collagen type I invasion was measured during the 24 h invasion assay, using parental HCT8/S11 cells (control) and their counterparts stably transfected by either PI3Kγ-wt, CAAX-PI3Kγ, or CAAX-K832R. Values shown are means ± SEM of three independent experiments.

have demonstrated that PI3Kα is a critical effector in cellular invasion mediated by these two pro-invasive factors in human colon epithelial cells.[3,33] Leptin and TFF3 also regulate several immune responses and inflammatory situations controlled by macrophages, neutrophils, eosinophils, and natural killer and dendritic

cells.[34,35] Similar results were obtained by using the HCT8/S11 cell line stably transfected with PI3Kγ-CAAX (not shown). Thus, cellular invasion promoted by leptin and TFF3 does not interfere with PI3Kγ signaling in this model. We found no additivity or synergy between endogenously activated PI3Ks and ectopic PI3Kγ-CAAX in HCT8/S11 cells.

We next examined the impact of pharmacological inhibitors targeting essential pro-invasive signaling elements, including PI3-kinases,[12,22] Rho-like GTPases, the Rho-Rho kinase (ROK) axis,[36] and MAPK on collagen type I invasion induced by PI3Kγ-CAAX in HCT8/S11 cells. As shown in Figure 3B, the PI3-kinase pan-inhibitor wortmannin, which inhibits all p110 isoforms to the same extent, abolished cellular invasion induced by p110γ-CAAX in HCT8/S11 cells. Neutralization of Rho-GTPases and the Rho-ROCK pathway by C3T or Y27632 blocked this cellular invasion, suggesting that p110γ-CAAX activates Rho-like GTPases in HCT8/S11 cells, and consequently actin polymerization, as shown in leukocytes.[25] In contrast, the PI3Kγ invasion pathway was insensitive to the MAPK inhibitor PD98059. In agreement, only the soluble, but not membrane-bound forms of PI3Kγ, were shown to activate MAPK pathways.[15]

Discussion

During adenoma formation and the neoplastic progression in human colon mucosa, loss and inversion in polarity gradients of proliferating, migrating, and apoptotic epithelial cells occurs along the crypt axis together with progressive disorganization of the mucosal architecture, leading to inappropriate and persistent release of paracrine and autocrine agents acting at illegitimate sites in the nascent tumor. Loss of several checkpoints at the cell proliferation cycle and alterations in the mechanisms of resistance to apoptosis are coordinated with the acquisition of the invasive and angiogenic potential in human solid tumors. Cancer cell

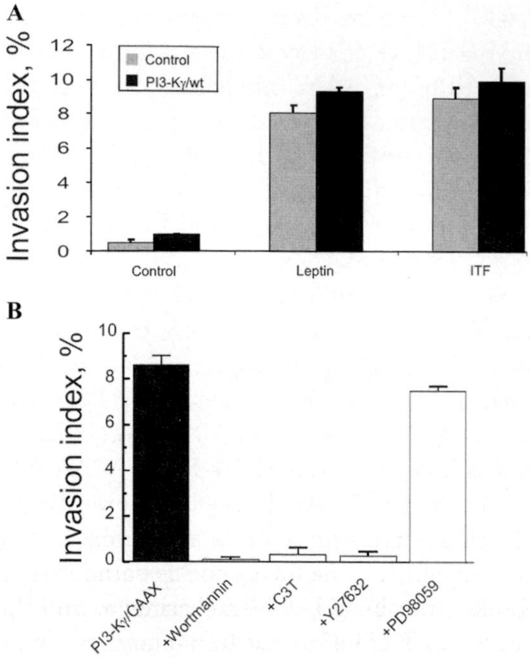

Figure 3. Impact of leptin, intestinal trefoil factor (TFF3) and pharmacological inhibitors targeting pro-invasive signaling pathways on collagen type I invasion by HCT8/S11 cells stably transfected by wt- or CAAX-PI3Kγ. **(A)** Cellular invasion induced by leptin (100 ng/mL) and TFF3 (100 nM) was measured in parental HCT8/S11 cells (control) and their counterparts stably transfected by the wild-type form of PI3Kγ. Data are means ± SEM of three independent experiments. **(B)** Effects of pharmacological inhibitors targeting PI3-kinase (wortmannin, 10 ng/mL), Rho-GTPases (C3T exoenzyme, 5 μg/mL), Rho-kinase ROK (Y27632, 10 μM), and p42/p44 MAPK (PD98059, 50 μM) on the invasive potential of HCT8/S11-CAAX-PI3Kγ cells. Data are means ± SEM of three independent experiments.

invasion and metastasis constitute the critical stages in the progression of human solid tumors, resulting in the death of cancer patients. In this context, initial studies based on the genetic inactivation of p110-PI3Kγ described the development of invasive colorectal adenocarcinomas in mice.[37] In contrast, we provided initial evidence that PI3Kγ does not behave like a tumor suppressor in the colon mucosa of transgenic mice, but instead induced several detrimental cellular functions associated with neoplastic progression, including cancer cell survival and invasion.[22] Our data were val-

idated later in a corrigendum suggesting that invalidation of PI3Kγ does not by itself cause colon cancer, but may require additional factors.[38] The present data demonstrate however that neither leptin nor TFF3 provides additional responses with wt-PI3Kγ in colon cancer cell invasion. In addition, we found that forced expression of wt-PI3Kγ was ineffective to collaborate with the oncogenic defects inherent to HCT8/S11 colon cancer cells. Notably, the present study provides further evidence that the constitutively activated p110γ induced by membrane targeting (CAAX-PI3Kγ) provokes cellular invasion through disruption of cell–cell adhesion and several canonical pro-invasive pathways, including PI3K-dependent signals, and the Rho GTPases–ROK axis. Our data are coherent with the contribution of PI3Kγ on directed movements in epithelial wounds of the rat cornea in response to endogenous electric fields (electrotaxis).[39] It is tempting to predict that tumorigenicity and metastasis of CAAX-PI3K-transformed HCT8/S11 cells would be greatly enhanced in nude mice. Obviously, further study is needed to address these concerns. In coherence with our initial study,[22] we found that wt-PI3Kγ and its lipid and protein kinase-deficient mutant CAAX-K832R are both inactive in cellular invasion, as expected. Indeed, the activation status of class IA and IB PI3Ks requires membrane targeting. For the PI3Kγ pathways, this priming state is induced through signaling responses via GPCR and their associated heterotrimeric subunits linked to Gβγ-dependent activation of p110γ via membrane targeting of the p101 adaptor, followed by Rac signaling via the cytosolic guanine-nucleotide exchange factor (GEF) P-Rex1, as well as direct activation of 110γ via Ras.[40] P-Rex1 is a GEF for the small GTPase Rac that is directly activated by Gβγ and the lipid second messenger PIP3 generated by PI3K. Both p101 and the newly discovered p110γ plasma membrane adaptor p87[PIKAP] seem to be required as regulatory subunits and priming scaffolds for subsequent activation of the class IB PI3K.[41] However, other studies have shown that

Gβγ-induced activation of 110γ occurs in the absence of p101,[42] suggesting that Gβγ exerts a dual role on membrane targeting and activation of 110γ in the presence and absence of p101. Thus, the upstream signaling requirements for membrane translocation and activation of p110γ are distinct from those of the α and δ isoforms. In addition, the constitutively activated BCR-ABL tyrosine kinase driving chronic myeloid leukemia also leads to increased expression and activity of the class IB catalytic subunit of PI3-kinase 110γ.[40] Thus, both GPCR and nonreceptor kinases are potentially involved in the initiation of functional cross-talk with 110γ and the determination of its selective expression and activity. Expression of the PI3-kinase 110γ isoform is therefore subjected to transcriptional signaling controls in hematopoietic cells[40] as well as to epigenetic silencing in human colon epithelial cells. To date, there is no convincing evidence for the expression of PI3-kinase 110γ in normal and transformed digestive epithelial cells.[22] Isolation and identification of the promoter and regulatory regions of class IB PI3Kγ should provide the molecular basis for its selective expression in the immune system, brain, and other peripheral tissues. The class IB PI3Kγ was initially discovered in neutrophils and subsequently in the hematopoietic and immune cell lineages, including dendritic cells, macrophages, and platelets. In agreement, PI3Kγ is now considered a key regulator of inflammatory responses, blood vessel and myocyte contractility, tumor angiogenesis, and drug resistance in chronic myeloid leukemia.[40,43]

The heterologous model of PI3Kγ-null HCT8/S11 human colon epithelial cells stably transfected with the wt-PI3Kγ, CAAX-PI3Kγ, and CAAX-K832R versions of PI3Kγ engineered in the present study will allow us to dissect and identify upstream and downstream signaling pathways driven by PI3Kγ in normal and pathological states, including cell survival and oncogenesis. In this connection, the expression and transforming role of the PI3Kγ adaptors and activators p101 and p87[PIKAP],[41]

as well as other molecular effectors interacting with PI3Kγ, can be further clarified. The extent to which downstream lipid and protein substrates are phosphorylated by the soluble and membrane-targeted forms of the serine-threonine kinase PI3Kγ, as well as their relative contribution to cancer progression in cellular systems expressing this dual kinase, need to be investigated in future studies.

Acknowledgments

This work was supported by INSERM, Faculty of Medicine and Health Sciences, UAE University and seed grants, Research Grants from the Association de la Recherche sur le Cancer (ARC), the Belgische Federatie tegen Kanker, the FORTIS Verzekeringen, and the Fund for Scientific Research Flanders (Brussels, Belgium). We thank Dr. Reinhard Weitzker and Prof. Matthias Wymann for providing the PI3Kγ expression vectors. We thank Drs. Bara Jacques and Nguyen Quang-De for providing technical help.

Conflicts of Interest

The authors declare no conflicts of interest.

References

1. Wymann, M.P. & L. Pirola. 1998. Structure and function of phosphoinositide 3-kinases. *Biochim. Biophys. Acta* **1436:** 127–150.

2. Royal, I. & M. Park. 1995. Hepatocyte growth factor-induced scatter of Madin-Darby canine kidney cells requires phosphatidylinositol 3-kinase. *J. Biol. Chem.* **270:** 27780–27787.

3. Attoub, S., V. Noe, L. Pirola, *et al.* 2000. Leptin promotes invasiveness of kidney and colonic epithelial cells via phosphoinositide 3-kinase-, rho-, and rac-dependent signaling pathways. *Faseb J.* **14:** 2329–2338.

4. Genot, E.M., C. Arrieumerlou, G. Ku, *et al.* 2000. The T-cell receptor regulates Akt (protein kinase B) via a pathway involving Rac1 and phosphatidylinositide 3-kinase. *Mol. Cell. Biol.* **20:** 5469–5478.

5. Rodriguez-Viciana, P., P.H. Warne, B. Vanhaesebroeck, *et al.* 1996. Activation of phosphoinositide

3-kinase by interaction with Ras and by point mutation. *EMBO J.* **15:** 2442–2451.

6. Burgering, B.M. & P.J. Coffer. 1995. Protein kinase B (c-Akt) in phosphatidylinositol-3-OH kinase signal transduction. *Nature* **376:** 599–602.

7. Frame, S. & P. Cohen. 2001. The renaissance of GSK3. *Nat. Rev. Mol. Cell. Biol.* **2:** 769–776.

8. Toker, A. & L.C. Cantley. 1997. Signalling through the lipid products of phosphoinositide-3-OH kinase. *Nature* **387:** 673–676.

9. Samuels, Y., Z. Wang, A. Bardelli, *et al.* 2004. High frequency of mutations of the PIK3CA gene in human cancers. *Science* **304:** 554.

10. Philp, A.J., I.G. Campbell, C. Leet, *et al.* 2001. The phosphatidylinositol 3'-kinase p85alpha gene is an oncogene in human ovarian and colon tumors. *Cancer Res.* **61:** 7426–7429.

11. Benistant, C., H. Chapuis & S. Roche. 2000. A specific function for phosphatidylinositol 3-kinase alpha (p85alpha-p110alpha) in cell survival and for phosphatidylinositol 3-kinase beta (p85alpha-p110beta) in de novo DNA synthesis of human colon carcinoma cells. *Oncogene* **19:** 5083–5090.

12. Kotelevets, L., V. Noe, E. Bruyneel, *et al.* 1998. Inhibition by platelet-activating factor of Src- and hepatocyte growth factor-dependent invasiveness of intestinal and kidney epithelial cells. Phosphatidylinositol 3'-kinase is a critical mediator of tumor invasion. *J. Biol. Chem.* **273:** 14138–14145.

13. Stoyanov, B., S. Volinia, T. Hanck, *et al.* 1995. Cloning and characterization of a G protein-activated human phosphoinositide-3 kinase. *Science* **269:** 690–693.

14. Stephens, L.R., A. Eguinoa, H. Erdjument-Bromage, *et al.* 1997. The G beta gamma sensitivity of a PI3K is dependent upon a tightly associated adaptor, p101. *Cell* **89:** 105–114.

15. Bondeva, T., L. Pirola, G. Bulgarelli-Leva, *et al.* 1998. Bifurcation of lipid and protein kinase signals of PI3Kgamma to the protein kinases PKB and MAPK. *Science* **282:** 293–296.

16. Lopez-Ilasaca, M., J.S. Gutkind & R. Wetzker. 1998. Phosphoinositide 3-kinase gamma is a mediator of Gbetagamma-dependent Jun kinase activation. *J. Biol. Chem.* **273:** 2505–2508.

17. Lopez-Ilasaca, M., P. Crespo, P.G. Pellici, *et al.* 1997. Linkage of G protein-coupled receptors to the MAPK signaling pathway through PI 3-kinase gamma. *Science* **275:** 394–397.

18. Cieslik, K., C.S. Abrams & K.K. Wu. 2001. Up-regulation of endothelial nitric-oxide synthase promoter by the phosphatidylinositol 3-kinase gamma/Janus kinase 2/MEK-1-dependent pathway. *J. Biol. Chem.* **276:** 1211–1219.

19. Stoyanova, S., G. Bulgarelli-Leva, C. Kirsch, *et al.* 1997. Lipid kinase and protein kinase activities of G-protein-coupled phosphoinositide 3-kinase gamma: structure-activity analysis and interactions with wortmannin. *Biochem. J.* **324**(Pt 2): 489–495.

20. Gershtein, E.S., V.A. Shatskaya, V.D. Ermilova, *et al.* 1999. Phospatidylinositol 3-kinase expression in human breast cancer. *Clin. Chim. Acta.* **287:** 59–67.

21. Krystal, G.W., G. Sulanke & J. Litz. 2002. Inhibition of phosphatidylinositol 3-kinase-Akt signaling blocks growth, promotes apoptosis, and enhances sensitivity of small cell lung cancer cells to chemotherapy. *Mol. Cancer Ther.* 913–922.

22. Barbier, M., S. Attoub, R. Calvez, *et al.* 2001. Weakening link to colorectal cancer? *Nature* **413:** 796.

23. Kang, S., A. Denley, B. Vanhaesebroeck, *et al.* 2006. Oncogenic transformation induced by the p110beta, -gamma, and -delta isoforms of class I phosphoinositide 3-kinase. *PNAS* **103:** 1289–1294.

24. Go, Y.M., H. Park, M.C. Maland, *et al.* 1998. Phosphatidylinositol 3-kinase gamma mediates shear stress-dependent activation of JNK in endothelial cells. *Am. J. Physiol.* **275**(5 Pt 2): H1898–H1904.

25. Rickert, P., O.D. Weiner, F. Wang, *et al.* 2000. Leukocytes navigate by compass: roles of PI3Kgamma and its lipid products. *Trends Cell Biol.* **10:** 466–473.

26. Han, J., K. Luby-Phelps, B. Das, *et al.* 1998. Role of substrates and products of PI 3-kinase in regulating activation of Rac-related guanosine triphosphatases by Vav. *Science* **279:** 558–560.

27. Graness, A., A. Adomeit, R. Heinze, *et al.* 1998. A novel mitogenic signaling pathway of bradykinin in the human colon carcinoma cell line SW-480 involves sequential activation of a Gq/11 protein, phosphatidylinositol 3-kinase beta, and protein kinase Cepsilon. *J. Biol. Chem.* **273:** 32016–32022.

28. Semba, S., N. Itoh, M. Ito, *et al.* 2002. Downregulation of PIK3CG, a catalytic subunit of phosphatidylinositol 3-OH kinase, by CpG hypermethylation in human colorectal carcinoma. *Clin. Cancer Res.* **8:** 3824–3831.

29. Boterberg, T., K.M. Vennekens, M. Thienpont, *et al.* 2000. Internalization of the E-cadherin/catenin complex and scattering of human mammary carcinoma cells MCF-7/AZ after treatment with conditioned medium from human skin squamous carcinoma cells COLO 16. *Cell Adhes. Commun.* **7:** 299–310.

30. Xie, Z. & D.D. Bikle. 2007. The recruitment of phosphatidylinositol 3-kinase to the E-cadherin-catenin complex at the plasma membrane is required for calcium-induced phospholipase C-gamma1 activation and human keratinocyte differentiation. *J. Biol. Chem.* **282:** 8695–8703.

31. Costa, C., L. Barberis, C. Ambrogio, *et al.* 2007. Negative feedback regulation of Rac in leukocytes from mice expressing a constitutively active phosphatidylinositol 3-kinase γ. *PNAS* **104:** 14354–14359.

32. Lee, H.Y., G.U. Bae, I.D. Jung, *et al.* 2002. Autotaxin promotes motility via G protein-coupled phosphoinositide 3-kinase gamma in human melanoma cells. *FEBS Letters* **515:** 137–140.

33. Emami, S., F. Le, N. loch, E. Bruyneel, *et al.* 2001. Induction of scattering and cellular invasion by trefoil peptides in src- and RhoA-transformed kidney and colonic epithelial cells. *FASEB J.* **15:** 351–361.

34. Emami, S., S. Rodrigues, C.M. Rodrigue, *et al.* 2004. Trefoil factors family (TFFs) peptides and cancer progression. *PEPTIDES* **25:** 885–898.

35. Lago, F., C. Dieguez, J. Gómez-Reino, *et al.* 2007. Adipokines as emerging mediators of immune response and inflammation. *Nat. Clin. Pract. Rheumatol.* 716–724.

36. Nguyen, Q.D., O. De Wever, E. Bruyneel, *et al.* 2005. Commutators of PAR-1 signaling in cancer cell invasion reveal an essential role of the Rho-Rho kinase axis and tumor microenvironment. *Oncogene* **24:** 8240–8251.

37. Sasaki, T., J. Irie-Sasaki, Y. Horie, *et al.* 2000. Colorectal carcinomas in mice lacking the catalytic subunit of PI(3)K^γ. *Nature* **406:** 897–902.

38. Sasaki, T., J. Irie-Sasaki, Y. Horie, *et al.* 2003. Colorectal carcinomas in mice lacking the catalytic subunit of PI(3)K^γ. *Nature* **426:** 584.

39. Zhao, M., B. Song, J. Pu, T. Wada, *et al.* 2006. Electrical signals control wound healing through phosphatidylinositol-3-OH kinase-gamma and PTEN. *Nature* **442:** 457–460.

40. Hickey, F.B. & T.G. Cotter. 2006. BCR-ABL regulates phosphatidylinositol 3-kinase-p110gamma transcription and activation and is required for proliferation and drug resistance. *J Biol. Chem.* **281:** 2441–2450.

41. Voigt, P., M.B. Dorner, M. Schaefer. 2006. Characterization of p87PIKAP, a novel regulatory subunit of phosphoinositide 3-kinase gamma that is highly expressed in heart and interacts with PDE3B. *JBC* **281:** 9977–9986.

42. Stoyanov, B., S. Volinia, T. Hanck, *et al.* 1995. Cloning and characterization of a G protein-activated human phosphoinositide-3 kinase. *Science* **269:** 690–693.

43. Hawkins, P.T. & L.R. Stephens. 2007. PI3Kgamma is a key regulator of inflammatory responses and cardiovascular homeostasis. *Science* **318:** 64–66.

Magnetic Resonance Imaging of Endometrial and Cervical Cancer

Anju Sahdev[a] and Rodney H. Reznek[b]

[a]*Department of Radiology, St. Bartholomew's Hospital, London, United Kingdom*

[b]*Cancer Imaging, St. Bartholomew's Hospital and the London School of Medicine and Dentistry, London, United Kingdom*

In this article we review the current and developing roles of magnetic resonance imaging (MRI) in endometrial and cervical cancer. In endometrial cancer, the purpose of MRI is to stage the primary tumor and in particular to identify myometrial and cervical invasion and extra-uterine disease, thereby informing preoperative surgical planning. MRI is also used to safely select young patients suitable for fertility-preserving medical management. In cervical cancer, MRI has an established role in local staging and in assessing proximal extension of tumors in young women for feasibility of fertility-preserving surgery. It is used to plan radiotherapy for primary tumors in cervical cancer and particularly for conformal radiotherapy to deliver optimal doses to the tumor sites, while limiting unwanted exposure of bowel and other pelvic organs. In both cancers, MRI is used for diagnosing nodal disease, surveillance, detection of recurrence, and evaluation of complications secondary to treatment.

Key words: cervical cancer; endometrial cancer; magnetic resonance imaging (MRI)

Introduction

The International Federation of Gynecology and Obstetrics (FIGO) recommends pretreatment imaging evaluation of endometrial and cervical cancer with conventional imaging techniques that include barium enema, chest X-ray, and intravenous urography. Transvaginal ultrasound (TVUS) for endometrial cancer, computed tomography (CT), magnetic resonance imaging (MRI), and 18-fluorodeoxyglucose positron emission tomography (FDG PET) have expanded the role of imaging in the management of patients with endometrial and cervical cancer but currently do not form part of the routine staging investigations. Imaging has become an important adjuvant to clinical and surgical evaluation. The role of imaging lies in tumor staging, treatment planning, assessing treatment response, and monitoring complications, as its excellent tissue contrast distinguishes between tumor and normal tissue. Unlike ultrasound MRI is not operator dependent, and unlike CT it has no radiation burden. Technical improvements in MR pelvic coils and acquisition software have made it easier to acquire quicker and better images of the pelvis. With breath hold fast spin-echo (FSE) T2-weighted and contrast enhanced spoiled gradient-echo T1-weighted sequences, image quality is significantly improved while acquisition times remain short. Consequently, MRI more than any other imaging modality has become essential in the management of women with gynecological cancer.

In this article we review its role and performance in endometrial cancer particularly in detecting myometrial and cervical invasion for predicting patients with low, intermediate, and high risk of nodal metastases. MRI has also recently been advocated for surveillance when young women with endometrial cancer have been treated with hormones alone for fertility

Address for correspondence: Anju Sahdev, MB BS, MRCP, FRCR, Department of Radiology, St. Bartholomew's Hospital, Dominion House, 59 Bartholomew's Close, London EC1A 7ED, UK. Voice: +442076018864; fax: +020-7601-8864/8329. anju.sahdev@bartsandthelondon.nhs.uk

Ann. N.Y. Acad. Sci. 1138: 214–232 (2008). © 2008 New York Academy of Sciences.
doi: 10.1196/annals.1414.028

preservation. In cervical cancer, MRI has an important role in assessing tumor volume, location, stage, proximal extension for fertility-preserving surgery (trachelectomy), planning radiotherapy, and detecting treatment complications and recurrent disease.

Endometrial Cancer

In 2006, The American Cancer Society estimated that endometrial cancer would account for 6% (approximately 41,000 cases) of all new female cancer cases and 3% (approximately 8200 cases) of all female cancer deaths. This makes it the eighth commonest female cancer and the fourth greatest cause of cancer fatality in the United States. The death rate for endometrial cancer has been declining since the 1950s, and the incidence rate is stable despite the increasing prevalence of obesity in the United States. The death rate for African American women is higher, 7 per 100,000 compared to 3.9 per 100,000 for white American women.[1] In 2002, 199,000 new cases and 50,000 deaths from endometrial cancer were reported worldwide, making it the 16th commonest cancer.[1–3]

Carcinoma of the endometrium occurs primarily in the 6th–7th decades. Only 25% occur in premenopausal women. Patients most commonly present with postmenopausal bleeding, indeed, endometrial cancer is the cause in 10–30% of patients with postmenopausal bleeding.[4] The precise etiology of endometrial cancer remains unknown but two mechanisms are thought to play a role: (1) unopposed estrogen stimulation causing endometrial hyperplasia, which progresses to carcinoma or (2) spontaneous carcinomas arising from atrophic endometrium. Tumors arising on a background of endometrial hyperplasia are well-differentiated (lower grade) and less likely to have deep myometrial invasion and nodal metastases, thereby carrying a better prognosis than spontaneous tumors, which are more poorly differentiated.[5] Recognized risk factors for endometrial cancer include nulliparity, un-

TABLE 1. Risk Groups for Pelvic and Para-aortic Nodal Disease in Endometrial Cancer

Risk group	Features
High group	Any age and all 3 features listed below:
	1. Grade 3 adenocarcinoma
	2. >50% deep myometrial invasion
	3. Lymphovascular space invasion
Intermediate groups	>50 years and any 2 of the above features
	>70 years and any 1 of the above features
Low	Grade 1 and 2 adenocarcinoma and no or superficial myometrial invasion

opposed estrogen replacement, and adenomatous endometrial hyperplasia. Relative risk factors are obesity, hypertension, diabetes mellitus, and long-term (>5 years) tamoxifen citrate treatment.

Ninety percent of endometrial carcinomas are adenocarcinomas, ranging from well-differentiated (grade 1) to undifferentiated (grade 3) carcinomas. The remaining 10% consist of adenosquamous, papillary serous, clear cell, and carcinosarcomas (malignant mixed Mullerian tumors). The rarer tumor types are associated with a poorer prognosis. The prognosis of endometrial cancer depends upon tumor grade, cell type, stage, and lymph-node status. Clinical staging understages 13–22% of carcinomas and, therefore, since 1988 the official FIGO staging combines surgical and histological findings.[6] Lymph-node metastases depend on the depth of myometrial invasion, cervical invasion, and tumor occupying greater than one-third of the endometrial cavity. Table 1 summarizes the risk factors for pelvic and para-aortic nodal metastases. Patients with grade 2 and grade 3 carcinoma have a 14% and 38% risk of para-aortic lymphadenopathy, respectively. Patients with no or only superficial myometrial invasion have a 5% prevalence of para-aortic nodal metastases, which rises to 46% in patients with deep (>50%) myometrial invasion.[7] The depth of myometrial invasion is the strongest prognostic factor with regard to the 5-year survival rate. Patients with

TABLE 2. MRI Findings Corresponding to the FIGO Staging of Endometrial Cancer

Stage	FIGO staging	MRI findings
Stage IA	Tumor limited to the endometrium	Normal or thickened endometrial stripe with diffuse or focal abnormal signal. Intact junctional zone
Stage IB	<50% myometrial invasion	Signal intensity of tumor extends into the <50% of myometrium. Partial or full thickness disruption of the junctional zone
Stage IC	>50% myometrial invasion	Signal intensity of tumor extends into >50% of myometrium. Full thickness disruption of the junctional zone
Stage IIA	Invasion of endocervix	Internal os and endo-cervical canal are widened. Low signal of cervical stroma remains undisrupted.
Stage IIB	Cervical stromal invasion	Disruption of low signal stroma
Stage IIIA	Invasion of serosa, adnexal, or positive peritoneal cytology	Disruption of continuity of outer myometrium. Irregular uterine configuration
Stage IIIB	Invasion of vagina	Segmental loss of hypointense vaginal wall
Stage IIIC	Pelvic or para-aortic lymphadenopathy	Regional or para-aortic nodes >1cm in short axis diameter
Stage IVA	Invasion of bladder or rectal mucosa	Tumor signal intensity disrupts normal bladder or rectal wall
Stage IVB	Distant metastases including intra-abdominal and inguinal lymphadenopathy	Tumor in distant sites or organs

stage 1A/B disease have been shown to have a 5-year survival rate of 90–100%, compared to 40–60% in stage 1C disease[8,9] (Table 2). It is not entirely clear whether cervical invasion per se diminishes survival, as it is more often associated with poorly differentiated tumor types.

Conventional treatment is by hysterectomy, and as 80% of tumors at presentation are confined to the uterus, this is a curative procedure.[10] In the remaining 20% there is regional or distant metastatic disease. Although the mainstay of treatment is hysterectomy with bilateral salpingo-oophrectomy, pelvic lymph-node sampling or lymphadenectomy is required in a subset of patients who have a higher risk of nodal metastases and an increased risk of relapse. The Gynecologic Oncology Group (GOG) has identified those groups of patients (high-risk patients) in whom they recommend that para-aortic and pelvic lymph nodes should be sampled.[11] If

- there is myometrial invasion greater than 50% regardless of tumor grade

- there is extension of tumor into the internal os or cervical stroma
- there are visible adnexal or other extra-uterine metastases
- there are visibly enlarged lymph nodes
- there is serous papillary, undifferentiated, clear cell, or squamous histology

The rationale underlying selective lymphadenectomy is that a more accurate assessment of the extent of disease allows for better individualization of adjuvant radiotherapy. Adjuvant radiotherapy can be prescribed to those found to have nodal metastases or other high-risk factors, while the vast majority without nodal metastases can be spared radiotherapy (Table 3). In a large retrospective analysis of the effect of the extent of selective lymphadenectomy on survival and morbidity in women with early-stage endometrial cancer, Cragun and colleagues[12] stratified patients into high-, intermediate-, and low-risk groups (Table 1). High-risk patients benefited from extended pelvic lymph-node dissection (>11 nodes resected). The 5-year overall survival rate

TABLE 3. The Proposed Use of Adjuvant Therapies in Cervical Cancer

FIGO stage	Risk	Subtypes*	Postoperative adjuvant therapy
Stage I	Low (5-year 5% locoregional relapse)	Stage IA ,Grade 1 + 2	None
		Stage IB, Grade 1	None
		Stage IB, Grade 2	None or vaginal brachytherapy
	High	>60 years	Node −ve vaginal brachytherapy
	(5-year 19% locoregional relapse, 20–30% distant relapse)	Stage IB, grade 3	Node +ve pelvic radiotherapy
		Stage IC, any grade	Vaginal brachytherapy +/− pelvic radiotherapy. Role of chemotherapy being investigated
Stage II		If full surgical staging shows no pelvic metastases	Pelvic radiotherapy Vaginal brachytherapy
Stage III		IIIA	Pelvic radiotherapy
		IIIB	Preoperative vaginal radiotherapy Extended field radiotherapy
Stage IV		IVA	Pelvic radiotherapy? chemotherapy
		IVB	Symptom management

*Lymphovascular space invasion (LVSI) places patients at high risk of nodal metastases. Patients managed surgically without lymphadenectomy should be treated with pelvic radiotherapy regardless of other risk factors.

was 82% compared with 64% in those with fewer than 11 nodes resected, and progression-free survival was 80% compared with 60%. In the low-risk group, no statistical survival benefit was observed in the extended pelvic lymphadenectomy group.[12] The first multicenter randomized trial to determine the value of lymphadenectomy for stage 1 and 2 endometrial carcinoma, the UK Medical Research Council-ASTEC study, is nearing completion and should provide definitive and unbiased information on the role of lymphadenectomy in intermediate- to high-risk endometrial cancer.

A significant number of women with endometrial cancer have comorbidities, increasing the risk of anesthesia and surgery. These include obesity, diabetes mellitus, hypertension, ischemic heart disease, and AIDS. It is prudent therefore to perform the most appropriate and expeditious procedure after consultation between the surgeon and anesthetists. Preoperative MRI allows accurate staging and surgical planning so that a straightforward hysterectomy and salpingo-oopherectomy is performed only when extended pelvic or para-aortic lymphadenectomy does not confer a survival ben-

efit, avoiding significantly increased morbidity and mortality associated with retroperitoneal and pelvic lymphadenectomy. Preoperative MRI identifies patients with deep myometrial invasion, cervical invasion, and extra-uterine pelvic disease who may benefit from referral to tertiary cancer centers for more extensive surgery and specifically to perform lymph-node sampling. The extent of sampling may be influenced by the preoperative knowledge of tumor extent.

Staging Endometrial Cancer

Endometrial biopsy establishes the diagnosis of endometrial cancer and shows an increase in endometrial width, heterogeneous echotexture, and an irregular poorly defined edge. As part of staging, TVUS has been used to evaluate the depth of myometrial and cervical invasion in endometrial cancer. TVUS, CT, and MRI have all been used to assess myometrial invasion. The performance of TVUS is variable and operator dependent. The reported accuracies for myometrial invasion vary between 77% and 91%.[13–15] CT, including newer

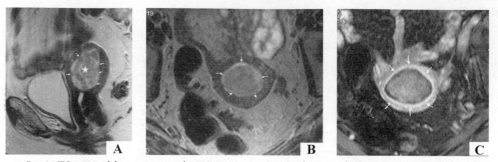

Figure 1. A 72-year-old woman with FIGO stage 1A endometrial carcinoma. **(A)** Sagittal FSE T2-weighted image showing the endometrial carcinoma (star) widening the endometrial cavity. There is a smooth tumor–myometrial interface (arrows) indicating no myometrial invasion. **(B)** Axial oblique FSE T2-weighted image providing a true axial view of the uterus and endometrial cavity. The smooth tumor–myometrial interface is retained circumferentially (arrows). **(C)** Axial oblique post gadolinium-enhanced, fat-saturated T1-weighted images showing the enhancing endometrial tumor. The submucosal stratum basale enhances avidly between 30–60 s, and its preservation precludes myometrial invasion (arrows).

multidetector CT, has poor sensitivity and specificity for myometrial and cervical invasion. For the detection of deep myometrial invasion, the sensitivity and specificity are 83% and 42%, respectively.[16] For the detection of cervical invasion, the sensitivity and specificity are 25% and 70%, respectively.[16] The overall staging accuracy of CT is between 58% and 76%.[17,18] CT is therefore of limited value for local staging and unlikely to affect management in early endometrial cancer. In more advanced disease with parametrial and pelvic side-wall disease, CT is highly accurate in detecting pelvic and abdominal spread beyond the uterus.[19]

Due to its excellent tissue contrast resolution, MRI has established its role in identifying deep myometrial invasion and thereby contributes to the preoperative decision regarding the need for lymphadenectomy. MRI is highly accurate in local staging and is recommended for patients in whom there is clinical suspicion of extra-uterine disease and in select histological subtypes, listed earlier. The MRI findings corresponding to the FIGO stage of the endometrial cancer are summarized in Table 2. With regards to myometrial invasion, the reported sensitivities and specificities are 84–87% and 91–94%, respectively. The positive predictive value (PPV) is 87% and the negative predictive value (NPV) is 91% for the identification

of myometrial invasion greater than 50%.[20,21] Intravenous injection of gadolinium can distinguish between viable tumor and debris and also highlights the tumor–myometrial junction, thereby improving the ability to assess the depth of myometrial invasion. Endometrial cancer typically has a lower signal intensity than myometrium after contrast medium enhancement providing greater contrast resolution than FSE T2-weighted images. The main error in determining myometrial invasion is an overestimation on both T2-weighted images and contrast-enhanced MRI.[20] In the study by Lee and colleagues,[21] T2-weighted sequences were more accurate in women with a normal thick myometrium and premenopausal women, while contrast-enhanced images were more accurate in postmenopausal women with thinned myometrium (Figs. 1–3). Contrast-enhanced MRI has been shown to significantly alter the pretest probability of myometrial invasion in all grades of adenocarcinoma. Frei and coworkers calculated the pretest probability for myometrial invasion for grade 1, 2, and 3 tumors as 13%, 35%, and 54%, respectively.[22] These increased to 60%, 84%, and 92%, respectively, when MRI suggested myometrial invasion and decreased to 1%, 5%, and 10%, respectively, for negative MRI. This confirms the high expected frequencies of deep myometrial

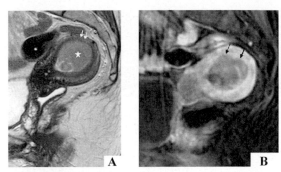

Figure 2. A 66-year-old woman with FIGO stage 1B endometrial carcinoma. **(A)** Sagittal FSE T2-weighted image showing the endometrial carcinoma (star) with early myometrial invasion and thinning of the junctional zone (arrows). **(B)** Sagittal post gadolinium-enhanced, fat-saturated T1-weighted images showing the endometrial tumor enhancing less than the myometrium. The tumor is seen infiltrating into the inner myometrium (arrows).

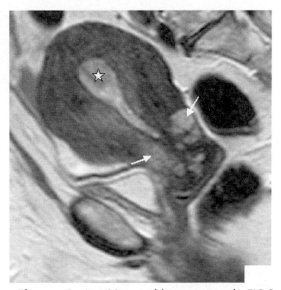

Figure 4. An 83-year-old woman with FIGO stage IIB endometrial carcinoma. Sagittal T2-weighted image showing an endometrial mass in the fundus of the uterus (star). Within the cervix, the normal low T2-signal intensity cervical stroma is replaced by high T2-signal intensity tumor (arrows) indicating stage IIB carcinoma.

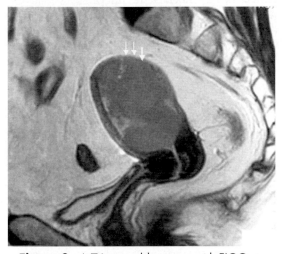

Figure 3. A 76-year-old woman with FIGO stage 1C endometrial carcinoma. Sagittal T2-weighted image demonstrating a large endometrial carcinoma with deep invasion of the posterior myometrium (arrows).

invasion in patients with grade 2 or 3 disease. MRI can reliably exclude deep myometrial disease in grade 1 and 2 disease and understages 10% of patients with grade 3 disease. These figures also show that if grade alone is considered, 13% of patients with grade 1 disease would be understaged and receive suboptimal surgery. In patients with grade 3 carcinoma, a positive MRI increases the probability for deep myome-

trial invasion from 54% to 92%. However, if all patients with grade 3 undergo lymphadenectomy, about 40% would undergo more invasive surgery than is necessary.[22] With preoperative MRI information there is little need for routine preoperative frozen sections.

MRI also performs particularly well in detection of cervical invasion, and sensitivity, specificity, accuracy, PPV, and NPV for cervical invasion are 80%, 96%, 92%, 89%, and 93%, respectively.[23] Several investigators have reported that macroscopic cervical invasion, detectable on MRI, imparts a worse prognosis than microscopic invasion.[24,25] Therefore preoperative assessment for cervical involvement may help in planning surgery and radiotherapy. For the detection of cervical invasion, FSE T2-weighted images are well suited (Fig. 4). The detection of cervical invasion utilizes the natural contrast between the low T2 signal of normal cervical stroma and the hyperintense T2-signal intensity of the invading endometrial carcinoma. In our

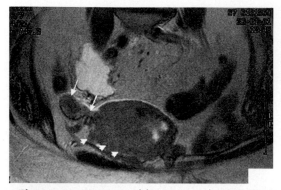

Figure 5. A 76-year-old woman with stage FIGO stage IIIA endometrial carcinoma. Axial oblique FSE T2-weighted image demonstrating a large endometrial carcinoma with deep myometrial invasion and tumor nodules on the serosal surface (arrow heads) and direct tumor invasion into the right fallopian tube and ovary (arrows).

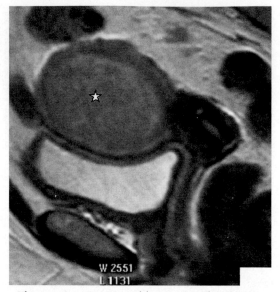

Figure 7. A 79-year-old woman with FIGO stage IC endometrial carcinoma. Sagittal T2-weighted image showing a large endometrial mass (star) in a patient with atrophy of the myometrium. The thin myometrium, particularly anteriorly, limits evaluation of myometrial invasion. On MRI the appearances were interpreted as early myometrial invasion but histology revealed deep myometrial invasion.

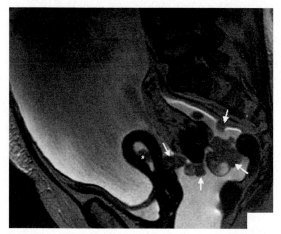

Figure 6. An 88-year-old woman with FIGO stage IIIC endometrial carcinoma. Sagittal T2-weighted image showing an endometrial mass in the body of the uterus (star). There is disseminated peritoneal disease with a large amount of ascites and peritoneal nodules in the pelvis (arrows).

experience contrast enhancement does not improve the detection of cervical invasion.

Also as part of MRI staging, extra-uterine disease in the form of tumor invasion of the serosal, adnexal, and peritoneal deposits in the Pouch of Douglas, omental disease, and pelvic or retroperitoneal lymphadenopathy is readily detected on MRI (Figs. 5 and 6).

To obtain optimum MRI performance described above, MRI technique should in-clude axial T1-weighted; axial, sagittal, and oblique FSE T2-weighted; and fat saturated gadolinium-enhanced dynamic T1-weighted sagittal and oblique images. The FSE T2-weighted oblique scans are obtained at a plane perpendicular to the long axis of the tumor-bearing uterus. Contrast-enhanced MRI has been shown to perform better than TVUS and CT in the detection and assessment of myometrial and cervical invasion.[16,23,26] Pitfalls in the staging of endometrial cancer on MRI include blood in the endometrial cavity due to recent dilation and curettage or tumor hemorrhage, extreme thinning of the myometrium, poor natural contrast between the tumor and myometrium, adenomyosis, and fibroids (Figs. 7–9). The tumor–myometrial interface in patients with adenomyosis and submucosal or inner myometrial fibroids becomes difficult to interpret. This interface may be abnormal without superficial myometrial invasion, and conversely deep myometrial invasion may not

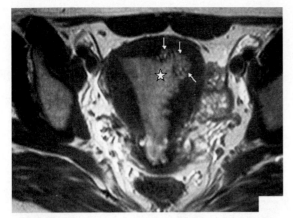

Figure 8. A 55-year-old woman with FIGO stage 1B endometrial carcinoma. Axial T2-weighted image demonstrating a focus of adenomyosis within the inner myometrium (arrows). Invasion of the myometrium by the endometrial carcinoma (star) is obscured by the adenomyosis.

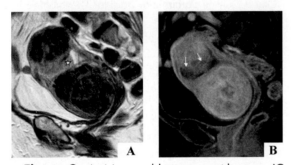

Figure 9. A 66-year-old woman with stage IC endometrial carcinoma **(A)** Sagittal T2-weighted image in a patient with multiple myometrial fibroids and an endometrial cancer within the distorted endometrial cavity (star). The fundal fibroid obscures the tumor–myometrial junction thereby limiting the assessment of myometrial invasion. **(B)** Sagittal post gadolinium-enhanced, fat-saturated T1-weighted image shows the endometrial carcinoma invading the underlying myometrial fibroid (arrows), but the depth of invasion is difficult to assess. Both sagittal and post gadolinium-enhanced images suggest superficial myometrial invasion, but the pathology specimen showed deep myometrial invasion around the fibroid.

be apparent due to underlying adenomyosis or fibroids. In stage 2A, widening of the endocervical canal may be caused by debris or mucus plugs, coexisting endocervical polyps, or endocervical mucosal hyperplasia.[27]

Although endometrial cancer is a disease of postmenopausal women, 25% of tumors oc-cur in younger, premenopausal women, with 3–5% presenting in patients under 40 years of age. In this subset of patients, the issue of fertility preservation poses a therapeutic dilemma for both patients and surgeons. Recent studies have shown grade 1, stage 1A tumors can be safely treated conservatively with hormonal therapy for a short time while the patient completes her family. Patients are treated with a high-dose progesterone regimen with endometrial sampling every 3 months until complete regression of the tumor is documented. MRI in these patients is performed during initial staging to exclude myometrial and cervical invasion, during surveillance, and after completion of treatment.[28–30] In long-term observational studies the recurrence rates were high even after complete pathological remission, and therefore close follow-up is recommended.[28]

Recurrent Endometrial Disease

The most important prognostic factor in endometrial cancer is stage: the expected 5-year survival rate of stage I is 87% and of stage II is 76%. The recurrence rate for stage I and II endometrial cancer is 4% in low-risk patients and up to 20% in patients with high-grade tumors, deep myometrial invasion, and lymphovascular space invasion.[31] The risk groups, their features, and recommended adjuvant therapies are summarized in Table 3. The table is constructed from the meta-analysis performed by Shaeffer and associates on the use of adjuvant therapy in endometrial cancer.[32] There remains controversy in the selection of adjuvant therapies, as most of the data available comprise small studies, but forthcoming reports from the PORTEC and ASTEC studies should clarify the role of adjuvant therapies.

MRI has also been advocated in detection of recurrent disease to evaluate surgical resectability. Recurrent endometrial cancer may present as a pelvic mass in the hysterectomy bed or as pelvic or retroperitoneal lymphadenopathy. Less frequently it may manifest as peritoneal

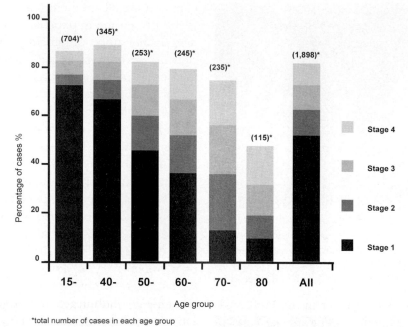

Graph 1. Variation in TNM stage with age group for cervical cancer cases. Cancers diagnosed 1991–1995. (Cancer Research UK.)

carcinomatosis. Distant metastases and early recurrent disease are usually associated with high-grade tumors and advanced stage at presentation.[33,34] CT performs well in detection of recurrent pelvic and distant disease, with an overall accuracy, sensitivity, and specificity of 92%, 92%, and 80%, respectively.[35] 18-FDG PET has been evaluated in small studies and reports promisingly high sensitivity of 96%, but a poor specificity of 57%. Correlation of 18-FDG PET with tumor markers and CT (18-FDG–PET-CT) minimizes false positive rates improving the specificity to 88%.[36] As 18-FDG-PET is a whole-body imaging technique, all comparative studies report a higher accuracy than CT and MRI in detection of upper abdominal disease and lung metastases.

Cervical Cancer

Carcinoma of the cervix remains a formidable problem, with the American Cancer Society estimating 9710 new cases and 3700 deaths in 2006. Worldwide in 2000, 471,000 new cases were estimated to have presented, making it the third commonest malignancy after breast and colorectal cancer in women.[1,37] The majority (42%) occur in 20- to 44-year-old women, and the incidence rate is an annual 8.8 per 100,000, with a life-time risk of 1:138. The stage distribution shows that 52% of cervical cancer cases are diagnosed while the cancer is confined to the cervix (stage 1), 34% are diagnosed after the cancer has spread to regional lymph nodes or directly beyond the primary site, and 9% are diagnosed with distant metastases. The corresponding 5-year relative survival rates are 92.0% for localized stage 1 disease, 55.5% for locoregional extension, and 14.6% for disease with distant metastatic spread. As is the case for endometrial cancer, cervical cancer is more often fatal in African American women than in white women, with death rates per 100,000 of 7.1 and 3.9, respectively.[37] In countries with national cervical cancer screening programs, younger women tend to present with earlier stages of the disease. Graph 1 summarizes the stage at presentation against the age at presentation in

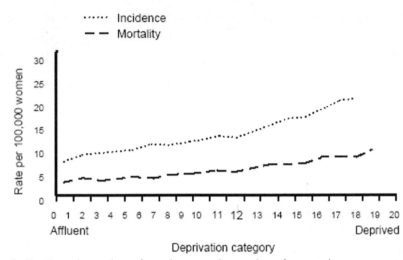

Graph 2. The relationship of incidence and mortality of cervical cancer against social deprivation score. (Cancer Research UK.)

women with cervical cancer in the West Midlands, United Kingdom. The rate of cervical cancer and mortality of the disease can be related to the Carstairs' deprivations score demonstrated in Graph 2, based on U.K. data.[38] These demographics—particularly the young age and early stage of presentation—are relevant to the role of MRI in cervical cancer.

Over the past several years, overwhelming evidence has accumulated for the role of MRI in the management of these patients. It is now an integral part of local staging, important in monitoring response and detection of recurrence, demonstrating complications of the disease itself and of treatment, determining feasibility of uterus-preserving surgery, and planning radiotherapy.

Staging of Cervical Cancer

Cervical cancer is confirmed histologically following clinical evaluation by cervical smear and cervical biopsy. The classic staging of cervical cancer uses the FIGO classification. The World Health Organization (WHO) tumor, nodal status, and metastases (TNM) classification is essentially based on the same criteria (Table 4). FIGO stages cervical cancer using the conventional techniques of chest X-ray, bar-

ium enema, and intravenous urography. However in many countries, these imaging studies are replaced by modern imaging techniques, such as CT and MRI. Official FIGO guidelines do not include cross-sectional imaging techniques in the staging of cervical cancer. This is mainly due to the principle that staging methods should be universally available, particularly as cervical cancer is more prevalent in the developing world where CT and MRI has limited availability.

Both CT and MRI have been used to stage cervical cancer. The cervical tumor is not seen on CT, but staging relies on identifying presence or absence of tumor in the parametrium. MRI is the most accurate imaging technique for preoperative staging of cervical cancer. For staging accuracy, MRI is significantly better than CT (86% versus 63%, respectively).[39] MRI is also cost effective as it can replace cystoscopy, sigmoidoscopy, barium enema, and intravenous urography.[40] The key role of MRI is to distinguish early stage (IA-IIA) disease from advanced disease. In early-stage tumors, the key role of MRI lies in detection of parametrial extension of tumor which renders the patient stage IIB or above. This is critical, as tumors below stage IIB in general are treated surgically, while those stage IIB and above are treated with radiotherapy alone or

TABLE 4. MRI Findings Corresponding to the FIGO and TNM Staging in Cervical Cancer

FIGO staging	TMN stage	MRI findings
IA	T1a preclinical invasive carcinoma	Normal
IB	T1b tumor greater than 5 mm deep and 8 mm wide	Tumor confined to the cervix. Low signal stroma surrounds the tumor
IB1-tumor < 4 cm		
IB2-tumor > 4 cm		
IIA	T2a upper two-thirds of the vagina. No parametrial invasion	Infiltrate the upper two-thirds of the vagina. Thickening or loss of normal low signal vaginal wall
IIB	T2b parametrial invasion	Parametrial invasion. Loss of the surrounding normal low signal stroma with tumor extension into the parametrium
IIIA	T3a lower third of the vagina not pelvic side-wall	Invasion of lower third of the vagina with thickening or loss of normal low signal of the vaginal wall
IIIB	T3b pelvic side-wall or hydroureter	Pelvic side-wall invasion including tumor extension into the vessels, muscles or utero–sacral ligaments Hydronephrosis
IVA	T4	Tumor invades bladder or rectal mucosa
IVB	M1	Distant metastases (including lymph nodes beyond the true pelvis)

combined with chemotherapy. The performance of MRI in early cervical tumors was evaluated in a meta-analysis by Bipat and colleagues[41] showing MRI had a sensitivity of 93% for tumor detection and an overall staging accuracy of 86%. By comparison, clinical FIGO staging performed poorly, with an overall accuracy of only 47%. More recently, the joint American College of Radiology Imaging Network (ACRIN) and Gynecology Oncology Group (GOG) study[42] reported much improved clinical FIGO staging results with a specificity, PPV, and NPV of 99%, 91%, and 84%, respectively. However in this study, final clinical staging was reported after CT and MRI findings were available, thereby strongly influencing and improving the clinical staging. As discussed in the ACRIN/GOG study and in our experience, CT—unlike MRI—does not visualize the extent of the primary cervical tumor. CT is therefore unsuitable in assessing suitability for trachelectomy or for planning modern conformal radiotherapy techniques particularly intensity modulated radiotherapy (IMRT).

The key feature when staging these early tumors on MRI is circumferential preservation

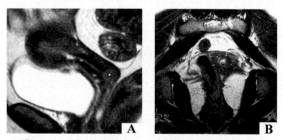

Figure 10. A 24-year-old woman with FIGO stage 1B1 carcinoma of the cervix. **(A)** Sagittal T2-weighted image showing the cervical carcinoma as high T2-signal intensity lesion in the posterior lip of the cervix (star). **(B)** Axial oblique T2-weighted image obtained perpendicular to the long axis of the cervix to provide a true axial image of the cervix. The high T2-signal intensity tumor (star) is surrounded by normal low T2-signal intensity cervical stroma. This preservation of the stroma (arrows) excludes parametrial invasion.

of normal cervical stroma around the tumor (Fig. 10). The assessment of parametrial invasion is best performed on axial oblique FSE T2-weighted sequences acquired perpendicular to the long axis of the cervix. In our experience and in that of others, preservation of normal low (black) T2-signal cervical stroma around intermediate T2-signal intensity tumor has a very high NPV, exceeding 96% for parametrial

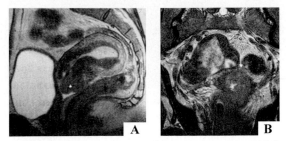

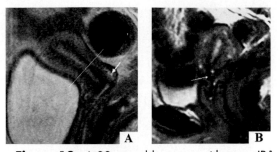

Figure 11. A 33-year-old woman with a FIGO stage IIB carcinoma of the cervix. **(A)** Sagittal T2-weighted image showing a large exophytic mass arising from the posterior lip of the cervix (star). **(B)** Axial oblique T2-weighted image showing the normal low T2-weighted cervical stroma is no longer preserved circumferentially. Tumor is noted extending into the parametrium posteriorly (arrow) in keeping with FIGO stage IIB carcinoma.

Figure 12. A 22-year-old woman with stage IB1 carcinoma of the cervix. **(A)** Sagittal T2-weighted image showing the small high T2-signal intensity carcinoma in the posterior lip of the cervix. This lies more than 1 cm distal to the internal os (solid line) indicating suitability for fertility-preserving trachelectomy. **(B)** Sagittal T2-weighted image showing the appearances of the residual uterus after trachelectomy. The utero-vaginal anastomosis is clearly seen (arrow) and carefully assessed for signs of early recurrent disease.

invasion.[43–45] Interruption of this low-signal stromal line indicates full thickness stromal invasion, either with or without parametrial invasion (Fig. 11). The PPV for parametrial invasion is therefore lower, between 82% and 86%.[46,47] In advanced tumors, staging depends on involvement of adjacent pelvic structures, pelvic side-wall, ureters, and vaginal wall. MRI criteria for pelvic side-wall invasion include tumor less than 3 mm away from the bony side-wall, vascular encasement by tumor, ureteric encasement or hydronephrosis, and tumor in obturator internus, piriformis, or levator ani.

The performance of MRI in the detection of bladder and rectal invasion has been extensively studied. The meta-analysis by Bipat and co-workers showed that MRI had a sensitivity of 91% for bladder invasion and 75% for rectal invasion.[41] In our own experience of 112 patients, by adopting a low threshold for bladder and rectal invasion, MRI had an NPV of 100%, thereby potentially negating the need for staging cystoscopy and sigmoidoscopy.[18]

Importance of Proximal Extension

One of the major uses of MRI is predicting proximal extension of tumor and thereby predicting feasibility for trachelectomy. In this pro-

cedure tumor-bearing cervix is removed and the cervical stump and uterine body are re-anastomosed to the vagina with insertion of a cerclage suture to maintain isthmic competency during pregnancy. In our institution, the technique is performed vaginally with laparoscopic lymph-node dissection.[49,50] An important criterion for surgery is that the proximal end of the tumor should be 1 cm or more distal to the internal os to permit tumor-free re-anastomosis (Fig. 12). Clinically, the internal os cannot be established by the examining gynecologist. MRI has been shown to be a reliable method of determining proximal extension of cervical cancer into the internal os, thus predicting the suitability for fertility-conserving surgery. For internal os tumor involvement, the sensitivity, specificity, PPV, and NPV have been shown to be 90%, 98%, 86%, and 98%, respectively.[47,51]

The prognostic importance of proximal extension of tumor has also been shown in patients with higher-stage disease undergoing radiotherapy (Fig. 13). In a study by Narayan and colleagues, in 70 patients the presence of proximal extension as seen on MRI increased the probability of nodal metastases to 75% versus 11% in patients without proximal

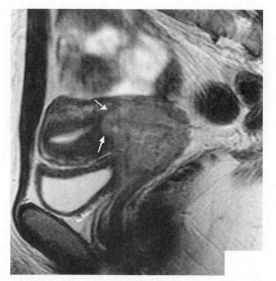

Figure 13. A 34-year-old woman with FIGO stage IIB carcinoma of the cervix. Sagittal T2-weighted image showing the tumor replaces the entire cervix and a barrel shaped tumor is seen. This extends to the level of the internal os and into the myometrium (arrow). This invasion of the myometrium is an indicator of poor prognostic.

extension.[52] Nodal metastases were diagnosed as tumor positive if they demonstrated positive tracer uptake on FDG-PET scans. The presence of nodal metastases had a significant negative association with disease-specific and disease-free survival.[52] A further recent PET study[53] reproduced these findings in 58 patients. Patients with endometrial invasion had a significantly higher rate of para-aortic and supraclavicular lymph-node metastases at presentation. Endometrial invasion was associated with decreased 2-year disease-free survival and overall survival. Proximal extension is therefore increasingly recognized as an important prognostic feature in patients presenting with both early and advanced stage cervical cancer.

Nodal Metastases

CT and MRI have comparable accuracies of 85–90% in detection of nodal metastases in cervical cancer.[54] The reported value of 18-FDG-PET is greater than that of either CT or MRI. The sensitivity and specificity of 18-FDG-PET are 100% and 96%, respectively, compared to MRI sensitivity and specificity of 83% and 73%, respectively.[55,56] The performance of MRI is greatly improved by the introduction of ultrasmall paramagnetic iron oxide particles (USPIOs), which are lymph-node specific intravenous contrast agents. These are administered to the patient intravenously at time of the staging MRI. The contrast agent is taken up by macrophages into lymph nodes. The paramagnetic effect of iron oxide particles results in loss of signal on T2-weighted sequences in normal, macrophage-laden nodes. In nodes replaced by tumor metastases, no loss of signal is seen after administration of US-PIOs. The use of USPIOs improves the sensitivity and specificity of MRI (using size criteria of nodes) from 29% and 98% to 93% and 97%, respectively.[57] Currently, FIGO staging does not include the assessment of lymph-node metastases. However, nodal metastases are recognized as indicative of poor disease prognosis.[58,59] Although there are controversies over the value of postoperative pelvic radiotherapy in patients with pelvic nodal metastases, improved survival has been reported irrespective of the number of nodes involved.[60] Pelvic and para-aortic nodal involvement is increasingly sought to identify patients suitable for adjuvant pelvic and extended field radiotherapy or chemotherapy.

Recurrent Disease

Approximately 30% of women with cervical cancer die of residual or recurrent cervical cancer after primary treatment.[61] The identification of recurrent disease is important, as secondary treatment with pelvic exenteration or further chemoradiotherapy has a 5-year survival rate of 46–52% compared to 5% in untreated recurrent disease.[62] The main treatment option in recurrent disease is radiotherapy alone or in combination with chemotherapy. Pelvic exenterative surgery is reserved for young women with low comorbidity

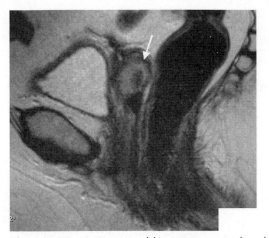

Figure 14. A 36-year-old woman treated with radical hysterectomy for stage IB2 carcinoma of the cervix. Sagittal T2-weighed image showing a recurrent mass at the vaginal vault, confirmed with a core biopsy (arrow). This patient had localized central recurrence only and would therefore be suitable for pelvic exenteration.

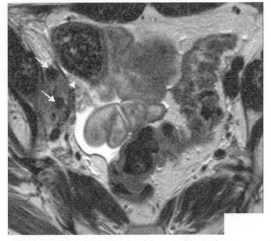

Figure 15. A 22-year-old woman with recurrent carcinoma of the cervix. Axial T2-weighted image demonstrating a recurrent right pelvic side-wall mass (arrow head). This encases the external iliac artery and vein (arrows) and extends to the bony cortex. This would not be suitable for pelvic exenteration.

and a localized central pelvic recurrence without peritoneal disease, pelvic side-wall vessel encasement, involvement of bony pelvic side-wall, distant extrapelvic disease, or nodal metastases.[63] The decision to perform local re-section, pelvic exenteration, or radiotherapy is largely based on the imaging findings. In our experience of recurrent cervical cancer, 30% had recurrent disease within 10 years, of which the majority (78%) recurred within 1 year. In patients receiving radiotherapy, 67% of recurrences were in the treated cervix while 87% of postsurgical recurrences were in the vaginal vault at the surgical resection margins. Only 13% of patients had recurrent disease outside the pelvis without evidence of pelvic recurrence.[64] The majority of the recurrences are therefore central, and as most patients with cervical cancer are young, MRI is increasingly used to select patients suitable for exentrative surgery (Fig. 14). Where surgery is planned and pelvic side-wall disease is suspected, MRI offers detailed anatomical information regarding the layers of the pelvic side-wall as only bony involvement and tumor extension into the pre-sacral space and sciatic notch are absolute contraindications to surgery (Fig. 15).[65]

Both CT and MRI have an important role in detection of recurrent disease. The accuracy of CT is up to 85%.[66] Its limitation is in differentiating postradiation fibrosis and edema from recurrent disease. The sensitivity of MRI for detecting recurrent pelvic disease is 90% and remains comparable to FDG-PET.[67,68] FDG-PET has a very high sensitivity for extrapelvic nodal disease (100%) but a relatively poor sensitivity (75%) and specificity (33%) for small-volume lung and bone disease.[67] False positive extrapelvic lesions include benign inflammatory lung disease and post radiotherapy fractures for bone disease. The performance of MRI versus FDG-PET in detecting distant chest and abdominal disease is difficult to directly evaluate as MRI and CT scans of the chest are not routinely performed. Consequently, sensitivity of FDG-PET in distant disease is higher,[67] as FDG-PET evaluates the entire body in one acquisition.

Planning Radiotherapy

In recent years the role of MRI in radiotherapy has expanded. The accuracy of MRI tumor volume measurements has been well established; increasing tumor volume confers poorer prognosis.[69] With accurate tumor location and volume measurements obtained by MRI, radiotherapy can be planned to be more localized to affected sites avoiding radiation injury to pelvic bowel and bladder. Although MRI has been shown to have a major impact on planning conventional radiotherapy for cervical cancer, in most institutions radiotherapy is delivered by CT-guided 3-D conformal planning. More recently, IMRT, a form of 3-D radiotherapy planning has been introduced. Here tumor and nodes are tracked out on either CT or MRI, and radiotherapy doses are delivered in a more focused way to affected tumor tissues only. This allows greater dose delivery to affected sites but also reduces radiation to unaffected pelvic structures, limiting unwanted affects. For effective use of IMRT, gross tumor volume (GTV) and affected lymph nodes need to be mapped out accurately. The present system of IMRT relies on tumor measurements on CT. However, in our experience, CT tends to overestimate the volume of the tumor, and it is crucial therefore that MRI be correlated with it to define the GTV.

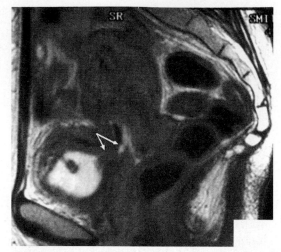

Figure 16. A 43-year-old woman treated with pelvic radiotherapy for stage IIB carcinoma of the cervix and presenting with a clinical vesicovaginal fistula. Sagittal T2-weighted image showing a thick-walled bladder, vagina, and radiotherapy changes in the cervix. There is also a high T2-signal intensity track between the posterior bladder wall and vagina (arrows). No recurrent mass is seen. The vesicovaginal fistula was secondary to radiotherapy changes only on MRI and confirmed by two biopsies of the fistula track, which revealed no recurrent malignancy.

Complications (Including Fistulae)

MRI is of value in patients undergoing radiotherapy treatment to distinguish the complications and effects of treatment from recurrent disease. The effects of radiotherapy on small bowel, bladder, bone, and muscle are well documented.[70,71] Among the most devastating complications is the formation of vaginal fistulae, which can occur as a result of recurrent disease or radiotherapy. MRI has been shown to correctly differentiate between fistulae secondary to recurrence and those secondary to radiotherapy effects. MRI is accurate in demonstrating the course, extent, and complexity of vaginal fistulae and in demonstrating associated active or recurrent disease (Fig. 16).[72]

Follow-up after Trachelectomy

MRI is routinely used for surveillance to detect early recurrence in women who have undergone trachelectomy.[73] Recurrence and death rates (4.2% and 2.8%, respectively) following trachelectomy seem to be comparable to classical radical abdominal hysterectomy and radiotherapy in early-stage cervical cancer.[74] It is important to be aware of the normal MRI postoperative appearances and to be able to discriminate between normal appearances and recurrent disease to avoid misinterpretation. We have observed three important appearances after trachelectomy that should be recognized as normal and not recurrent disease. First, in 56% of the patients there was posterior extension of the vaginal wall mimicking a vaginal fornix. This retains the normal low T2-signal intensity of the vaginal wall, in contrast with recurrent disease which has an intermediate-to-high T2-signal intensity. Second, in 6% diffuse thickening of the vaginal wall with intermediate T2-signal intensity was persistent up to 1 year after surgery and slowly resolved without treatment. Third, 4% of patients had slowly resolving hematomas with high T1-signal intensity and low/intermediate T2-signal intensity in the vaginal wall. Suture artifacts also occur from the uterovaginal anastomotic and cerclage sutures used during the procedure. To date, these have not limited the diagnostic ability of the MRI. Pelvic lymphoceles and concurrent benign disease (endometriosis and adenomyosis) were also common findings.[74]

Conclusion

In this article we review the ever-increasing role of MRI in two common gynecological malignancies. The ultimate goal is to obtain accurate staging and early disease detection to provide optimal treatment and minimize morbidity and mortality. In endometrial cancer, MRI provides accurate preoperative evaluation of myometrial and cervical invasion allowing selective preoperative scheduling of lymphadenectomy. In cervical cancer the applications of MRI are several, including distinguishing early from advanced disease and thereby deciding whether the patient is to be managed surgically or with radiotherapy. MRI is important in selecting patients suitable for trachelectomy and providing prognostic information regarding proximal tumor extension and nodal metastases. In our experience it has become essential in the management of patients with endometrial and cervical cancer. With continuing research and technical advances in MRI, its role will continue to grow.

Conflicts of Interest

The authors declare no conflicts of interest.

References

1. American Cancer Society. www.cancer.org/docroot/PRO/content/PRO_1_1_Cancer_Statistics_2006 (accessed Feb. 7, 2007).

2. UK National Statistics Office. http://www.statistics.gov.uk/statbase (accessed Feb. 7, 2007).

3. Parkin, D.M., F. Bray, J. Ferlay & P. Pisani. 2005. Global Cancer statistics, 2002. *CA Cancer J. Clin.* **55**(2): 74–108.

4. Smith-Bindman, R., K. Kerlikowske, V.A. Feldstein, *et al.* 1998. Endovaginal ultrasound to exclude endometrial cancer and other endometrial abnormalities. *JAMA* 4;**280:** 1510–1517.

5. Ohkawara, S., T. Jobo, R. Sato & H. Kuramoto. 2000. Comparison of endometrial carcinoma coexisting with and without endometrial hyperplasia. *Eur. J. Gynaecol. Oncol.* **21:** 573–577.

6. Shepherd, J.H. 1989. Revised FIGO staging for gynaecological cancer. *Br. J. Obstet. Gynaecol.* **96:** 889–892. Erratum in: *Br J Obstet Gynaecol* 1992; **99:** 440.

7. Piver, M.S., S.B. Lele, J.J. Barlow & L. Blumenson. 1982. Paraaortic lymph node evaluation in stage I endometrial carcinoma. *Obstet. Gynecol.* **59:** 97–100.

8. Larson, D.M., G.P. Connor, S.K. Broste, *et al.* 1996. Prognostic significance of gross myometrial invasion with endometrial cancer. *Obstet. Gynecol.* **88:** 394–398.

9. Chen, S.S. & L. Lee. 1983. Retroperitoneal lymph node metastases in Stage I carcinoma of the endometrium: correlation with risk factors. *Gynecol. Oncol.* **16:** 319–325.

10. International Federation of Gynaecology and Obstetrics. 1985. *Annual Report on the Results of Treatment in Gynaecologic Cancer.* FIGO. Stockholm.

11. Boronow, R.C., C.P. Morrow, W.T. Creasman, *et al.* 1984. Surgical staging in endometrial cancer: clinical-pathologic findings of a prospective study. *Obstet. Gynecol.* **63:** 825–832.

12. Cragun, J.M., L.J. Havrilesky, B. Calingaert, *et al.* 2005. Retrospective analysis of selective lymphadenectomy in apparent early-stage endometrial cancer. *J. Clin. Oncol.* **23:** 3668–3675.

13. Weber, G., E. Merz, F. Bahlmann, *et al.* 1995. Assessment of myometrial infiltration and preoperative staging by transvaginal ultrasound in patients with endometrial carcinoma. *Ultrasound Obstet. Gynecol.* **6:** 362–367.

14. Fishman, A., M. Altaras, J. Bernheim, *et al.* 2000. The value of transvaginal sonography in the preoperative assessment of myometrial invasion in high and low grade endometrial cancer and in comparison to frozen section in grade 1 disease. *Eur. J. Gynaecol. Oncol.* **21:** 128–130.

15. Gordon, A.N., A.C. Fleischer & G.W. Reed. 1990. Depth of myometrial invasion in endometrial cancer: preoperative assessment by transvaginal ultrasonography. *Gynecol. Oncol.* **39:** 321–327.

16. Hardesty, L.A., J.H. Sumkin, C. Hakim, *et al.* 2001. The ability of helical CT to preoperatively stage endometrial carcinoma. *AJR* **176:** 603–606.

17. Kim, S.H., H.D. Kim, Y.S. Song, *et al.* 1995. Detection of deep myometrial invasion in endometrial carcinoma: comparison of transvaginal ultrasound, CT, and MRI. *J. Comput. Assist. Tomogr.* **19:** 766–772.

18. Connor, J.P., J.I. Andrews, B. Anderson & R.E. Buller. 2000. Computed tomography in endometrial carcinoma. *Obstet. Gynecol.* **95:** 692–696.

19. Kinkel, K., Y. Kaji, K.K. Yu, *et al.* 1999. Radiological staging in patients with endometrial cancer: a meta-analysis. *Radiology* **212:** 711–718.

20. Sironi, S., E. Colombo & G. Villa. 1992. Myometrial invasion by endometrial carcinoma: Assessment with plain and gadolinium-enhanced MR imaging. *Radiology* **185:** 207–212.

21. Lee, E.J., J.Y. Byun, B. Kim, *et al.* 1999. Staging of early endometrial carcinoma: assessment with T2-weighted and gadolinium-enhanced T1-weighted MR imaging. *Radiographics* **19:** 937–945.

22. Frei, K.A., K. Kinkel, H.M. Bonel, *et al.* 2000. Prediction of deep myometrial invasion in patients with endometrial cancer: clinical utility of contrast-enhanced MR imaging-a meta-analysis and Bayesian analysis. *Radiology* **216:** 444–449.

23. Manfredi, R., P. Mirk & G. Maresca. 2004. Local-regional staging of endometrial carcinoma: role of MR imaging in surgical planning. *Radiology* **231:** 372–378.

24. Elia, G., D.A. Garfinkel, G.L. Goldberg, *et al.* 1995. Surgical management of patients with endometrial cancer and cervical involvement. *Eur. J. Gynaecol. Oncol.* **16:** 169–172.

25. Rubin, S.C., W.J. Hoskins & P.E. Saigo. 1992. Management of endometrial carcinoma with cervical involvement. *Gynaecol. Oncol.* **45:** 294–298.

26. Yamashita, Y., H. Mizutani & M. Torashima. 1993. Assessment of myometrial invasion by endometrial carcinoma: transvaginal sonography vs contrast-enhanced MR imaging. *AJR Am. J. Roentgenol.* **161:** 595–599.

27. Kinkel, K. 2006. Pitfalls in staging uterine neoplasm with imaging: a review. *Abdom Imaging* **31:** 164–173.

28. Niwa, K., K. Tagami, Z. Lian, *et al.* 2005. Outcome of fertility preserving treatment in young women with endometrial carcinomas. *BJOG* **112:** 317–320.

29. Benshushan, A. 2004. Endometrial adenocarcinoma in young patients: evaluation and fertility-preserving treatment. *Eur. J. Obstet. Gynecol. Reprod. Biol.* **117:** 132–137.

30. Ben-Shacher, I., K.M. Vitellas & D.E. Cohn. 2004. The role of MRI in the conservative management of endometrial cancer. *Gynecol. Oncol.* **93:** 233–237.

31. Morrow, C.P., B.N. Bundy, R.J. Kumar, *et al.* 1991. Relationship between surgical-pathological risk factors and outcome in clinical stages I and II carcinoma of the endometrium: a gynaecologic oncology group study. *Gynecol. Oncol.* **40:** 55–56.

32. Shaeffer, D.T. & M.E. Randall. 2005. Adjuvant radiotherapy in endometrial carcinoma. *Oncologist* **10:** 623–631.

33. Sohaib, S.A., S.L. Houghton, R. Meroni, *et al.* 2007. Recurrent endometrial cancer: patterns of recurrent disease and assessment of prognosis. *Clin. Radiol.* **62:** 28–34; discussion 35–36.

34. Creasman, W.T., C.P. Morrow, B.N. Bundy, *et al.* 1987. Surgical pathologic spread patterns of endometrial cancer. A Gynecologic Oncology Group Study. *Cancer* 15(8 Suppl): 2035–2041.

35. Franchi, M., A. La Fianza, L. Babilonti, *et al.* 1989. Clinical value of computerized tomography (CT) in assessment of recurrent uterine cancers. *Gynecol. Oncol.* **35:** 31–37.

36. Saga, T., T. Higashi & T. Ishimori. 2003. Clinical value of FDG-PET in the follow up of post-operative patients with endometrial cancer. *Ann. Nucl. Med.* **17:** 197–203.

37. National Cancer Institute. www.seer.cancer.gov/statfacts/html/cervix (accessed June 9, 2007).

38. Cancer Research UK. www.cancerresearchuk.org/aboutcancer/statistics/statstables/cervicalcancer (accessed June 9, 2007).

39. Pannu, H.K., F.M. Corl & E.K. Fishman. 2001. CT evaluation of cervical cancer: spectrum of disease. *Radiographics* **21:** 1155–1168.

40. Hricak, H., C.B. Powell, K.K. Yu, *et al.* 1996. Invasive cervical carcinoma: role of MR imaging in pretreatment work-up–cost minimization and diagnostic efficacy analysis. *Radiology* **198:** 403–409.

41. Bipat, S., A.S. Glas, J. Van Der Velden, *et al.* 2003. Computed tomography and magnetic resonance imaging in staging of uterine cervical carcinoma: a systematic review. *Gynecol. Oncol.* **91:** 59–66.

42. Hricak, H., C. Gatsonis & D.S. Chi. 2005. Role of Imaging in pre-treatment evaluation of early invasive cervical cancer: results of the intergroup study American College of Radiology Imaging Network 6651-Gynecology Oncology Group 183. *J. Clin. Oncol.* **23:** 9329–9337.

43. Janus, C.L., D.S. Mendelson, S. Moore, *et al.* 1989. Staging of cervical carcinoma: accuracy of magnetic resonance imaging and computed tomography. *Clin. Imaging* **13:** 114–116.

44. Cobby, M., J. Browing, A. Jones, *et al.* 1990. Magnetic resonance imaging, computed tomography and endosonography in staging of carcinoma of the cervix. *Br. J. Radiol.* **63:** 673–679.

45. Subak, L.L., H. Hricak, C.B. Powell, *et al.* 1995. Cervical carcinoma: computed tomography and

magnetic resonance imaging for preoperative staging. *Obstet. Gynecol.* **86:** 43–50.

46. Kaji, Y., K. Sugimura, M. Kitao & T. Ishida. 1994. Histopathology of uterine cervical carcinoma: diagnostic comparison of endorectal surface coil and standard body coil MRI. *J. Comput. Assist. Tomogr.* **18:** 785–792.

47. Sahdev, A., S.A. Sohaib, A.E. Wenaden, *et al.* 2007. The performance of magnetic resonance imaging in early cervical carcinoma: a long-term experience. *Int. J. Gynecol. Cancer.* **17:** 629–636.

48. Rockall, A.G., S. Ghosh & F. Alexander-Sefre. 2006. Can MRI rule out bladder and rectal invasion in cervical cancer to help select patients for limited EUA? *Gynecol. Oncol.* **101:** 244–249.

49. Shepherd, J.H., R.A. Crawford & D.H. Oram. 1998. Radical trachelectomy: a way to preserve fertility in the treatment of early cervical cancer. *Br. J. Obstet. Gynaecol.* **105:** 912–916.

50. Shepherd, J.H. 2005. Uterus conserving surgery for invasive cervical cancer. *Best Pract. Res. Clin. Obstet. Gynaecol.* **19:** 577–590.

51. Peppercorn, P.D., A.R. Jeyarajah & R. Woolas. 1999. Role of MR imaging in the selection of patients with early cervical carcinoma for fertility-preserving surgery: initial experience. *Radiology* **212:** 395–399.

52. Narayan, K., A.F. McKenzie, R.J. Hicks, *et al.* 2003. Relation between FIGO stage, primary tumor volume, and presence of lymph node metastases in cervical cancer patients referred for radiotherapy. *Int. J. Gynecol. Cancer.* **13:** 657–663.

53. Hope, A.J., P. Saha & P.W. Grigsby. 2006. FDG-PET in carcinoma of the uterine cervix with endometrial extension. *Cancer* **106:** 196–200.

54. Yang, W.T., W.W. Lam, M.Y. Yu, *et al.* 2000. Comparison of dynamic helical CT and dynamic MR imaging in the evaluation of pelvic lymph nodes in cervical carcinoma. *AJR* **175:** 759–766.

55. Narayan, K., R.J. Hicks, T. Jobling, *et al.* 2001. A comparison of MRI and PET scanning in surgically staged loco-regionally advanced cervical cancer: potential impact on treatment. *Int. J. Gynecol. Cancer.* **11:** 263–271.

56. Reinhardt, M.J., C. Ehritt-Braun, D. Vogelgesang, *et al.* 2001. Metastatic lymph nodes in patients with cervical cancer: detection with MR imaging and FDG PET. *Radiology* **218:** 776–782.

57. Rockall, A.G., S.A. Sohaib & M.G. Harisinghani. 2005. Diagnostic performance of nanoparticle-enhanced magnetic resonance imaging in the diagnosis of lymph node metastases in patients with endometrial and cervical cancer. *J. Clin. Oncol.* **23:** 2813–2821.

58. Zaino, R.J., S. Ward, G. Delgado, *et al.* 1992. Histopathologic predictors of the behavior of surgi-cally treated stage IB squamous cell carcinoma of the cervix. A Gynecologic Oncology Group study. *Cancer* **69:** 1750–1758.

59. Lanza, A., A. Re, F. D'Addato, *et al.* 1989. Lymph nodal metastases and pathological patterns in cervical cancer: a critical review. *Eur. J. Gynaecol. Oncol.* **10:** 3–8.

60. Tan, R., C.H. Chung, M.T. Liu, *et al.* 1991. Results of postoperative radiotherapy for clinical stage Ib uterine cervical carcinoma with evidence of microscopic involvement of surgical margin, parametrium and/or lymph node metastasis. *J. Formos. Med. Assoc.* **90:** 836–839.

61. Hawnaur, J. 2004. Uterine and cervical tumours. In *Imaging in Oncology*, 2nd ed. J.E. Husband & R.H. Reznek, Eds.: 467–496. Taylor and Frances. London.

62. Shepherd, J.H., H.Y. Ngan, P. Neven, *et al.* 1994. Multivariate analysis of factors affecting survival in pelvic exenteration. *Int. J. Gynecol. Cancer.* **4:** 361–370.

63. Popovich, M.J., H. Hricak, K. Sugimura & J.L. Stern. 1993. The role of MR imaging in determining surgical eligibility for pelvic excenteration. *AJR* **160:** 525–531.

64. Babar, S.A., A.G. Rockall, A. Googe, *et al.* 2004. MRI appearances of recurrent cervical cancer. *Eur. Radiol.* **14:** 429.

65. Suaris, T.D., A. Sahdev, R.H. Reznek & A. Rockall. 2007. Where is the pelvic sidewall? An anatomical depiction with radiological and surgical correlates. *European Congress of Radiology*, Vienna (C-369). [Abstract.]

66. Heron, C.W., J.E. Husband, M.P. Williams, *et al.* 1988. The value of CT in the diagnosis of recurrent carcinoma of the cervix. *Clin. Radiol.* **39:** 496–501.

67. Yen, T.C., L.C. See & T.C. Chang. 2004. Defining the priority of using 18F-FDG PET for recurrent cervical cancer. *J. Nucl. Med.* **45:** 1632–1639.

68. Sakurai, H., Y. Suzuki & T. Nonaka. 2006. FDG-PET in the detection of recurrence of uterine cervical carcinoma following radiation therapy-tumour volume and FDG uptake value. *Gynecol. Oncol.* **100:** 601–607.

69. Toita, T., Y. Kakinohana & S. Shinzato. 1999. Tumor diameter/volume and pelvic node status assessed by magnetic resonance imaging (MRI) for uterine cervical cancer treated with irradiation. *Int. J. Radiat. Oncol. Biol. Phys.* **43:** 777–782.

70. Blomlie, V., E.K. Rofstad, C. Trope & H.H. Lien. 1997. Critical soft tissues of the female pelvis: serial MR imaging before, during, and after radiation therapy. *Radiology* **203:** 391–397.

71. Blomlie, V., E.K. Rofstad, K. Tvera & H.H. Lien. 1996. Noncritical soft tissues of the

female pelvis: serial MR imaging before, during, and after radiation therapy. *Radiology* **199:** 461–468.

72. Healy, J.C., R.R. Phillips, R.H. Reznek, *et al.* 1996. The MR appearance of vaginal fistulas. *AJR* **167:** 1487–1489.

73. Sahdev, A., J. Jones, J.H. Shepherd & R.H. Reznek.

2005. Post-surgical MR imaging appearances of the female pelvis following trachelectomy. *Radiographics* **25:** 41–52.

74. Dursun, P., E. Leblanc & M.C. Nogueira. 2007. Radical vaginal trachelectomy (Dargent's operation): a critical review of the literature. *Eur. J. Surg. Oncol.* **33:** 933–941.

New Developments in the Surgical Therapy of Cervical Carcinoma

Nadja Dornhöfer and Michael Höckel

Department of Obstetrics and Gynecology, University of Leipzig, Leipzig, Germany

For almost a century abdominal radical hysterectomy has been the standard surgical treatment of early-stage macroscopic carcinoma of the uterine cervix. The excessive parametrial resection of the original procedures of Wertheim, Okabayashi, and Meigs has later been "tailored" to tumor extent. Systematic pelvic and eventually periaortic lymph node dissection is performed to identify and treat regional disease. Adjuvant (chemo)radiation therapy is liberally added to improve locoregional tumor control when histopathological risk factors are present. The therapeutic index of the current surgical treatment, particularly if combined with radiation, appears to be inferior to that of primary chemoradiation as an oncologically equivalent therapeutic alternative. Several avenues of new conceptual and technical developments have been used since the 1990s with the goal of improving the therapeutic index. These are: surgical staging, including sentinel node biopsy and nodal debulking; minimal access and recently robotic radical hysterectomy; fertility-preserving surgery; nerve-sparing radical hysterectomy; total mesometrial resection based on developmentally defined surgical anatomy; and supraradical hysterectomy. The superiority of these new developments over the standard treatment remains to be demonstrated by controlled prospective trials. Multimodality therapy including surgery for locally advanced disease represents another area of clinical research. Both neoadjuvant chemotherapy followed by radical surgery, with or without adjuvant radiation, and completion surgery after (chemo)radiation are feasible and have to be compared to primary chemoradiation as the new nonsurgical treatment standard. Surgical treatment of postirradiation persisting or recurrent cervical carcinoma has been traditionally limited to pelvic exenteration for central disease. Applying the principle of developmentally derived anatomical compartments increases R0 resectability. The laterally extended endopelvic resection allows even the extirpation of a subset of visceral pelvic side wall tumors with clear margins. Many questions regarding the indication for these "ultraradical" operations, the surgery of irradiated tissues, and the optimal reconstructive procedures are still open and demand multiinstitutional controlled trials to be answered.

Key words: cervical carcinoma; radical hysterectomy; fertility preservation; minimal access surgery; autonomic nerve sparing; pelvic exenteration

Introduction

On a global scale, carcinoma of the uterine cervix is still a serious health problem, with approximately 490,000 new cases and 270,000 deaths per year.[1] This neoplasm is less prevalent and its incidence continues to decrease in developed countries due to cancer screening, education about risk factors, and probably as a consequence of changes in sexual behavior. In Europe and North America, about 60,000 and 15,000 women, respectively, developed cervical cancer, and 30,000 and 6000, respectively, died from the disease in 2002.[1] It is suggested that human papillomavirus vaccination, which in recent trials has proven to be successful in preventing the precursor lesions, will have a

Address for correspondence: Michael Höckel, MD, PhD, Professor and Chairman, Department of Ob/Gyn, Liebigstr. 20a, 04103 Leipzig, Germany. Voice: +341-9723400; fax. +341-9723409. michael.hoeckel@uniklinik-leipzig.de

Ann. N.Y. Acad. Sci. 1138: 233–252 (2008). © 2008 New York Academy of Sciences.
doi: 10.1196/annals.1414.029

major impact on further reducing cervical cancer in the future.[2,3] However, if successful, this effect will need at least 1–2 decades to become epidemiologically apparent. Although the incidence rank of cervical cancer in the developed world is in the middle range, the socioeconomic impact of this malignant disease is much higher since patients are affected at a relative young age. As the median age at diagnosis is in the fifth decade and appropriately 20% are diagnosed before the age of 40 years, the number of life-years lost due to cervical carcinoma is significantly surpassed only by breast cancer.

The current standard in the management of this disease is staging according to the International Federation of Gynecology and Obstetrics (FIGO) and stage-adjusted treatment with surgery or/and (chemo)radiation.[4] A significant drawback of the present treatment practice is the relatively high morbidity from radical hysterectomy, particularly if combined with adjuvant (chemo)radiation. Severe vaginal dysfunction, late sequelae of tissue fibrosis and necrosis, and secondary neoplasms are of special concern for young women treated with primary (chemo)radiation. Several new developments in surgical therapy of cervical carcinoma are based on the application of minimal access and recently robotic techniques focusing on surgical staging and the treatment of small-volume disease. The new era of fertility preservation in the treatment of cervical cancer began with the pioneering work of Daniel Dargent introducing "radical trachelectomy." Autonomic nerve sparing is no longer an issue for Japanese gynecologic oncologists only. However, many questions remain unresolved. The superiority of concepts and techniques using minimal access compared to open surgery are yet unproven. Moreover, all the new nerve-sparing and fertility-preserving surgical procedures rely on historical foundations of surgical anatomy in the female pelvis and of local tumor spread. We have translated insights of female genital tract anatomy and cervical cancer spread from the perspective of human embryology into new surgical techniques. This appears

to improve the therapeutic index in the management of early and intermediate stage disease and provides local control of advanced and recurrent disease, which has often proved difficult to achieve.

Methodology of Search and Selection

We searched four computerized databases:

- MEDLINE was searched by PubMed from 1990–2007
- COCHRANE Database of Systematic Reviews was searched from inception to 2007
- POPLINE was searched from inception to 2007
- LILCAS was searched from inception to 2007

The following terms were used to search the databases:

- Trials on surgical staging: *surgical staging* and *cervical cancer.*
- Trials on sentinel biopsy: *sentinel biopsy* and *cervical cancer.*
- Trials on laparoscopic staging: *laparoscopic staging* and *cervical cancer.*
- Trials on laparoscopically assisted radical vaginal hysterectomy (LARVH): *LARVH* and *cervical cancer, laparoscopic assisted radical vaginal hysterectomy* and *cervical cancer.* Trials comparing results of LARVH with the standard abdominal approach were included.
- Trials on laparoscopic radical hysterectomy (LRH): *laparoscopic radical hysterectomy* and *cervical cancer, laparoscopic hysterectomy* and *cervical cancer.*
- Trials on radical trachelectomy: *trachelectomy.* Trials reporting on obstetrical and/or oncologic outcome were included.
- Trials on nerve-sparing radical hysterectomy: *nerve sparing* and *radical hysterectomy* and *cervical cancer* or *autonomic nerve*

and *radical hysterectomy* and *cervical cancer* or *hypogastric plexus* and *radical hysterectomy*.

- Trials on robotic surgery: *robotic radical hysterectomy* and *cervical cancer*, *robotic surgery* and *cervical cancer*, *robotic surgery* and *gynecology*.
- Trials on fertility-sparing surgical therapy: *fertility-sparing surgical therapy* and *cervical cancer*.
- Trials on neoadjuvant chemotherapy: *neoadjuvant chemotherapy* and *cervical cancer*.
- Trials on neoadjuvant chemoradiation: *neoadjuvant chemoradiation* and *cervical cancer*.
- Trials on intraoperative radiotherapy: *IORT* and *cervical cancer*, *CORT* and *cervical cancer*.
- Trials on suprarenal lymph node dissection: *suprarenal lymph node* and *cervical cancer*.

The reference lists of articles identified by this strategy were searched, and additional relevant publications were selected. Only English-language trials were included (exception: Mathevet *et al.*[5]).

Staging

Following the histopathological diagnosis of cervical carcinoma staging of the disease is mandatory to establish a treatment plan. According to FIGO, cervical cancer staging of macroscopic disease has to be exclusively clinical and based on inspection, palpation, cystoscopy, rectoscopy, and limited radiographic studies (chest radiograph, skeletal radiograph, barium enema, and intravenous pyelogram). The initial FIGO stage should never be changed, additional information from other diagnostic procedures and surgery must not influence the stage but may have therapeutic implications. To date it has not been proven in randomized prospective trials that the additional use of advanced imaging techniques, such as CT, MRI, and PET to develop a treatment plan improves the outcome. The results of a recent multicenter trial by the American College of Radiology Imaging Network addressing

the relevance of CT and MRI have shown that MRI is superior to CT and clinical examination for detecting uterine body involvement and estimating tumor size, but cervical stroma was not accurately evaluated by either method.[6] Using MRI with an endovaginal coil appears to improve the accuracy in detecting the volume and extent of small tumors, which may be of particular importance concerning indications for minimal access and fertility-preserving treatment options.[7,8] Extracervical local tumor spread is generally poorly established and not better predicted by advanced imaging than by clinical assessment.[9] Both MRI and transvaginal sonography scoring systems may improve diagnostic accuracy for bladder and rectum involvement.[10,11] Lymph node metastases cannot be ascertained noninvasively with acceptable accuracy to date. Several recent trials demonstrated that FDG-PET has little value in pelvic and periaortic lymph node staging, particularly in early-stage disease.[12–14] MRI after intravenous application of iron oxide nanoparticles, which provide a negative image of metastases due to storing defects, appears to improve the preoperative detection of lymphatic spread.[15]

Because of the limitations of clinical and radiologic staging, there is an ongoing discussion about the potential benefit of surgical staging. The protagonists also refer to observational and noncontrolled studies that have claimed a place for the resection of bulky pelvic lymph node metastases prior to radiation and argue that the demonstration of periaortic lymph node metastases would lead to a radiation field extension with a higher probability of locoregional tumor control.[16–22]

Laparoscopical surgical staging is recommended by some for selecting either minimal access surgical therapy of small volume (<2 cm) cancers without lymph node metastases or individualized (chemo)radiation for larger and/or nodal-positive tumors as main treatment alternatives.[22–33] Within the context of this treatment philosophy sentinel lymph node biopsy substitution for systematic lymph node dissection is currently investigated.[34–55] The sentinel

TABLE 1. Comparison of Laparoscopic-assisted Radical Vaginal Hysterectomy (LARVH) versus Radical Abdominal Hysterectomy (RAH)

Procedure	Malur et al., 2001[75]		Nam et al., 2004[76]		Steed et al., 2004[77]		Jackson et al., 2004[78]		Sharma et al., 2006[79]		Morgan et al., 2007[80]	
	LARVH	RAH	LARVH	RAH	LARVH	RAH	LARVH	RAH	LARVH	RAH	LARVH	RAH
Treatment period	1994–1999	1991–1994	1997–2002		1996–2003		1996–2003		1999–2005		2000–2005	
Median follow-up (months)	NR	NR	35	44	17	21	52	49	34*	42*	31*	31*
# of patients	70	70	47	96	71	205	50	50	27	28	30	30
Histology (%)												
SCC	76	79	77	79	44	54	66	66	67	57	80	53
Adeno-Ca	23	19	21	17	56	46	34	34	33	39	20	37
Other	1	2	2	4						4		10
FIGO Stage (%)												
IA1	4	1			20	14					30	6
IA2	19	1			14	5						
IB1	59	73	100	100	65	72	94	94	100	82	70	80
IB2					1	9	2	2		18		
IIA	4	7										
IIB	13	16										
III	1	1										
IV	0	1										
Mean tumor volume (cm³)	NR	NR	2.8	2.9	NR	NR	NR	NR	0.1	5.0	NR	NR
Mean tumor size (cm)	NR	NR	NR	NR	2.3	2.6	1.6	1.7	NR	NR	NR	NR
pN1 (%)	NR	NR	6	6	7	9	2	2	0	7	0	17
Intraoperative												
OR time (min)	293	210	233	239	210	150	180	120	160	132	187	131
Blood loss (mL)	NR	NR	NR	NR	300	500	350	875	479	715	NR	NR
Complication rate (%)	11	1	2	1	13	4	8	6	NR	NR	13	23

Continued

TABLE 1. *Continued*

Procedure	Malur et al., 2001[75]		Nam et al., 2004[76]		Steed et al., 2004[77]		Jackson et al., 2004[78]		Sharma et al., 2006[79]		Morgan et al., 2007[80]	
	LARVH	RAH	LARVH	RAH	LARVH	RAH	LARVH	RAH	LARVH	RAH	LARVH	RAH
Treatment period	1994–1999	1991–1994	1997–2002		1996–2003		1996–2003		1999–2005		2000–2005	
Postoperative hospital stay (days)	11	23	16	23	1	5	5	8	5	10	6	8
Adjuvant treatment (%)												
Chemotherapy	NR	0	17	19	0	0	0	0			NR	NR
Chemo-radiation	NR	0	4	4	22	21	0	0		7	NR	NR
Radiation	NR	100	0	2	0	0	14	4			NR	NR
Recurrence (%)												
Locoregional	NR	NR	6	2	6	6	2	2	7	7	6	3
Distant	NR	NR	2				0	0				3
Both	NR	NR	0				2	2				
Disease-free survival	NR	NR	87 (3y)	99 (3y)	94 (2y)	94 (2y)	NR	NR	NR	NR	NR	NR
Overall survival (%)	NR	NR	NR	NR	NR	NR	94 (4y)	96 (4y)	NR	NR	NR	NR

NR, not reported; y, years; * , mean follow-up.

Fertlity-preserving Surgery

Radical vaginal trachelectomy exploits the LARVH technique for fertility preservation in patients with small-volume cervical cancer and a strong desire for future child bearing. The uterine cervix, proximal vagina, and parts of the paracervix and paracolpia are resected, but the uterine corpus with its blood supply from the uterine and ovarian arteries is retained and anastomosed to the middle part of the vagina. Cervical function is substituted by a permanent cerclage. Delivery is achieved by primary cesarean section. Following the pioneering work of Dargent and coworkers,[89] vaginal radical trachelectomy combined with laparoscopic lymph node dissection has been performed in several centers since the 1990s.[5,90–104] More recently an abdominal version has been developed claiming the resection of more paracervical tissue.[105–109] Published oncologic results on vaginal and abdominal radical trachelectomy are summarized in Table 2a. If patients with small (<2 cm), nodal-negative tumors are selected, surgery-related parameters, such as operating time, complications, blood loss, and postoperative hospital stay, correspond to the LARVH. The question of oncologic safety is not definitively settled. Most studies report only the recurrence rates of the successfully executed cases. However, approximately 10% of planned trachelectomies have to be abandoned. According to Plante and colleagues,[101] the recurrence rate of the abandoned cases has been 30%. In order to correctly estimate the oncologic results of the procedures, the recurrence rate of all patients treated with the intention to perform radical trachelectomy needs to be reported.

The second aspect of fertility-preserving surgery relates to obstetrical outcome. Its current status is compiled in Table 2b. Forty-five percent of the patients with a strong desire to preserve their fertility despite the diagnosis of cervical cancer tried to get pregnant after treatment with radical trachelectomy, and 28% of the whole group conceived. The most important obstetrical outcome parameter is the rate of very premature infants related to the overall number of babies born, which is 15%. Despite major medical progress, children born at 24–28 weeks of gestation are still at a significant risk to develop cognitive and motoric deficiencies,[110] and the treatment costs for these infants are very high. In order to minimize the rate of very premature infants after radical trachelectomy, the preservation of at least 1 cm of residual cervical tissue is mandatory. Because of this contribution of central cervical tissue for obstetrical reasons the advisability of resecting parametrial tissue has been questioned. Less radical procedures, including conization with or without neoadjuvant chemotherapy, are currently being tested in controlled prospective trials.[111,112]

Autonomic Nerve-sparing Surgery

Radical hysterectomy techniques with the preservation of the autonomic nerve system have a longer tradition in China and Japan.[113] Following our first publication of liposuction-assisted, nerve-sparing, extended radical hysterectomy,[113] several other groups reported successful autonomic nerve-sparing radical hysterectomy procedures either with open surgery or laparoscopically.[81,114–127] Adhering to the traditional view of surgical anatomy, the concept of tailored paracervical resection exposition and preservation of the inferior hypogastric plexus and its vesical branches in the more extended resection obviously reduces the bladder and vaginal dysfunction to that obtained with only proximal parametrectomy.[125,126,128] Contrary to earlier fears, nerve-sparing does not interfere with oncologic safety according to published retrospective studies. Utilizing the developmental view on surgical anatomy of the female pelvis, which is the basis for the TMMR (see below), the autonomic nerve system, except the uterine branches of the inferior hypogastric plexus, is principally preserved as it does not belong to the uterovaginal morphogenetic unit.

TABLE 2a. Oncologic Outcome of Published Studies Using Vaginal Radical Trachelectomy (VRT) or Abdominal Radical Trachelectomy (ART)

Author	Covens[99,100]	Mathevet[5]	Burnett[96]	Schlaerth[97]	Plante[101]	Ungar[108]	Shepherd[104]	Hertel[103]	TOTAL
Procedure	VRT	VRT	VRT	VRT	VRT	ART	VRT	VRT	
Time period	1994–2003	1987–2002	1995–2001	1995–1999	1991–2003	1997–2004	1994–2005	1995–2005	
Median follow-up	30	76	32	48	60	47	45	29	
# of patients									
Planned RT (IT)	93	108	21	12	82	33	123	108	N = 580
Abandoned RT	0	12	2	2	10	3	11*	8	8%
Performed RT (ET)	93	95	19	10	72	30	112	100	N = 531
Histology (%)									
SCC	48	80	57	40	58	86	67	69	66%
Adeno-Ca	52	20	43	50	38	7	27	31	32%
Other				10	4	7	6		2%
FIGO Stage (%)									
IA1	42	14			5	33		17	14%
IA2	24	15	5	80	32	33	2	19	19%
IB1	33	58	95	20	60	50	98	64	63%
IB2	1	1			0	17			1%
IIA	0	7			3				2%
IIB	0	5			0				1%
Tumor size < 2 cm (%)	91	70	100	100	89	70	NR	100	87%
pN1 (%)	2	3	NR	0	1	0	6	4	3%
Intraoperative									
OR time (min.)	180	161	318	NR	252	226	NR	253	216
Blood loss (ml)	300	NR	293	203	254	NR	NR	NR	257
Postoperative									
Hospital stay (days)	1	NR	3	3	3	14	NR	8	4
Recurrence (%)	7 (7/93)	4 (4/95)	0	0	4 (3/72)	0	3 (3/112)	4 (4/100)	4%
Locoregional		4			3		3	4	
Distant					1				
Both									
5-y disease-free surv.	NR	NR	NR	NR	95	NR	NR	97	

NR, not reported; IT, intention to treat; ET, executed treatment.
* 11 patients received completion therapy, 2 of these 11 patients had recurrence (18%).

TABLE 2b. Obstetrical Outcome of Published Studies Using Vaginal Radical Trachelectomy (VRT) or Abdominal Radical Trachelectomy (ART)

Author	Mathevet[5]	Burnett[96]	Schlaerth[97]	Bernardini[98]	Ungar[108]	Plante[102]	Shepherd[104]	
Procedure	VRT	VRT	VRT	VRT	ART	VRT	VRT	
Time period	1987–2002	1995–2001	1995–1999	1994–2002	1997–2004	1991–2003	1994–2005	TOTAL
# of patients (ET)	95	19	10	80	30	72	112	418
# pt. attempting pregnancy	42	NR	NR	39	5	34	63	183
# pt. conceiving	33	3	4	18	3	31	26	118
# pregnancies	56	3	4	22	3	50	55	193
# viable newborns	34	3	2	18[b]	2	36	28	123
# very premature newborn (24–28 weeks)	NR	2[a]	2	4[b]	0	2	5	15[c]

NR, not reported; ET, executed treatment.
[a] Twins.
[b] Two sets of twins.
[c] Including the three sets of twins.

Total Mesometrial Resection

Standard surgical treatment of cervical cancer and all new developments in this field introduced in this review are based on an uterocentric and ligament-focused view of surgical anatomy and the assumption of undirected intra- and transcervical tumor spread.[129] The uterocentric perspective is misleading as it does not distinguish tissues integral to the uterovaginal tract from those that are only attached or connected to it. The ligament-focused view is also misleading, as prominent structures, such as the cardinal ligament and the posterior leaf of the vesicouterine ligament, do not exhibit any suspensory functions at all. Moreover, the sagittal pelvic curvature is usually not considered, with the pretence of a transverse location of the dorsally directed uterovaginal attachments in the deep pelvis. As a consequence of the concept of undirected transcervical tumor spread, the resection of all paracervical tissues is claimed to be necessary for the unrestricted radicality of the surgical treatment.[58–60] Tailoring paracervical resection to the estimated tumor extent[61–63] necessitates additional local treatment by adjuvant radiation in a high percentage of patients after primary surgery. Moreover, R1 and 2 resection rates usually exceed 10%.[64–67]

We have proposed that local tumor spread is not completely random but may be confined for an extended phase in malignant progression to a permissive compartment, which can be morphologically deduced from the embryologic development of the organ from which the neoplasm arises. Although tumor propagation is usually undirected within that compartment, the neoplasm respects the compartment borders for extended phases in its malignant progression. Adjacent compartments of different embryologic origin are invaded only late in the disease process, and even at these late stages a hierarchy of embryologic kinship is maintained.[130] The logic from this developmental view is compartment resection as a new principle of surgical radicality for local tumor control. Depending on tumor features surgical radicality may be reduced to sub- or intracompartment resection or may have to be extended to supra- and multicompartment resection. Compartment resection should result in a high local tumor control rate without additional radiation. As tissues of different embryologic origin may be left *in situ* despite their close proximity to a malignant tumor, treatment-related morbidity should be significantly less than that of conventional radical resection. We have deduced the Müllerian morphogenetic unit in the adult female from the study of uterovaginal development and demonstrated that its distal part represents the permissive compartment for the local spread of cervical carcinoma.[131]

TMMR has been developed to remove the complete Müllerian compartment except parts of the vagina.[131,132] With respect to the vagina the resection is intracompartmental and, therefore, a resection margin of 1.5–2 cm microscopically tumor-free tissue is regarded as obligatory. Otherwise, the presence of an intact bordering lamella represents radical tumor resection. Contrary to traditional radical hysterectomy, the paracervical and paravaginal resection of FIGO IB and IIA cases is not "tailored" to the tumor extension, but generally the complete Müllerian compartment is removed. Non-Müllerian tissues such as the mesorectum, inferior hyogastric plexus, and "mesobladder" with the vesical vessels and autonomic nerves remain *in situ* despite their possible proximity to the tumor. For regional tumor control, TMMR is supplemented by therapeutic pelvic lymph node dissection sparing the autonomic nerves (hypogastric nerves and superior hypogastric plexus). Staged, nerve-sparing, periaortic lymph node dissection is performed in the case of intraoperatively detected pelvic lymph node metastases.

From July 1998 to December 2006, 163 patients with cervical carcinoma, FIGO stages IB1 ($n = 94$), IB2 ($n = 21$), IIA ($n = 14$), and IIB ($n = 34$) have been treated with TMMR and nerve-sparing therapeutic lymph node dissection. Twenty-five patients received neoadjuvant chemotherapy. No patient underwent adjuvant radiotherapy although 95 patients (58%) would have needed this additional modality if conventional radical hysterectomy had been performed because of their high-risk histopathological tumor features. At a median follow-up time of 45 months (3–104 months), recurrence-free and disease-specific overall survival is 93% and 96%, respectively. Maximum treatment-related morbidity according to the Franco-Italian score[133] has been grade 2 in 12 patients (8%).

From these results we conclude that the developmental view of local tumor spread and surgical anatomy holds great promise for improving the therapeutic index of surgical cervical cancer therapy and challenges the uterocentric/ligament-focused perspective as well as tailored paracervical resection. Participation in a prospective multi-institutional trial for the evaluation of TMMR without adjuvant radiation for cervical cancer FIGO stages IB-IIA irrespective of histopathological risk factors is encouraged.

Advanced and Recurrent Disease

Standard Treatment

Forty-four percent of patients with cervical cancer are treated for locally advanced primary disease corresponding to the FIGO stages IIB, IIIA, IIIB, and IVA, according to the recent FIGO Annual Report.[134] The current treatment standard is chemoradiation, that is, the combination of percutaneous pelvic radiation, brachytherapy of the cervix and upper vagina, and platinum-based systemic chemotherapy.[135] Radical hysterectomy eventually followed by adjuvant (chemo)radiation as an alternative therapy for FIGO stage IIB cervical carcinoma is controversial. There is no evidence that tumor control is improved with this treatment but its excessive morbidity is well proven.[67] FIGO stage IB2 tumors are considered advanced disease by some authors. A recent study revealed that primary radical hysterectomy eventually followed by adjuvant (chemo)radiation provides a similar outcome to neoadjuvant chemotherapy followed by radical hysterectomy ± adjuvant radiation or primary chemoradiation but is the most cost effective of the three treatment options.[136] Pelvic exenteration, which has been mainly employed for central pelvic recurrences after primary radiotherapy (see below), may also be indicated for mobile, locally advanced, primary disease if radiation therapy is regarded as being suboptimal, for example due to vesicovaginal or rectovaginal fistulae in FIGO stage IVA cancer. In the majority of cases with bladder and/or rectal infiltration the tumors also involve the pelvic side wall and, hence, are considered unresectable.

Recurrent carcinoma of the uterine cervix is diagnosed in the pelvis, at distant site(s) or both in the pelvis and at distant site(s). Recurrence rates are 10–20% in FIGO stages IB/IIA cervical cancers and 50–70% in locally advanced cases (FIGO IIB, III, IVA).[4] Tumor persistence or recurrence within the pelvis is the major cause of death in patients suffering from carcinoma of the uterine cervix. Both persistent and locally recurrent pelvic tumors are characterized by an advanced malignant progression and often exhibit an anatomically complex topography rendering curative treatment very difficult and rarely successful.

With regard to current treatment modalities, persistent or locally recurrent tumors are classified as central or pelvic side wall disease. Whereas central disease is a relatively homogenous entity of tumors originating from the retained cervix and vagina following primary radiation, or from the vaginal cuff and central scar after surgical therapy, side wall disease is more heterogeneous. We propose a classification discriminating between parietal and visceral side wall disease. Parietal disease represents regional lymph node metastases, and tumors are mostly located above the level of the obturator nerve. Visceral pelvic side wall disease originates from the paracervix/paracolpium or from the scars of the paracervical resection and is usually located below the level of the obturator nerve. Visceral pelvic side wall disease is the most frequent relapse type irrespective of primary treatment.[137] According to present consensus, patients with recurrent cervical cancer in the pelvis after surgical therapy should be treated with (chemo)radiation and only central pelvic relapses following (primary or adjuvant) radia-

tion should undergo surgery.[138] Whereas radical hysterectomy may be adequate for selected smaller lesions, most irradiated patients with central disease will need pelvic exenteration for resection with clear margins.[139] Patients with a pelvic side wall component of their recurrent tumor in an irradiated pelvis—representing the most common situation of failure—are no longer considered for curative therapy.

Supraradical Hysterectomy and Extended Periaortic Lymph Node Dissection

Extending both paracervical resection and lymph node dissection is not new. Its potential has not been systematically explored by prospective controlled trials. The lateral extension of the parametrectomy with inclusion of the internal iliac vessels with the visceral branches, and thus exposure of the sacral plexus, was already performed in the mid 20th century by Mibayashi in Japan.[140] Ungar and Palfalvi applied laterally extended parametrectomy to treat patients with FIGO IB cervical carcinomas with intraoperatively detected pelvic lymph node metastases and those with FIGO IIB cancer. From their results with 146 patients they concluded the feasibility of the procedure and claimed that it may be a surgical alternative to chemoradiation.[141,142] Suprarenal periaortic lymph node dissection can be performed to supplement upper (infrarenal) periaortic lymphonodectomy in the presence of metastases either through open access or laparoscopically.[143,144] The impact of extended periaortic lymph node dissection is not known.

Multimodality Therapy Including Surgery for Locally Advanced Primary and Recurrent Disease

Neoadjuvant intravenous cisplatinum-based chemotherapy followed by radical hysterectomy, pelvic/para-aortic lymph node dissection, and eventually postoperative adjuvant radiation has been compared with primary radiation for squamous cell carcinoma of the uterine cervix, FIGO stages IB2, IIA (>4 cm), IIB, and III in prospective randomized trials.[145,146] A survival benefit of the combined surgical treatment modality for FIGO stages IB2 and IIB was observed, whereas an advantage for stage III cervical cancers was not obvious. The intra-arterial application of cisplatinum-containing neoadjuvant chemotherapy followed by radical hysterectomy, pelvic/para-aortic lymph node dissection, and eventually adjuvant radiation for locally advanced cervical carcinoma has been tested in several small studies.[147] The treatment appeared to be feasible and led to promising preliminary results. However, whether it may be superior to intravenous neoadjuvant chemotherapy is not known and cannot be anticipated based on the results reported to date.

A systematic Cochrane meta-analysis of all prospective randomized study data updated to February 2006 confirmed a survival benefit of neoadjuvant chemotherapy followed by radical surgery compared to radiotherapy alone.[148] Applying dose-dense cisplatinum (>25 mg/m^2/week) and chemotherapy cycle lengths of shorter than 14 days, a 14% absolute gain in 5-year survival was obtained. Limitations of the analysis are the relatively low overall patient numbers, use of different chemotherapy regimens (intravenous, intra-arterial), and the inclusion of patients with early (IB1, IIA) disease. All trials used radiation therapy alone in the standard arm. As concurrent chemoradiation has meanwhile been generally accepted as the new standard therapy for locally advanced cervical cancer, due to its proven superior results with respect to disease-free and overall survival, new trials comparing neoadjuvant chemotherapy followed by radical surgery with concurrent chemoradiation are mandatory. A randomized study with FIGO stage IB cases with mean tumor size >4 cm treated with radical hysterectomy and eventually adjuvant radiation showed fewer lymph node metastases, less parametrial and vascular space in-

volvement, and better disease-free and overall survival in patients who received neoadjuvant cisplatin and 5-Fluorouraci.[149] The optimal regimen for neoadjuvant chemotherapy in cervical cancer needs to be determined. The combination of cisplatin with ifosfamide and cisplatin with ifosfamide and paclitaxel appear to increase the response rate but also the rate of severe complications without a significant effect on overall survival so far.[150] Various other combined regimens are currently being evaluated.[151-153]

Preoperative chemoradiation with cisplatinum-containing regimens up to a total pelvic dose of 45 Gy followed by radical surgery 4–6 weeks later, with or without additional intraoperative electron beam radiotherapy, for locally advanced primary cancer has been investigated in recent phase I–II trials. High local control rates are reported at a 15–20% rate of severe complications, mostly urinary.[154-157] The studies do not allow conclusions regarding a definite benefit as compared to standard primary chemoradiation. A small comparative study of neoadjuvant chemoradiation versus neoadjuvant chemotherapy and eventually adjuvant chemoradiation and radical hysterectomy for stage IB and IIB bulky (>4 cm) cervical cancer did not demonstrate significant differences.[158] Current clinical experience indicates that both intraoperative radiation (IORT) and the combined operative and radiation treatment (CORT), that is the application of guide tubes for postoperative brachytherapy and protective pelvic wall plasty, necessitate complete (R0) tumor resection for local control.[155,159,160] Whether the addition of both forms of site-directed radiation improves treatment results for advanced primary and recurrent disease over surgery alone has not been shown.

Multicompartmental and Laterally Extended Endopelvic Resection

If cervical cancer recurs in an irradiated pelvis, the prognosis is mainly influenced by three features: (i) the existence of metastases, (ii) relapse size, and (iii) R0 resectability.[161] Distant metastases, with very few exceptions, exclude a chance of cure, whereas regional metastases significantly decrease, but—particularly in low number—do not completely abolish a curative treatment option. Tumor size >5 cm is usually no longer compatible with long-term survival despite resection with tumor-free margins. Parietal pelvic side wall disease (i.e., lymph node metastases) can only be surgically controlled if the lymph node capsule is respected, otherwise R0 resection is no longer possible.

In order to increase R0 resectability of locally advanced and recurrent gynecologic tumors, we have adjusted the dissection planes of pelvic exenteration to the borders of the combined developmentally defined compartments of the pelvic organs.[161,162] Pelvic exenteration is thus performed as multimesovisceral excision by combining total mesorectal excision[163] and TMMR[131] with resection of the ureterovesical compartment. For R0 resection of tumors fixed to the lower pelvic side wall up to the level of the obturator nerve anteriorly, and up to the level of the ischial spine posteriorly thus excluding the sciatic foramen, the laterally extended endopelvic resection (LEER) has been introduced.[164,165] LEER is a composite exenteration characterized by the resection of the complete pelvic visceral compartments *en bloc* with any of the following endopelvic parietal structures: paravisceral fat pad, internal iliac vessel system, obturator internus muscle, and pubococcygeus, iliococcygeus, and coccygeus muscles. The logic for LEER follows from the topography of local tumor spread. Locally advanced and recurrent tumors of the lower female genital tract generally respect the bordering surface between visceral and parietal compartments, that is, the endopelvic fascia to which these tumors may be broadly fixed. Lateral dissection by including the layer of striated muscle into the specimen will keep the tumor adhering fascia intact.

The R0 resection rate of a series of 74 patients treated with these new pelvic exentera-

tion techniques is 97%, although no treatment was intraoperatively aborted due to pelvic side wall involvement and 56 patients were clinically and radiologically diagnosed with side wall disease. Two patients (3%) with advanced age and extensive comorbidity, respectively, died during the early postoperative period. Moderate and severe treatment-related morbidity was 66%. At a median follow-up period of 29 months (1–112 months) 5-year overall and recurrence-free survival probabilities are 56% (95% CI: 42–69) and 56% (42–70), respectively. Disease progression occurred locally and regionally in the pelvis in six patients, in the pelvis and simultaneously at extrapelvic sites in five patients, and exclusively at extrapelvic sites in 14 patients. Morbidity, disease control, and survival did not differ in patients with pelvic side wall disease treated with the LEER when compared with patients having central disease who underwent multimesovisceral excision. Multicompartmental pelvic surgery has significant potential to salvage selected patients with locally advanced and recurrent gynecologic malignancies, including those with pelvic side wall disease traditionally not considered for surgical therapy.

Acknowledgments

This work has been supported in part by an unrestricted grant from Fresenius-Kabi, Germany (M. Höckel) and by a grant of the Else Kröner-Fresenius-Foundation (N. Dornhöfer). The manuscript was produced by readypress* Dr. Susanne Höckel, Munich, Germany.

Conflicts of Interest

The authors declare no conflicts of interest.

References

1. Kamangar, F., G.M. Dores & W.F. Anderson. 2006. Patterns of cancer incidence, mortality, and prevalence across five continents: defining priorities to

reduce cancer disparities in different geographic regions of the world. *J. Clin. Oncol.* **24:** 2137–2150.

2. Koutsky, L.A. *et al.* 2002. A controlled trial of a human papillomavirus type 16 vaccine. *N. Engl. J. Med.* **347:** 1645–1651.

3. Harper, D.M. *et al.* 2004. Efficacy of a bivalent L1 virus-like particle vaccine in prevention of infection with human papillomavirus types 16 and 18 in young women: a randomised controlled trial. *Lancet* **364:** 1757–1765.

4. Waggoner, S.E. 2003. Cervical cancer. *Lancet* **361:** 2217–2225.

5. Mathevet, P., L.E. de Kaszon & D. Dargent. 2003. La preservation de la fertilité dans les cancers du col uterin de stade precoce. *Gynecol. Obstet. Fertil.* **31:** 706–712.

6. Mitchell, D.G. *et al.* 2006. Early invasive cervical cancer: tumor delineation by magnetic resonance imaging, computed tomography, and clinical examination, verified by pathologic results, in the ACRIN 6651/GOG 183 Intergroup Study. *J. Clin. Oncol.* **24:** 5687–5694.

7. deSouza, N.M. *et al.* 2006. Cervical cancer: value of an endovaginal coil magnetic resonance imaging technique in detecting small volume disease and assessing parametrial extension. *Gynecol. Oncol.* **102:** 80–85.

8. Akata, D. *et al.* 2005. Efficacy of transvaginal contrast-enhanced MRI in the early staging of cervical carcinoma. *Eur. Radiol.* **15:** 1727–1733.

9. Hricak, H. *et al.* 2005. Role of imaging in pretreatment evaluation of early invasive cervical cancer: results of the Intergroup Study American College of Radiology Imaging Network 6651- Gynecologic Oncology Group 183. *J. Clin. Oncol.* **23:** 9329–9337.

10. Rockall, A.G. *et al.* 2006. Can MRI rule out bladder and rectal invasion in cervical cancer to help select patients for limited EUA? *Gynecol. Oncol.* **101:** 244–249.

11. Huang, W.-C. *et al.* 2006. Ultrasonographic characteristics and cystoscopic correlates of bladder wall invasion by endophytic cervical cancer. *Ultrasound Obstet. Gynecol.* **27:** 680–686.

12. Chou, H.-H. *et al.* 2006. Low value of [^{18}F]-fluoro-2-deoxy-D-glucose positron emission tomography in primary staging of early-stage cervical cancer before radical hysterectomy. *J. Clin. Oncol.* **24:** 123–128.

13. Roh, J.-W. *et al.* 2005. Role of positron emission tomography in pretreatment lymph node staging of uterine cervical cancer: a prospective surgicopathologic correlation study. *Eur. J. Cancer* **41:** 2086–2092.

14. Wright, J.D. *et al.* 2005. Preoperative lymph node staging of early-stage cervical carcinoma by [^{18}F]-fluoro-2-deoxy-D-glucose positron emission tomography. *Cancer* **104:** 2484–2491.

15. Rockall, A.G. *et al.* 2005. Diagnostic performance of nanoparticle-enhanced magnetic resonance imaging in the diagnosis of lymph node metastases in patients with endometrial and cervical cancer. *J. Clin. Oncol.* **23:** 2813–2821.

16. Hughes, R.R. *et al.* 1980. Extended field irradiation for cervical cancer based on surgical staging. *Gynecol. Oncol.* **9:** 153–161.

17. Varia, M.A. *et al.* 1998. Cervical carcinoma metastatic to para-aortic nodes: extended field radiation therapy with concomitant 5-fluorouracil and cisplatin chemotherapy: a Gynecologic Oncology Group study. *Int. J. Radiat. Oncol. Biol. Phys.* **42:** 1015–1023.

18. Haie, C. *et al.* 1988. Is prophylactic para-aortic irradiation worthwhile in the treatment of advanced cervical carcinoma? Results of a controlled clinical trial of the EORTC radiotherapy group. *Radiother. Oncol.* **11:** 101–112.

19. Querleu, D., E. Leblanc & B. Castelain. 1991. Laparoscopic pelvic lymphadenectomy in the staging of early carcinoma of the cervix. *Am. J. Obstet. Gynecol.* **164:** 579–581.

20. Rotman, M. *et al.* 1995. Prophylactic extended-field irradiation of para-aortic lymph nodes in stages IIB and bulky IB and IIA cervical carcinomas. Ten-year treatment results of RTOG 79–20. *JAMA* **274:** 387–393.

21. Stryker, J.A. & R. Mortel. 2000. Survival following extended field irradiation in carcinoma of cervix metastatic to para-aortic lymph nodes. *Gynecol. Oncol.* **79:** 399–405.

22. Marnitz, S. *et al.* 2005. Is there a benefit of pretreatment laparoscopic transperitoneal surgical staging in patients with advanced cervical cancer? *Gynecol. Oncol.* **99:** 536–544.

23. Chu, K.K. *et al.* 1997. Laparoscopic surgical staging in cervical cancer—preliminary experience among Chinese. *Gynecol. Oncol.* **64:** 49–53.

24. Cosin, J.A. *et al.* 1998. Pretreatment surgical staging of patients with cervical carcinoma: the case for lymph node debulking. *Cancer* **82:** 2241–2248.

25. Goff, B.A. *et al.* 1999. Impact of surgical staging in women with locally advanced cervical cancer. *Gynecol. Oncol.* **74:** 436–442.

26. Odunsi, K.O. *et al.* 2001. The impact of pre-therapy extraperitoneal surgical staging on the evaluation and treatment of patients with locally advanced cervical cancer. *Eur. J. Gynaecol. Oncol.* **22:** 325–330.

27. Hasenburg, A. *et al.* 2002. Evaluation of patients after extraperitoneal lymph node dissection and subsequent radiotherapy for cervical cancer. *Gynecol. Oncol.* **84:** 321–326.

28. Vergote, I. *et al.* 2002. Laparoscopic lower para-aortic staging lymphadenectomy in stage IB2, II, and III cervical cancer. *Int. J. Gynecol. Cancer* **12:** 22–26.

29. Sonoda, Y. *et al.* 2003. Prospective evaluation of surgical staging of advanced cervical cancer via a laparoscopic extraperitoneal approach. *Gynecol. Oncol.* **91:** 326–331.

30. Kohler, C. *et al.* 2004. Introduction of transperitoneal lymphadenectomy in a gynecologic oncology center: analysis of 650 laparoscopic pelvic and/or paraaortic transperitoneal lymphadenectomies. *Gynecol. Oncol.* **95:** 52–61.

31. Schneider, A. & H. Hertel. 2004. Surgical and radiographic staging in patients with cervical cancer. *Curr. Opin. Obstet. Gynecol.* **16:** 11–18.

32. Querleu, D. *et al.* 2005. Staging of advanced cervical cancer. *Int. J. Radiat. Oncol. Biol. Phys.* **62:** 614.

33. Denschlag, D. *et al.* 2005. Evaluation of patients after extraperitoneal lymph node dissection for cervical cancer. *Gynecol. Oncol.* **96:** 658–664.

34. Malur, S. *et al.* 2001. Sentinel lymph node detection in patients with cervical cancer. *Gynecol. Oncol.* **80:** 254–257.

35. Barranger, E. *et al.* 2003. Laparoscopic sentinel lymph node procedure using a combination of patent blue and radioisotope in women with cervical carcinoma. *Cancer* **97:** 3003–3009.

36. Buist, M.R. *et al.* 2003. Laparoscopic detection of sentinel lymph nodes followed by lymph node dissection in patients with early stage cervical cancer. *Gynecol. Oncol.* **90:** 290–296.

37. Lambaudie, E. *et al.* 2003. Laparoscopic identification of sentinel lymph nodes in early stage cervical cancer: prospective study using a combination of patent blue dye injection and technetium radiocolloid injection. *Gynecol. Oncol.* **89:** 84–87.

38. Plante, M. *et al.* 2003. Laparoscopic sentinel node mapping in early-stage cervical cancer. *Gynecol. Oncol.* **91:** 494–503.

39. van Dam, P.A. *et al.* 2003. Intraoperative sentinel node identification with technetium-99m-labeled nanocolloid in patients with cancer of the uterine cervix: a feasibility study. *Int. J. Gynecol. Cancer.* **13:** 182–186.

40. Barranger, E. *et al.* 2004. Value of intraoperative imprint cytology of sentinel nodes in patients with cervical cancer. *Gynecol. Oncol.* **94:** 175–180.

41. Barranger, E. *et al.* 2004. Histopathological validation of the sentinel node concept in cervical cancer. *Ann. Oncol.* **15:** 870–874.

42. Marchiole, P. *et al.* 2004. Sentinel lymph node biopsy is not accurate in predicting lymph node status for patients with cervical carcinoma. *Cancer* **100:** 2154–2159.

43. Martinez-Palones, J.M. *et al.* 2004. Intraoperative sentinel node identification in early stage cervical cancer using a combination of radiolabeled albumin injection and isosulfan blue dye injection. *Gynecol. Oncol.* **92:** 845–850.

44. Hauspy, J. *et al.* 2007. Sentinel lymph nodes in early stage cervical cancer. *Gynecol. Oncol.* **105:** 285–290.

45. Bats, A.S. *et al.* 2007. Sentinel lymph node biopsy improves staging in early cervical cancer. *Gynecol. Oncol.* **105:** 189–193.

46. Schwendinger, V. *et al.* 2006. Sentinel node detection with blue dye technique in early cervical cancer. *Eur. J. Gynaecol. Oncol.* **27:** 359–362.

47. Popa, I. *et al.* 2006. Negative sentinel lymph node accurately predicts negative status of pelvic lymph nodes in uterine cervix carcinoma. *Gynecol. Oncol.* **103:** 649–653.

48. Wydra, D. *et al.* 2006. Sentinel node identification in cervical cancer patients undergoing transperitoneal radical hysterectomy: a study of 100 cases. *Int. J. Gynecol. Cancer* **16:** 649–654.

49. Wang, H.Y. *et al.* 2006. Micrometastases detected by cytokeratin 19 expression in sentinel lymph nodes of patients with early-stage cervical cancer. *Int. J. Gynecol. Cancer* **16:** 643–648.

50. Marnitz, S. *et al.* 2006. Topographic distribution of sentinel lymph nodes in patients with cervical cancer. *Gynecol. Oncol.* **103:** 35–44.

51. Rob, L. *et al.* 2005. Study of lymphatic mapping and sentinel node identification in early stage cervical cancer. *Gynecol. Oncol.* **98:** 281–288.

52. Barranger, E. *et al.* 2005. Sentinel node biopsy is reliable in early-stage cervical cancer but not in locally advanced disease. *Ann. Oncol.* **16:** 1237–1242.

53. Silva, L.B. *et al.* 2005. Sentinel node detection in cervical cancer with (99m) Tc.phytate. *Gynecol. Oncol.* **97:** 588–595.

54. Lin, Y.S. *et al.* 2005. Sentinel node detection with radiocolloid lymphatic mapping in early invasive cervical cancer. *Int. J. Gynecol. Cancer* **15:** 273–277.

55. Angioli, R. *et al.* 2005. Role of sentinel lymph node biopsy procedure in cervical cancer: a critical point of view. *Gynecol. Oncol.* **96:** 504–509.

56. Lai, C.H. *et al.* 2003. Randomized trial of surgical staging (extraperitoneal or laparoscopic) versus clinical staging in locally advanced cervical cancer. *Gynecol. Oncol.* **89:** 160–167.

57. Clement, P. & R. Young. 2000. *Atlas of Gynecologic Surgical Pathology.* W. B. Brothers. Philadelphia. pg. 99.

58. Wertheim, E. 1912. The extended abdominal operation for carcinoma uteri (based on 500 operative cases). *Am. J. Obstet. Dis. Women Child* **66:** 169–232.

59. Okabayashi, H. 1921. Radical abdominal hysterectomy for cancer of the cervix uteri. *Surg. Gynecol. Obstet.* **33:** 335–341.

60. Meigs, V. 1951. Radical hysterectomy with bilateral pelvic lymph node dissections: a report of 100 patients operated on five or more years ago. *Am. J. Obstet. Gynecol.* **62:** 854–870.

61. Piver, M.S., F. Rutledge & J.P. Smith. 1974. Five classes of extended hysterectomy for women with cervical cancer. *Obstet. Gynecol.* **44:** 265–272.

62. Symmonds, R.E. 1975. Some surgical aspects of gynecologic cancer. *Cancer* **36:** 649–660.

63. Massi, G., L. Savino & T. Susini. 1996. Three classes of radical hysterectomy. *Am. J. Obstet. Gynecol.* **175:** 1576–1585.

64. Hellebrekers, B.W. *et al.* 1999. Surgically-treated early cervical cancer: prognostic factors and the significance of depth of tumor invasion. *Int. J. Gynecol. Cancer* **9:** 212–219.

65. Sedlis, A. *et al.* 1999. A randomized trial of pelvic radiation therapy versus no further therapy in selected patients with stage IB carcinoma of the cervix after radical hysterectomy and pelvic lymphadenectomy: a Gynecologic Oncology Group Study. *Gynecol. Oncol.* **73:** 177–183.

66. Peters, W.A. *et al.* 2000. Concurrent chemotherapy and pelvic radiation therapy compared with pelvic radiation therapy alone as adjuvant therapy after radical surgery in high-risk early-stage cancer of the cervix. *J. Clin. Oncol.* **18:** 1606–1613.

67. Landoni, F. *et al.* 1997. Randomised study of radical surgery versus radiotherapy for stage Ib-IIa cervical cancer. *Lancet* **350:** 535–540.

68. Low, J.A., G.M. Mauger & J.A. Carmichael. 1981. The effect of Wertheim hysterectomy upon bladder and urethral function. *Am. J. Obstet. Gynecol.* **139:** 826–834.

69. Sekido, N., K. Kawai & H. Akaza. 1997. Lower urinary tract dysfunction as persistent complication of radical hysterectomy. *Int. J. Urol.* **4:** 259–264.

70. Bergmark, K. *et al.* 1999. Vaginal changes and sexuality in women with a history of cervical cancer. *N. Engl. J. Med.* **340:** 1383–1389.

71. Barnes, W. *et al.* 1991. Manometric characterization of rectal dysfunction following radical hysterectomy. *Gynecol. Oncol.* **42:** 116–119.

72. Dargent, D. 1987. A new future for Schauta's operation through presurgical retroperitoneal pelviscopy. *Eur. J. Gynaecol. Oncol.* **8:** 292–296.

73. Sardi, J. *et al.* 1999. Laparoscopically assisted Schauta operation: learning experience at the Gynecologic Oncology Unit, Buenos Aires University Hospital. *Gynecol. Oncol.* **75:** 361–365.

74. Hertel, H. *et al.* 2003. Laparoscopic-assisted radical vaginal hysterectomy (LARVH): prospective evaluation of 200 patients with cervical cancer. *Gynecol. Oncol.* **90:** 505–511.

75. Malur, S., M. Possover & A. Schneider. 2001. Laparoscopically assisted radical vaginal versus radical abdominal hysterectomy type II in patients with cervical cancer. *Surg. Endosc.* **15:** 289–292.

76. Nam, J.H. *et al.* 2004. Comparative study of laparoscopico-vaginal radical hysterectomy and abdominal radical hysterectomy in patients with early cervical cancer. *Gynecol. Oncol.* **92:** 277–283.

77. Steed, H. *et al.* 2004. A comparison of laparascopic-assisted radical vaginal hysterectomy and radical abdominal hysterectomy in the treatment of cervical cancer. *Gynecol. Oncol.* **93:** 588–593.

78. Jackson, K.S. *et al.* 2004. Laparoscopically assisted radical vaginal hysterectomy vs. radical abdominal hysterectomy for cervical cancer: a match controlled study. *Gynecol. Oncol.* **95:** 655–661.

79. Sharma, R. *et al.* 2006. Laparoscopically assisted radical vaginal hysterectomy (Coelio-Schauta): a comparison with open Wertheim/Meigs hysterectomy. *Int. J. Gynecol. Cancer* **16:** 1927–1932.

80. Morgan, D.J. *et al.* 2007. Is laparoscopically assisted radical vaginal hysterectomy for cervical carcinoma safe? A case control study with follow up. *BJOG* **114:** 537–542.

81. Querleu, D. *et al.* 2002. Modified radical vaginal hysterectomy with or without laparoscopic nerve-sparing dissection: a comparative study. *Gynecol. Oncol.* **85:** 154–158.

82. Canis, M. *et al.* 1990. Does endoscopic surgery have a role in radical surgery of cancer of the cervix uteri? *J. Gynecol. Obstet. Biol. Reprod.* **19:** 921.

83. Nezhat, C.R. *et al.* 1992. Laparoscopic radical hysterectomy with paraaortic and pelvic node dissection. *Am. J. Obstet. Gynecol.* **166:** 864–865.

84. Spirtos, N.M. *et al.* 2002. Laparoscopic radical hysterectomy (type III) with aortic and pelvic lymphadenectomy in patients with stage I cervical cancer: surgical morbidity and intermediate follow-up. *Am. J. Obstet. Gynecol.* **187:** 340–348.

85. Ramirez, P.T. *et al.* 2006. Total laparoscopic radical hysterectomy and lymphadenectomy: the M.D. Anderson Cancer Center experience. *Gynecol. Oncol.* **102:** 252–255.

86. Li, G. *et al.* 2006. A comparison of laparoscopic radical hysterectomy and pelvic lymphadenectomy and laparotomy in the treatment of Ib-IIa cervical cancer. *Gynecol. Oncol.* **105:** 176–180.

87. Lanfranco, A.D. *et al.* 2004. Robotic surgery. A current perspective. *Ann Surg.* **239:** 14–21.

88. Sert, B.M. & V.M. Abeler. 2006. Robotic-assisted laparoscopic radical hysterectomy (Piver type III) with dissection—case report. *Eur. J. Gynaecol. Oncol.* **27:** 531–533.

89. Dargent, D., J. Brun & M. Roy. 1994. La trachelectomie elargie (T.E.). Une alternative à l'hysterectomie radicale dans le traitement des cancers infiltrants developpés sur la face du col uterin. *J. Obstet. Gynecol.* **2:** 292–295.

90. Roy, M. & M. Plante. 1998. Pregnancies after radical vaginal trachelectomy for early-stage cervical cancer. *Am. J. Obstet. Gynecol.* **179:** 1491–1496.

91. Shepherd, J.H., R.A. Crawford & D.H. Oram. 1998. Radical trachelectomy: a way to preserve fertility in the treatment of early cervical cancer. *Br. J. Obstet. Gynaecol.* **105:** 912–916.

92. Covens, A. *et al.* 1999. Is radical trachelectomy a safe alternative to radical hysterectomy for patients with stage IA-B carcinoma of the cervix? *Cancer* **86:** 2273–2279.

93. Dargent, D. *et al.* 2000. Laparoscopic vaginal radical trachelectomy: a treatment to preserve the fertility of cervical carcinoma patients. *Cancer* **88:** 1877–1882.

94. Shepherd, J.H., T. Mould & D.H. Oram. 2001. Radical trachelectomy in early stage carcinoma of the cervix: outcome as judged by recurrence and fertility rates. *Br. J. Obstet. Gynaecol.* **108:** 882–885.

95. Hertel, H. *et al.* 2001. Fertility after radical trachelectomy in patients with early stage cervical cancer. *Geburtsh. Frauenheilk.* **61:** 117–120.

96. Burnett, A.F. *et al.* 2003. Radical vaginal trachelectomy and pelvic lymphadenectomy for preservation of fertility in early cervical carcinoma. *Gynecol. Oncol.* **88:** 419–423.

97. Schlaerth, J.B., N.M. Spirtos & A.C. Schlaerth. 2003. Radical trachelectomy and pelvic lymphadenectomy with uterine preservation in the treatment of cervical cancer. *Am. J. Obstet. Gynecol.* **188:** 29–34.

98. Bernardini, M. *et al.* 2003. Pregnancy outcomes in patients after radical trachelectomy. *Am. J. Obstet. Gynecol.* **189:** 1378–1382.

99. Covens, A. 2003. Preserving fertility in early stage cervical cancer with radical trachelectomy. *Contemp. Obstet. Gynaecol.* **108:** 882–885.

100. Steed, H. & A. Covens. 2003. Radical vaginal trachelectomy and laparoscopic pelvic lymphadenectomy for preservation of fertility. *Postgrad. Obstet. Gynecol.* **23:** 1–6.

101. Plante, M. *et al.* 2004. Vaginal radical trachelectomy: an oncologically safe fertility-preserving surgery. An updated series of 72 cases and review of the literature. *Gynecol. Oncol.* **94:** 614–623.

102. Plante, M. *et al.* 2005. Vaginal trachelectomy: a valuable fertility-preserving option in the management of early-stage cervical cancer. A series of 50 pregnancies and review of the literature. *Gynecol. Oncol.* **98:** 3–10.

103. Hertel, H. *et al.* 2006. Radical vaginal trachelectomy (RVT) combined with laparoscopic pelvic lymphadenectomy: Prospective multicenter study of 100 patients with early cervical cancer. *Gynecol. Oncol.* **103:** 506–511.

104. Shepherd, J.H. *et al.* 2006. Radical vaginal trachelectomy as a fertility-sparing procedure in women with early-stage cervical cancer – cumulative pregnancy rate in a series of 123 women. *BJOG* **113:** 719–724.

105. Smith, J.R. *et al.* 1997. Abdominal radical trachelectomy: a new surgical technique for the conservative management of cervical carcinoma. *Br. J. Obstet. Gynaecol.* **104:** 1196–1200.

106. Rodriguez, M., O. Guimares & P.G. Rose. 2001. Radical abdominal trachelectomy and pelvic lymphadenectomy with uterine conservation and subsequent pregnancy in the treatment of early invasive cervical cancer. *Am. J. Obstet. Gynecol.* **185:** 370–374.

107. Del Priore, G. *et al.* 2003. Abdominal radical trachelectomy for fertility preservation in cervical cancer. *Obstet. Gynecol.* **101**(Suppl 4): 3S–4S.

108. Ungar, L. *et al.* 2005. Abdominal radical trachelectomy: a fertility-preserving option for women with early cervical cancer. *BJOG* **112:** 366–369.

109. Abu-Rustum, N.R. *et al.* 2006. Fertility-sparing radical abdominal trachelectomy for cervical carcinoma: technique and review of the literature. *Gynecol. Oncol.* **103:** 807–813.

110. Marlow, N. *et al.* 2005. Neurologic and developmental disability at six years of age after extremely preterm birth. *N. Engl. J. Med.* **352:** 9–19.

111. Kobayashi, Y., F. Akiyama & K. Hasumi. 2006. A case of successful pregnancy after treatment of invasive cervical cancer with systemic chemotherapy and conization. *Gynecol. Oncol.* **100:** 213–215.

112. Rob, L. *et al.* 2007. Less radical fertility-sparing surgery than radical trachelectomy in early cervical cancer. *Int. J. Gynecol. Cancer* **17:** 304–310.

113. Höckel, M., M.A. Konerding & C.P. Heussel. 1998. Liposuction-assisted nerve-sparing extended radical hysterectomy: oncologic rationale, surgical anatomy, and feasibility study. *Am. J. Obstet. Gynecol.* **178:** 971–976.

114. Possover, M. *et al.* 2000. Identification and preservation of the motoric innervation of the bladder in radical hysterectomy type III. *Gynecol. Oncol.* **79:** 154–157.

115. Trimbos, J.B. *et al.* 2001. A nerve-sparing radical hysterectomy: guidelines and feasibility in Western patients. *Int. J. Gynecol. Cancer* **11:** 180–186.

116. Kato, T., G. Murakami & Y. Yabuki. 2003. A new perspective on nerve-sparing radical hysterectomy: nerve topography and over-preservation of the cardinal ligament. *Jpn. J. Clin. Oncol.* **33:** 589–591.

117. Ercoli, A. *et al.* 2003. Classical and nerve-sparing radical hysterectomy: an evaluation of the risk of injury to the autonomous pelvic nerves. *Surg. Radiol. Anat.* **25:** 200–206.

118. Maas, C.P. *et al.* 2003. Nerve sparing radical hysterectomy: latest developments and historical perspective. *Crit. Rev. Oncol. Hematol.* **48:** 271–279.

119. Possover, M. 2003. Technical modification of the nerve-sparing laparoscopy-assisted vaginal radical hysterectomy type 3 for better reproducibility of this procedure. *Gynecol. Oncol.* **90:** 245–247.

120. Ito, E. & T. Saito. 2004. Nerve-preserving techniques for radical hysterectomy. *Eur. J. Surg. Oncol.* **30:** 1137–1140.

121. Raspagliesi, F. *et al.* 2004. Nerve-sparing radical hysterectomy: a surgical technique for preserving the autonomic hypogastric nerve. *Gynecol. Oncol.* **93:** 307–314.

122. Possover, M., J. Quakernack & V. Chiantera. 2005. The LANN technique to reduce postoperative functional morbidity in laparoscopic radical pelvic surgery. *J. Am. Coll. Surg.* **201:** 913–917.

123. Katahira, A. *et al.* 2005. Intraoperative electrical stimulation of the pelvic splanchnic nerves during nerve-sparing radical hysterectomy. *Gynecol. Oncol.* **98:** 462–466.

124. Sakuragi, N. *et al.* 2005. A systematic nerve-sparing radical hysterectomy technique in invasive cervical cancer for preserving postsurgical bladder function. *Int. J. Gynecol. Cancer* **15:** 389–397.

125. Raspagliesi, F. *et al.* 2006. Type II versus type III nerve-sparing radical hysterectomy: comparison of lower urinary tract dysfunctions. *Gynecol. Oncol.* **102:** 256–262.

126. Todo, Y. *et al.* 2006. Urodynamic study on postsurgical bladder function in cervical cancer treated with systematic nerve-sparing radical hysterectomy. *Int. J. Gynecol. Cancer* **16:** 369–375.

127. Charoenkwan, K. *et al.* 2006. Nerve-sparing class III radical hysterectomy: a modified technique to spare the pelvic autonomic nerves without compromising radicality. *Int. J. Gynecol. Cancer* **16:** 1705–1712.

128. Trimbos, J.B. 2007. Nerve-sparing radical hysterectomy. International symposium on radical hysterectomy dedicated to Hidekazu Okabayashi. The 16th Annual Review Course on Gynecologic Oncology and Pathology. Kyoto, Japan.

129. Landoni, F. *et al.* 1995. Cancer of the cervix, FIGO stages IB and IIA: patterns of local growth and paracervical extension. *Int. J. Gynecol. Cancer* **5:** 329–334.

130. Höckel, M. & N. Dornhöfer. 2005. The Hydra phenomenon of cancer: why tumors recur locally after microscopically complete surgical resection. *Cancer Res.* **65:** 2997–3002.

131. Höckel, M., L.-C. Horn & H. Fritsch. 2005. Local tumour spread in stage IB-IIB cervical carcinoma is confined to the mesenchymal compartment of uterovaginal organogenesis. *Lancet Oncol.* **6:** 751–756.

132. Höckel, M. *et al.* 2003. Total mesometrial resection: High resolution nerve-sparing radical hysterectomy based on developmentally defined surgical anatomy. *Int. J. Gynecol. Cancer* **13:** 791–803.

133. Chassagne, D. *et al.* 1993. A glossary for reporting complications of treatment in gynecological cancers. *Radiother. Oncol.* **26:** 195–202.

134. Quinn, M.A. *et al.* 2006. FIGO Annual Report, Vol. 26. Carcinoma of the cervix uteri. *Int. J. Gynecol. Obstet.* **95**(Suppl. 1): S43–S103.

135. Green, J.A. *et al.* 2001. Survival and recurrence after concomitant chemotherapy and radiotherapy for cancer of the uterine cervix: a systematic review and meta-analysis. *Lancet* **358:** 781–786.

136. Rocconi, R.P. *et al.* 2005. Management strategies for stage IB2 cervical cancer: a cost-effectiveness analysis. *Gynecol. Oncol.* **97:** 387–394.

137. Höckel, M. 1999. Pelvic recurrences of cervical cancer. Relapse pattern, prognostic factors, and the role of extended radical treatment. *J. Pelv. Surg.* **5:** 255–266.

138. Friedlander, M. & M. Grogan. 2002. Guidelines for the treatment of recurrent and metastatic cervical cancer. *Oncologist* **7:** 342–347.

139. Brunschwig, A. 1948. Complete excision of pelvic viscera for advanced carcinoma. *Cancer* **1:** 177–183.

140. Mibayashi, R. 1962. Results in the treatment of cervical cancer at the Kyoto University obstetrical and gynecological clinic. *Jpn. Obstet. Gynecol. Soc.* **14:** 471–472.

141. Ungar, L. & L. Palfalvi. 2003. Surgical treatment of lymph node metastases in stage IB cervical cancer: the laterally extended parametrectomy (LEP) procedure. *Int. J. Gynecol. Cancer* **13:** 647–651.

142. Palfalvi, L. & L. Ungar. 2003. Laterally extended parametrectomy (LEP), the technique for radical pelvic side wall dissection: feasibility, technique and results. *Int. J. Gynecol. Cancer* **13:** 914–917.

143. Vasilev, S.A. 1995. A modified incision and technique for total retroperitoneal access and lymph node dissection. *Gynecol. Oncol.* **56:** 226–230.

144. Possover, M. *et al.* 1998. Left-sided suprarenal retrocrural para-aortic lymphadenectomy in advanced cervical cancer by laparoscopy. *Gynecol. Oncol.* **71:** 219–222.

145. Sardi, J. *et al.* 1998. Neoadjuvant chemotherapy in cervical carcinoma stage IIB: a randomized controlled trial. *J. Gynecol. Cancer* **8:** 441–450.

146. Benedetti-Panici, P. *et al.* 2002. Neoadjuvant chemotherapy and radical surgery versus exclusive

radiotherapy in locally advanced squamous cell cervical cancer: results from the Italian multicenter randomized study. *J. Clin. Oncol.* **20:** 179–188.

147. Yamakawa, Y. *et al.* 2000. Neoadjuvant intraarterial infusion chemotherapy in patients with stage IB2-IIIB cervical cancer. *Gynecol. Oncol.* **77:** 264–270.

148. Neoadjuvant Chemotherapy for Cervical Cancer Meta-analysis Collaboration (NACCCMA) Collaboration. Neoadjuvant chemotherapy for locally advanced cervix cancer. *Cochrane Database of Systematic Review 2004.* Issue 1, Art. No: CD001774. DO1: 10.1002/14651858CD001774.pub2.

149. Cai, H.B., H.Z. Chen & H.H. Yin. 2006. Randomized study of preoperative chemotherapy versus primary surgery for stage IB cervical cancer. *J. Obstet. Gynaecol. Res.* **32:** 315–323.

150. Buda, A. *et al.* 2005. Randomized trial of neoadjuvant chemotherapy comparing paclitaxel, ifosfamide, and cisplatin with ifosfamide and cisplatin followed by radical surgery in patients with locally advanced squamous cell cervical carcinoma: The SNAP01 (Studio Neo-Adjuvante Portio) Italian collaborative study. *J. Clin. Oncol.* **23:** 4137–4145.

151. Choi, C.H. *et al.* 2007. Phase II study of neoadjuvant chemotherapy with mitomycin-c, vincristine and cisplatin (MVC) in patients with stages IB2-IIB cervical carcinoma. *Gynecol. Oncol.* **104:** 64–69.

152. Tanak, T., K. Kokawa & N. Umesaki. 2005. Preoperative chemotherapy with irinotecan and mitomycin for FIGO stage IIIb cervical squamous cell carcinoma: a pilot study. *Eur. J. Gynaecol. Oncol.* **26:** 605–607.

153. Nagao, S. *et al.* 2005. Combination chemotherapy of docetaxel and carboplatin in advanced or recurrent cervix cancer. A pilot study. *Gynecol. Oncol.* **96:** 805–809.

154. Mancuso, S. *et al.* 2000. Phase I-II trial of preoperative chemoradiation in locally advanced cervical carcinoma. *Gynecol. Oncol.* **78:** 324–328.

155. Martinez-Monge, R. *et al.* 2001. Intraoperative electron beam radiotherapy during radical surgery for locally advanced and recurrent cervical cancer. *Gynecol. Oncol.* **82:** 538–543.

156. Disraefano, M. *et al.* 2005. Preoperative chemoradiotherapy in locally advanced cervical cancer: long-term outcome and complications. *Gynecol. Oncol.* **99:** S166–S170.

157. Classe, J.M. *et al.* 2006. Surgery after chemoradiotherapy and brachytherapy for the treatment of advanced cervical cancer: morbidity and outcome: results of a multicenter study of the GCCLCC (Groupe des Chirurgiens de Centre de Lutte Contre le Cancer). *Gynecol. Oncol.* **102:** 523–529.

158. Modarress, M. *et al.* 2005. Comparative study of chemoradiation and neoadjuvant chemotherapy effects before radical hysterectomy in stage IB-IIB bulky cervical cancer and with tumor diameter greater than 4 cm. *Int. J. Gynecol. Cancer* **15:** 483–488.

159. Del Carmen, M.G. *et al.* 2000. Intraoperative radiation therapy in the treatment of pelvic gynecologic malignancies: a review of fifteen cases. *Gynecol. Oncol.* **79:** 457–462.

160. Höckel, M. *et al.* 1996. Five-year experience with combined operative and radiotherapeutic treatment of recurrent gynecologic tumors infiltrating the pelvic wall. *Cancer* **77:** 1918–1933.

161. Höckel, M. & N. Dornhöfer. 2006. Pelvic exenteration for gynaecologic tumours: achievements and unanswered questions. *Lancet Oncol.* **7:** 837–847.

162. Höckel, M. 2006. Ultra-radical compartmentalized surgery in gynaecological oncology. *Eur. J. Surg. Oncol.* **32:** 859–865.

163. Heald, R.J., E.M. Husband & R.D.H. Ryall. 1982. The mesorectum in rectal cancer surgery: the clue to pelvic recurrence? *Br. J. Surg.* **62:** 613–616.

164. Höckel, M. 1999. Laterally extended endopelvic resection: surgical treatment of infrailiac pelvic wall recurrences of gynecologic malignancies. *Am. J. Obstet. Gynecol.* **180:** 306–312.

165. Höckel, M. 2003. Laterally extended endopelvic resection. Novel surgical treatment of locally recurrent cervical carcinoma involving the pelvic side wall. *Gynecol. Oncol.* **91:** 369–377.

Cervical Cancer Prevention in the Human Papilloma Virus Vaccine Era

Saad Ghazal-Aswad

Department of Obstetrics and Gynaecology, Tawam Hospital,
Al Ain, United Arab Emirates

Globally, cervical cancer is second only to breast cancer as the leading cause of cancer in women, with a global prevalence of 2.3 million. It is the third most common cause of female cancer-related mortality worldwide, and 82% of new cervical cancer cases occur in developing countries. As stated by WHO, "without screening programs, cervical cancer is detected too late and leads to death in almost all cases." However, even in Europe, the United States, and Canada, where most women have access to routine screening, approximately 30,000 women die each year. Infection with oncogenic types of HPV 16 and 18 is the most significant risk/causative factor in cervical cancer etiology, and worldwide HPV positivity in cervical carcinoma has been documented to be 99.7%. In 2006 Merck's quadrivalent vaccine was approved by FDA. It targets four HPV types (6, 11, 16, and 18) that are involved in cervical cancer, high and low grade squamous intraepithelial lesions,, and anogenital warts. Results from combined Phase II/III studies show that the efficacy of vaccine was 95–100% against LGSIL and HGSIL related to HPV 16 and 18 and vaccine use led to a 99% reduction in the incidence of genital warts (related to HPV 6 and 11). Due to morbidity associated with infection with HPV types 6, 11, 16, and 18, a prophylactic quadrivalent HPV vaccine targeting these four HPV types is expected to substantially reduce the burden of HPV-related disease.

Key words: HPV (human papilloma virus); cervical cancer; quadrivalent vaccine

Introduction

Globally, cervical cancer is second only to breast cancer as a leading cause of cancer death in women,[1] with global prevalence of 2.3 million cases[2] and annual incidence of around half a million.[1] It accounts for nearly 10% of all cancers,[3] and approximately 275,000 women die from this disease every year throughout the world.[1] In Europe, cervical cancer has had a significant impact on women's health, with more than 33,000 women affected by the disease annually, and almost 16,000 women die every year from the disease.[1] In the UAE, cancer is the third greatest cause of death in the population, and cervical cancer is the second most common cancer in women after breast cancer.[4] It is very important to recognize that cervical cancer affects women at a younger age than breast cancer, as reflected by the fact that life productivity lost from cervical cancer is almost the same as from breast cancer. According to data obtained from GLOBACAN 2002, 82% of new cervical cancer cases occur in developing countries[1] where no screening program is available. The World Health Organization states, "without screening programs, cervical cancer is detected too late and leads to death in almost all cases."[2] However, even in Europe, the United States, and Canada, where most women have access to routine screening, approximately 30,000 women die every year from cervical cancer.

Address for correspondence: Dr. Saad Ghazal-Aswad, Chair, Dept of Obstetrics and Gynaecology, Tawam Hospital, P.O. Box 15258, Al Ain, UAE. Voice: +00971-3-7677 444. saswad@tawam-hosp.gov.ae

Ann. N.Y. Acad. Sci. 1138: 253–256 (2008). © 2008 New York Academy of Sciences.
doi: 10.1196/annals.1414.030

Epidemiology of Human Papilloma Virus and Its Role in Cervical Cancer Development

In many case-controlled studies, it has been evident that cervical cancer is associated with many risk factors, in particular, early sexual intercourse, multiple sexual partners, smoking, and low social class. Nevertheless, infection with the human papilloma virus (HPV) high-risk group (oncogenic types) is thought to be the most significant risk factor in cervical cancer etiology, and it has become clearer that cervical cancer is caused by HPV.[5,6]

HPVs are very common viruses and according to the Center for Disease Control (USA), 50% of the female population will be infected with HPV at some stage in their lifetime.[7] Although HPV is mainly implicated in cervical cancer, it is also responsible for many other diseases. The type of disease is dependent on the type of HPV and the tissues infected. So the oncogenic types 16 and 18 are implicated in lower genital tract (cervix, vaginal, and vulva as well as anus and penis) precancer and cancer. On the other hand, the benign subgroup, in particular types 6 and 11, is implicated in genital warts as well as other benign head and neck diseases. In many parts of the world HPV16 is the predominant subtype in squamous cell carcinoma of the cervix (46–63%) followed by HPV18 (10–14%), and according to Walboomers and colleagues (1999) and based on data obtained from 932 patients with cervical cancer worldwide, HPV was found to be present in cervical carcinoma tissue samples in 99.7% of patients.[6]

Vaccine Development and Its Efficacy

In June 2006, Merck Sharp & Dohme (Whitehouse Station, NJ) quadrivalent vaccine (Gardasil®) was approved by the FDA and subsequently was made available in many parts in the world. It protects against infection with HPV types 6, 11, 16, and 18 and the subsequent diseases arising from this infection. HPV types 16 and 18 account for more than 70% of cervical cancer and cervical high-grade squamous intraepithelial lesions, whereas HPV subtypes 6 and 11 are associated with approximately 90% of anogenital warts. In all, these four types are responsible for over 40% of low-grade cervical lesions.[8] Results from the phase III "Future I" study indicated that the quadrivalent vaccine efficacy in protecting from HPV 6/11/16/18–related cervical intraepithelial neoplasia (CIN) and endocervical glandular lesions at 3 years was 100% (95% CI, 94–100).[9] In addition, the Phase III "Future II" study confirmed that the protection against HPV 16/18–related CIN 2/3 or worse was 98% at 3 years (95% CI, 86–100).[10] Moreover, clinical efficacy results suggest reductions in the incidence of vulval and vaginal lesions (VIN 2 and 3, VAIN 2 and 3) by 71% (95% CI, 37–88).[11] In addition, the vaccine led to a 99% reduction in the incidence of genital warts related to HPV 6 and 8.[11]

Gardasil is a prophylactic vaccine. It is a non-infectious, recombinant, quadrivalent vaccine containing the disease-causing capsule, but not the infectious virus itself. It combines highly purified virus-like particles (VLPs) and adjuvant amorphous aluminum hydroxyl phosphate sulphate (AAHS). The VLPs present in the vaccine mimic natural infection with the disease-causing agent but without the possibility of causing any disease. While the AAHS focuses and enhances the immune response to produce the specific antibody. Clinical studies have shown that the VLPs and the AAHS adjuvant induce strong immune memory.[12]

Who Will Be Vaccinated with Gardasil?

Recommendations regarding who should receive the vaccine will be determined by the health authority in each country. In the United States, the Centers for Disease Control (CDC) recommended that all young females should receive the vaccine routinely between the ages of 9–15, a catch-up program is indicated for those up to the age of 26. The vaccine should be given as three injections at the following intervals: 0, 2, and 6 months. In all studies, the vaccine was generally well-tolerated, with a slightly higher number of subjects in the vaccine group reporting one or more injection-site adverse experiences. It is anticipated that vaccination of adolescent and young females will greatly reduce the burden of cervical cancer and all genital neoplasia and genital warts over the next one to two decades.

The Role of HPV Vaccination and Cervical Cancer Screening

Over the last few decades, screening for cervical cancer has been largely responsible for a significant reduction (40–50%) in the incidence of cervical cancer in Europe, America, and Canada. The Pap test normally enables clinicians to detect cervical abnormality before it progresses to cancer, and organized screening with high coverage and good quality control have reduced the incidence, morbidity, and mortality related to cervical cancer but have not eradicated it completely.

In the UAE, there is no organized cervical cancer screening program, and more than 80% of our patients with cervical cancer present at a late stage when treatment offers little chance of cure. Although there have been many attempts to organize screening programs, these were hindered by many technical and logistic problems. In 2004 a national cervical cancer prevention workshop was organized in the presence of five international experts in the field. This workshop called for a national screening program and proposed all the necessary arrangements.[13] Although the final report was published and copies were sent to the responsible authorities, no action has been taken as yet regarding the initiation of the screening program. As such, there is a strong feeling that while still waiting to start the organized screening program in the UAE, we should vaccinate our female population as primary prevention for cervical cancer. This vaccination, hand-in-hand with screening, hopefully will help with a significant reduction, and possibly eradication, of morbidity and mortality attributable to cervical cancer in the next two decades.

Conclusion

Due to the high morbidity associated with infection with HPV types 6, 11, 16, and 18, the prophylactic quadrivalent HPV vaccine tackling these four HPV types is expected to substantially reduce the burden of HPV-related disease, in particular lower genital tract neoplasia and cancer. The need to establish a screening program in the UAE is essential at this stage, but the recommendation to review screening guidelines with implementation of the vaccine will be needed once we have more information about the combined interaction of the screening program and vaccination.

Conflicts of Interest

The author declares no conflicts of interest.

References

1. Ferlay, J., F. Bray, P. Pisani, D.M. Parkin, GLOBO-CAN 2002. 2004. Cancer incidence, mortality and prevalence worldwide, version 2.0. IARC Cancer Base No. 5. IARC Press. Lyon, France.
2. World Health Organization. 2003. *State of the Art of New Vaccines Research and Development: Initiative for Vaccine Research.* 1–74. World Health Organization. Geneva, Switzerland.
3. Franco, E.L. & D.M. Harper. 2005. Vaccination against human papillomavirus infection: a new paradigm in cervical cancer control. *Vaccine* **23:** 2388–2394.
4. Ministry of Health, UAE Statistics. http://www.uae.gov.ae/moh/statistics.htm (accessed July 12, 2004).
5. Muñoz, N. 2000. Human papillomavirus and cancer: the epidemiological evidence. *J. Clin. Virol.* **9:** 1–5.

6. Walboomers, J.M.M., M.V. Jacobs, M.M. Manos, *et al.* 1999. Human papillomavirus is a necessary cause of invasive cervical cancer worldwide. *J. Pathol.* **189:** 12–19.

7. Koutsky, L. 1997. Epidemiology of genital human papillomavirus infection. *Am. J. Med.* **102:** 3–8.

8. Smith, J.S., L. Lindsay, B. Hoots, *et al.* 2007. Human papillomavirus type distribution in invasive cervical cancer and high-grade cervical lesions: a meta-analysis update. *Int. J. Cancer* **121:** 621–632.

9. Garland, S.M., M. Hernandez-Avila, C.M. Wheeler, *et al.* 2007. Females United to Unilaterally Reduce Endo/Ectocervical Disease (FUTURE) I Investigators. Quadrivalent vaccine against human papillomavirus to prevent anogenital diseases. *N. Engl. J. Med.* **356:** 1928–1943.

10. FUTURE II Study Group. 2007. Quadrivalent vaccine against human papillomavirus to prevent high-grade cervical lesions. *N. Engl. J. Med.* **356:** 1915–1927.

11. Joura, E.A., S. Leodolter, M. Hernandez-Avila, *et al.* 2007. Efficacy of a quadrivalent prophylactic human papillomavirus (types 6, 11, 16, and 18) L1 virus-like-particle vaccine against high-grade vulval and vaginal lesions: a combined analysis of three randomised clinical trials. *Lancet* **369:** 1693–1702.

12. Olsson, S.E., L.L. Villa, R.L. Costa, *et al.* 2007. Induction of immune memory following administration of a prophylactic quadrivalent human papillomavirus (HPV) types 6/11/16/18 L1 virus-like particle (VLP) vaccine. *Vaccine* **25:** 4931–4939.

13. Ghazal-Aswad, S., H. Gargash, P. Badrinath, *et al.* 2005. National Workshop for Cervical Cancer prevention and control in the United Arab Emirates, Abu Dhabi, September 2004. *Emirates Med. J.* **23:** 71–75.

Recent London Improvements in Curative Radiation Therapy for Relevant Early Prostate Cancer

P. N. Plowman

Department of Clinical Oncology, St. Bartholomew's Hospital, London, United Kingdom

Since the advent of PSA screening, the detection of early (organ confined) prostate cancer has improved. Although some indolent cancers in the elderly may be safely watched, the early diagnosis in younger men requires curative treatment. Two exciting modernized radiation therapy methods provide alternatives to major surgery and lead to cure rates equivalent to surgery. Modern intensity modulated external beam radiotherapy (IMRT) allows high-dose treatment to the prostate (+/− seminal vesicles) while maximally sparing the rectum (due to the extraordinary capability of creating a concavity in a high-dose radiation therapy volume). This has allowed escalation in the therapy dose to the prostate and improved cure rates. We have recently compared two different IMRT methods. Our introduction of "axial limits" rectal definition allows more accurate quantitation of relevant rectal sparing. Prostate radiation seed brachytherapy (Seattle 125-iodine method) provides a sophisticated, single-session radiation therapy method that has become the most popular curative method by busy men who want minimum interruption to their lives. The implant is "tailored" for the individual's gland size and shape, and in the London adaptation of the method there is interoperative monitoring of seed implantation, such that if any seed is slightly misplaced the information of deposition site is relayed back to a computer, which reconfigures the deposition of all subsequent seeds such that an ideal plan is achieved—dynamic, iterative, computer assisted implantation. The popularity of these two radiation techniques is largely due to the lesser rate of morbidity compared to surgery and the usual fast return to everyday life.

Key words: intensity modulated external beam radiotherapy (IMRT); prostate cancer

Prostate specific antigen (PSA) testing was introduced to routine clinical practice over 10 years ago, and the screening serum measurement has led to an enormous increase in the diagnosis of early prostate cancer.[1] It is true that many, particularly older patients, will die with the disease rather than from the disease, and the much-quoted incidence-to-prevalence and -to-death ratios highlight and emphasize this point. Nevertheless, otherwise fit patients with a decade or more of life expectancy or intermediate to higher risk features are advantaged (with respect to survival chances) by active, radical (curative) therapy, which should be recommended. Unquestionably, PSA screening has assisted in the diagnosis of these relevant early cases of prostate cancer. The concept of relevant early prostate cancer is an important one that I emphasize often; it refers to an early, organ-confined prostate cancer, the existence of which is perceived (from the prognosticators available) to threaten life expectancy.

External beam radiotherapy for early prostate cancer has been available as curative treatment for several decades, but the results were probably inferior to those published more recently, probably because the diagnosis was made (on average) later and current radiation techniques allow the dose prescription to be

Address for correspondence: Dr. Nicholas Plowman, Consultant in Radiotherapy, Senior Clinical Oncologist, St. Bartholomew's Hospital, West Smithfield, London EC1A 7BE, UK. Nick.Plowman@bartsandthelondon.nhs.uk

Ann. N.Y. Acad. Sci. 1138: 257–266 (2008). © 2008 New York Academy of Sciences.
doi: 10.1196/annals.1414.031

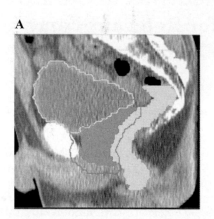

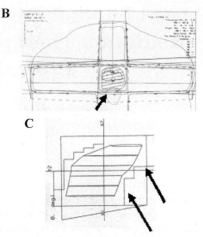

Figure 1. (A) Pelvic CT reconstruction in the sagittal plane, demonstrating the prostate and seminal vesicles in red, the rectum in blue, and the bladder outlined by a thin yellow line. Note that the seminal vesicles cause the volume for radiotherapy to extend posteriorly in the superior region. **(B)** The isodosimetric plan for conformal radiotherapy to the prostate. Note the horizontal posterior border to the high-dose zone (arrowed). The consequence of this is that, inferiorly, more rectum is encompassed in the primary beam of the lateral portals. **(C)** The lateral portal in conformal radiotherapy, with two MLC leaves (arrowed) placed to shield the inferoposterior section of the portal where rectum is bowing anteriorly. (In color in *Annals* online.)

safely escalated. The word "probably" has been inserted in the foregoing sentence because the diagnosis of cure and relapse was also more crude 20 years ago since the current definition of relapse (based on biochemical/PSA rise) was unavailable and consequently the definition of relapse was less stringent. Flattering 5- and 10-year overall survival statistics obfuscated the analysis of local control and cure by radiation therapy.[2] In those days of 20 years ago, doses to the prostate of 66–70 Gy fractionated in 1.8–2.0 daily fractions were advised; shielding to square or rectangular portals (usually an open anterior and wedged laterals) was not routine. With regard to the morbidity of radiotherapy from that era, Haffermann[2] reported rates of 4% for small bowel injury, 5% for moderately severe late proctitis, and 2% severe proctitis rates. The overall incidence of significant morbidity increased from 6% to 11% when patients received more than 65 Gy.[3]

With improvements in radiation therapy in the 1990s, including CT planning and the introduction of multileaf collimation into routine usage, the portals could be adapted (usually by

effecting screening to the infero-posterior corners of the lateral portals) to shield some rectum and minor other adaptations to create a more conformal plan (Fig. 1).

The integral rectal dose was thus lowered and it became safer to escalate dosage to the prostate. This last opportunity gained importance when many studies demonstrated an improved cure rate for prostate cancer when the prescription dose exceeded 72 Gy of conventionally fractionated radiotherapy.[4–6] The introduction of the multileaf collimator into linear accelerator design was further advanced when the concept of intensity modulated radiotherapy (IMRT) was born. Here, the multileaf collimation (MLC) leaves adopted different configurations during the therapy dose to an individual treatment portal, allowing the fluence of the beam to be changed in two dimensions. During therapy in the currently favored dynamic IMRT, the leaves slide across the therapy beam during therapy to influence the dose received by different segments of the portal. With this development the radiotherapist was able to create low-dose areas/volumes within the

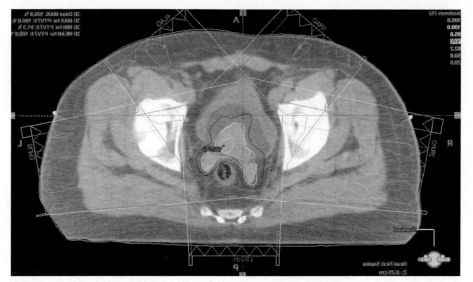

Figure 2. Axial CT scan through pelvis with an IMRT isodosimetric plan superimposed and the high-dose regions dose-washed in turquoise and red. Note the ability of the IMRT technique to cause a concavity in the high-dose region such that the rectum (pink) is spared from the high-dose radiotherapy. (In color in *Annals* online.)

target volume and—very importantly in so many areas of radiotherapy where an organ at risk is adjacent to the tumor volume—a concavity in the high-dose isodose contour. This methodology allowed further sparing of rectal dose during the treatment course and once again proved to be an advance in terms of being able to more safely escalate the dose to the prostate without increased rectal toxicity (Fig. 2).

Tomotherapy (TomoTherapy Incorporated, Madison, Wisconsin) represents a further development in the quest for optimal IMRT/conformal radiotherapy. This new 6 MV linear accelerator is mounted on a gantry ring and rotates through 360° during therapy. A narrow fan beam (1.0–2.5 cm wide) is emitted and may be modified in shape during therapy by 32 pairs of multileaf collimators. One leaf of MLC is considered to have 51 beamlets associated with it during one gantry rotation. Last, the treatment couch is translated/pitched in a direction perpendicular to the rotating beam, concurrent with beam exposure and at a constant rate. The target volume is therefore treated by a spiral beam and there are tens of

thousands of beamlet configurations available to "intensity modify" the dose within the targeted volume. This intricate rotational method of IMRT delivery may improve dose conformity of a treatment plan (dose-sparing adjacent organs at risk) compared to IMRT by standard linear accelerator technology (Fig. 3). However, in a recent head-to-head dosimetric study of Linac IMRT with Tomotherapy for radical therapy of prostate cancer, our group found very similar dosimetry, although we were able to show slightly improved (subtle) coverage of the seminal vesicles to 66 Gy during deposition of 74 Gy (median dose) to the prostate.[7]

The introduction of IMRT has led to a low incidence of rectal complications despite dose escalation of the prostate prescription.[8]

In this recent work from our unit, it became clear to us that the optimal assessment of the organ at risk was now a high priority in the quest for improved conformal/IMRT methods of prostate radiotherapy. Most of the current conformal/IMRT methods will achieve good and comparable coverage of the target volume, but the quality of organ-at-risk avoidance still

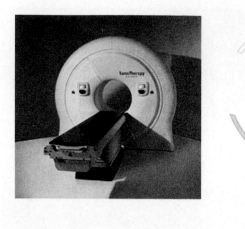

Figure 3. *Left panel*: TomoTherapy Machine. *Right panel*: Figurative demonstration of Tomotherapy linac arcing around patient while patient is translated through the beam on the treatment couch. (In color in *Annals* online.)

separates (in a qualitative dosimetric sense) the various techniques.

In radical high-dose radiotherapy to the prostate, the organ at risk is the rectum, or more specifically the front half of the rectum, between the superior and inferior (cranial and caudal) axial limits of the targeted organ (the prostate). This front rectal wall is where damage is later manifest in the small percentage of cases that suffer late morbidity. This is the main concern to the clinician who prescribes high doses of 74 Gy or more to prostate.

We noted that all publications that had studied the rectal dosimetry during prostate radiotherapy had taken the whole rectum as the organ at risk—as though rectal tolerance was dependent on the total, integral organ dose received. By anatomical definition, this accepted the rectum as extending from the dentate line inferiorly to the peritoneal reflection superiorly and therefore was a much longer volume than that between the axial limits of the target prostate (that is, the high-dose volume). The rectal dose–volume histograms therefore included irrelevant rectum, and it was consequently difficult to distinguish between the dosimetric quality of conformal/IMRT techniques

of similar (but not quite equal) quality. By studying the rectum between the axial limits of the targeted prostate, we not only studied the relevant rectum at risk of morbidity but the rectal dose–volume histogram only reflected relevant anterior rectal wall for the higher doses and it became possible to accurately compare different conformal/IMRT techniques for small dosimetric differences/improvements. In this recent work from London, we have been best able to demonstrate small but important differences in the quality of modern conformal techniques which otherwise demonstrated similar abilities to cover the target prostate volume (Fig. 4).[9]

In summary, we currently have available to us conformal and two IMRT techniques (dynamic MLC linear accelerator and Tomotherapy) for curatively treating early prostate cancer. With these methods we may more safely take the prostate to very high doses of conventionally fractionated radiotherapy (a median dose of 74 Gy leads to some parts of the targeted volume receiving 78 Gy) with higher expectations of cure than ever before. IMRT is now the preferred methodology. Added to this, we have recently improved the definition

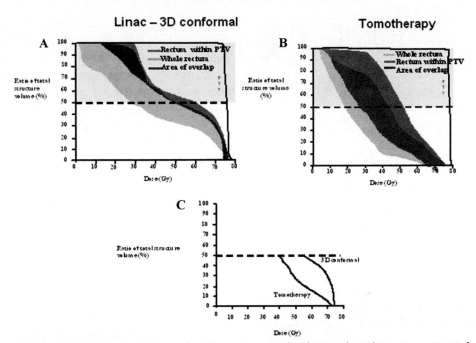

Figure 4. Upper panels **(A and B)** demonstrating the dose–volume histograms (DVH) for rectal dose during prostate radiotherapy utilizing the conformal technique shown in Figure 1 — range DVH for nine patients. Note that the graphs for rectum between the upper and lower limits of the prostate volume (rectum within the PTV) lie to the right of the whole rectum graphs and, we argue, are the relevant ones to study in this situation. By so doing, and taking the mid-range lines from the upper panels and plotting them in panel **C**, we see the graphical demonstration of the superiority of IMRT (here: TomoTherapy) over conformal radiotherapy with regard to rectal sparing. The graph for TomoTherapy more gently approaches maximum dose than that for the conformal technique, quantifying exactly the smaller amount of anterior rectal wall that receives this high dose with IMRT/TomoTherapy. PTV, planning tumor volume.

of organ avoidance with regard to the adjacent rectum (rectal morbidity risk has been the brake on prostate dose escalation), and by so doing, we have demonstrated how to qualitatively distinguish subtly better conformal/IMRT techniques.

The term "brachytherapy" is derived from the Greek root meaning "close proximity" and relies on the fact that when a radioisotope source is implanted within a tumor or organ, an intense radiation dose is deposited around the radiation source, but the dose falls off with distance from the source, according to the inverse square law (such as in the familiar example that when a ship doubles the distance between itself and a lighthouse, the intensity of the light diminishes fourfold). The consequence and advantage of radiation brachytherapy is that the clinician may deliver an intensely high dose of radiation therapy to a tumor while sparing adjacent normal tissues from maximal dose, because of this fast fall off in dose at the perimeter of the tumor under therapy.

Prostate brachytherapy utilizing low-dose rate Iodine-125 seeds has now become a fine art. The technique commenced with the introduction of high-quality transrectal ultrasound with the anesthetized patient in a Trendelenberg position. This allowed the operator to directly visualize the implanting needle tips by virtue of their echogenicity. Needles are inserted transperineally through a template placed against the perineum and perforated with holes of 0.5 cm spacing on x and y axes, thus creating a "checker board" pattern (Fig. 5).

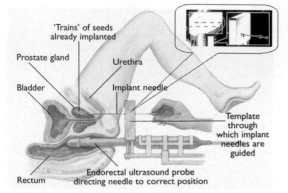

Figure 5. Sagittal view of the Seattle low-dose radiation seed implant technique for prostate cancer with the transrectal probe *in situ* and the implant taking place via the transperineal route through a template (seen "side-on" in the main diagram but "en face" in the "bubble," top right), with the depth coordinate being called by the rectal ultrasound probe. (In color in *Annals* online.)

With the template against the perineum, accurate implantation by grid reference was possible, as the template coordinates were also projected on the transrectal ultrasound viewing screen. The transrectal probe is inserted in a graduated fashion at 0.5-cm depths into the rectum (while viewing the prostate in a perpendicularly forward direction) so the prostate can be mapped—from base to apex—in 0.5-cm steps, and exact x,y coordinates located for any point. The prostate is therefore reduced to a series of slices—like a loaf of sliced bread—of 0.5 cm thickness, and this information is relayed to a planning computer. The computer then creates a radiation seed deposition formation tailored to the individual's gland and designed to deliver a minimum dose to the margin of the gland (+3 mm margin). Each seed has x, y, and z coordinates for its deposition.

During insertion of needles, the transrectal probe is placed at one of the 0.5-cm steps—called retraction planes—from the prostate base to apex, and this gives the (third plane) z coordinate to the stereotactic deposition of each seed. By inserting each needle into the correct x,y coordinate hole on the transperineal template and advancing the needle until its echogenic tip shows up as a bright star on the transrectal ultrasound viewing screen—the correct z coordinate—the seed (or train of seeds) can be deposited at any desired/prescribed x,y,z coordinate with great accuracy. An arrow marker on the ultrasound viewing screen is placed on the correct coordinate and the clinician's job is to find that exact spot with the needle tip before deposition of the seed (or seed train) (Fig. 6).

For several reasons, this low-dose brachytherapy system has gained great popularity. The large number of seeds that are deposited means that each individual seed contributes less to the whole isodose plan and the technique is therefore more forgiving with respect to occasional seed misplacement. In this regard the system has an advantage over the critical placement requirements of the high-dose catheter implant technique, which often requires external beam radiotherapy in combination to improve coverage of the gland. Furthermore, the low-dose seed system allows more flexibility in conformal dose planning for irregularly shaped glands (such as those with odd median lobes) because the placement of many individually sited seeds allows better fine tuning with respect to "dose shaping," creating better tailoring of the dose to prostate margins.

The London team has now 8 years of operative experience in the technique and has fairly faithfully followed the pioneering method of the Seattle group, whose 5-, 10-, and now 15-year cure rates have proved equivalent to those from surgical and external beam radiotherapy series.[10] Ragde and co-workers analyzed data on disease-free status of 769 patients that they had implanted at their institution using permanent low-dose-rate radioisotope seeds.[10] Very interestingly, their data on 3-, 5-, 10-, and 13-year disease-free survival rates (as assessed by biochemical lack of PSA progression) were: 84, 79, 76, and 76%, respectively, for 441 perceived low-risk cases and 87, 82, 80, and 80% for perceived intermediate and higher risk cases. The similarity of the data for two groups is of great interest as this technique had previously been confined to patients with

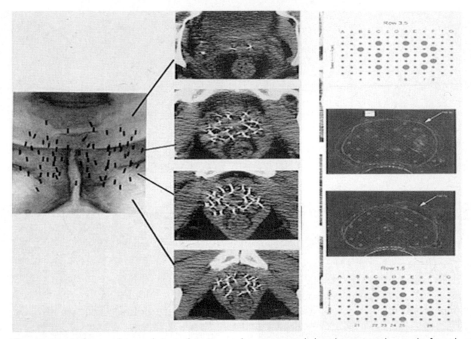

Figure 6. Left panel is a plain pelvis X-ray showing seed distribution at the end of implant. The middle panel shows the axial CT cuts through the prostate at various levels from base to apex demonstrating the deposited seeds around the urethra. The right panel demonstrates the template coordinates, through which holes the needles were inserted to achieve this distribution, the middle two pictures showing these coordinates superimposed on ultrasound pictures. (In color in *Annals* online.)

good prognostic features only: PSA less than 15, Gleason grade less than 7, small glands, and good urinary function. Since then, and with corroborative outcome data from the Guildford group in the United Kingdom, there is now an established role for low-dose radiation seed implant brachytherapy as monotherapy (that is without the preceding external beam radiotherapy to a wider volume) for the intermediate risk patients. This has further increased the scope for the technique.

The technique of brachytherapy has evolved considerably over the last 10 years. At first, an initial planning session was performed with the anesthetized patient in the lithotomy position—just as he would be on the treatment day—in order to map the prostate in 0.5-cm slices, from base to apex, as described above. This information was then used by the physics team to produce an optimal dose (seed deposition) plan, which was then performed at a sep-

arate therapy session some time later (perhaps some weeks later).

The development of seeds in trains held in place by a polyglycerin filament strand, bearing up to five seeds, as required (Rapidstrand; Oncura Ltd, Berkshire, UK), has been an advance both with regard to ease of implantation of large numbers of seeds and for stabilizing the implant within the gland (and indeed stabilizing seeds that may be placed just outside the capsule of the gland). While there have been occasions when the seed trains have stuck within the implanting needles, this has now become a rarity and the trains of seeds may be smoothly deposited with 1-cm spacing between seeds in the base-to-apex direction.

The need for two separate sessions was inconvenient for the patient and labor intensive. Next came the one-step process in which the transrectal ultrasound mapping process and the planning were performed sequentially on

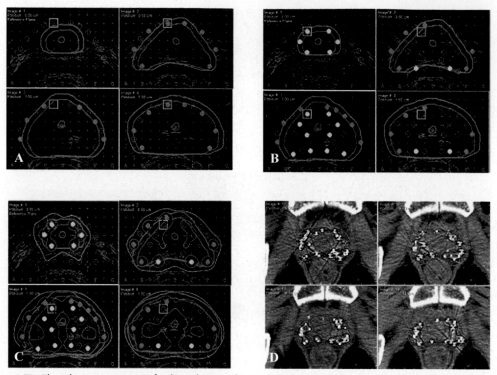

Figure 7. The planning process for low-dose radiation seed implantation. In panel **A**, the first phase of the process is shown in terms of template needles (shown as red dots) to be inserted in a peripheral "horseshoe" distribution around the perimeter of the gland. In panel **B**, the needle coordinates for the second phase of the implant are shown in green and the composite plan, with the 145 Gy isodose line circumnavigating the gland, is shown figuratively in panel **C** and actually on a CT scan slice in panel **D**. (In color in *Annals* online.)

the same day, under the same anesthetic (usually general anesthetic, but epidural where the patient or concomitant medical condition dictated this to be optimal). This was undoubtedly an advance.

Following the lead from the Seattle group and a perceived desire to broaden the volume of cover of the radiation dose, many operators used a more peripheral loading technique, in which a higher proportion of peripheral needles/seeds were implanted (and fewer central prostate seeds) giving a slightly more generous margin of coverage around the prostate's margins, although still respecting the anterior rectal wall. This alteration in technique also reduced the V150—the very high "hot spots" within the prostate volume that received 150% or more of the prescribed dose to the margin of the gland. The dose to urethra was lowered by this alteration in technique, and this

has now been widely adopted. Once again, the Rapidstrand trains of seeds are more stable, and when there are extracapsular seeds—usually toward the base and apex where the gland is less bulbous—the midgland Rapidstrand filament that lies within gland helps to anchor these extracapsular seeds.

As a consequence of this last modification of technique, the peripheral needle distribution bears a great similarity among all patients' plans, for any particular size. Thus there is a fairly uniform plan with respect to the peripheral seed distribution for 25-cm^3, 35-cm^3, and 45-cm^3 glands, and in any axial section of the gland, this resembles a "horseshoe" distribution around the gland's perimeter (Fig. 7).

Recent developments of the technique from our unit in London have been first to have the physics team not only in theater throughout the procedure but active throughout

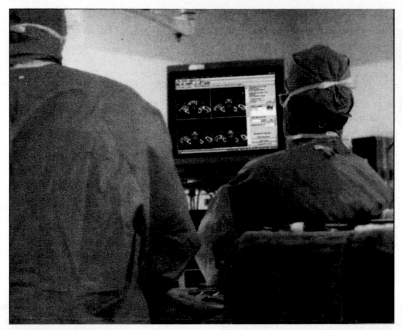

Figure 8. The physics team in the theater, working with the clinical team, throughout the implant provides the facility to alter the computer-derived needle deposition plan dynamically and iteratively as the implant proceeds. (In color in *Annals* online.)

(Fig. 8). In other words, the physics team no longer produces the plan and then leaves matters to the implanting clinician to effect the desired dose plan. Instead, the physicists rapidly produce a "Phase 1" horseshoe plan of peripherally placed seeds, which, as I have just described, is a fairly constant distribution for all patients with similar sized glands, varying somewhat in spacing and number for patients with different sized glands. This is done quickly, and this Phase 1 plan is given to the clinical implant team to implant. While the implant team is at work with this phase of the operation, the physics team works on the second phase of the implant in which they evaluate the seed implant distribution for the central regions of the gland and tailor the implant to the patient's particular gland shape—a slightly longer job (Fig. 8). By so doing, the anesthetic/operation time has been halved.

However, the major advance that we have introduced (and acknowledgement for this should be made here to one of our physicists: John Pettingell) is the ability to be dynamic and interactive throughout the implant. Thus, at any time during the implant, the clinician is monitoring the accurate deposition of the seeds, which is a straightforward job as the seeds themselves give an echo at the x,y,z coordinate of deposition and so an echogenic focus should remain at the arrow tip after the needle is removed. With such sophistication of monitoring of seed deposition, it is not uncommon that there are minor variations from the ideal, prescribed seed position. We now have in place the immediate notification to the physics team of any significant (0.5 cm) misplacement in any individual seed. The physics team is then in a position to register this on the plan, which the computer immediately reconfigures based on this new seed (seed train) position. The consequence is that, with no delay, the subsequent seed positions are optimized to allow for this unexpected small variation in position of the previously implanted seed(s). By this means, we have produced an iterative, dynamic, computer-based implant that allows for optimization during the procedure. The decline in PSA following brachytherapy

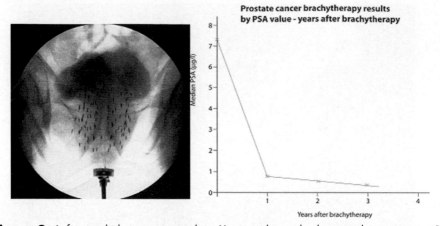

Figure 9. Left panel demonstrates plain X-ray with seeds deposited in prostate. Right panel demonstrates the median PSA serum values with time after low-dose 125-Iodine seed implantation by the technique described here. (In color in *Annals* online.)

attests to the usefulness of the technique (Fig. 9), which is now becoming the most popular method of curing prostate cancer among informed patients with early, organ-confined disease.

Conflicts of Interest

The author declares no conflicts of interest.

References

1. Barry, J. 2001. Prostate specific antigen testing for early diagnosis of prostate cancer. *N. Eng. J. Med.* **344:** 1373–1377.
2. Haffermann, M.D. 1986. Cancer of prostate—external radiotherapy. In *Clinics in Oncology*, Vol. 2. G.P. Murphy, Ed.: 371–405. WB Saunders. Philadelphia.
3. Hanks, G.E., J.M. Krall, K.L. Martz, *et al.* 1988. The outcome of 313 patients with T1 (UICC) prostate cancer treated with external beam irradiation. *Int. J. Radiat. Oncol. Biol. Phys.* **14:** 243–248.
4. Zelfesky, M.J., S.A. Leibel & P.B. Gaudin. 1998. Dose escalation with 3D conformal radiation therapy affects the outcome in prostate cancer. *Int. J. Radiat. Oncol. Biol. Phys.* **41:** 491–500.
5. Pollack, A., G.K. Zagars & G. Starkschall. 2002. Prostate cancer radiation dose: results of the MD Anderson phase 111 randomised trial. *Int. J. Radiat. Oncol. Biol. Phys.* **53:** 1097–1105.
6. Dearnley, D.P., E. Hall & D. Lawrence. 2005. Phase 111 pilot study of dsoe escalation using conformal radiotherapy in prostate cancer. *Br. J. Cancer* **92:** 488–498.
7. Whitelaw, G.L., I. Blasiak-Wal, K. Cooke, *et al.* 2008. A dosimetric comparison of two intensity modulated radiotherapy techniques: TomoTherapy versus linear accelerator. *Brit. J. Radiol.* **81:** 333–340.
8. Zelefsky, M.J., Z. Fuks & M. Hunt. 2002. High dose intensity modulated radiation therapy for prostate cancer: early toxicity and biochemical outcome in 772 patients. *Int. J. Radiat. Oncol. Biol. Phys.* **553:** 1111–1116.
9. O'Donnell, H., K. Finnegan, H. Eliades, *et al.* 2008. Re-defining rectal volume and DVH for analysis of rectal morbidity risk after radiotherapy for early prostate cancer. *Brit. J. Radiol.* **81:** 327–332.
10. Ragde, H., G.L. Grado & B.S. Nadir. 2001. Brachytherapy for clinically localised prostate cancer: thirteen year disease free survival of 769 consecutive prostate cancer patients treated with permanent implants alone. *Arch. Esp. Urol.* **54:** 739–747.

Radical Prostatectomy

Oncological Outcomes

Fayez T. Hammad

Department of Surgery, Faculty of Medicine and Health Sciences,
UAE University, Al Ain, United Arab Emirates

The first radical prostatectomy was performed in 1904. Since then, it has become one of the main treatment options for patients with prostate cancer, especially those with organ-confined disease. As it is the case in all types of malignancies, the treatment choice for the patient with prostate cancer depends on several considerations, the most important of which is the ability of the treatment modality to control disease. This review provides a brief comparison between radical prostatectomy and other main treatment options of prostate cancer, such as "watchful waiting" and radiation therapy, in terms of cancer control. In addition, an overview is provided of the oncological outcomes following various techniques and approaches of radical prostatectomy including open retropubic, perineal, laparoscopic, and robot-assisted surgery.

Key words: **radical prostatectomy; prostate cancer; oncological outcomes**

Introduction

Radical prostatectomy (RP) was first performed through a perineal approach in 1904 by Young, who reported the details of the procedure in 1905.[1] Subsequently, few modifications of the technique were introduced; the most important of which was the use of intersphincteric approach by Belt in 1939.[2] In 1945, Millin described, for the first time, the transabdominal retroperitoneal approach to access the prostate. This approach was used to perform simple prostatectomies,[3] and it was not until 1949 that Memmelaar used the same approach to perform retropubic RP for the first time.[4] Initially the procedure was fraught with a high incidence of complications, namely impotence, incontinence, and excessive hemorrhage and it was not until the early 1980s that Walsh and colleagues described the anatomic nerve-sparing technique with a much lower incidence of postoperative erectile dysfunction.[5,6]

The first laparoscopic RP was performed by Schuessler through a transperitoneal approach in 1991, and described in the literature in 1997.[7] Subsequently, Guillonneau *et al.* defined the Montsouris technique in 1999.[8] In 2001, Bollens *et al.* described the extraperitoneal laparoscopic RP which is sometimes called extraperitoneal endoscopic RP.[9] The robot-assisted RP using the ad Vinci Surgical System (Intuitive Surgical, Sunnyvale, CA) was first performed about the year 2000.[10] In 2007, it is estimated that approximately 63% of RP for localized prostate cancer will be performed using the robot-assisted approach, 36% by an open approach, and less than 1% by the pure laparoscopic technique.[11]

The technical details of the various techniques and approaches of RP are beyond the scope of this review, but the commonest indication for this procedure is early or organ-confined prostate cancer. In addition, RP is sometimes performed in patients with locally advanced prostate cancer in an attempt to debulk the tumor and facilitate adjuvant

Address for correspondence: Fayez T. Hammad, FRCS, PhD, FRACS (Urology), Department of Surgery, FMHS, UAE University, PO Box 17666, Al Ain, UAE. Voice: +971-50-4880021; fax: +971-4-2719340.
fayez@mail2doctor.com

Ann. N.Y. Acad. Sci. 1138: 267–277 (2008). © 2008 New York Academy of Sciences.
doi: 10.1196/annals.1414.032

therapies. The aim of this article is to review the oncological outcomes of RP in both early and locally advanced prostate cancer by comparing the oncological outcomes of this operation with those of other treatment options. Prior to this, a brief review of the oncological outcome parameters commonly used in prostate cancer will be provided.

Post-radical Prostatectomy Cancer Control Parameters

Similar to all cancer types, the ultimate measure of cancer control following RP is survival. In this context, the most frequently reported types of survival are cancer (disease)-specific survival and overall survival. The later is an estimate of the probability of surviving all causes of death. Cancer-specific survival is the probability of surviving cancer in the absence of other causes of death. It is a measure that is not influenced by changes in mortality from other causes and, therefore, provides a useful measure for tracking survival across time and comparisons between racial/ethnic groups or between different registries. In addition, other types of survival, such as metastasis-free survival, are sometimes reported.

Similar to survival, the incidences of distant metastasis and local recurrence are also used as parameters to measure the efficiency of RP in terms of cancer control. The importance of these two parameters arises from the fact that they not only shorten survival but also affect the patient's quality of life following RP. Because local recurrence and distant metastasis may take a long time to occur following RP, other parameters have been used as "surrogates" for cancer control post-RP, especially in studies that have a short duration of postoperative follow-up. The two common parameters used in this regard are the status of the surgical margin and biochemical recurrence.

There are several definitions of positive surgical margin in the RP specimen. The details of these definitions are beyond the scope of this review; however, the majority of investigators define positive surgical margin as extension of the tumor to the inked surface of the resected specimen.[12–16] The status of the surgical margin has been shown to be a reliable predictor of cancer control. Indeed it is the only predictor that is influenced by the surgical technique, making it a very suitable parameter to report especially in comparative trials with a short duration of postoperative follow-up. Prostate cancer patients with positive surgical margins are more likely to progress biochemically,[12,13,17–20] locally,[13,18,20] and systematically,[13,18–20] which ultimately affects cancer-specific mortality. For example, Hull and colleagues have shown that the 10-year progression-free probability in margin-positive patients was 36%, compared to 80% in margin-negative cases.[21] Similar findings were also reported by Swindle and colleagues.[22] The 10-year prostate specific antigen (PSA) progression-free probability in margin-positive and margin-negative patients was 58% and 81%, respectively.

Biochemical recurrence is another important outcome measure of cancer control following RP and other interventional modalities. Following RP, the PSA level should become undetectable within 6 weeks after surgery, as its source of production is removed. Thus, a detectable PSA following RP indicates the presence of residual prostate tissue, local recurrence, or distant metastasis.[23] The PSA level that indicates disease recurrence after RP has been poorly defined.[24] In their recent review of the literature, the American Urological Association Prostate Cancer Guidelines Panel found more than 50 definitions of biochemical recurrence following RP.[25] There was a wide range of definitions with different values and patterns of PSA rise. The most common definition found was a PSA level of >0.2 ng/mL or a slight variation thereof. The panel acknowledged the need for a strict definition for biochemical recurrence to identify men at risk for disease progression and to allow meaningful comparisons among patients treated similarly. For the time being their recommended definition of biochemical recurrence is an initial serum PSA level of ≥ 0.2 ng/mL, with a second confirmatory level of PSA of >0.2 ng/mL. The first postoperative PSA should be obtained between 6 weeks and 3 months following therapy. The date of failure should be defined as the date of the first detectable PSA level once this value has been confirmed.

In addition to the actual occurrence of biochemical recurrence, the time to this biochemical recurrence has also been shown to correlate with the outcome following RP. In this regard, Pound and co-workers have shown that the time to development of distant metastasis and thus metastasis-free survival was dependent on the time of PSA elevation following RP.[26] For example, the actuarial likelihood of metastasis-free survival 10 years following PSA recurrence was 25% and 61% when the biochemical recurrence occurred ≤ 2 or >2 years following RP, respectively.

Obviously, in addition to the parameters just discussed, there are other prognostic factors that determine the cancer-control outcome following RP, such as preoperative PSA level, clinical stage, biopsy Gleason grade, pathologic stage (organ confined, extra capsular extension, and seminal vesicle and lymph nodes involvement), and Gleason score of the RP specimen.[21,27] However, these parameters are mainly determined by the inherent tumor characteristics and may not be very helpful in comparing the treatment efficacy of various treatment options and techniques.

Radical Prostatectomy for Localized Prostate Cancer

Localized prostate cancer constitutes the main indication for RP. However, patients with localized prostate cancer have other treatment options, which mainly include "watchful waiting," radiotherapy (external beam radiotherapy and brachytherapy), and other new therapeutic modalities, such as cryotherapy and HIFU (High Intensity Focused Ultrasound).

Therefore, the oncological outcome of RP is best studied by comparing the results of RP with those of other treatment options. However, a comparison between the cancer-control efficiency of RP and the new therapeutic modalities such as HIFU will not be provided in this review due to the lack of well-designed studies, as these modalities are still considered investigational by many urologists.

Unfortunately, there are very few well-designed randomized controlled studies that compare the oncological outcomes of the various treatment options of organ-confined prostate cancer. Indeed, there is only one randomized controlled study that compares the outcome of RP with "watchful waiting."[28] Fortunately, however, some large-scale comparative studies are ongoing. These include the Veterans Affairs Prostate Cancer Intervention versus Observation (PIVOT) trial, the recruitment of which will hopefully be completed in 2009. In addition, the ongoing U.K. Prostate Testing for Cancer and Treatment Study (Protect) will randomize men with prostate cancer to receive radiation, undergo RP, or remain in observation. Study accrual is estimated to be completed in 2008. Therefore, until the results of these and other randomized studies are available, retrospective observational, and especially case-matched, studies may provide insight into important clinical questions related to the cancer control of RP.

Radical Prostatectomy versus Watchful Waiting

There is a growing body of evidence to suggest a survival benefit with RP over "watchful waiting," at least in some patients. This is supported by the results of studies with different levels of evidence. For example, in a retrospective study, Tewari and colleagues studied the data of more than 3000 men, 75 years or younger, with biopsy-confirmed, clinically localized prostate cancer diagnosed between 1980 and 1997.[29] The patients were treated

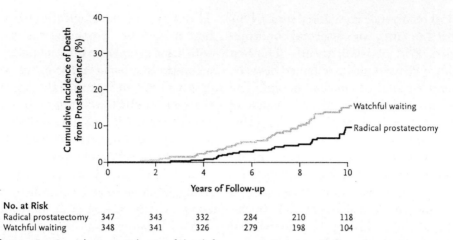

Figure 1. Cumulative incidence of death from prostate cancer in the radical prostatectomy and "watchful waiting" groups. Reproduced with permission from Bill-Axelson *et al.*[30]

either conservatively or with definitive treatment (RP or external beam radiotherapy). After adjusting for age, race, tumor grade, comorbid diseases, income status, and year of diagnosis, the overall survival rate at 15 years was 35% for conservative treatment compared to 65% for RP (adjusted relative risk of 0.4 for RP, $P < 0.001$).

The only randomized prospective study that compared RP with "watchful waiting" was reported by the Scandinavian Prostate Cancer Group, published initially in 2002[28] and later in 2005[30] with an additional 3 years of follow-up. This study, which deserves some detailed description, accrued 695 men from 14 centers from 1989 to 1999, included patients with clinical stage T1 or T2 prostate cancer, a PSA level of <50 ng/mL, and negative bone scans. The patients were randomly assigned to undergo either RP ($n = 347$) or watchful waiting ($n = 348$). Analysis was by "intention to treat," with a 5% cross-over in the RP group and a 10% cross-over in the "watchful waiting" group. During a median follow-up of 8.2 years, there were significant advantages in the RP group in terms of death from prostate cancer (30 versus 50 men, $P < 0.01$) (Fig. 1) and deaths from any cause (83 versus 106 men, $P < 0.04$). Importantly, although there was no difference in the incidence of distant metastases in the two groups during the first 5 years of follow-up, an addi-

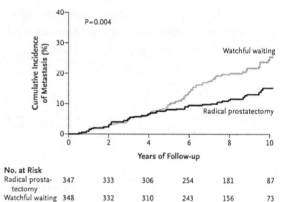

Figure 2. Cumulative incidence of metastasis from prostate cancer in the radical prostatectomy and "watchful waiting" groups. Reproduced with permission from Bill-Axelson *et al.*[30]

tional 3-year follow-up yielded an absolute risk reduction of 10% in favor of the RP group, with a relative risk of 0.60 (Fig. 2). Likewise, the difference in cumulative incidence of local progression, although statistically significant at 5 years of follow-up, increased markedly in the additional 3 years, with a relative risk of 0.33 in the RP group. Thus, this study has shown a better oncological outcome of RP over "watchful waiting" in terms of cancer-specific mortality, overall mortality, distant metastases, and local progression.

Whether older men would also benefit from RP is still not very clear, with different conclusions from various studies. In the Scandinavian

Prostate Cancer Group study, subgroup analysis revealed no significant advantage of RP in men older than 65 years.[30] The study, however, was not powered to analyze subgroups and the analysis was exploratory. The authors, thus, concluded that this result should be taken with caution before implementing it in clinical practice.

In an attempt to address this important gap in the current knowledge, Wong and colleagues have recently addressed this issue with a well-designed observational study with population-based linked data from the National Cancer Institute's Surveillance, Epidemiology, and End Results (SEER) program and Medicare.[31] The authors studied more than 40,000 men aged 65–80 years with organ-confined, well- or moderately differentiated prostate cancer. They found a significant survival advantage associated with RP (hazard ratio, 0.50; 95% CI 0.47–0.53). Because observational studies cannot completely adjust for potential selection bias and confounding, these results must be interpreted with caution. Therefore, and until a more clear-cut answer from a randomized study especially designed to address this issue, physicians should apply the above provocative findings judiciously and individualize treatment counseling according to each patient.

Radical Prostatectomy versus Radiotherapy

There is a lack of well-designed randomized controlled trials that compare RP with radiotherapy. Several problems could be encountered with head-to-head comparisons between the two treatment options. Among these is selection bias such that patients with more comorbidity are offered for radiotherapy rather than RP. In addition, radiotherapy series include patients who were treated with either adjuvant, neoadjuvant, or both therapies, making it difficult to make a direct comparison between radiotherapy with those different protocols and RP. Moreover, the exact definition of biochemical recurrence following RP and radiotherapy

are different and the implications of this difference is not fully understood. Finally, the introduction of the newer radiotherapy techniques, such as the conformal radiotherapy, as opposed to the traditional technique adds to the difficulty in comparing these techniques to RP.

In their retrospective review of men with localized prostate cancer, and after adjusting for age, race, tumor grade, comorbid disease, income status, and year of diagnosis, Tewari and colleagues reported a 92% 15-year prostate cancer–specific survival in RP patients compared to 87% in the group with external beam radiotherapy (relative risk ratio of cancer-specific mortality is 0.60, $P = 0.018$).[29] Despite the potential bias and other confounding factors in this retrospective study, it showed a slight but statistically significant advantage of RP over external beam radiotherapy. Whether this benefit is clinically relevant is unclear and certainly was not shown by other retrospective studies. For instance, Potters and colleagues reviewed a cohort of more than 1800 consecutively treated patients with clinical stage T1-T2 prostate cancer who received monotherapy treatment without additional adjuvant therapy.[32] After a median follow-up of 58 months, the freedom from biochemical recurrence was not different in patients who received external beam radiotherapy and those who underwent RP (77% versus 79%). Thus, and until the results of randomized studies are available, it appears that there is only little advantage, if any, of RP over external beam radiotherapy in localized prostate cancer.

Similar to external beam radiotherapy, there are no randomized controlled trials comparing brachytherapy with RP in terms of cancer-control efficiency. In the absence of such studies, clinically useful data can be obtained by comparing survival data in cohorts of men with comparable tumor characteristics treated with RP or brachytherapy during similar time periods. For example, Han and associates have reported their 15-year survival data for a group of more than 2400 men who underwent RP between 1982 and 1999.[27] Similarly, the

Northwest Hospital (Seattle) experience was reported with 12-year data for men undergoing brachytherapy.[33] In spite of the several caveats that must be considered when comparing these survival data reports, such as the difference between the definitions of the biochemical recurrence–free survival in surgical and radiation therapy series, it appears that the 10-year disease-free, biochemical recurrence–free survival is slightly different in the two series with a possible minimal advantage of RP (74% for RP and 60% for brachytherapy).

Comparative data regarding RP and brachytherapy come also from the few retrospective or nonrandomized trials in this field. Borchers and colleagues studied 132 patients with low-risk, clinically localized prostate cancer who were treated with either RP or ^{125}I-seed brachytherapy.[34] After a relatively short median follow-up of 27 months, there was a PSA relapse in 2 of the 80 patients in the RP group and 6 of the 52 patients who received brachytherapy (2.5% versus 11.5%, $P = 0.04$). Because of the small numbers of patients in each arm and the relatively short duration of follow-up, the results of this study must be interpreted with caution. Potters and colleagues, on the other hand, after a median follow-up of 58 months did not show any significant difference between the freedom from biochemical recurrence following either RP or brachytherapy (74% versus 79%, respectively).[32] Therefore, and from the available data, it appears that there is no strong evidence to suggest greater efficacy of RP over brachytherapy in terms of cancer control.

Radical Prostatectomy for Locally Advanced Prostate Cancer

Despite downward stage migration of prostate cancers in the PSA era,[35] there are still a significant number of men presenting with locally advanced disease.[36] As already discussed in this review, for patients with organ-confined prostate cancer, both surgery[37,38] and

radiation[39–41] monotherapies provide relatively excellent cancer control. However, high-risk tumor characteristics, such as clinical stage ≥T2b, PSA ≥10 ng/mL, or Gleason score 7–10 render patients at greater risk for local recurrence after definitive therapy and are associated with a greater risk of harboring occult metastasis.[37,38,42] Unfortunately, neither RP,[37,43] external beam radiotherapy,[40,44,45] nor brachytherapy[41,44–46] alone has shown excellent biochemical relapse–free survival in such patients. In an attempt to produce more promising cancer control for this population, various combination therapies have been developed. Such approaches include RP or radiotherapy combined with androgen deprivation, and external beam radiotherapy with brachytherapy boost. Although randomized comparisons of neoadjuvant androgen deprivation plus RP to RP alone have produced a reduced likelihood of positive margins with the use of androgen deprivation, these trials have not demonstrated improved disease-specific survival with neoadjuvant androgen deprivation plus RP.[47,48] However, neoadjuvant and adjuvant androgen deprivation in the context of external beam radiotherapy have been shown to improve disease-specific survival in men with high-risk prostate cancer.[49–52] Similar survival rates have been published for multimodality radiotherapy protocols with and without neoadjuvant androgen deprivation.[41,53,54] In this review, a trial to compare RP and various radiotherapy techniques with or without androgen deprivation therapy will be attempted.

Unfortunately, there are very few randomized studies with long-term follow-up to address this issue. The randomized trial by Akakura and co-workers[55] was designed to compare RP combined with pelvic lymph node dissection versus external beam radiotherapy in patients with stage B2 and C prostate cancer. Both neoadjuvant and adjuvant androgen deprivation were used in both groups. The median follow-up period was 58 months, and survival analysis revealed progression-free survival rates of 91% in the RP group versus 81% in the external beam radiotherapy ($P = 0.044$). This study, however, was limited by small sample size (a total of 95 patients in both groups). Thus, caution must be taken in interpreting the results of this study.

A larger, retrospective, multi-institutional comparison of RP, external beam radiotherapy, and brachytherapy was reported by D'Amico and colleagues.[44] The patients were stratified into low, intermediate, or high risk for post-therapy PSA failure based on pretreatment PSA level, biopsy Gleason score, and clinical stage. In the high-risk cohort (stage T2c, PSA >20 ng/mL, or Gleason ≥8), the relative risk of PSA recurrence of various treatment options compared to RP were as follows: external beam radiotherapy (0.9, $P = 0.26$), brachytherapy alone (3.0, $P = 0.0002$), and brachytherapy plus androgen deprivation therapy (2.2, $P = 0.02$). Therefore, this study has clearly shown an oncological advantage of RP over brachytherapy with or without androgen deprivation in high-risk patients. This study, however, did not address some treatment options, such as combination therapy using external beam radiotherapy plus brachytherapy boost, which may have greater efficacy than either modality alone in high-risk patients.[56,57] Furthermore, this study reported radiotherapy techniques that are no longer state of the art in both technique and dose. Finally, no matching of clinical, pathologic, or biochemical features between patients was performed.

In a trial to address this issue, Fletcher and colleagues have recently reported on case-matched retrospective analysis of data from 409 men with PSA ≥10, Gleason score 7–10, or stage ≥T2b cancer treated uniformly at one institute between March 1988 and December 2000.[58] Patients had undergone RP, brachytherapy implant alone, or external beam radiotherapy with brachytherapy boost with short-term neoadjuvant and adjuvant androgen deprivation therapy. Estimated 4-year biochemical relapse–free survival rates were superior for patients treated with external beam radiotherapy with brachytherapy boost with short-term neoadjuvant and adjuvant androgen deprivation therapy (72%) when compared to brachytherapy implant alone (25%) and RP (53%), ($P < 0.001$). Matched analysis confirmed these results.

Collectively, these data suggest a survival benefit for a combination of external beam radiotherapy, brachytherapy, and neoadjuvant and adjuvant androgen deprivation over RP. However, there appears to be no advantage of either external beam radiotherapy or brachytherapy with or without androgen deprivation over RP. In fact, as demonstrated above, there may be some survival advantage of RP over the latter two treatment modalities.

Oncological Outcome of Various Techniques of Radical Prostatectomy

All available surgical techniques of RP share the common goal of curing the patient by removing the prostate gland and seminal vesicles—and sometimes the pelvic lymph nodes—while at the same time preserving continence and sexual function.[59,60] They differ primarily in the extent of invasiveness. Of the two open surgical approaches, namely retropubic RP and perineal RP, the perineal approach is considered less invasive than the retropubic approach, although it is less widely used.[61]

Since 1997, a minimally invasive approach has been available in the form of laparoscopic RP, and more recently surgical robotic systems have been used as an additional tool for laparoscopic RP. Like all minimally invasive approaches, laparoscopic RP is expected to decrease patient blood loss and postoperative recovery time. In theory, laparoscopic approaches should provide improved visualization of the pelvic anatomy with possibly better preservation of anatomical structures, which could lead to improvements in continence and potency. It is also accepted that the laparoscopic approaches are technically difficult with a significant learning curve, and uncertainty exists regarding the number of procedures required to achieve acceptable competence in the procedure.[60,62–65]

Regardless of the technical details of these approaches, which are beyond the scope of this review, there appear to be no well-designed randomized controlled trials to compare between these various approaches in terms of cancer control. Any comparison between the various techniques is potentially confounded by several factors including the fact that both pure laparoscopic and robot-assisted RP are relatively new techniques with a lack of long-term follow-up. In addition, and as with all other newly developed techniques, there is always exceptional physicians' enthusiasm and selection bias such that healthier and more enthusiastic patients are usually chosen for these techniques, at least in the early phase. Furthermore, the newer laparoscopic techniques tend to have long learning curves, with earlier results showing less efficacy. Nonetheless, there are several nonrandomized studies that compare the various techniques. However, the vast majority of these studies have small numbers of patients in each arm with relatively short-term follow-up.

In an attempt to compare open retropubic RP with perineal RP, Lance and colleagues reported on a retrospective review of 190 patients who were matched by race, preoperative PSA level, clinical stage, and biopsy Gleason score to eliminate selection bias as much as possible.[66] The patients were operated upon in the same center. There were no significant differences in the margin-positive (39% versus 43%) or biochemical recurrence rates (12.9% versus 17.6%) at a mean follow-up of 47.1 versus 42.9 months, respectively. Similar findings were obtained by Korman and associates in their retrospective study of 60 patients who underwent retropubic RP and 40 patients who underwent perineal RP by the same surgeon.[67] The two groups had comparable clinical stage and Gleason grades. Although, there was no long-term follow-up, there was no significant difference in the positive margin rate in the retropubic and perineal procedures (16% and

22%, $P = 0.53$). Other studies have shown similar results.[68] Therefore, it can be concluded that both approaches of open RP result in similar oncological outcomes.

Similar to the open approaches, the various approaches and techniques of laparoscopic RP appear to have similar cancer-control efficacy. In their recent review, Tooher and co-workers reviewed the literature in this regard up to December 2004.[69] They identified nine studies, none of which was randomized and controlled, comparing different laparoscopic approaches with a total of 1148 patients. For example, when comparing transperitoneal laparoscopic RP with extraperitoneal laparoscopic RP, the rates of positive margin were 15–23% (median 20) versus 10–30% (median 16), respectively. The recurrence-free survival in the two approaches was also found to be comparable, ranging from 97% to 100% in all the studies, taking into consideration the relatively short and variable duration of follow-up. The comparison between the pure laparoscopic and the robot-assisted technique also revealed comparable outcomes. The rates of positive surgical margin were 25 (all studies) versus 6–25 (median 17.5), respectively. The recurrence-free survival was found to be 95% for transperitoneal pure laparoscopic RP and 98% for robot-assisted RP.

In the same review, Tooher and co-workers[69] found that various laparoscopic approaches of RP have similar oncological outcomes to the open RP. For example, the rates of positive surgical margin in the transperitoneal laparoscopic RP were 11–50% (median 23) compared to 20–34% (median 29) for retropubic open RP. In the two studies that compared the two techniques, recurrence-free survival rates were 84% and 99% in the transperitoneal laparoscopic RP versus 75% and 97% in the open retropubic RP.

More recent studies confirmed the findings of Tooher and associates. For instance, Dahl and colleagues compared the clinicopathologic data of 286 men who had laparoscopic RP with those of 714 men who underwent open

RP performed at the same institute from 2001 to 2005.[70] The rates of positive surgical margin were 15.0% and 17.4%, respectively. The two groups had a comparable mean age, mean preoperative PSA, clinical stage, biopsy and RP specimen Gleason score, average prostate weight, and pathologic stage.

In conclusion, there is a paucity of randomized controlled trials that compare the oncological outcomes of RP versus other treatment options or outcomes of various approaches and techniques of RP. For localized prostate cancer, the available data suggests some degree of "superiority" of RP over "watchful waiting." The "superiority" of RP over radiotherapy, especially external beam radiotherapy, in some studies is yet to be proven by well-designed randomized controlled trials. Moreover, it appears that the various approaches and techniques of RP result in similar oncological outcomes. Therefore, the final treatment choice of patients with early prostate cancer should also depend on treatment complications or side effects, the patient's preferences, the surgeon's experience, and treatment availability in that particular setting.

For locally advanced prostate cancer, available studies suggest a survival benefit for a combination of external beam radiotherapy, brachytherapy, and neoadjuvant and adjuvant hormone ablation over RP. However, there appears to be no advantage of either external beam radiotherapy or brachytherapy with or without hormone ablation over RP. In fact, there may be some survival advantage of RP over the latter two treatment modalities.

Conflicts of Interest

The author declares no conflicts of interest.

References

1. Young, H. 1905. The early diagnosis and radical cure of carcinoma of the prostate. Being a study of 40 cases and presentation of a radical operation which was carried out in four cases. *Johns Hopkins Hosp. Bull.* **16:** 315.

2. Belt, E.E., C.E. Ebert & A.C. Surber Jr. 1939. A new approach in perineal prostatectomy. *J. Urol.* **41:** 482–497.

3. Millin, T. 2002. Retropubic prostatectomy: a new extravesical technique report on 20 cases. 1945. *J. Urol.* **167**(2 pt 2): 976–979.

4. Memmelaar, J. 1949. Total prostatovesiculectomy: Retropubic approach. *J. Urol.* **62**(3): 340–348.

5. Walsh, P.C. & P.J. Donker. 1982. Impotence following radical prostatectomy: insight into etiology and prevention. *J. Urol.* **128:** 492–497.

6. Walsh, P.C., H. Lepor & J.C. Eggleston. 1983. Radical prostatectomy with preservation of sexual function: anatomical and pathological considerations. *Prostate.* **4:** 473–485.

7. Schuessler, W.W. *et al.* 1997. Laparoscopic radical prostatectomy: initial short-term experience. *Urology* **50:** 854–857.

8. Guillonneau, B. *et al.* 1999. Laparoscopic radical prostatectomy: technical and early oncological assessment of 40 operations. *Eur. Urol.* **36:** 14–20.

9. Bollens, R. *et al.* 2001. Extraperitoneal laparoscopic radical prostatectomy. Results after 50 cases. *Eur. Urol.* **40:** 65–69.

10. Abbou, C.C. *et al.* 2000. [Remote laparoscopic radical prostatectomy carried out with a robot. Report of a case]. *Prog. Urol.* **10:** 520–523.

11. Menon, M. 2007. American Urological Association (AUA) lecture: The future of robotics in Urology. *Presented at the 22nd Annual Congress of the European Association of Urology.* Berlin, March 23.

12. Watson, R.B., F. Civantos & M.S. Soloway. 1996. Positive surgical margins with radical prostatectomy: detailed pathological analysis and prognosis. *Urology* **48:** 80–90.

13. Paulson, D.F. 1994. Impact of radical prostatectomy in the management of clinically localized disease. *J. Urol.* **152**(5 Pt 2): 1826–1830.

14. Ackerman, D.A. *et al.* 1993. Analysis of risk factors associated with prostate cancer extension to the surgical margin and pelvic node metastasis at radical prostatectomy. *J. Urol.* **150:** 1845–1850.

15. Ohori, M. *et al.* 1995. Prognostic significance of positive surgical margins in radical prostatectomy specimens. *J. Urol.* **154:** 1818–1824.

16. Wieder, J.A. & M.S. Soloway. 1998. Incidence, etiology, location, prevention and treatment of positive surgical margins after radical prostatectomy for prostate cancer. *J. Urol.* **160:** 299–315.

17. Smith, R.C. *et al.* 1996. Extended followup of the influence of wide excision of the neurovascular bundle(s) on prognosis in men with clinically localized prostate cancer and extensive capsular

perforation. *J. Urol.* **156**(2 Pt 1): 454–457; discussion 457–8.

18. Epstein, J.I., G. Pizov & P.C. Walsh. 1993. Correlation of pathologic findings with progression after radical retropubic prostatectomy. *Cancer* **71:** 3582–3593.

19. Paulson, D.F. *et al.* 1986. Radical prostatectomy: anatomical predictors of success or failure. *J. Urol.* **136:** 1041–1043.

20. Catalona, W.J. & D.S. Smith. 1994. 5-year tumor recurrence rates after anatomical radical retropubic prostatectomy for prostate cancer. *J. Urol.* **152**(5 Pt 2): 1837–1842.

21. Hull, G.W. *et al.* 2002. Cancer control with radical prostatectomy alone in 1,000 consecutive patients. *J. Urol.* **167**(2 Pt 1): 528–534.

22. Swindle, P. *et al.* 2005. Do margins matter? The prognostic significance of positive surgical margins in radical prostatectomy specimens. *J. Urol.* **174:** 903–907.

23. Moul, J.W. 2000. Prostate specific antigen only progression of prostate cancer. *J. Urol.* **163:** 1632–1642.

24. Amling, C.L. *et al.* 2001. Defining prostate specific antigen progression after radical prostatectomy: what is the most appropriate cut point? *J. Urol.* **165:** 1146–1151.

25. Cookson, M.S. *et al.* 2007. Variation in the definition of biochemical recurrence in patients treated for localized prostate cancer: the American Urological Association Prostate Guidelines for Localized Prostate Cancer Update Panel report and recommendations for a standard in the reporting of surgical outcomes. *J. Urol.* **177:** 540–545.

26. Pound, C.R. *et al.* 1999. Natural history of progression after PSA elevation following radical prostatectomy. *JAMA* **281:** 1591–1597.

27. Han, M. *et al.* 2001. Long-term biochemical disease-free and cancer-specific survival following anatomic radical retropubic prostatectomy. The 15-year Johns Hopkins experience. *Urol. Clin. North Am.* **28:** 555–565.

28. Holmberg, L. *et al.* 2002. A randomized trial comparing radical prostatectomy with watchful waiting in early prostate cancer. *N. Engl. J. Med.* **347:** 781–799.

29. Tewari, A. *et al.* 2006. Long-term survival probability in men with clinically localized prostate cancer treated either conservatively or with definitive treatment (radiotherapy or radical prostatectomy). *Urology* **68:** 1268–1274.

30. Bill-Axelson, A. *et al.* 2005. Radical prostatectomy versus watchful waiting in early prostate cancer. *N. Engl. J. Med.* **352:** 1977–1984.

31. Wong, Y.N. *et al.* 2006. Survival associated with treatment vs observation of localized prostate cancer in elderly men. *JAMA* **296:** 2683–2693.

32. Potters, L. *et al.* 2004. Monotherapy for stage T1-T2 prostate cancer: radical prostatectomy, external beam radiotherapy, or permanent seed implantation. *Radiother Oncol.* **71:** 29–33.

33. Korb, L.J. & M.K. Brawer. 2001. Modern brachytherapy for localized prostate cancers: the Northwest Hospital (Seattle) experience. *Rev. Urol.* **3:** 51–62.

34. Borchers, H. *et al.* 2004. Permanent I^{125}-seed brachytherapy or radical prostatectomy: a prospective comparison considering oncological and quality of life results. *BJU Int.* **94:** 805–811.

35. Noldus, J. *et al.* 2000. Stage migration in clinically localized prostate cancer. *Eur. Urol.* **38:** 74–78.

36. Meng, M.V. *et al.* 2005. Treatment of patients with high risk localized prostate cancer: results from cancer of the prostate strategic urological research endeavor (CaPSURE). *J. Urol.* **173:** 1557–1561.

37. Catalona, W.J. & D.S. Smith. 1998. Cancer recurrence and survival rates after anatomic radical retropubic prostatectomy for prostate cancer: intermediate-term results. *J. Urol.* **160**(6 Pt 2): 2428–2434.

38. Walsh, P.C. 2000. Radical prostatectomy for localized prostate cancer provides durable cancer control with excellent quality of life: a structured debate. *J. Urol.* **163:** 1802–1807.

39. Blasko, J.C. *et al.* 2000. Palladium-^{103} brachytherapy for prostate carcinoma. *Int J. Radiat. Oncol. Biol. Phys.* **46:** 839–850.

40. Pollack, A. *et al.* 2002. Prostate cancer radiation dose response: results of the M. D. Anderson phase III randomized trial. *Int. J. Radiat. Oncol. Biol. Phys.* **53:** 1097–1105.

41. Ragde, H. *et al.* 2000. Modern prostate brachytherapy. Prostate specific antigen results in 219 patients with up to 12 years of observed follow-up. *Cancer* **89:** 135–141.

42. Partin, A.W. *et al.* 2001. Contemporary update of prostate cancer staging nomograms (Partin Tables) for the new millennium. *Urology* **58:** 843–848.

43. Cheng, W.S. *et al.* 1993. Radical prostatectomy for pathologic stage C prostate cancer: influence of pathologic variables and adjuvant treatment on disease outcome. *Urology* **42:** 283–291.

44. D'Amico, A.V. *et al.* 1998. Biochemical outcome after radical prostatectomy, external beam radiation therapy, or interstitial radiation therapy for clinically localized prostate cancer. *JAMA* **280:** 969–974.

45. Zelefsky, M.J. *et al.* 1999. Comparison of the 5-year outcome and morbidity of three-dimensional conformal radiotherapy versus transperineal permanent iodine-125 implantation for early-stage prostatic cancer. *J. Clin. Oncol.* **17:** 517–522.

46. Stone, N.N. & R.G. Stock. 1999. Prostate brachytherapy: treatment strategies. *J. Urol.* **162:** 421–426.

47. Soloway, M.S. *et al.* 2002. Neoadjuvant androgen ablation before radical prostatectomy in cT2bNxMo prostate cancer: 5-year results. *J. Urol.* **167:** 112–116.

48. Klotz, L.H. *et al.* 2003. Long-term followup of a randomized trial of 0 versus 3 months of neoadjuvant androgen ablation before radical prostatectomy. *J. Urol.* **170:** 791–794.

49. Laverdiere, J. *et al.* 1997. Beneficial effect of combination hormonal therapy administered prior and following external beam radiation therapy in localized prostate cancer. *Int. J. Radiat. Oncol. Biol. Phys.* **37:** 247–252.

50. Pilepich, M.V. *et al.* 1997. Phase III trial of androgen suppression using goserelin in unfavorable-prognosis carcinoma of the prostate treated with definitive radiotherapy: report of Radiation Therapy Oncology Group Protocol 85-31. *J. Clin. Oncol.* **15:** 1013–1021.

51. Pilepich, M.V. *et al.* 2005. Androgen suppression adjuvant to definitive radiotherapy in prostate carcinoma—long-term results of phase III RTOG 85-31. *Int. J. Radiat. Oncol. Biol. Phys.* **61:** 1285–1290.

52. Bolla, M. *et al.* 1997. Improved survival in patients with locally advanced prostate cancer treated with radiotherapy and goserelin. *N Engl. J. Med.* **337:** 295–300.

53. Coblentz, T.R. *et al.* 2002. Multimodality radiotherapy and androgen ablation in the treatment of clinically localized prostate cancer: early results in high risk patients. *Prostate Cancer Prostatic Dis.* **5:** 219–225.

54. Copp, H., E.A. Bissonette & D. Theodorescu. 2005. Tumor control outcomes of patients treated with trimodality therapy for locally advanced prostate cancer. *Urology* **65:** 1146–1151.

55. Akakura, K. *et al.* 1999. Long-term results of a randomized trial for the treatment of Stages B2 and C prostate cancer: radical prostatectomy versus external beam radiation therapy with a common endocrine therapy in both modalities. *Urology* **54:** 313–318.

56. Dattoli, M. *et al.* 1996. 103Pd brachytherapy and external beam irradiation for clinically localized, high-risk prostatic carcinoma. *Int. J. Radiat. Oncol. Biol. Phys.* **35:** 875–879.

57. Sylvester, J.E. *et al.* 2003. Ten-year biochemical relapse-free survival after external beam radiation and brachytherapy for localized prostate cancer: the Seattle experience. *Int. J. Radiat. Oncol. Biol. Phys.* **57:** 944–952.

58. Fletcher, S.G. *et al.* 2006. Case-matched comparison of contemporary radiation therapy to surgery in patients with locally advanced prostate cancer. *Int. J. Radiat. Oncol. Biol. Phys.* **66:** 1092–1099.

59. Richie, J.P. 1997. Localized prostate cancer: overview of surgical management. *Urology* **49**(3A Suppl): 335–357.

60. Hasan, W.A. & I.S. Gill. 2004. Laparoscopic radical prostatectomy: current status. *BJU Int.* **94:** 7–11.

61. Salomon, L. *et al.* 2004. Open versus laparoscopic radical prostatectomy: part I. *BJU Int.* **94:** 238–243.

62. Salomon, L. *et al.* 2004. Open versus laparoscopic radical prostatectomy: Part II. *BJU Int.* **94:** 244–250.

63. Rassweiler, J. *et al.* 2001. Laparoscopic radical prostatectomy with the Heilbronn technique: an analysis of the first 180 cases. *J. Urol.* **166:** 2101–2108.

64. Stolzenburg, J.U. & M.C. Truss. 2003. Technique of laparoscopic (endoscopic) radical prostatectomy. *BJU Int.* **91:** 749–757.

65. Link, R.E. *et al.* 2004. Making ends meet: a cost comparison of laparoscopic and open radical retropubic prostatectomy. *J. Urol.* **172:** 269–274.

66. Lance, R.S. *et al.* 2001. A comparison of radical retropubic with perineal prostatectomy for localized prostate cancer within the Uniformed Services Urology Research Group. *BJU Int.* **87:** 61–65.

67. Korman, H.J. *et al.* 2002. A centralized comparison of radical perineal and retropubic prostatectomy specimens: is there a difference according to the surgical approach? *J. Urol.* **168:** 991–994.

68. Frank, I. & R. Parra. 2002. Radical perineal prostatectomy: an update. *AUA Update Series* **21:** 18.

69. Tooher, R. *et al.* 2006. Laparoscopic radical prostatectomy for localized prostate cancer: a systematic review of comparative studies. *J. Urol.* **175:** 2011–2017.

70. Dahl, D.M. *et al.* 2006. Pathologic outcome of laparoscopic and open radical prostatectomy. *Urology* **68:** 1253–1256.

Cancer Pain and Analgesia

Paul J. Christo and Danesh Mazloomdoost

*Department of Anesthesiology & Critical Care Medicine, Division of Pain Medicine,
The Johns Hopkins University School of Medicine, Baltimore, Maryland, USA*

Pain ranges in prevalence from 14–100% among cancer patients and occurs in 50–70% of those in active treatment. Cancer pain may result from direct invasion of tumor into nerves, bones, soft tissue, ligaments, and fascia, and may induce visceral pain through distension and obstruction. Cancer pain is multifaceted. Clinicians may describe cancer pain as acute, chronic, nociceptive (somatic), visceral, or neuropathic. Despite implementation of the WHO guidelines, reports of undertreatment of cancer pain persist in various clinical settings and in spite of decades of work to reduce unnecessary discomfort. Substantial obstacles to adequate pain relief with opioids include specific concerns of patients themselves, their family members, physicians, nurses, and the healthcare system. The WHO analgesic ladder serves as the mainstay of treatment for the relief of cancer pain in concert with tumoricidal, surgical, interventional, radiotherapeutic, psychological, and rehabilitative modalities. This multidimensional approach offers the greatest potential for maximizing analgesia and minimizing adverse effects. Primary therapies are directed at the source of the cancer pain and may enhance a patient's function, longevity, and comfort. Adjuvant therapies include nonopioids that confer analgesic effects in certain medical conditions but primarily treat conditions that do not involve pain. Nonopioid medications (over-the-counter agents) are useful in the management of mild to moderate pain, and their continuation through step 3 of the WHO ladder is an option after weighing a drug's risks and benefits in individual patients. Symptomatic treatment of severe cancer pain should begin with an opioid, regardless of the mechanism of the pain. They are very effective analgesics, titrate easily, and offer a favorable risk/benefit ratio. Cancer pain remains inadequately controlled despite the diagnostic and therapeutic means of ensuring that patients feel comfortable during their illness. Therefore, all practitioners need to make control of cancer pain a professional duty, even if they can only use the most basic and least expensive analgesic medications, such as morphine, codeine, and acetaminophen, to reduce human suffering.

Key words: cancer; pain; analgesia; opioids; addiction; barriers to pain relief; cancer pain; adjuvant therapies; nonopioid therapies; co-analgesics; malignancy; therapies; WHO 3-step analgesic ladder

Scope of the Problem

Pain ranges in prevalence from 14–100% among cancer patients[1] and occurs in 50–70% of those in active treatment.[2] The literature reports pain figures as high as 60–90% for patients with advanced stages of cancer.[2–4] Two-thirds of this pain in advanced disease is due to tumor infiltration, and almost one-fourth is a consequence of cancer treatments. No cures exist for many patients with advanced systemic cancers; yet, pain therapies do exist that can ease the suffering related to an individual's course of illness. This knowledge is critically important to communicate given that patients with advanced cancer commonly experience and fear pain. The World Health Organization (WHO) recognized the global need

Address for correspondence: Paul J. Christo, M.D., M.B.A., Assistant Professor, Director, Multidisciplinary Pain Fellowship Director, Pain Treatment Center, Department of Anesthesiology & Critical Care Medicine, Division of Pain Medicine, The Johns Hopkins University School of Medicine, 550 N. Broadway, Suite 301, Baltimore, MD 21205. Voice: +410-955-1818; fax: +410-502-6730. pchristo@jhmi.edu

Ann. N.Y. Acad. Sci. 1138: 278–298 (2008). © 2008 New York Academy of Sciences.
doi: 10.1196/annals.1414.033

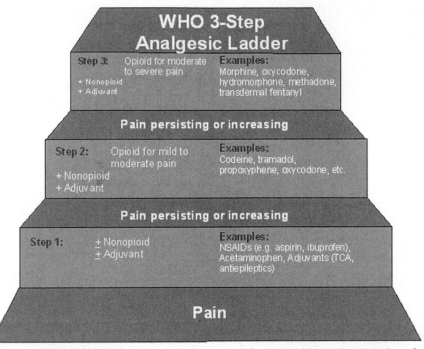

Figure 1. World Health Organization 3-Step Analgesic Ladder with examples of analgesics. Adapted from Management of Cancer Pain: Clinical Practice Guideline Number 9. Rockville, MD: U.S. Department of Health and Human Services; 1994, AHCPR Pub No. 94-0592.

to establish guidelines for basic pain control in cancer patients and thereby developed an elemental "3-step analgesic ladder" in 1986 for use among practitioners.[5] The WHO made an important step in disseminating critical concepts of pain management through education and opioid availability. Increasingly, patients, healthcare providers, and healthcare accreditation bodies are demanding greater attention to the burden of pain and, in particular, cancer-related pain. However, despite application of the WHO "3-step analgesic ladder" (Fig. 1), advancing pain research, and expansive interventional modalities, as many as 50% of cancer patients with pain may remain undertreated.[6] In response to the significant problem of unrelieved pain in cancer and other disease states, the Joint Commission on Accreditation of Health Organizations, an independent, nonprofit organization that evaluates and accredits healthcare organizations in the United States, created comprehensive standards for pain management in 1999. Health-

care institutions must fulfill these standards in order to meet the requirements for reaccreditation. Perhaps this initiative will move clinicians closer to the overarching goal that, "no cancer patient should live or die with unrelieved pain."[7]

The following review will discuss important principles of managing pain in malignant disease. Concepts relating to the sources of pain in cancer, types of pain in cancer, barriers to effective pain control, measuring pain in cancer patients, and pharmacotherapeutic approaches to pain control will be discussed.

Sources of Cancer Pain

Cancer pain may result from direct invasion of tumor into nerves, bones, soft tissue, ligaments, and fascia, and may induce visceral pain through distension and obstruction (Table 1). While over two-thirds of cancer pain usually results from the tumor burden, a quarter of pain experienced by cancer

TABLE 1. Sources of Cancer Pain

Direct invasion
   Bone
   Soft tissue
   Nerves
   Ligaments
   Fascia
Metastases
Treatment side effects
   Surgery
   Radiation
   Chemotherapy

TABLE 2. Types of Cancer Pain

Examples of neuropathic pain
   Tumor compression of plexi
   Tumor invasion into nerves
   Tumor invasion into spinal cord
   Chemotherapy-induced neuritis
   Radiation-induced nerve injury
Examples of somatic/nociceptive pain
   Tumor invasion into bone
   Pathologic fracture
   Postsurgical pain
Examples of visceral pain
   Tumor invasion into organs
   Obstruction (e.g., biliary, intestinal)
   Organ rupture (e.g., bowel, bladder)

patients can be attributed to the cancer-related treatments.[3] For instance, surgery, radiation, and chemotherapeutics may all elicit acute pain that diminishes in time, while other therapies may cause chronic pain conditions.[8] Radiation treatment frequently causes acute muscle stiffness and aching, but carries the risk of chronic pain secondary to nerve injury, chronic inflammation, osteoradionecrosis, or myofascial injury. Surgery-associated pain may result from direct nerve injury, inflammation, postamputation phantom pain conditions, and even the development of Complex Regional Pain Syndrome. Many chemotherapeutic agents are known to cause pain. Several classes, such as the alkaloids, platinum-based compounds, and the antimitotics, are known to contribute to peripheral neuropathies.

Types of Pain

Cancer pain is multifaceted, as illustrated in Table 2. Clinicians may describe cancer pain as acute, chronic, nociceptive (somatic), visceral, or neuropathic. Alternatively, some have proposed just three prime categories of cancer pain: nociceptive, neuropathic, and psychogenic.[9] Furthermore, multiple taxonomies of pain exist including a research-oriented and treatment-oriented classification of pain that groups together patients with similar pain mechanisms.[10] Clearly, no individual classification is optimal in truly capturing the multidimensional phenomenon of cancer pain. Clin-

ically, patients experience pain with varying degrees of intensity, frequency, anatomic location, duration, and body system involvement. Further, they may describe features of both nociceptive and neuropathic pain rather than distinctive elements of a single process. It is instructive, nevertheless to understand common terminology often applied to cancer pain. For instance, nociceptive pain arises from activation of nociceptors (free nerve terminals of primary afferent fibers that respond to painful stimuli) that are located in all tissues except the central nervous system. Neuropathic pain results from a primary lesion or dysfunction in the central or peripheral nervous system.[11] The following terms help distinguish varying physiological types of cancer pain.[12]

> **Nociceptive pain**—associated with tissue injury from surgery, trauma, inflammation, or tumor. The pain is caused by stimulation of pain receptors in cutaneous and deeper musculoskeletal structures. It is often proportional to the degree of nociceptor activation. Both somatic and visceral pain conditions may be characterized as nociceptive.
> **Somatic pain**—arising from direct injury to bones, tissue, or tendons. Some consider somatic and nociceptive pain to be synonymous. Somatic pain is described as aching or dull and sometimes stabbing.

It tends to be very focal. This category often includes metastatic bone pain, postsurgical incisional pain, and musculoskeletal inflammation and spasm.

Visceral pain—arising from organ damage or tumor infiltration, compression, or distortion of organs within the pelvis, abdomen, or thorax. It is described as a pressure-like sensation, internal squeezing, or crampiness. It tends to be vague and diffuse and may be associated with distension/stretching of organs, nausea, vomiting, and sweating. The pain may be referred to superficial locations that are distant from the affected organ.

Neuropathic pain—may be directly related to the malignant disease, such as tumor infiltration of peripheral nerves, plexi, roots, or spinal cord. It may arise from efforts to treat the disease, such as surgery, chemotherapy, or other drug-induced neuropathy or neuritis, and even from radiation-induced injury to peripheral nerves and the spinal cord. This type of pain is invariably associated with sensory changes caused by injury to the central or peripheral nervous system and may be incompletely responsive to opioid therapy. Patients typically describe this pain as burning, shooting, pins/needles, electrical, or numbness, and it tends to radiate over dermatomal distributions.

Barriers to Treating Pain

Despite implementation of the WHO guidelines and in spite of decades of work to reduce unnecessary discomfort, reports of undertreatment of cancer pain persist in various clinical settings.[13] Substantial obstacles to adequate pain relief with opioids include specific concerns of patients themselves, their family members, physicians, nurses, and the healthcare system.[14–17] Many of these barriers focus on psychosocial factors related to the fear of opioid addiction and physical dependence, concerns about adverse effects of medications, and patient fears of disappointing their physician by reporting pain.[18–20] Healthcare providers, patients, and their families report distinct but sometimes overlapping concerns.

Healthcare Providers as Barriers to Pain Relief

Physicians are often reluctant to prescribe opioids and nurses may express concern about administering opioids to patients. Physicians tend to feel that managing pain with opioids and other controlled substances leads to documentation woes, entails frequent prescription refills, requires onerous telephone calls, and exposes themselves to intense regulatory scrutiny.[21] Moreover, many healthcare professionals still lack appropriate knowledge of analgesic (primarily opioid) pharmacology with respect to dosing, timing, alternative routes of administration (such as rectal, subcutaneous, epidural, intrathecal), and converting from intravenous to oral therapies. Coupled with an over-exuberant fear of respiratory compromise and a pervasive fear of addiction, physicians and other healthcare providers leave many patients inadequately treated.

While understandable, fears of opioid adverse effects and complications related to respiratory depression need not paralyze practitioners from prescribing opioids. Opioids do affect both the rate and depth of respiration. Data from studies on mice indicate that both the analgesic and respiratory depressive features of morphine are linked to the mu opioid receptor[22,23] in a dose-dependent fashion (that is, increasing the dose produces greater analgesia and greater depression of respiration). A recent acute-pain study in healthy human volunteers shows similar effects and notes that respiratory depression is possible irrespective of concomitant severe pain.[24] In contrast, many clinicians find that respiratory depression rarely precedes analgesia when administering opioids to relieve chronic pain. That is, physicians treating chronic pain patients with opioids report that patients typically feel comfortable before experiencing respiratory compromise. This clinical phenomenon provides some comfort in escalating doses of opioids in patients who continue to experience pain. Further, cancer pain may in fact more accurately mimic chronic rather than acute pain models, thereby attenuating the risk of respiratory depression in this population. Nonetheless, serious adverse effects can be mitigated by attention to dosing, frequency of dosing, duration of pain (periodic or constant), co-administration of psychoactive substances (such as benzodiazepines, barbiturates, alcohol, other opioids), and proper supervision of patients on chronic opioid therapy. Practitioners can safely tailor opioid therapy in cancer patients by considering the delicate balance between depression of respiration (from factors such as opioid therapy, sleep deprivation, and sedation from co-administered sedatives) and stimulation of respiration (from pain, arousal, stress, anxiety, inflammation, and other causes).

A myriad of healthcare providers use the risk of opioid addiction as justification for minimizing or withholding appropriate opioid therapy. Three medical societies (The American Society of Addiction Medicine, The American Pain Society, and The American Academy of Pain Medicine) define addiction as "a primary, chronic, neurobiological disease, with genetic, psychosocial, and environmental factors influencing the development and manifestations. It is characterized by behaviors that include one of more of the following: impaired control over drug use, compulsive use, continued use despite harm, and craving."[25] In the context of treating patients in chronic pain with opioids, addiction may be viewed as a combination of observations that suggest maladaptive behaviors rather than pharmacologic phenomena, such as tolerance, physical dependence, and dose escalation. These latter conditions are expected to occur during the course of pain treatment. Accordingly, addiction may be more specifically defined in patients on chronic opioid therapy as a series of behavioral observations that suggest: adverse consequences due to the use of

TABLE 3. Warning Signs of Addiction among Patients Treated with Opioids

Apathy to adverse consequences
Loss of control
Preoccupation with opioids despite psychological dependence
Aberrant drug-related behaviors
Manipulation of healthcare provider
Seeking drugs from other providers
Use of unsanctioned drugs

drugs, loss of control over drug use, preoccupation with obtaining opioids despite the presence of adequate analgesia, evidence of psychological dependence, and demonstration of aberrant drug-related behaviors, such as obtaining additional drug by manipulating the treating physician or medical system, procuring drugs from other medical or nonmedical sources, and use of unsanctioned drugs during opioid therapy (see Table 3).[26,27]

Regrettably, overestimation of addiction in cancer patients treated with opioids has led to widespread undertreatment of pain in this population.[28] Unfortunately, some countries have even enacted laws and regulations that impede the availability of opioids for medical purposes because of this excessive fear of addiction.[29] It is difficult to interpret the results of many studies designed to estimate prevalence of addiction in cancer patients on long-term opioid therapy because few studies exist and many fail to clearly define the terms used to evaluate addiction. However, the evidence thus far suggests that addiction or related problematic opioid use ranges in prevalence from 0–7.7% in cancer patients.[30–33] One of these studies found an addiction rate as low as 0.2%.[33] These rates suggest that cancer-pain patients should receive sufficient opioid treatment to relieve their discomfort without an undue fear of addiction. In chronic, nonmalignant-pain patients, the risk of addiction requires continuous monitoring during the course of treatment with opioids. As the longevity of cancer patients grows due to improvements in chemotherapy and other antineoplastic agents, their pain conditions will become longer-lasting and in fact may mimic those of the chronic, nonmalignant-pain population receiving opioid therapy. Therefore, rational use of opioids in cancer patients who receive opioids for chronic treatment demands continual monitoring for addictive behaviors, notwithstanding the low rates of addiction in this group.

Other barriers to effective pain control in cancer patients include insufficient education of adjuvant analgesics, such as tricyclic antidepressants (TCAs) and anticonvulsants. Both of these classes of agents may be may be useful at many stages of disease and especially in easing the symptoms associated with neuropathic pain. Finally, educational efforts that expose the entire healthcare team (including physicians, nurses, social workers, and pharmacists) to the array of targeted interventional therapies for cancer pain would help to deconstruct another barrier to pain relief in patients suffering from cancer.

Patients and Families as Barriers to Pain Relief

Patients and their families may also present obstacles to proper pain control (Table 4). For instance, patients worry that alerting physicians to their pain may divert attention away from their cancer treatment, and that "good" patients do not complain of pain. Furthermore, some patients and their families share a mistaken belief that neither medications nor interventions can alleviate their discomfort.

More specific evidence of these beliefs comes from work by Ward and colleagues in their survey of 270 patients with cancer. This investigation focused on reasons that patients may be to reluctant to report pain or use pain-relieving medications.[20] Almost 80% of patients cited fear of addiction with pain medications as a prime concern, and up to 85% reported believing that side effects of pain medications can not be controlled. Approximately 60% of patients stated that a choice needed to be made between treating the pain and treating the dis-

TABLE 4. Patient Barriers to Pain Control

Fear of addiction
Fear of developing tolerance
Fear of masking disease progression
Fear of physician fatigue or annoyance

ease. An equally high percentage felt that pain medication should be reserved for severe pain; otherwise, it might be ineffective when needed. Finally, nearly half of the patients feared annoyance from the physician if they complained of pain. Clearly, healthcare providers must address the need to dispel these myths. Educating both patients and families on the proper use of pain medications and communicating the truth about their risks should be the duty of all clinical practitioners. Addiction concerns can be addressed with patients and their families in a way that reflects the known risk and describes methods of minimizing that risk through assessment, evaluation, and monitoring. Likewise, clinicians can share treatment options (including pharmacologic and holistic) for possible side effects of pain medications with patients and their families.

Treatment of Cancer Pain with Medications

Advances in Past Decades

Prior to the discovery of opioid receptors in the central nervous system in 1973, only theories of their existence permeated the literature. Physicians inconsistently incorporated opioids into pain therapy for cancer patients and rarely in patients with noncancer pain. Unfortunately, many cancer patients died in severe pain despite a developing scientific base and improvements in therapeutic approaches. New methods of drug delivery were introduced in the 1980s, such as continuous subcutaneous, intravenous, epidural, and intrathecal infusions of opioids. The latter two techniques permitted more precise placement of opioids to their receptors and offered alternative means of analgesia. Computerized tomography imaging gave physicians the ability to more clearly inspect cancerous lesions that may be a source of pain.[34] The introduction of the WHO 3-step analgesic ladder in 1986 provided a concrete tool for physicians worldwide to use in combating cancer pain with oral medications ranging from acetaminophen to morphine. Progress in opioid delivery systems has led to a variety of sustained-release preparations that permit transdermal dosing every 3 days or oral dosing twice daily or even once daily. This has produced more stable blood levels of medication, thereby enabling better pain control and increased compliance with therapy. Other routes of opioid delivery including patient-controlled analgesic pumps, epidural catheters, and intrathecal (implantable) pumps have dramatically improved our ability to achieve better pain control in patients with cancer pain.

WHO Cancer Pain "Ladder"

The WHO analgesic ladder serves as the mainstay of treatment for the relief of cancer pain in concert with tumoricidal, surgical, interventional, radiotherapeutic, psychological, and rehabilitative modalities. This multidimensional approach offers the greatest potential for maximizing analgesia and minimizing adverse effects. In fact, it is estimated that 70–90% of cancer pain is relieved when clinicians apply the WHO ladder appropriately.[5] Although several studies have validated the effectiveness of this tool in managing cancer pain,[5,35–37] few controlled clinical trials have been performed to support its effectiveness 20 years after its initial release.[37] Given the imperative for high-quality, evidence-based guidelines in medicine, it is important to analyze the effectiveness of analgesics and adjuvants recommended by the WHO pain relief ladder. Only in this way, can clinicians draw the most accurate conclusions about the value of each step of the ladder and compare the steps to other analgesic treatments. Until controlled, clinical trials suggest more effective analgesic therapies for cancer

pain, clinicians must continue to implement the WHO analgesic ladder in order to meet the basic, global need for treating cancer pain adequately.

This stepwise approach to using pain-relieving medications suggests that clinicians begin with a nonopioid (such as acetaminophen or ibuprofen) and progress from weaker to stronger opioids for incremental pain states (Fig. 1). It is commonly recommended to consider adjuvant medications (that is, drugs that are primarily indicated for nonpainful conditions that can produce analgesia in certain painful conditions) at any step of the ladder. WHO advises that clinicians use acetaminophen or a nonsteroidal anti-inflammatory drug (NSAID) for mild pain (step 1); combination products, such as acetaminophen or aspirin plus codeine, hydrocodone, propoxyphene, or oxycodone, for moderate pain (step 2); and morphine, hydromorphone, oxycodone, methadone, or transdermal fentanyl for severe pain (step 3). In practice, new opioid formulations that include sustained-release preparations of codeine, oxycodone, morphine, tramadol, fentanyl, buprenorphine, or oxymorphone are given to patients at appropriate doses for moderate to severe pain. Generally, pain is more effectively controlled if the clinician evaluates the correct analgesic agent, dose, and timing while simultaneously assessing and managing side effects.[38,39] Some practitioners have moved to algorithm-based approaches for treating cancer pain,[40] and others have incorporated an interventional/procedural "fourth step" to the ladder because cancer pain rarely progresses in a stepwise fashion as indicated by the WHO ladder. Irrespective of the specific strategy employed, an overview of typical therapies to consider for the treatment of cancer pain is essential for clinical practitioners.

Primary Therapies

These treatments are directed at the source of the cancer pain and may enhance a patient's function, longevity, and comfort. Analgesic agents are often needed in conjunction with these primary therapies.

Vertebroplasty: This procedure involves the injection of methylmethacrylate into a pain-sensitive vertebral body under radiographic guidance. The active agent stabilizes bony metastasis by solidifying the lesion and can achieve rapid resolution of pain with restoration of spine stability in 1–3 days.[41] Physicians trained in this technique treat cancer patients with osteolytic lesions of the vertebral body who do not have disruption of the posterior body wall, may or may not have vertebral body collapse, and suffer from severe pain.

Radiofrequency tumor ablation: This therapy may produce significant pain relief from certain cancerous conditions, such as liver cancer, pelvic tumor recurrences, pancreatic cancer, vertebral metastases, and renal and adrenal tumors. The anecdotal literature mostly supports this approach, and several thousand case reports demonstrate its promise in hepatic cancer therapy.[42]

Surgery: Surgery can be invaluable in relieving painful symptoms from hollow organ obstruction, neural compression, and unstable bony structures.[43,44] When cancerous conditions induce pain from obstruction of the esophagus, colon, biliary tract, or ureters, stenting of these structures may offer needed relief.[45,46]

Radiotherapy: Substantial data support the effectiveness of radiotherapy in reducing the pain associated with bone metastases, epidural neoplasm, and headaches caused by cerebral metastases.[47]

Chemotherapy: There is a strong clinical belief that an inverse relationship exists between cancer shrinkage from chemotherapy and analgesia, though there are virtually no data to illustrate the specific analgesic benefits of chemotherapy.[48] There are reports of pain reduction without tumor shrinkage,[49] but most clinicians relate pain relief to the likelihood of tumor response to chemotherapy.

Antibiotics: When pain is a manifestation of infection, antibiotics can serve an analgesic role. For instance, antibiotics are essential in treating pelvic abscess, chronic sinus infections, and cellulitis. Pain may also dissipate when empiric treatment of occult infections is initiated with antibiotic therapy.

Adjuvant Therapies (Co-analgesics)

These medications include nonopioids that confer analgesic effects in certain medical conditions, but primarily treat conditions that do not involve pain. Clinicians typically prescribe adjuvants for the treatment of neuropathic pain like postherpetic neuralgia or painful diabetic neuropathy. The evidence for their effectiveness derives from studies in the nonmalignant pain population rather than the cancer pain population. However, the pathologic processes of neuropathic pain are assumed to be similar in both groups of patients; therefore, these agents are successfully used in treating neuropathic pain in cancer patients. Medications, such as corticosteroids, topical local anesthetics, antidepressants, anticonvulsants, bisphosphonates, and radiopharmaceuticals, are included among the group of agents viewed as adjuvants.

Corticosteroids: These medications inhibit prostaglandin synthesis and reduce neural tissue edema.[50,51] They represent a widely used group of adjuvant therapies for cancer pain[52] and commonly treat the following conditions: increased intracranial pressure headache, superior vena cava syndrome, acute spinal cord compression, neuropathic pain due to nerve compression or infiltration, metastatic bone pain, hepatic capsular distention from metastasis, painful cancer plexopathies, and symptomatic lymphedema. Dexamethasone is the drug of choice given its low mineralocorticoid effect and consequent reduction in risk of Cushing's syndrome. Doses range from 1–2 mg twice daily to 100 mg daily followed by tapered doses in cases of acute and severe pain.[52] The standard dose of dexamathesone is 16–24 mg per day and can be administered once daily because of its extended half-life.[53]

Topical local anesthetics: Painful lesions of the mucosa and skin may respond to lidocaine preparations. For instance, patients find that viscous lidocaine eases the discomfort associated with oropharyngeal ulcerations, though the risk of aspiration and dysphagia from anesthesia should be considered since the numbing effect can inhibit airway protective reflexes.

Antidepressants: Antidepressant medications can help treat neuropathic pain and offer analgesic effects independent of their antidepressant effects.[54,55] The strongest level of evidence for analgesic efficacy exists for the TCAs and specifically, the tertiary amines (including doxepin and amitriptyline).[54] The secondary amines (such as nortriptyline and desipramine) produce analgesia and a more favorable adverse effect profile, especially if there is concern about sedation, anticholinergic effects, and dysrhythmias. Clinicians tend to use TCAs in cancer patients for pain linked to surgery, chemotherapy, radiation therapy, or malignant nerve infiltration. The TCAs may also be useful adjunctively as anxiolytics and sedatives, and often promote sleep. The selective serotonin reuptake inhibitors (SSRIs) provide little analgesia based on clinical experience, and the literature demonstrates mixed results in randomized controlled trials (RCTs). Some clinicians do use the SSRIs in managing neuropathic pain in patients who fail TCAs because they have a lowered risk of adverse events.[56]

Anticonvulsants: Certain anticonvulsants may be effective for various types of neuropathic pain. They typically ease shooting, stabbing, burning, and electric-like sensations associated with a dysfunctional nervous system. Gabapentin, for instance, could be considered a first-line agent for treating neuropathic pain. High quality evidence from RCTs supports its analgesic effect, safety, good tolerability, and absence of drug–drug interactions.[57–59] Pregabalin may also be regarded as a principal anticonvulsant for use in neuropathic pain given strong evidence for its analgesic effect, rapid titration schedule, and tolerability.[60,61] Interestingly, small, open-label studies suggest that gabapentin may be effective in alleviating neuropathic pain induced by cancer treatment. Newer agents, such as topiramate, oxcarbazepine, and lamotrigine, hold promise in treating neuropathic pain as well.

Bisphosphonates: As a group, these substances inhibit osteoclast activity, adhere strongly to bone, demonstrate a long half-life, and can effectively reduce bone pain. For example, bisphosphonates, such as pamidronate and clodronate, have been shown in controlled trials to reduce bone pain in patients with advanced cancer.[62] Moreover, studies confirm their efficacy in treating bone pain from multiple myeloma and metastases from other cancers.[63,64]

Radiopharmaceuticals: Painful and diffuse metastatic bone disease can also be well treated with radiolabeled agents that areas of high bone turnover absorb. These agents deposit radiation directly to the affected region of the bone. The most commonly used and best-studied radiopharmaceutical is strontium-89.[65] Samarium-153 lexidronam, a radiopharmaceutical linked to a bisphosphonate compound has produced a positive clinical response,[66] and both strontium and samarium can reduce pain for 6 months or more in 60–80% of patients with metastatic breast and prostate cancers.[67-69]

Nonopioid Therapy/ Over-the-Counter Agents

The WHO analgesic ladder recommends nonopioids beginning at step 1. These medications are useful in the management of mild to moderate pain and their continuation through step 3 is an option after weighing a drug's risks and benefits in individual patients. The two prime agents include the NSAIDS and acetaminophen. Both types have a "ceiling effect" or maximum therapeutic dose beyond which no further benefit is achieved and at which the risk of toxicity increases.

Acetaminophen: Acetaminophen produces analgesia and reduces fever (antipyretic activity) without clinically meaningful peripheral anti-inflammatory activity.[70] Clinicians often combine this agent with short-acting opioids if initial therapy is unsuccessful. Combining acetaminophen with opioids can offer a dose-sparing effect that not only may reduce the amount of opioid required for analgesia, but may limit opioid-induced adverse effects (examples include sedation, nausea and vomiting, constipation, dry mouth, and cognitive dysfunction). Healthcare providers must be mindful of the risk of acetaminophen hepatotoxicity at sustained doses of 4 g per day in adults[71,72] and note that a pending recommendation exists to limit the toxic dose to 3 g per day. Practitioners should also assess the number and dose of multi-ingredient products (such as cold/flu remedies and analgesics) containing acetaminophen that patients may be taking as treatment for pain or other conditions

NSAIDS: NSAIDS are commonly used to reduce inflammatory pain caused by cancer, such as metastatic bone pain and soft tissue infiltration. They have a well-established role in treating mild cancer pain as monotherapy and in conjunction with opioids in reducing moderate to severe pain.[73,74] Like acetaminophen, NSAIDS offer the benefit of an opioid-sparing effect.[75] In cancer patients, clinicians should consider the adverse effects of NSAIDS (mainly gastrointestinal and renal) and especially a patient's co-existing conditions (such as thrombocytopenia orneutropenia) when selecting a particular medication. NSAIDs inhibit the cyclooxygenase (COX) enzyme, which converts arachidonic acid to prostaglandins[76]; prostaglandins mediate renal plasma flow,[76] gastric mucosal protection,[76] platelet aggregation, and pain and inflammation. The COX-2 selective agents confer the same effectiveness as the nonselective agents with less risk of gastrointestinal damage and bleeding.[76] Care should be taken when using NSAIDS in the neutropenic population because the antipyretic and anti-inflammatory properties may mask signs and symptoms of infection.

Opioid Therapy

Symptomatic treatment of severe cancer pain should begin with an opioid, regardless of the mechanism of the pain. Opioids are very effective analgesics, titrate easily, and offer a favorable risk/benefit ratio. They reduce pain by binding to specific receptors located in the central and peripheral nervous system. Most of the commonly used opioids exert their effect through mu opioid receptors, though some bind to kappa or delta receptors. No compelling evidence supports the use of one opioid over another in managing cancer pain. The goal of

TABLE 5. Drug Enforcement Agency (DEA) Schedule of Controlled Substances

Schedule	Criteria	Examples
Schedule I	High potential for abuse	Heroin
	No accepted medical use	Mescaline
		LSD
Schedule II	High potential for abuse	Codeine
	Accepted medical use ± severe restrictions	Morphine
	Abuse may lead to severe psychological or physical dependence	Fentanyl
		Hydromorphone
		Meperidine
		Methadone
		Oxycodone
		Oxymorphone
		Amphetamines
		Cocaine
Schedule III	Potential for abuse less than Schedules I and II	Combined codeine or hydrocodone w/ NSAID or acetaminophen
	Accepted medical use	Ketamine
	Abuse → moderate/low physical dependence or high psychological dependence	Buprenorphine
Schedule IV	Low potential for abuse	Propoxyphene
	Accepted medical use	Benzodiazepines
	Abuse → limited physical dependence or psychological dependence	Long-acting barbiturates
Schedule V	Lower potential for abuse than Schedule IV	Opioid preparations used to treat diarrhea or cough
	Accepted medical use	
	Abuse → limited physical dependence or psychological dependence which is less than Schedule IV	

Adapted from DEA, Title 21, Section 812 and Principles of Addiction Medicine, 3rd Edition.

minimizing adverse effects while maximizing analgesia remains paramount when selecting among opioids. Classification schemes include whether the opioid is a full agonist (morphine, oxycodone), partial agonist (buprenorphine), or mixed agonist-antagonist (nalbuphine, pentazocine); whether the opioid provides short- or long-term relief based on formulation (oxycodone versus sustained-release oxycodone); and where the opioid ranks on the federal schedule of controlled drugs (Table 5) according to their medical importance and abuse potential, from Schedule I (high abuse potential and no medical use) to Schedule V (low abuse potential and accepted medical use).

Tramadol: Tramadol is a centrally acting analgesic that shares properties of both opioids and TCAs. This agent binds weakly to the mu opioid receptor, inhibits the reuptake of serotonin and norepinephrine, and promotes neuronal serotonin release. The WHO places tramadol on step 2 of the ladder as an option for treating mild to moderate cancer pain. It is often used for its opioid-like analgesic effects in the cancer population, although it may be incorporated into the armamentarium of drugs considered for neuropathic pain. For instance, a recent RCT of tramadol compared to placebo demonstrated efficacy in controlling neuropathic pain in patients with cancer.[77] Furthermore, high-quality studies in patients with nonmalignant neuropathic pain[78,79] confirm its efficacy in treating this painful condition. Clinicians feel comfortable using tramadol because it is not listed on the federal schedule of controlled drugs, has low abuse liability,[33] and is associated with low risk of respiratory depression.[80] Adverse effects resemble those of opioids and caution is advised when using tramadol with SSRIs, monoamine oxidase inhibitors, or TCAs given the potential for serotonin syndrome. Tramadol is available in immediate-release form or in combination with acetaminophen, and now in a controlled-release preparation.[81]

Morphine: Morphine remains the most commonly used opioid for treating severe cancer pain (step 3 of the WHO ladder). No other drug has demonstrated greater analgesic efficacy, though no controlled studies have proven morphine's superiority over other opioids. Morphine's wide availability, cost effectiveness, and multiple formulations (including oral, rectal, intravenous, intranasal, epidural, subcutaneous, intrathecal, and sustained-release) illustrate its preferred status for managing cancer pain. Oral administration is the preferred and simplest route. Morphine is metabolized in the liver, producing morphine-3-glucuronide (M3G) and morphine-6-glucuronide (M6G). Although M3G is inactive, M6G is an active metabolite that exceeds morphine in potency and half-life. Both metabolites are excreted by the kidneys; however, patients with renal dysfunction may experience prolonged morphine effects, including respiratory depression from accumulation of M6G. Clinicians should consider small doses of immediate-release morphine and/or reducing the dosing frequency when prescribing morphine to patients with renal impairment. Some have advocated the avoidance of morphine altogether in patients with renal failure due to the risks of managing adverse effects of the metabolites.[82] A novel liposomal delivery system that carries morphine epidurally to targeted sites has been shown to provide 48 h of postoperative pain relief,[83] and this system holds exciting applications for future analgesic delivery in cancer patients.

Codeine: The WHO places codeine on step 2 of the analgesic ladder to be used for mild–moderate pain. Codeine is available as a combination product with acetaminophen or aspirin. The liver metabolizes codeine once absorbed and 90% of its metabolites are primarily excreted as inactive forms in the urine. Only about 10% of codeine is demethylated (converted) to morphine, which accounts for its analgesic properties as well as its recommendation for the control of only mild–moderate cancer pain. It is important to remember that genetic differences in the enzyme responsible for the conversion of codeine to morphine lead to the inability to produce morphine in about 10% of the Caucasian population.[84] Hence, codeine is rendered ineffective in these patients. Similarly, Chinese people convert less morphine from codeine and demonstrate less sensitivity to the effects of morphine.[85] Accordingly, clinicians should consider rotating to other opioids in the event that certain patients fail to experience adequate relief from codeine. Unique receptors that bind codeine exclusively may explain its significant antitussive effects.[86] Practitioners should avoid using codeine in patients with renal failure because its active metabolites accumulate[87] and can cause significant adverse effects.[88,89]

Hydromorphone: Hydromorphone (step 3 of the WHO ladder) is a semisynthetic derivative of morphine that is about 6 times more potent. It binds to both the mu and, to a lesser degree, the delta opioid receptor.[90] Hydromorphone is available in oral (immediate-release and controlled-release [not available in the United States]), parenteral (intravenous, intramuscular, subcutaneous), and intraspinal preparations. RCTs support the drug's efficacy and tolerability in patients with cancer pain.[91,92] Therefore, it is included in clinical practice guidelines for the management of cancer pain.[53,93] Studies report that hydromorphone shares equivalency with morphine in analgesic efficacy and adverse effects.[92] Hydromorphone seems to have active, nonanalgesic metabolites which may cause neuroexcitatory effects (myoclonus, allodynia, seizures, confusion) at high doses or in the setting of renal failure.[94,95] Therefore, patients who present with increased pain, confusion, and myoclonus should rotate to another opioid or reduce the dose and frequency of administration.

Fentanyl: Initially used as an intraoperative anesthetic, fentanyl's use has evolved into a popular transdermal, controlled systemic delivery formulation. The data support the effectiveness of transdermal fentanyl (fentanyl patch) for treating cancer pain,[96–98] and most clinicians would place the drug on step 3 of the WHO analgesic ladder. The fentanyl patch serves as a viable alternative to oral opioids, especially when cancer or adverse treatment effects preclude the oral administration of analgesics. Fentanyl is 100 times more potent than morphine[99] and is very lipid soluble, which affords easy passage of the drug through the skin and mucous membranes en route to systemic circulation. As an opioid for patient-controlled analgesia infusions of short duration, fentanyl has a relatively short time to peak analgesic effect and a quick termination of effect after small bolus doses; it provides marked cardiovascular stability (fentanyl releases no histamine).[99] The transdermal system usually requires 12–24 h be-

fore serum levels stabilize when starting the patch or changing the dose.[100] Recommended dosing is every 72 h, though some patients report an attenuated analgesic response by the 3rd day and request a shortened dosing interval to every 48 h. Many clinicians prescribe the patch to patients who display stable pain symptomatology due to the longer time needed to increase the dose to therapeutic levels.[101] In addition to its transdermal formulation, fentanyl is administered intravenously, orally (lollipop, lozenge, buccal tablet), intravenously, epidurally, and intrathecally. An innovative delivery system called the fentanyl iontophoretic transdermal system shows promise in treating postoperative pain[102,103] and may have future value in treating breakthrough pain among chronic cancer pain sufferers. This system represents a noninvasive, transdermal method of drug delivery in which an electrical field drives small charged lipophilic particles across the skin.[104] The liver and to a lesser extent the duodenum metabolize fentanyl to inactive metabolites. Based on limited data, clinicians can use fentanyl in patients with renal failure, but should monitor patients for evidence of gradual accumulation of the opioid.[82]

Oxycodone: Oxycodone may be useful as a step 2 or step 3 analgesic on the cancer pain ladder. It binds to both the mu[105,106] and kappa[107] opioid receptors, and is often used in combination with acetaminophen, aspirin, or ibuprofen as a short-acting analgesic. Oxycodone is primarily used orally in both immediate-release (capsule, liquid, tablet) and controlled-release forms to manage pain. Several RCTs document oxycodone's ability in controlled-release preparation to provide effective pain relief in moderate to severe cancer pain compared to sustained-release morphine.[108–110] Further, patients in these studies reported fewer hallucinations with oxycodone as well as less pruritus and nausea compared to morphine.[109,110] Controlled-release formulations of oxycodone and other opioids have greatly facilitated the provision of stable dosing and pain relief for patients with cancer pain. Controlled-release oxycodone, for example, provides sustained relief for 12 h and offers faster onset of relief than sustained-release morphine.[111] In the elderly, oxycodone may be a desirable alternative to morphine if patients are sensitive to morphine-induced sedation and mental status changes. The liver metabolizes oxycodone to small amounts of oxymorphone, the only active metabolite, and oxymorphone does accumulate in renal failure along with the parent drug.[112] Although the data are sparse, one case reports sedation and central nervous system toxicity in patients with renal failure given oxycodone.[113] Hence, clinicians should prescribe oxycodone cautiously and carefully monitor symptoms of toxicity in patients with renal compromise.

Meperidine: This opioid binds predominantly to the mu opioid receptor and is used most often as an intraoperative analgesic. Small, single doses are effective for postoperative shivering as well. The drug may produce an anticholinergic response in the form of tachycardia and acts as a weak local anesthetic. Oral and parenteral formulations are available for clinical use. Most clinicians avoid meperidine for the treatment of chronic pain and cancer pain due to its short duration of action and concerns over metabolic toxicity. In fact, The Agency for Health Care Policy and Research recommends its use for no longer than 48 h and in doses that do not exceed 600 mg per day.[114] Hence, this drug is rarely recommended as a therapeutic agent listed on the WHO analgesic ladder. Meperidine is metabolized to normeperidine which is eliminated by both the liver and the kidney; therefore, hepatic or renal dysfunction can lead to metabolite accumulation. Normeperidine toxicity manifests as shakiness, muscle twitches, myoclonus, dilated pupils, and seizures.[115] Renal failure greatly elevates the risk of normeperidine neurotoxicity, therefore clinicians should avoid its use in patients with kidney disease. Furthermore, co-administering monoamine oxidase inhibitors with meperidine can yield serious reactions, such as delusions, hyperpyrexia, respiratory depression or excitation, and convulsions.

Buprenorphine: Typically used as a step 3 agent for cancer pain, buprenorphine is a partial agonist at the mu opioid receptor and an antagonist at the kappa and delta receptors.[116–118] It has a high affinity for and slow dissociation from the mu receptor and may produce less analgesia than a full mu agonist. Aside from its analgesic properties, buprenorphine is approved for the treatment of opioid dependence disorders in a combination product with naloxone.[119] New data indicate that buprenorphine causes limited respiratory depression compared to fentanyl and probably other opioids.[120] In fact, buprenorphine may also have a ceiling effect for respiratory depression at high doses that is independent of its analgesic effect.[121] It is 25–50 times more potent than morphine, and is available in parenteral, sublingual, and transdermal formulations. A recent study of transdermal buprenorphine in cancer and non-cancer patients showed that almost half of the patients reported satisfactory pain relief and over a one-third experienced good pain relief.[122] Evidence from other studies demonstrates that buprenorphine provides improvement in pain, enhanced quality of life, and stable dosing in cancer pain patients.[123–125] In addition, this opioid shows promise in treating neuropathic pain, which can often manifest in cancer pain conditions.[40,126,127] Adverse effects, such as constipation and patch-related erythema and pruritis, appear at lower rates with buprenorphine than other opioids. For instance, constipation rates range from 0.97% to 6.7% in studies of transdermal buprenorphine.[128-130] In contrast, transdermal fentanyl produces constipation at rates between 9% and 28%.[131,132] Buprenorphine requires no dose adjustment in patients with renal failure, which confers substantial advantage to vulnerable populations like cancer patients and older adults.[122] The liver metabolizes buprenorphine to norbuprenorphine, which represents its major, weakly active metabolite. This metabolite, along with others, passes into the bile and then into the feces which bypasses any accumulation in patients with renal dysfunction. The safe administration of buprenorphine in patients with renal impairment[133,134] offers a unique alternative to many other opioids that may accumulate and cause severe adverse events.

Methadone: Methadone (step 3 agent on the WHO ladder) is a long-acting mu and delta opioid receptor agonist that shares similar efficacy and comparable adverse effect profile with morphine. It also causes monoamine reuptake inhibition. Further, methadone has N-methyl-D-aspartate (NMDA) antagonist properties based on animal studies.[135-137] This unique feature may make methadone a particularly useful choice for the treatment of neuropathic pain, though no trial evidence supports a role in alleviating neuropathic pain of malignant origin.[138] The available data suggest that methadone is an effective analgesic in patients with cancer pain.[138] However, it displays complex and erratic pharmacokinetics requiring extreme vigilance in initiation and dose titration—methadone's plasma half-life is about 24 h,[137,139] whereas its analgesic half-life if only 4–6 h.[140] Moreover, significant variability in plasma half-life between individuals has been observed in clinical practice.[141] Methadone firmly binds to extravascular binding sites and is released slowly back into plasma, resulting in a characteristically long half-life. Therefore, clinicians must be aware of the potential for delayed toxicity (including respiratory depression) from drug accumulation in tissues. Repeat administration ("by the clock" as proposed by the WHO) in treating cancer pain, coupled with a prolonged half-life, increases the risk of overdose in two vulnerable populations, those with cancer pain and older adults. Infrequent (two to three times daily), low, and slow dosing along with vigilant monitoring can lend a margin of safety to clinicians when prescribing methadone. Caution is advised when rotating to methadone, especially from high doses of a previous opioid given its variable conversion ratio.[142] Available formulations exist for oral, rectal, and parenteral administration. Patients taking monoamine oxidase inhibitors should not concurrently use methadone. Clinicians should be mindful of possible QT prolongation and torsades de pointes associated with higher doses of methadone (300 mg and above), and methadone use in concert with certain antidepressants, severe hypokalemia or hypomagnesemia, and congestive heart failure.[143,144] The liver transforms methadone to inactive metabolites[145] that are excreted in the urine and mainly in the bile (feces). Renal dysfunction does not seem to impair clearance of the drug, so clinicians may consider methadone in patients with renal failure.[146] Despite its hazards, methadone can serve as an ally in easing pain among gravely ill patients.[139,147,148] For example, methadone produces a rapid onset of analgesic effect (about 30 min), has high oral bioavailability (85%), has a long half-life, induces tolerance slowly, produces no active metabolites, and costs little.

Oxymorphone: Oxymorphone, a metabolite of oxycodone, may reflect a new treatment option for cancer patients suffering from moderate-to-severe pain (step 3). Formerly available only as a parenteral or rectal agent, oxymorphone has recently been developed as immediate-release and sustained-release formulations. Its analgesic effects are mediated through mu and delta opioid receptors.[90] In a pilot study, Sloan and colleagues found that oxymorphone produced equivalent analgesia to extended-release morphine or extended-release oxycodone in patients with moderate-to-severe cancer pain.[149] In fact, patients taking sustained-release oxymorphone required less breakthrough medication than those taking extended-release morphine. The half-life of the immediate-release formulation of oxymorphone (approximately 7–9 h[150]) exceeds that of many short-acting formulations of opioids including morphine, oxycodone, and hydromorphone. Furthermore, a 6-h dosing interval is recommended, which is longer than most immediate-release opioids. Consequently, clinicians may find this shorter-acting form of oxymorphone an attractive option for limiting episodes of breakthrough pain. The liver biotransforms oxymorphone into oxymorphone 3-glucoronide and 6-hydroxyoxymorphone. The latter metabolite has been shown to have analgesic bioactivity in animals.[150] Oxymorphone is renally excreted and accumulates in renal failure,[112] so clinicians should consider increasing the dosing interval and/or lowering the dose in the setting of renal dysfunction.

Conclusion

Cancer pain remains inadequately controlled despite the diagnostic and therapeutic means of ensuring that patients feel comfortable during their illness. More effective methods of ensuring that physicians and healthcare providers apply the WHO cancer pain analgesic ladder must be developed. Further, educational tools that deconstruct the barriers to providing adequate pain care to cancer patients require initiation and implementation; otherwise, patterns of ignorance will prevail and patients will suffer in pain needlessly. Concerns about opioid compliance, diversion, abuse, and addiction all contribute to an inadequate level of interest in treating cancer patients with opioids. The available evidence suggests that rates of problematic opioid use in this population are low; therefore, patients should not be denied opioid therapy for fear of inducing substance abuse. Clinicians should consider the range of medical therapies (primary, adjuvant, nonopioid, and opioid) available for patients suffering from cancer pain, and incorporate them into a treatment strategy that maximizes analgesia and minimizes adverse effects. Importantly, an array of short- and long-acting opioids now exists and should be prescribed for cancer pain. Each opioid confers a unique set of analgesic properties and adverse effects which need to be considered before use in any cancer patient. Moreover, clinicians must pay special attention to active opioid metabolites in patients with renal disease. Uncontrolled pain is incompatible with a satisfactory quality of existence, and multiple studies highlight the deleterious impact of persistent pain on daily life and social interaction. Accordingly, all practitioners must make control of cancer pain a professional duty, even if they can use only the most basic and least expensive analgesic medications, such as morphine, codeine, and acetaminophen, to reduce human suffering.

Conflicts of Interest

The authors declare no conflicts of interest.

References

1. NIH. 2002. NIH State of the Science Statement on symptom management in cancer: pain, depression, and fatigue. in NIH Con. *State of the Sci. Statm.* 1–29.
2. Keefe, F.A., AP Abernethy & CL Campbell. 2005. Psychological approaches to understanding and treating disease related pain. *Annual Rev. Psychol.* **56:** 1–22.
3. Bonica, J. 1990. *The Management of Pain*. Vol. 1. Lea & Febiger. Philadelphia.
4. ESMO. 2007. Management of cancer pain: ESMO Clinical Recommendations. *Annals of Oncology* **18**(Suppl 2): ii92–ii94.
5. Jadad, A.R. & G.P. Browman. 1995. The WHO analgesic ladder for cancer pain management. Stepping up the quality of its evaluation. *JAMA* **274:** 1870–1873.
6. Azevedo, S.L.F., M. Kimura & M. Jacobsen Teizeira. 2006. The WHO analgesic ladder for cancer pain control, twenty years of use. How much pain relief does one get from using it? *Support Care Cancer*.
7. Levy, M. 1999. Pain control in patients with cancer. *Oncology (Williston Park)* **13**(5 Suppl 2): 9–14.
8. Polomano, R.C. & J.T. Farrar. 2006. Pain and neuropathy in cancer survivors. *Am. J. Nurs.* **106**(3 Suppl): 39–47.
9. Portenoy, R.K. 1989. Mechanisms of clinical pain. Observations and speculations. *Neurol. Clin. North Am.* **7:** 205–230.
10. Loeser, J. 2001. *Bonica's Management of Pain*, 3rd edn.: 19–21. Lippincott, Williams & Wilkins. Philadelphia.
11. LeBel, A.A. 2002. *The Massachusetts General Hospital Handbook of Pain Management*, 2 edn. J.C. Ballantyne, Ed.: Lippincott Williams & Wilkins. Philadephia.
12. Foley, K. 1998. Pain assessment and cancer pain syndromes. In *Oxford Textbook of Palliative Medicine*. H.G. Doyle D & N. MacDonald, Eds.: 310–331. Oxford University Press. Oxford.
13. American Pain Society Quality of Care Committee. 1995. Quality improvement guidelines for the treatment of acute pain and cancer pain. *JAMA* **274:** 1874–1880.
14. Baltic, T.E., M.B. Whedon, T.A. Ahles & G. Fanciullo. 2002. Improving pain relief in a rural cancer center. *Cancer Pract.* **10**(Suppl 1): S39–S44.
15. Lasch, K. 2002. Why study pain? A qualitative analysis of medical and nursing faculty and students' knowledge of and attitudes to cancer pain management. *J. Palliat Med.* **5:** 57–71.
16. Payne, R. 2000. Chronic pain: challenges in the assessment and management of cancer pain. *J. Pain Symptom Manage.* **19**(1 Suppl): S12–S15.
17. Ward, S. 2001. Patient education in pain control. *Support Care Cancer* **9:** 148–155.
18. Gunnarsdottir, S. 2002. Patient-related barriers to pain management: the Barriers Questionnaire II (BQ-II). *Pain* **99:** 385–396.
19. Ward, S. & J. Gatwood. 1994. Concerns about reporting pain and using analgesics. A comparison of persons with and without cancer. *Cancer Nurs.* **17:** 200–206.
20. Ward, S.E., N. Goldberg, V. Miller-McCauley, *et al.* 1993. Patient-related barriers to management of cancer pain. *Pain* **52:** 319–324.
21. Phillips, D.M. 2000. JCAHO pain management standards are unveiled. Joint Commission on Accreditation of Healthcare Organizations. *JAMA* **284:** 428–429.
22. Dahan, A. 2001. Anesthetic potency and influence of morphine and sevoflurane on respiration in mu-opioid receptor knockout mice. *Anesthesiology* **94:** 824–832.
23. Romberg, R. 2003. Comparison of morphine-6-glucuronide and morphine on respiratory depressant and antinociceptive responses in wild type and mu-opioid receptor deficient mice. *Br J. Anaesth* **91:** 862–870.
24. Dahan, A. 2004. Simultaneous measurement and integrated analysis of analgesia and respiration after an intravenous morphine infusion. *Anesthesiology* **101:** 1201–1209.
25. American Society of Addiction Medicine. 1998. Public policy statement on definitions related to the use of opioids in pain treatment. *J. Addict. Dis.* **17:** 129–133.
26. Portenoy, R.K. 1990. Chronic opioid therapy in nonmalignant pain. *J. Pain Symptom Manage.* **5**(1 Suppl): S46–S62.
27. Sees, K.L. & H.W. Clark. 1993. Opioid use in the treatment of chronic pain: assessment of addiction. *J. Pain Symptom Manage.* **8:** 257–264.
28. McQuay, H. 1999. Opioids in pain management. *Lancet* **353:** 2229–2232.
29. *Cancer pain relief. With a guide to opioid availability*. 1996, World Health Organization.
30. Macaluso, C., D. Weinberg & K.M. Foley. 1988. Opioid abuse and misuse in a cancer pain population. *J. Pain Symptom Manage.* **3:** S24.

31. Passik, S.D., K.L. Kirsh, M.V. McDonald, S. Ahn, *et al.* 2000. A pilot survey of aberrant drug-taking attitudes and behaviors in samples of cancer and AIDS patients. *J. Pain Symptom Manage.* **19:** 274–286.

32. Passik, S.D., J. Schreiber & K.L. Kirsh. 2000. A chart review of the ordering of urine toxicology screen in a cancer center: do they influence on pain management. *J. Pain Symptom Manage.* **19:** 44.

33. Schug, S.A., D. Zech, S. Grond, *et al.* 1992. A long term survey of morphine in cancer pain patients. *J. Pain Symptom Manage.* **7:** 259–266.

34. Foley, K.M. & N. Sundaresan. 1985. Management of cancer pain. In *Cancer: Principles and Practice of Oncology.* Vol. 2. V.T. DeVita, Jr., S. Hellman & S.A. Rosenberg, Eds.: 1940–1962. JB Lippincott Company. Philadelphia.

35. Mercadante, S. 1999. Pain treatment and outcomes for patients with advanced cancer who receive follow-up care at home. *Cancer* **85:** 1849–1858.

36. Ventafridda, V. 1987. A validation study of the WHO method for cancer pain relief. *Cancer* **59:** 850–856.

37. Zech, D.F. 1995. Validation of World Health Organization Guidelines for cancer pain relief: a 10-year prospective study. *Pain* **63:** 65–76.

38. Quigley, C. 2005. The role of opioids in cancer pain. *BMJ* **331:** 825–829.

39. Twycross, R. & A. Wilcock 2001. *Symptom Management in Advanced Cancer*, 3rd edn. Radcliffe Medical Press. Oxford.

40. Miaskowski, C., J. Cleary, R. Burney, *et al.*, Eds. 2005. *Guideline for the Management of Cancer Pain in Adults and Children*, Vol. Clinical Practice Guidelines Series, No. 3. American Pain Society. Glenview, IL.

41. Fourney, D.R. 2003. Percutaneous vertebroplasty and kyphoplasty for painful vertebral body fractures in cancer patients. *J. Neurosurg.* **98**(1 Suppl): 21–30.

42. Neeman, Z. & B.J. Wood. 2002. Radiofrequency ablation beyond the liver. *Tech. Vasc. Interv. Radiol.* **5:** 156–163.

43. Krouse, R. 2004. Advances in palliative surgery for cancer patients. *J. Support Oncol.* **2:** 80–87.

44. McCahill, L. & B. Ferrell. 2002. Palliative surgery for cancer pain. *West J. Med.* **176:** 107–110.

45. Amersi, F., M.J. Stamos & C.Y. Ko. 2004. Palliative care for colorectal cancer. *Surg. Oncol. Clin. North Am.* **13:** 67–77.

46. Homs, M.Y. 2004. Quality of life after palliative treatment for oesophageal carcinoma—a prospective comparison between stent placement and single dose brachytherapy. *Eur. J. Cancer* **40:** 1862–1871.

47. Nielsen, O.S., S.M. Bentzen & E. Sandberg. 1998. Randomized trial of single dose versus fractionated palliative radiotherapy of bone metastases. *Radiother Oncol.* **47:** 233–240.

48. Bang, S.M. 2005. Changes in quality of life during palliative chemotherapy for solid cancer. *Support Care Cancer* **13:** 515–521.

49. Burris, H.A. 3rd. 1997. Improvements in survival and clinical benefit with gemcitabine as first-line therapy for patients with advanced pancreas cancer: a randomized trial. *J. Clin. Oncol.* **15:** 2403–2413.

50. Ettinger, A.B. & R.K. Portenoy. 1988. The use of corticosteroids in the treatment of symptoms associated with cancer. *J. Pain Symptom Manage.* **3:** 99–103.

51. Watanabe, S. & E. Bruera. 1994. Corticosteroids as adjuvant analgesics. *J. Pain Symptom Manage.* **9:** 442–445.

52. Rousseau, P. 2001. The palliative use of high-dose corticosteroids in three terminally ill patients with pain. *Am. J. Hosp. Palliat Care* **18:** 343–346.

53. Jacox, A., D.B. Carr & R. Payne. 1994. New clinical-practice guidelines for the management of pain in patients with cancer. *N. Engl. J. Med.* **330:** 651–655.

54. McQuay, H.J. 1996. A systematic review of antidepressants in neuropathic pain. *Pain* **68:** 217–227.

55. Sindrup, S.H. & T.S. Jensen. 1999. Efficacy of pharmacological treatments of neuropathic pain: an update and effect related to mechanism of drug action. *Pain* **83:** 389–400.

56. Mattia, C. 2002. New antidepressants in the treatment of neuropathic pain. A review. *Minerva Anestesiol.* **68:** 105–114.

57. Backonja, M. 1998. Gabapentin for the symptomatic treatment of painful neuropathy in patients with diabetes mellitus: a randomized controlled trial. *JAMA* **280:** 1831–1836.

58. Bennett, M.I. & K.H. Simpson. 2004. Gabapentin in the treatment of neuropathic pain. A review. *Palliat Med.* **18:** 5–11.

59. Rice, A.S. & S. Maton. 2001. Gabapentin in postherpetic neuralgia: a randomised, double blind, placebo controlled study. *Pain* **94:** 215–224.

60. Dworkin, R.H. 2003. Advances in neuropathic pain: diagnosis, mechanisms, and treatment recommendations. *Arch. Neurol.* **60:** 1524–1534.

61. Freynhagen, R. 2005. Efficacy of pregabalin in neuropathic pain evaluated in a 12-week, randomised, double-blind, multicentre, placebo-controlled trial of flexible- and fixed-dose regimens. *Pain* **115:** 254–263.

62. Wong, R & P.J. Wiffen. 2002. Bisphosphonates for the relief of pain secondary to bone metastases (Cochrane Review). *Cochrane Database Syst Rev* **2:** CD002068.

63. Berenson, J.R. 1996. Efficacy of pamidronate in reducing skeletal events in patients with advanced multiple myeloma. Myeloma Aredia Study Group. *N. Engl. J. Med.* **334:** 488–493.

64. Bloomfield, D.J. 1998. Should bisphosphonates be part of the standard therapy of patients with multiple myeloma or bone metastases from other cancers? An evidence-based review. *J. Clin. Oncol.* **16:** 1218–1225.

65. Gunawardana, D.H. 2004. Results of strontium-89 therapy in patients with prostate cancer resistant to chemotherapy. *Clin. Nucl. Med.* **29:** 81–85.

66. Sartor, O. 2004. Samarium-153-Lexidronam complex for treatment of painful bone metastases in hormone-refractory prostate cancer. *Urology* **63:** 940–945.

67. Robinson, R.G., D.F. Preston, K.G. Baxter, R.W. Dusing & J.A. Spicer. 1993. Clinical experience with Strontium-89 in prostatic and breast cancer patients. *Seminars in Oncology* **20:** 44–48.

68. Rogers, C.L., B.L. Speiser & P.C. Ram. 1998. Efficacy and toxicity of intravenous strontium-89 for symptomatic osseous metastases. *J. of Brachytherapy International* **14:** 133–142.

69. Sciuto, R., C.L. Maini & A. Tofani. 1996. Radiosensitization with low-dose carboplatin enhances pain palliation in radioisotope therapy with strontium-89. *Nucl. Med. Commun.* **17:** 799–804.

70. Watson, A.C., S.T. Brookes, J.R. Kirwan & A. Faulkner. 2000. Non-aspirin, non-steroidal anti-inflammatory drugs for osteoarthritis of the knee. *Cochrane Database of Systematic Reviews* 2.

71. Makin, A.J., J. Wendon & R. Williams. 1995. A 7-year experience of severe acetaminophen-induced hepatotoxicity (1987-1993). *Gastroenterology* **109:** 1907–1916.

72. Schiodt, F.V. 1997. Acetaminophen toxicity in an urban county hospital. *N. Engl. J. Med.* **337:** 1112–1117.

73. Grond, S. 1991. The importance of non-opioid analgesics for cancer pain relief according to the guidelines of the World Health Organization. *Int. J. Clin. Pharmacol. Res.* **11:** 253–260.

74. McNicol, E. 2004. Nonsteroidal anti-inflammatory drugs, alone or combined with opioids, for cancer pain: a systematic review. *J. Clin. Oncol.* **22:** 1975–1992.

75. Mercadante, S., F. Fulfaro & A. Casuccio. 2002. A randomised controlled study on the use of anti-inflammatory drugs in patients with cancer pain on morphine therapy: effects on dose-escalation and a pharmacoeconomic analysis. *Eur. J. Cancer.* **38:** 1358–1363.

76. Simon, L., A. Lipman, A. Jacox, M. Caudill-Slosberg, *et al.* 2002. *Guideline for the management of pain in osteoarthritis, rheumatoid arthritis, and juvenile chronic arthritis.* American Pain Society. Glenview, IL.

77. Arbaiza, D. & O. Vidal. 2007. Tramadol in the treatment of neuropathic cancer pain: a double-blind, placebo-controlled study. *Clin. Drug. Investig.* **27:** 75–83.

78. Boureau, F., P. Legallicier & M. Kabir-Ahmadi. 2003. Tramadol in post-herpetic neuralgia: a randomized, double-blind, placebo-controlled trial. *Pain* **104:** 323–331.

79. Harati, Y. 1998. Double-blind randomized trial of tramadol for the treatment of the pain of diabetic neuropathy. *Neurology* **50:** 1842–1846.

80. Shipton, E.A. 2000. Tramadol—present and future. *Anaesth Intensive Care* **28:** 363–374.

81. Babul, N. 2004. Efficacy and safety of extended-release, once-daily tramadol in chronic pain: a randomized 12-week clinical trial in osteoarthritis of the knee. *J. Pain Symptom Manage.* **28:** 59–71.

82. Dean, M. 2004. Opioids in renal failure and dialysis patients. *J. Pain Symptom Manage.* **28:** 497–504.

83. Viscusi, E.R. 2005. Forty-eight hours of postoperative pain relief after total hip arthroplasty with a novel, extended-release epidural morphine formulation. *Anesthesiology* **102:** 1014–1022.

84. Eichelbaum, M. & B. Evert. 1996. Influence of pharmacogenetics on drug disposition and response. *Clin. Exp. Pharmacol. Physiol.* **23:** 983–985.

85. Caraco, Y., J. Sheller & A.J. Wood. 1999. Impact of ethnic origin and quinidine coadministration on codeine's disposition and pharmacodynamic effects. *J. Pharmacol. Exp. Ther.* **290:** 413–422.

86. Gutstein, H. & A. Huda. 2006. *Goodman & Gilman's The Pharmacological Basis of Therapeutics, 11 edn. Opioid Analgesics.* P. Laurence & L. Brunton, Eds.: 566. McGraw-Hill. New York, New York.

87. Guay, D.R.P., W.M. Awni & J.W.A. Findaly. 1988. Pharmacokinetics and pharmacodynamics of codeine in end-state renal disease. *Clin. Pharmacol. Ther.* **43:** 63–71.

88. Matzke, G.R., G.L.C. Chan & P.A. Abraham. 1986. Codeine dosage in renal failure. *Clinical Pharmacy* **5**(letter): 15–16.

89. Talbott, G.A. 1997. Respiratory arrest precipitated by codeine in a child with chronic renal failure. *Clin Pediatr (Phila)* **36:** 171–173.

90. Ananthan, S. 2004. Identification of opioid ligands possessing mixed micro agonist/delta antagonist activity among pyridomorphinans derived from naloxone, oxymorphone, and hydromorphone [correction of hydropmorphone]. *J. Med. Chem.* **47:** 1400–1412.

91. Junker, U. & V. Figge. 2005. Controlled-release hydromorphone in elderly patients with severe

pain of different etiologies. Results of an observational study. *MMW Fortschr. Med.* **147**(Suppl 3): 91–96.

92. Quigley, C. 2002. Hydromorphone for acute and chronic pain. *Cochrane Database of Systematic Reviews* **1**(CD003447).

93. World Health Organization. 1990. *Report on cancer pain relief and palliative care*. World Health Organization. Geneva.

94. Hagen, N.A. & R. Swanson. 1997. Strychnine-like multifocal myoclonus and seizures from extremely high dose opioids: treatment strategies. *J. Pain Symptom Manage.* **14:** 51–58.

95. Smith, M. 2000. Neuroexcitatory effects of morphine and hydromorphone: evidence implicating the 3-glucuronide metabolites. *Clin. Exp. Pharmacol. Physiol.* **27:** 524–528.

96. Ahmedzai, S. & D. Brooks. 1997. Transdermal fentanyl versus sustained-release oral morphine in cancer pain: preference, efficacy, and quality of life. The TTS-Fentanyl Comparative Trial Group. *J. Pain Symptom Manage.* **13:** 254–261.

97. Donner, B. 1998. Long-term treatment of cancer pain with transdermal fentanyl. *J. Pain Symptom Manage.* **15:** 168–175.

98. Radbruch, L. 2001. Transdermal fentanyl for the management of cancer pain: a survey of 1005 patients. *Palliat Med.* **15:** 309–321.

99. Gutstein, H. & A. Huda. 2006. *Goodman & Gilman's The Pharmacological Basis of Therapeutics, 11 edn. Opioid Analgesics*. P. Laurence & L. Brunton, Eds.: 571. McGraw-Hill. New York, New York.

100. Muijsers, R.B. & A.J. Wagstaff. 2001. Transdermal fentanyl: an updated review of its pharmacological properties and therapeutic efficacy in chronic cancer pain control. *Drugs* **61:** 2289–2307.

101. Hanks, G.W. 2001. Morphine and alternative opioids in cancer pain: the EAPC recommendations. *Br. J. Cancer* **84:** 587–593.

102. Hartrick, C.T. 2006. Fentanyl iontophoretic transdermal system for acute-pain management after orthopedic surgery: a comparative study with morphine intravenous patient-controlled analgesia. *Reg. Anesth. Pain Med.* **31:** 546–554.

103. Viscusi, E.R. 2004. Patient-controlled transdermal fentanyl hydrochloride vs intravenous morphine pump for postoperative pain: a randomized controlled trial. *JAMA* **291:** 1333–1341.

104. Viscusi, E.R. & T.A. Witkowski. 2005. Iontophoresis: the process behind noninvasive drug delivery. *Reg. Anesth. Pain Med.* **30:** 292–294.

105. Monory, K. 1999. Opioid binding profiles of new hydrazone, oxime, carbazone and semicarbazone derivatives of 14-alkoxymorphinans. *Life Sci.* **64:** 2011–2020.

106. Yoburn, B.C. 1995. Supersensitivity to opioid analgesics following chronic opioid antagonist treatment: relationship to receptor selectivity. *Pharmacol. Biochem. Behav.* **51:** 535–539.

107. Prommer, E. 2006. Oxymorphone: a review. *Support Care Cancer* **14:** 109–115.

108. Bruera, E. 1998. Randomized, double-blind, cross-over trial comparing safety and efficacy of oral controlled-release oxycodone with controlled-release morphine in patients with cancer pain. *J. Clin. Oncol.* **16:** 3222–3229.

109. Heiskanen, T. & E. Kalso. 1997. Controlled-release oxycodone and morphine in cancer related pain. *Pain* **73:** 37–45.

110. Mucci-LoRusso, P. 1998. Controlled-release oxycodone compared with controlled-release morphine in the treatment of cancer pain: a randomized, double-blind, parallel-group study. *Eur. J. Pain.* **2:** 239–249.

111. Curtis, G.B., G.H. Johnson & P. Clark. 1999. Relative potency of controlled-release oxycodone and controlled-release morphine in a postoperative pain model. *Eur. J. Clin. Pharmacol.* **55:** 425–429.

112. Kirvela, M. 1996. The pharmacokinetics of oxycodone in uremic patients undergoing renal transplantation. *J. Clin. Anesth.* **8:** 13–18.

113. Fitzgerald, J. 1991. Narcotic analgesics in renal failure. *Conn. Med.* **55:** 701–704.

114. Acute Pain Management in Infants, Children, and Adolescents: Operative and Medical Procedures, in U.S. Dept. of Health and Human Services. 1992. Agency for Health Care Policy and Research. p. Rockville, MD.

115. Hershey, L. 1983. Meperidine and central neurotoxicity. *Ann. Intern. Med.* **98:** 548–549.

116. Cowan, A., J.W. Lewis & I.R. Macfarlane. 1977. Agonist and antagonist properties of buprenorphine, a new antinociceptive agent. *Br. J. Pharmacol.* **60:** 537–545.

117. Lee, K.O. *et al.* 1999. Differential binding properties of oripavines at cloned mu- and delta-opioid receptors. *Eur. J. Pharmacol.* **378:** 323–330.

118. Lewis, J.W. & S.M. Husbands. 2004. The orvinols and related opioids-high affinity ligands with diverse efficacy profiles. *Curr. Pharm. Des.* **10:** 717–732.

119. Gutstein, H. & A. Huda. 2006. *Goodman & Gilman's the Pharmacological Basis of Therapeutics, 11 edn. Opioid Anaglesics*. P. Laurence & L. Brunton, Eds.: 576. McGraw-Hill. New York, New York.

120. Dahan, A. 2006. Opioid-induced respiratory effects: new data on buprenorphine. *Palliat Med.* **20**(Suppl 1): s3–s8.

121. Cowan, A. 2003. Buprenorphine: new pharmacological aspects. *Int. J. Clin. Pract. Suppl.* 3–8; discussion 23–4.

122. Likar, R., H. Kayser & R. Sittl. 2006. Long-term management of chronic pain with transdermal buprenorphine: a multicenter, open-label, follow-up study in patients from three short-term clinical trials. *Clin. Ther.* **28:** 943–952.

123. Pace, M.C., M.B. Passavanti, E. Grella, *et al.* 2007. Buprenorphine in long term control of chronic pain in cancer patients. *Front Biosci.* **1:** 1291–1299.

124. Sittl, R., M. Nuijten & B.P. Nautrup. 2006. Patterns of dosage changes with transdermal buprenorphine and transdermal fentanyl for the treatment of non-cancer and cancer pain: a retrospective data analysis in Germany. *Clin Ther.* **28:** 1144–1154.

125. Sorge, J. & R. Sittl. 2004. Transdermal buprenorphine in the treatment of chronic pain: results of a phase III, multicenter, randomized, double-blind, placebo-controlled study. *Clin Ther.* **26:** 1808–1820.

126. Christoph, T. 2005. Broad analgesic profile of buprenorphine in rodent models of acute and chronic pain. *Eur. J. Pharmacol.* **507:** 87–98.

127. Likar, R. & R. Sittl. 2005. Transdermal buprenorphine for treating nociceptive and neuropathic pain: four case studies. *Anesth. Analg.* **100:** 781–785.

128. Griessinger, N., R. Sittl & R. Likar. 2005. Transdermal buprenorphine in clinical practice—a post-marketing surveillance study in 13,179 patients. *Curr. Med. Res. Opin.* **21:** 1147–1156.

129. Likar, R., H. Kayser & R. Sittl. 2005. Transdermal buprenorphine for long-term management of chronic cancer and non-cancer pain. Results of an open-label, multicentre, follow up study. Book of Abstracts, International Forum on Pain Medicine. (Sofia).

130. Sittl, R. 2006. Transdermal buprenorphine in cancer pain and palliative care. *Palliat Med.* **20**(Suppl 1): s25–s30.

131. Mystakidou, K. 2003. Long-term management of noncancer pain with transdermal therapeutic system-fentanyl. *J. Pain* **4:** 298–306.

132. Nugent, M. 2001. Long-term observations of patients receiving transdermal fentanyl after a randomized trial. *J. Pain Symptom Manage.* **21:** 385–391.

133. Filitz, J. 2006. Effects of intermittent hemodialysis on buprenorphine and norbuprenorphine plasma concentrations in chronic pain patients treated with transdermal buprenorphine. *Eur. J. Pain.* **10:** 743–748.

134. Summerfield, R.J., M.C. Allen & R.A. Moore. 1985. Buprenorphine in end-stage renal failure. *Anaesthesia* **40**(Letter): 914.

135. Bulka, A. 2002. Reduced tolerance to the anti-hyperalgesic effect of methadone in comparison to morphine in a rat model of mononeuropathy. *Pain* **95:** 103–109.

136. Bulka, A., Z. Wiesenfeld-Hallin & X.J. Xu. 2002. Differential antinociception by morphine and methadone in two sub-strains of Sprague-Dawley rats and its potentiation by dextromethorphan. *Brain Res.* **942:** 95–100.

137. Davis, M. & D. Walsh. 2001. Methadone for relief of cancer pain: a review of pharmacokinetics, pharmacodynamics, drug interactions and protocols of administration. *Support Care Cancer* **9:** 73–83.

138. Nicholson, A. 2004. Methadone for cancer pain. Cochrane Database of Systematic Reviews, (1): p. Art. No.: CD003971. DOI: 10.1002/14651858. CD003971. pub2.

139. Fainsinger, R., T. Schoeller & E. Bruera. 1993. Methadone in the management of cancer pain: a review. *Pain* **52:** 137–147.

140. Grochow, L. 1989. Does intravenous methadone provide longer lasting analgesia than intravenous morphine? A randomized, double-blind study. *Pain* **38:** 151–157.

141. Ripamonti, C., E. Zecca & E. Bruera. 1997. An update on the clinical use of methadone for cancer pain. *Pain* **70:** 109–115.

142. Bryson, J. 2006. Methadone for treatment of cancer pain. *Curr. Oncol. Rep.* **8:** 282–288.

143. Reddy, S.F., M. Fisch & E. Bruera. 2004. Oral methadone for cancer pain: no indication of Q-T interval prolongation or torsades de pointes. *J. Pain Symptom Manage.* **28:** 301–303.

144. Roden, M. 2004. Drug-induced prolongation of the QT-interval. *N. Engl. J. Med.* **350:** 1015–1022.

145. Kreek, M.J. & C.L. Gutjahr. 1976. Drug interactions with methadone. *Ann. N.Y. Acad. Sci.* **281:** 350–370.

146. Kreek, M.J. & A.J. Schecter. 1980. Methadone use in patients with chronic renal disease. *Drug Alcohol Dep.* **5:** 197–205.

147. Hanks, G.W.C. & N. Cherny. 1998. Opioid analgesic therapy. In *Oxford Text of Palliative Medicine*. H.G. Doyle D & N. MacDonald, Eds.: 331–351. Oxford University Press. Oxford.

148. Twycross, R., A. Wilcock & S. Thorpe. 1998. *Palliative Care Formulary*. Radcliffe Medical Press. Oxford.

149. Sloan, P., N. Slatkin & H. Ahdieh. 2005. Effectiveness and safety of oral extended-release oxymorphone for the treatment of cancer pain: a pilot study. *Support Care Cancer* **13:** 57–65.

150. Adams, M.A. & H. Ahdieh. 2005. Single and multiple dose pharmacokinetic and dose proportionality study of oxymorphone immediate release tablets. *Drugs RD* **6:** 91–99.

Interventional Pain Treatments for Cancer Pain

Paul J. Christo and Danesh Mazloomdoost

Department of Anesthesiology & Critical Care Medicine, Division of Pain Medicine,
The Johns Hopkins University School of Medicine, Baltimore, Maryland, USA

Cancer pain is prevalent and often multifactorial. For a segment of the cancer pain population, pain control remains inadequate despite full compliance with the WHO analgesic guidelines including use of co-analgesics. The failure to obtain acceptable pain or symptom relief prompted the inclusion of a fourth step to the WHO analgesic ladder, which includes advanced interventional approaches. Interventional pain-relieving therapies can be indispensable allies in the quest for pain reduction among cancer patients suffering from refractory pain. There are a variety of techniques used by interventional pain physicians, which may be grossly divided into modalities affecting the spinal canal (e.g., intrathecal or epidural space), called neuraxial techniques and those that target individual nerves or nerve bundles, termed *neurolytic techniques*. An array of intrathecal medications are infused into the cerebrospinal fluid in an attempt to relieve refractory cancer pain, reduce disabling adverse effects of systemic analgesics, and promote a higher quality of life. These intrathecal medications include opioids, local anesthetics, clonidine, and ziconotide. Intrathecal and epidural infusions can serve as useful methods of delivering analgesics quickly and safely. Spinal delivery of drugs for the treatment of chronic pain by means of an implantable drug delivery system (IDDS) began in the 1980s. Both intrathecal and epidural neurolysis can be effective in managing intractable cancer-related pain. There are several sites for neurolytic blockade of the sympathetic nervous system for the treatment of cancer pain. The more common sites include the celiac plexus, superior hypogastric plexus, and ganglion impar. Today, interventional pain-relieving approaches should be considered a critical component of a multifaceted therapeutic program of cancer pain relief.

Key words: cancer; pain; analgesia; opioids; nerve blocks; epidural; intrathecal; infusion therapies; implantable drug delivery systems; intrathecal pumps; pain pumps; programmable pumps; external epidural catheter; external intrathecal catheter; neuraxial therapies; neurolytic blocks; chemical neurolysis; celiac plexus; superior hypogastric plexus; ganglion impar; ganglion of Walther; cancer pain; nonopioid therapies; malignancy; WHO 3-step analgesic ladder; palliative care

Overview

Cancer pain is prevalent and often multifactorial (Table 1). Though estimates vary, severe and chronic cancer pain occurs in approximately 33% of patients in active therapy and in 67% of patients with advanced disease.[1–3] In an era of multimodal approaches to reducing pain, it is notable that 46% of dying patients lack adequate pain treatment at death, as reported by family members.[4] Improving pain control has been a topic of interest for numerous agencies including the Joint Commission on Accreditation of Health Organizations (JCAHO), with its memoranda on Cancer Pain published in 1999[5] and the World Health Organization (WHO) in its publication entitled *Cancer Pain Release*[6] in 1988.

Address for correspondence: Paul J. Christo, M.D., M.B.A., Assistant Professor, Director, Multidisciplinary Pain Fellowship, Director, Pain Treatment Center, Department of Anesthesiology & Critical Care Medicine, Division of Pain Medicine, The Johns Hopkins University School of Medicine, 550 N. Broadway, Suite 301, Baltimore, MD 21205. Voice: +410-955-1818; fax: +410-502-6730. pchristo@jhmi.edu

Ann. N.Y. Acad. Sci. 1138: 299–328 (2008). © 2008 New York Academy of Sciences.
doi: 10.1196/annals.1414.034

TABLE 1. Cancer Type and Its Association with Pain

Cancer type	Patients with pain (%)
Bone	85
Oral Cavity	80
Genitourinary (Men/Women)	75–78
Breast	52
Lung	45
Gastrointestinal	40
Lymphoma	20
Leukemia	5

Source: Warfield CA, Manual of Pain Management, Philadelphia, PA: JB Lippincott Co. 1991: 145.
Reprinted with permission.

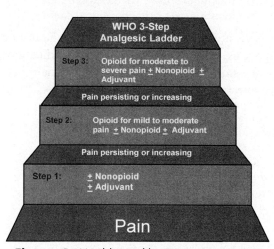

Figure 1. World Health Organization 3-Step Analgesic Ladder. Source: Management of Cancer Pain: Clinical Practice Guideline Number 9. Rockville, MD: US Dept. of Health and Human Services; 1994, AHCPR Pub No. 94-0592. Reprinted with permission.

In 1986, the WHO published a 3-tiered ladder as a guideline for managing cancer pain (Fig. 1). Prospective trials have demonstrated the ladder's widespread efficacy, and the latest trial reports 76% satisfaction with systemic medications in a 10-year follow-up of 2118 cancer patients.[7] Yet, nearly 50% of these patients have reached the final tier of the WHO ladder in order to control their pain, and some yearn for another step of the ladder that would enhance the quality of their remaining life.

Opioid therapy remains the mainstay of cancer pain control,[8] and adherence to the WHO analgesic ladder reportedly manages pain in the majority of cancer patients.[9] In some patients however, the adverse-effect profile of opioids prevents them from benefiting maximally from opioid therapy and leads to needless suffering.[4,10] For instance, gastrointestinal side effects may include both constipation and nausea. Constipation requires stool softeners and laxatives in proportion to the dosage and gastrointestinal effect of opioid use. The incidence of nausea as a result of opioid use is estimated to range from 10–40%.[11] Fortunately, tolerance to opioid-induced nausea usually develops over 3–5 days of continual use.[12] Patients with metastatic cancer frequently complain of fatigue as well as pain. Opioids can exacerbate fatigue, depress consciousness, and even hasten depressive symptoms. Some of these symptoms can be managed with psychostimulants like methylphenidate.[13] Opioid-induced respiratory depression, delirium, or confusion may occur, though other causes of these conditions should be investigated in cancer patients.

For a segment of the cancer pain population, pain control remains inadequate despite full compliance with the WHO algorithm including use of co-analgesics. For example, about 14% of cancer pain patients suffer from significant unrelieved pain even when clinicians apply the WHO analgesic guidelines.[14] Patients may experience side effects of medical therapy that severely attenuate the analgesic effects of the medication and reduce compliance.[15] Moreover, persistent adverse effects have been reported in one of every four treatment days with WHO recommended medications.[7] Further, pain in some patients simply fails to respond to dose escalation of opioids or co-analgesics. In these patients, opioid rotation may provide inadequate relief or may more effectively control pain at the expense of intolerable adverse effects.[16,17]

The failure to obtain acceptable pain or symptom relief prompted the addition of a fourth step to the WHO analgesic ladder,[18] which includes advanced interventional approaches. Interventional pain-relieving therapies can be indispensable allies in the quest for pain reduction among cancer patients suffering from refractory pain. These techniques represent a welcome addition to the pain management armamentarium. The more commonly performed procedural interventions for control of cancer pain are discussed in the substance of this article. These procedural approaches include epidural and intrathecal infusion therapies; implantable drug delivery systems (IDDSs); neuraxial neurolytic interventions; and celiac plexus, superior hypogastric plexus (SHP), and ganglion impar blocks and neurolysis.

Interventional Pain-Relieving Techniques

There are a variety of techniques used by interventional pain physicians that may be grossly divided into modalities affecting the spinal canal (e.g., intrathecal or epidural space), called neuraxial techniques, and those that target individual nerves or nerve bundles, termed *neurolytic techniques*.[19] Neurolytic techniques can be applied to both the neuraxial canal and to specific nerves or nerve bundles.

Neuraxial Techniques

Neuraxial techniques focus on regions of the spinal cord, that correspond to the distribution of pain. By placing medication in close proximity to the entrance of nociceptive (pain) afferent fibers, interneurons, and ascending fibers of the spinal cord, physicians are able to maximize pain relief while minimizing medication toxicity. Neuraxial drugs can bind to neuroreceptors in the dorsal horn of spinal cord, such as N-methyl-D-aspartate (NMDA), opioid, and calcium channels, that modulate the sensation of pain. Other medications lyse or rupture neuronal axons to quell the transmission of pain until axonal regeneration. Clinicians subdivide neuraxial techniques into epidural or intrathecal approaches, depending on the anatomic site of medication delivery.

Epidural Infusion Therapy

Anatomy. The epidural space is located within the spinal canal, between the dura and connective tissues covering the vertebrae and ligamentum flavum (Fig. 2). Within the epidural space, lymphatics, arteries, and a meshwork of veins travel sporadically within a layer of loose adipose and connective tissue. No free fluid exists in the epidural space. Pain medicine specialists and anesthesiologists use this anatomic space as a repository for delivering medications that modulate pain transmission and pain perception. Epidural catheters can be inserted under sterile conditions, tunneled subcutaneously, and attached to filters. A bag containing analgesic medications is then connected to the system, which establishes the epidural infusion therapy.

Efficacy. Reducing the pain of labor or cesarean section is a common role for epidural analgesia; yet, epidurals are used to effectively treat cancer pain as well. For instance, two studies report that epidural analgesia can provide successful pain relief in 100%[20] and 76%[21] of cancer patients receiving this therapy. One study reported greater pain relief from epidurals placed in the lower half of the body for low thoracic, abdominal, pelvic, or leg pain, though sufficient pain relief was also achieved in over 50% of patients with epidurals placed for upper extremity, neck, or shoulder pain.[21] In our experience, percutaneous epidural analgesia can provide substantial relief in treating severe cancer pain, especially at the end of life.

Cost and Complications. When considering long-term epidural catheter therapy for delivery of analgesic medications, clinicians should weight the higher costs of epidural therapy beyond 3 months compared to IDDS

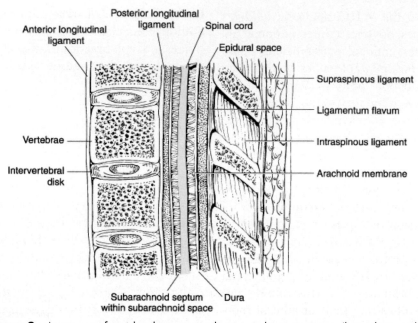

Figure 2. Anatomy of epidural space and surrounding structures (lateral view through lumbar vertebrae). *Source:* Morgan GE, Mikhail MS, & Murray MJ: *Clinical Anesthesiology,* 4th Edition, 1996, McGraw-Hill: http://www.accessmedicine.com *Reprinted with permission of The McGraw-Hill Companies.*

therapy[22] and the risk of complications. Epidural catheter infusions require greater drug dose and volume compared to intrathecal infusions. This typically leads to increased cost and more frequent violations of the sterile catheter system to refill the medication bag and exchange the filters. Consequently, infection rates may escalate as a result of more frequent breaks in the sterile system. For instance, one study describes complications occurring in 69% of cancer patients with epidural analgesia,[20] and another study reports complications in 43% of patients with epidural catheter infusions.[21] Many of these complications included catheter dysfunction, superficial and deep tissue infections, and medication-induced adverse effects, such as nausea/emesis, drowsiness, and constipation. Moreover, technical complications (such as infection and catheter dislocation and obstruction) are reported as more frequent with long-term (greater than 1 month) epidural therapy than with long-term intrathecal infusions (55% complication rate compared to 5%, respectively).[23]

Compared to intrathecal opioid administration, epidural opioids may carry a reduced risk of respiratory depression. However, epidural opioids generally result in a higher rate of systemic opioid absorption (about 80–90%) and require a higher dose of administration. Furthermore, epidural catheters may lead to dural fibrosis, which can inhibit effective spread of epidural solutions, require escalating doses and volume of drugs (until the analgesia effects attenuate or the catheter obstructs), and impede drug diffusion to the intrathecal space.[23,24]

Intrathecal Infusion Therapy

Anatomy. The intrathecal or subarachnoid space refers to the area between the spinal cord's arachnoid membrane and pia mater in which the cerebrospinal fluid circulates. Local anesthetics, opioids, and other agents can be effectively placed into this space in an effort to reduce severe cancer pain. Tunneled and externalized intrathecal catheters can be inserted under sterile conditions and used for short- or long-term treatment of both malignant and nonmalignant pain.

External Delivery of Intrathecal Medication. Trepidation concerning heightened risks of infection and other complications has directed pain clinicians away from the application of externalized intrathecal catheters for delivering analgesic medications. However, specialists have safely used these catheters for 1–2 months and even as long as to 1.5 years[25] in alleviating intractable cancer and noncancer pain conditions.[25–28] Clinical data support the safety and efficacy of externalized intrathecal analgesia for use in advanced cancer pain,[29,30] and evidence suggests that intrathecal catheters are safer than epidural catheters if required for greater than 3 weeks of treatment.[31,32] Furthermore, clinical studies demonstrate that intrathecal morphine can provide more satisfactory pain relief with fewer adverse effects than epidural administration of morphine.[33–35] In contrast to epidural catheters, externalized intrathecal catheters require smaller drug dose and volume, which permits more compact, portable external infusion devices and more extended periods before refilling the device (medication bag) is necessary. Both ambulatory patients and home health refill teams often consider less frequent refills an advantage. Furthermore, home therapy with externalized intrathecal catheters may provide more acceptable analgesia and improved quality of life in advanced cancer pain than treatment with epidural catheters.[30]

Complications. A small number of case reports demonstrate the formation of intrathecal granulomas in patients receiving continuous subarachnoid opioids or admixtures.[36] Most of these cases involved noncancer pain patients who were exposed to the drugs at high doses and/or over a sustained period of time. Other reports show catheter tip masses occurring in patients receiving infusions for almost 1.5 years or having exposure to morphine at high doses.[37–39] Most externalized intrathecal infusion therapies are offered to cancer patients as a method to control their

TABLE 2. Spinal (Subarachnoid and/or Epidural) Medications

Pain Type	Medication
Visceral and somatic	*Opioids:*
	Morphine
	Hydromorphone
	Fentanyl
	Sufentanil
	Buprenorphine
	Local Anesthetics:
	Lidocaine
	Bupivacaine
	Tetracaine
	Ropivacaine
Neuropathic	*Local Anesthetics:*
	Lidocaine
	Bupivacaine
	Tetracaine
	Ropivacaine
	N-type Calcium channel blocker:
	Ziconotide
	Alpha-2 agonists:
	Clonidine
	Dexmedetomidine
	Antispasmodics:
	Baclofen

Source: Adapted from Miguel, R., Interventional treatment of cancer pain: the fourth step in the World Health Organization analgesic ladder? Cancer Control, 2000. 7(2): 149–56.

Reprinted with permission.

extreme pain at the end of life; therefore, granuloma formation is less likely to occur in this population. Notwithstanding the presumed lower risk of granuloma development in cancer patients, consensus recommendations for reducing risk include administering the lowest opioid dose and concentration for the longest period of time and assessing pathologic symptoms, such as diminishing pain relief and evidence of spinal cord compression.[36]

A number of agents can be infused in the intrathecal space (Table 2), though very few are actually approved for use by the Food and Drug Administration (FDA). An IDDS represents an increasingly popular form of delivering intrathecal medications for the relief of cancer pain.

Intrathecal Medications and Implantable Drug Delivery Systems

History

Intrathecal administration of analgesic medications probably began in 1885 when J.L. Corning discovered that intrathecal cocaine produced limb paralysis in dogs, and induced anesthesia in humans.[40] The earliest application of morphine for intrathecal use was reported in 1900, and then for epidural use in cancer and postoperative pain in 1979.[41] Spinal delivery of drugs for the treatment of chronic pain by means of an IDDS began in the 1980s. This form of drug delivery used a fixed, continuous rate of infusion and offered clinicians the ability to use lower doses of drug that would generally produce fewer adverse effects (such as sedation, cognitive deficits, fatigue, and constipation). By 1991, battery-powered, externally programmable IDDS pumps entered the U.S. market[42] permitting noninvasive dose changes of drug with an external programmer. Previously, dose changes could only be made by refilling the constant flow rate pumps with different concentrations of medication.[42,43] Today, clinicians typically implant programmable pumps when frequent dosage changes are likely. The cancer pain population reflects the broader group of chronic pain patients who often require changes to their analgesic therapies in response to the dynamic features of their pain condition.[43] Hence, many physicians implant programmable pumps for ease of dose changes in both cancer and chronic noncancer pain patients.

When the WHO analgesic "ladder" is applied fully, as many as 20% of cancer patients in pain fail to attain adequate pain or symptom control.[2,14,44] This group of patients suffering from intractable pain should be considered for interventional pain-relieving therapies, including IDDSs. One randomized controlled trial (RCT) even suggests that earlier implementation of intrathecal therapy may lead to improved outcomes, such as enhanced survival.[45] Delivery of medication intrathecally usually consists of placing a needle or small catheter into the cerebrospinal fluid where a drug can bind directly onto specific receptors in the spinal cord. Several agents, such as opioids, local anesthetics, clonidine, and ziconotide, have been infused by the intrathecal route to successfully reduce cancer pain. The intrathecal route of drug delivery holds substantial value in permitting a 300-fold reduction in opioid dose compared to the oral route.[42,46] This dose reduction often alleviates the impact of certain toxicities associated with high-dose oral opioid therapy, such as cognitive disturbance, excessive sedation, and severe constipation. Moreover, clinical evidence suggests that intrathecal drug administration can provide more effective analgesia than systemically administered drug.[45]

Intrathecal Medications

An array of intrathecal medications are infused into the cerebrospinal fluid in an attempt to relieve refractory cancer pain, reduce disabling adverse effects of oral or transdermal analgesics, and promote a higher quality of life. Morphine represents the only opioid approved by the FDA for intrathecal use. Many pain specialists and researchers consider morphine the gold standard intraspinal opioid against which all other opioids are compared. For instance, morphine has been shown to be safe and effective for long-term administration based on preclinical and human studies.[42] In practice, hydromorphone, fentanyl, and sufentanil are used as alternatives to morphine in patients who are less responsive to morphine's analgesic properties or who demonstrate intolerable adverse effects to morphine. In fact, guidelines from the 2004 Polyanalgesic Consensus Conference (an expert group that updates clinical guidelines for the use of intraspinal drug infusion in pain management) recommends hydromorphone along with morphine as a first line agent for consideration among pain practitioners.[47]

Clonidine, an alpha-2 agonist with analgesic efficacy, is FDA approved for epidural use in the management of cancer pain. A large, well-designed study performed by Eisenach and colleagues reported the beneficial effects of epidural clonidine for the management of severe cancer pain with neuropathic features.[48] Further, Coombs and colleagues reported the effectiveness of intrathecal clonidine in combination with hydromorphone for the treatment of intractable cancer pain.[49] Clonidine's role as a monotherapy is often dwarfed by its more common use as a dual intrathecal agent with morphine or hydromorphone. Clinically, clonidine seems to simultaneously enhance analgesia and reduce opioid-related toxicity. Practitioners also consider clonidine a useful agent in concert with local anesthetics. Used alone or in combination with opioids or local anesthetics, clonidine can be beneficial in treating patients who exhibit a neuropathic component to their pain.[50]

When pain becomes refractory to singular treatment with intrathecal opioids, it may respond to the addition of local anesthetic. Though bupivacaine is not approved by the FDA for intrathecal use, substantial clinical experience and several reports in the literature support its application for treating cancer pain. Moreover, both the Polyanalgesic Consensus Conference[47] and the Cancer Pain Best Practices Algorithm[51] recommend intrathecal bupivacaine as either a first- or second-line agent for the control of refractory cancer pain. Most clinical reports of intrathecal bupivacaine describe combination therapy with morphine, though hydromorphone or other opioids can be substituted for morphine. Bupivacaine used in concert with morphine can behave synergistically to reduce severe cancer pain and attenuate opioid-related toxicity. For instance, the addition of intrathecal bupivacaine to morphine permits a lowered dose of morphine while potentiating treatment efficacy in patients with refractory cancer pain.[26,52] Clinical experience with bupivacaine demonstrates its effectiveness for controlling neuropathic pain or mixed neuropathic and nociceptive pain associated with malignancy.[26,47,51] This parallels the application of intrathecal clonidine to both neuropathic and mixed cancer pain conditions.

Intrathecal ziconotide is approved by the FDA for the treatment of refractory cancer pain or AIDS, and data demonstrate its analgesic capability.[53] Moreover, some patients with opioid-resistant pain or with intolerable opioid adverse effects may experience relief with ziconotide.[53] The most recent guidelines from the Polyanalgesic Consensus Conference (2007) place ziconotide on a par with morphine and hydromorphone as a first-line agent for the management of pain.[54] Given its blockade of the N-type voltage-sensitive calcium channels in the spinal cord,[55] ziconotide does not induce a withdrawal syndrome upon discontinuation.[56] However, significant cognitive impairment and psychiatric changes can be associated with dose escalation; therefore, clinicians should increase this drug slowly and carefully in order to avoid these drug-limiting effects. Due to its adverse effect profile, ziconotide has yet to gain wide acceptance as an effective analgesic agent for managing cancer pain.

IDDS Overview

An IDDS consists of a small, hockey puck–sized electronic pump that delivers drug(s) to the intrathecal space through a catheter (Fig. 3). Physicians implant the pump subcutaneously in the anterior wall of the abdomen and tunnel the catheter across the flank to the intrathecal space. A reservoir containing the drug is refilled through a port, which is accessed by a needle inserted through the skin. Practitioners program the pump (for instance increase or decrease the dose) by an external, hand-held device, which controls the rate of infusion, delivers bolus doses, and provides information about the pump's functional status. The battery life of state-of-the-art programmable pumps can reach 7 years. Consequently, most cancer patients with advanced disease will not require surgical pump replacement during their average lifetime. Advantages of IDDS over tunneled, externalized intrathecal or epidural catheters used for pain control include patient

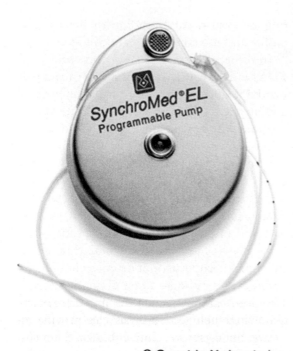

Figure 3. Implantable drug delivery system (IDDS).

mobility, ease of use, lower maintenance, and cost-effectiveness.[22] Potential complications of an IDDS reported in studies include pump malposition, wound infection, nausea/emesis, pruritus, urinary retention, and hardware malfunction.[57]

Cost Effectiveness

Compared to medical management or to an exteriorized epidural catheter for treating chronic pain, IDDS has been shown to offer cost savings over time.[22,58] For instance, de Lissovoy and associates studied the cost effectiveness of IDDSs infusing morphine for failed back surgery syndrome. The research group compared intrathecal morphine therapy to medical management and determined that IDDS therapy was cost effective for patients when the duration of therapy exceeded 12–22 months.[58] Furthermore, in comparing IDDSs to epidural morphine delivery with an external pump, Bedder and colleagues showed that the costs of therapy are equivalent at 3 months (the break-even point), despite the

higher upfront costs associated with intrathecal pump implantation. At 1 year, the costs of epidural morphine treatment were twice those of IDDS therapy.[22]

Selection Criteria

No uniform protocol exists for selecting patients with malignant pain for intrathecal therapy. Generally, pain specialists consider patients for IDDSs if they suffer from chronic, intractable cancer pain, report insufficient pain relief or intolerable adverse effects from systemic agents, respond favorably to a screening trial, and have a life expectancy of at least 3 months.[42,45] Both the patient and pain specialist should carefully assess the decision to proceed with long-term intrathecal therapy because the device requires ongoing management and responsible care.

Trialing Protocol

Techniques for trialing intrathecal agents range from a single injection of drug to continuous infusion of medication with a catheter. There is no consensus that a particular screening protocol leads to a more successful outcome, so techniques vary according to physician preference. All clinicians should assess patients during the trial and include elements of pain, function, mood, and adverse effects.[42,59] Many practitioners interpret a 50% decrement in pain along with a favorable side-effect profile as predictive of sustained success with an IDDS[60]; however, no studies provide outcome-based data that support the type or level of improvement necessary for successful IDDS treatment. Regular monitoring of pain relief, functional status, and medication-related adverse effects should be initiated once chronic intrathecal therapy has begun. Physicians and patients must also consider the logistics of ongoing pump maintenance, including refills of drug and dose changes. For example, both unplanned interruptions in therapy that may cause withdrawal symptoms and improper dose escalations can pose serious health risks to a medically vulnerable population of patients.

Oncologists typically refer patients for intrathecal therapy when patients with cancer pain fail comprehensive medical management or experience unacceptable adverse effects from conventional delivery (oral, parenteral, or transdermal) of analgesic medications. A growing number of physicians now refer such patients for intrathecal therapy when the oral route of drug delivery is unreliable. For instance, patients with substantial pain who may be undergoing an aggressive chemotherapeutic regimen may be ideal candidates for the intrathecal approach.

Efficacy of IDDS

Several cohort studies have demonstrated the efficacy of IDDSs for alleviating intractable cancer pain since their inception in 1991.[34,61 66] Stronger evidence for effectiveness derives from a multicenter, RCT of over 200 refractory cancer pain patients. In this study, Smith and co-workers compared IDDS therapy (opioid $+/-$ bupivacaine) plus medical management (opioids $+/-$ adjuvants) to medical management alone.[45] At 4 weeks, the IDDS plus medical management group reported greater reduction in pain and drug-related toxicity, a significant decrease in fatigue, and an elevated level of consciousness. Further, 60% of IDDS patients compared to 42% of medical management patients reported a visual analog scale score of less than 4, which represents mild pain-interference and improved function.[67] Even more striking was the finding of improved survival at 6 months among IDDS patients—54% of IDDS patients alive at 6 months versus 37% of patients alive in the medical management alone group. IDDS therapy may have contributed to longevity by allowing patients to enhance their level of activity, reduce the risk of pulmonary embolism, improve their nutrition, and develop a greater "will to live."[68]

Chemical Neurolysis

In general, neurolysis describes intentional injury to a nerve or group of nerves by chemical (e.g., alcohol or phenol), thermal (heat), surgical, or cryogenic (freezing) methods with the intent to relieve pain. The effects of neurolytic therapy typically persist between 3–6 months, although the response can vary widely. Many pain specialists apply neurolytic techniques to discrete clinical conditions in which patients suffer from refractory cancer pain and have otherwise failed previous analgesic and complementary approaches. Neurolysis is less commonly invoked for nonmalignant pain due to its risks of neuritis, neurologic deficit, damage to non-neural tissue (such as skin or organs) or nontargeted neural structures, and impermanent effects. Additionally, the therapy can render incomplete pain relief due to existing adhesions, tumor burden, or nerve regeneration. Nonetheless, neurolysis can provide effective analgesia and life-enhancing benefits when applied appropriately. For instance, alcohol neurolysis for irreversible abdominal pain from pancreatic cancer can provide significant analgesia for up to 6 months and improve survival ($P < 0.0001$).[69] There are several sites for neurolytic blockade of the sympathetic nervous system for the treatment of cancer pain (Table 3; Fig. 4). Sympathetically mediated pain associated with gastrointestinal and genitourinary cancers tends to respond to celiac plexus, SHP, or ganglion impar neurolytic blocks.

Neurolytic techniques more effectively treat discrete, well-circumscribed pain that patients can identify easily (such as hemithoracic pain from malignancy). Interestingly, visceral pain—often diffuse and vague generally—responds to neurolysis despite its broadly based clinical features. For instance, celiac plexus or splanchnic neurolysis is often considered in patients with abdominal and referred back pain secondary to visceral or retroperitoneal malignancy in the abdomen, and SHP neurolysis can effectively reduce pelvic pain due to visceral pelvic cancers. Empirical data suggest that visceral and somatic pain respond more favorably to neurolytic therapy than does neuropathic pain.

gallbladder, stomach, spleen, kidneys, intestines, adrenals, and all abdominal vessels except the left colon, rectum, and pelvis.[86] Accordingly, pain caused by pathologic conditions of these anatomic structures can be interrupted by neurolytic blockade at the level of the celiac plexus or splanchnic nerves.

Techniques. There are several techniques to access the celiac plexus: percutaneous using fluoroscopy or computed tomographic (CT) imaging, surgical, and endoscopic ultrasound. Only the percutaneous approaches are reviewed in this article.

The first percutaneous technique was associated with a relatively high incidence of neurologic complications from excessive posterior spread of agent.[87] However, subsequent methods have become safer by better limiting the spread of the neurolytic solution to the celiac plexus exclusively, often with the aid of CT guidance.[88] Four common percutaneous techniques are listed. Three of these represent posterior approaches (transcrural, retrocrural, and transaortic), and one is an anterior technique (anterior approach). Fluoroscopy or CT imaging can be used for all except the anterior approach, which requires CT scan or ultrasound.

Generally, all patients remain in the prone position for 20–30 min after neurolytic injection to reduce the risk of posterior spread of lytic agent and subsequent injury to the spinal canal or neuroforamina. Patients are monitored for symptoms of bleeding, hypotension, or vascular or neurologic injury. Coagulation studies and platelet count should be carefully reviewed prior to the procedure and found to be within normal limits. Needles should be flushed with saline or local anesthetic prior to removal to avoid depositing neurolytic agent along the needle track.

Transcrural Approach. The transcrural approach to the celiac plexus represents one of the earliest attempts to target this structure by placing a needle anterior to the diaphragm in the plane of the aorta. This technique was discovered after evaluating CT images of a needle's trajectory toward the celiac plexus after avoiding the renal parenchyma, major vessels, vertebral body, and lung parenchyma.[81] This procedure requires the patient to lie prone with a pillow beneath the abdomen to reduce the natural lumbar lordosis. Two needles (frequently 22 gauge and 5–7 inches in length) are often used under fluoroscopic guidance or CT imaging (Fig. 10A). The left side needle is inserted 4 cm lateral to midline with the tip approaching the anterolateral aspect of the aorta. The right side needle is inserted 5–10 cm lateral to midline and is directed between the inferior vena cava and the aorta. Each needle traverses the diaphragmatic crus, and eventually lies anterior to this structure. Proper needle location is confirmed with radiographic contrast followed by a test dose of local anesthetic with epinephrine to ensure nonvascular uptake and a non-neuraxial injection. Next, a reasonable volume (for example, 16–20 mL) of local anesthetic is used as a diagnostic block prior to injecting a neurolytic agent (10% phenol or approximately 20–25 mL of 80–100% alcohol). This technique offers a more focused distribution of neurolytic agent and has reduced the incidence of major nerve damage associated with larger volumes and spread of active agent.[82]

Retrocrural Approach. The retrocrural approach can be slightly modified from the classic technique[84,85] to include bilateral needle insertion that initially contacts the T12 or L1 vertebral bodies and is ultimately advanced to the anterolateral surface of T12. Essentially, the retrocrural technique blocks the thoracic splanchnic, vagal, and sensory afferent fibers that compose the celiac plexus.[89] This block is often considered when tumor burden is extensive in the pre-aortic region, thus limiting adequate spread of neurolytic agent over the celiac ganglia. Two 20–22 gauge, 5–7 inch needles are inserted bilaterally, inferior to the 12th rib, and no more than 7.5 cm lateral to midline. Once the needles contact the vertebral body, they each can be "walked-off" and advanced 1–3 cm or until aortic pulsations are transmitted to the left side needle. Appropriate needle course is guided by fluoroscopy or CT imaging.

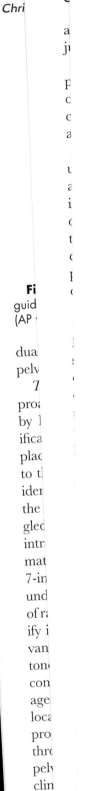

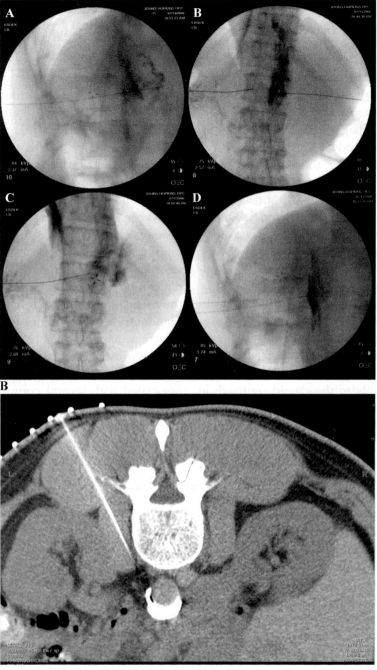

Figure 10. (A) Fluoroscopically guided celiac plexus neurolytic block (AP and lateral views). (B) CT-guided celiac plexus neurolytic block (transaortic approach).

CT guidance will demonstrate the needles' location with respect to pertinent structures, such as the vertebral body, aorta, inferior vena cava, kidney, and diaphragm. Both needles remain posterior to the diaphragmatic crura. Splanchnic nerve blocks require passing the needle to the lateral edge of the middle to superior aspect of the T12 vertebral body.[84] Near the

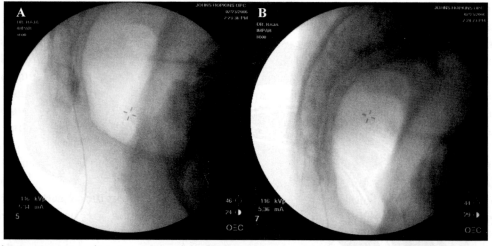

Figure 14. Ganglion impar neurolytic block, anococcygeal approach, fluoroscopically guided (lateral views).

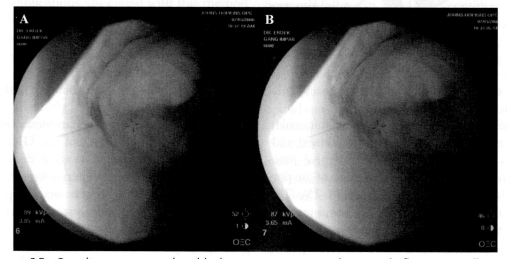

Figure 15. Ganglion impar neurolytic block, trans-sacrococcygeal approach, fluoroscopically guided (lateral views).

future, this technique may hold promise for alleviating pain of malignant origin while reducing the risk of complications associated with chemical neurolysis.

Anococcygeal Approach. This approach was first described by Plancarte in 1990 using a bent needle technique[71,123] (Figs. 13 and 14). With the patient in the lateral decubitus position and knees bent against the abdomen, the anococcygeal ligament is palpated inferior to the coccyx. A 60° curved, 22 gauge, 3.5-inch needle is placed through the anococcygeal ligament and directed cephalad with a slightly posterior an-

gle to minimize the risk of rectal perforation. Proper position of the needle is noted when the tip has reached the sacrococcygeal junction. The practitioner may perform a continuous rectal exam to confirm the integrity of the rectum. A similar technique has been modified with the patient in a frog-legged position to extend the distance from the anococcygeal ligament to the impar in order to eliminate the need for needle angulation.[132]

Trans-Sacrococcygeal Approach. The sacrococcygeal approach was first described by Wemm and colleagues in 1995.[133] In this technique, the patient is placed in the lateral decubitus position with both knees flexed, and fluoroscopy is used to identify the sacrococcygeal joint (Fig. 15). A 22-gauge, 3.5-inch needle is used to penetrate midline through the sacrococcygeal ligament and into the retroperitoneal space. Local anesthetic or neurolytic agent is injected in a quantity sufficient to cover the sacrococcygeal joint and to ensure blockade of the GI.

Intercoccygeal Approach. This technique has been described most recently (2006) and entails the insertion of a 22-gauge, 2-inch needle through the space between the first and second coccygeal bones.[124,125] After proper spread of radiographic contrast, 1 mL of 4% lidocaine is deposited as a prognostic test prior to injecting 4 mL of 100% alcohol.

Coccygeal Transverse Approach. In 2004, Huang reported this technique as an alternative to the sacrococcygeal approach.[134] Needle entry is inferior to the transverse process of the coccyx. The patient is placed in the prone or lateral position, and a bent or curved 22-gauge, 3.5-inch needle is directed superiorly and medially toward the sacrococcygeal junction. If the coccyx is encountered, the needle is repositioned inferiorly and walked off the bone. The needle is inserted near the anterior surface of the coccyx until it reaches the sacrococcygeal junction. Local anesthetic and/or neurolytic agent can be injected after correct needle position is verified by fluoroscopy.

Side Effects and Complications. There are currently no reported complications in the literature[105,135]; however, theoretical risks include needle breakage, failure of the block/neurolysis (e.g., secondary to tumor spread), rectal perforation, periosteal injection, sacral nerve root injury, epidural injection, and motor, sexual, bowel, or bladder dysfunction from accidental spread of neurolytic agent.[126,131]

Clinical Effectiveness. Two prospective studies have reported good efficacy of neurolytic blockade of the GI using 6% phenol for unremitting perineal pain due to cancer.[123,136] In another

study, the effects of radiofrequency ablation of the GI produced a 50% decrease in pain scores, with average duration of 2.2 months and no complications.[131]

Failures. Failures can be attributed to the variable anatomic location of the GI and incomplete understanding of visceral nociceptive processing and specific neural connections that lead to and from the GI.[131]

Conclusion

A significant number of patients with cancer may suffer from considerable pain at some point during their disease. Application of the WHO analgesic guidelines is a critical component to managing cancer pain effectively. However, healthcare professionals must consider the array of interventional pain-relieving strategies currently available that can substantially improve the quality of life of patients suffering from cancer pain. These procedural interventions include epidural and intrathecal infusion therapies, IDDS, and neuraxial interventions, such as celiac plexus, SHP, and GI neurolytic blocks. Many of these procedures offer rapid and effective analgesia with less toxicity than oral or parenteral agents, permit dose reductions of systemic analgesics, serve as an alternative to cases of refractory pain, and enhance performance status and quality of life of patients with cancer pain. Some interventions (such as IDDS and celiac plexus neurolysis) even confer a survival benefit among those patients treated with the therapy.[45,69] Clearly, pain practitioners face complex clinical challenges while treating cancer pain patients. Today, interventional pain-relieving approaches should be considered as a critical component of a multifaceted therapeutic program of cancer pain relief.

Conflicts of Interest

The authors declare no conflicts of interest.

References

1. Brescia, F.J. *et al.* 1992. Pain, opioid use, and survival in hospitalized patients with advanced cancer. *J. Clin. Oncol.* **10:** 149–155.

2. Cleeland, C.S. *et al.* 1994. Pain and its treatment in outpatients with metastatic cancer. *N. Engl. J. Med.* **330:** 592–596.

3. Portenoy, R.K. *et al.* 1992. Pain in ambulatory patients with lung or colon cancer. Prevalence, characteristics, and effect. *Cancer* **70:** 1616–1624.

4. Tolle, S.W. *et al.* 2000. Family reports of barriers to optimal care of the dying. *Nurs. Res.* **49:** 310–317.

5. Berry, P.H. & J.L. Dahl. 2000. The new JCAHO pain standards: implications for pain management nurses. *Pain. Manag. Nurs.* **1:** 3–12.

6. WHO. 1998. Cancer Pain Release. Available from: http://www.whocancerpain.wisc.edu/ (accessed Nov. 9, 2007).

7. Zech, D.F. *et al.* 1995. Validation of World Health Organization Guidelines for cancer pain relief: a 10-year prospective study. *Pain* **63:** 65–76.

8. Committee, W.E. 1990. Cancer pain relief and palliative care. In World Health Organ. Tech. Rep. Ser., W.H. Organization, Editor. 1–75.

9. Levy, R.M. 1996. Pharmacologic treatment of cancer pain. *N. Engl. J. Med.* **335:** 1124–1132.

10. Cherny, N.I. & K.M. Foley. 1997. Nonopioid and opioid analgesic pharmacotherapy of cancer pain. *Otolaryngol. Clin. North Am.* **30:** 279–306.

11. Pappagallo, M. 2001. Incidence, prevalence, and management of opioid bowel dysfunction. *Am. J. Surg.* **182**(5A Suppl): 11S–18S.

12. Walsh, T.D. 1990. Prevention of opioid side effects. *J. Pain Symptom. Manage.* **5:** 362–367.

13. Bruera, E. *et al.* 1992. The use of methylphenidate in patients with incident cancer pain receiving regular opiates. A preliminary report. *Pain* **50:** 75–77.

14. Meuser, T. *et al.* 2001. Symptoms during cancer pain treatment following WHO-guidelines: a longitudinal follow-up study of symptom prevalence, severity and etiology. *Pain* **93:** 247–157.

15. Miaskowski, C. *et al.* 2001. Lack of adherence with the analgesic regimen: a significant barrier to effective cancer pain management. *J. Clin. Oncol.* **19:** 4275–4279.

16. Bruera, E. *et al.* 1996. Opioid rotation in patients with cancer pain. A retrospective comparison of dose ratios between methadone, hydromorphone, and morphine. *Cancer* **78:** 852–857.

17. de Stoutz, N.D., E. Bruera & M. Suarez-Almazor. 1995. Opioid rotation for toxicity reduction in terminal cancer patients. *J. Pain Symptom. Manage.* **10:** 378–384.

18. Miguel, R. 2000. Interventional treatment of cancer pain: the fourth step in the World Health Organization analgesic ladder? *Cancer Control.* **7:** 149–156.

19. Agency for Health Care Policy and Research Rockville, Maryland. 1994. Management of cancer pain guideline overview. *J. Natl. Med. Assoc.* **86:** 571–573, 634.

20. Hogan, Q. *et al.* 1991. Epidural opiates and local anesthetics for the management of cancer pain. *Pain* **46:** 271–279.

21. Smitt, P.S. *et al.* 1998. Outcome and complications of epidural analgesia in patients with chronic cancer pain. *Cancer* **83:** 2015–2022.

22. Bedder, M.D., K. Burchiel & A. Larson. 1991. Cost analysis of two implantable narcotic delivery systems. *J. Pain Symptom. Manage.* **6:** 368–373.

23. Crul, B.J. & E.M. Delhaas. 1991. Technical complications during long-term subarachnoid or epidural administration of morphine in terminally ill cancer patients: a review of 140 cases. *Reg. Anesth.* **16:** 209–213.

24. Bahar, M., M. Rosen & M.D. Vickers. 1984. Chronic cannulation of the intradural or extradural space in the rat. *Br. J. Anaesth.* **56:** 405–410.

25. Baker, L. *et al.* 2004. Evolving spinal analgesia practice in palliative care. *Palliat. Med.* **18:** 507–515.

26. Sjoberg, M. *et al.* 1991. Long-term intrathecal morphine and bupivacaine in "refractory" cancer pain. I. Results from the first series of 52 patients. *Acta Anaesthesiol. Scand.* **35:** 30–43.

27. Nitescu, P. *et al.* 1992. Bacteriology, drug stability and exchange of percutaneous delivery systems and antibacterial filters in long-term intrathecal infusion of opioid drugs and bupivacaine in "refractory" pain. *Clin. J. Pain.* **8:** 324–337.

28. Nitescu, P. *et al.* 1998. Continuous infusion of opioid and bupivacaine by externalized intrathecal catheters in long-term treatment of "refractory" nonmalignant pain. *Clin. J. Pain.* **14:** 17–28.

29. Nitescu, P. *et al.* 1991. Long-term, open catheterization of the spinal subarachnoid space for continuous infusion of narcotic and bupivacaine in patients with "refractory" cancer pain. A technique of catheterization and its problems and complications. *Clin. J. Pain.* **7:** 143–161.

30. Nitescu, P. *et al.* 1990. Epidural versus intrathecal morphine-bupivacaine: assessment of consecutive treatments in advanced cancer pain. *J. Pain Symptom. Manage.* **5:** 18–26.

31. Penn, R.D. *et al.* 1984. Cancer pain relief using chronic morphine infusion. Early experience with a programmable implanted drug pump. *J. Neurosurg.* **61:** 302–306.

32. Sjoberg, M. *et al.* 1992. Neuropathologic findings after long-term intrathecal infusion of morphine and bupivacaine for pain treatment in cancer patients. *Anesthesiology* **76:** 173–186.

33. Dahm, P. *et al.* 1998. Efficacy and technical complications of long-term continuous intraspinal infusions of opioid and/or bupivacaine in refractory nonmalignant pain: a comparison between the epidural and the intrathecal approach with externalized or implanted catheters and infusion pumps. *Clin. J. Pain.* **14:** 4–16.

34. Gestin, Y., A. Vainio & A.M. Pegurier. 1997. Long-term intrathecal infusion of morphine in the home care of patients with advanced cancer. *Acta Anaesthesiol. Scand.* **41**(1 Pt 1): 12–17.

35. Krames, E.S. & R.M. Lanning. 1993. Intrathecal infusional analgesia for nonmalignant pain: analgesic efficacy of intrathecal opioid with or without bupivacaine. *J. Pain Symptom. Manage.* **8:** 539–548.

36. Hassenbusch, S. *et al.* 2002. Management of intrathecal catheter-tip inflammatory masses: a consensus statement. *Pain Med.* **3:** 313–323.

37. Cabbell, K.L., J.A. Taren & O. Sagher. 1998. Spinal cord compression by catheter granulomas in high-dose intrathecal morphine therapy: case report. *Neurosurgery* **42:** 1176–1180; discussion 1180–1181.

38. Langsam, A. 1999. Spinal cord compression by catheter granulomas in high-dose intrathecal morphine therapy: case report. *Neurosurgery* **44:** 689 691.

39. McMillan, M.R., T. Doud & W. Nugent. 2003. Catheter-associated masses in patients receiving intrathecal analgesic therapy. *Anesth. Analg.* **96:** 186–190, table of contents.

40. Corning, J. 1885. Spinal anaesthesia and local medication of the cord. *N. Y. Med. J.* **42:** 483–485.

41. Brill, S., G.M. Gurman & A. Fisher. 2003. A history of neuraxial administration of local analgesics and opioids. *Eur. J. Anaesthesiol.* **20:** 682–689.

42. Wallace, M. & T.L. Yaksh. 2000. Long-term spinal analgesic delivery: a review of the preclinical and clinical literature. *Reg. Anesth. Pain Med.* **25:** 117–157.

43. Prager, J.P. 2002. Neuraxial medication delivery: the development and maturity of a concept for treating chronic pain of spinal origin. *Spine* **27:** 2593–2605; discussion 2606.

44. Vainio, A. & A. Auvinen. 1996. Prevalence of symptoms among patients with advanced cancer: an international collaborative study. symptom prevalence group. *J. Pain Symptom. Manage.* **12:** 3–10.

45. Smith, T.J. *et al.* 2002. Randomized clinical trial of an implantable drug delivery system compared with comprehensive medical management for refractory cancer pain: impact on pain, drug-related toxicity, and survival. *J. Clin. Oncol.* **20:** 4040–4049.

46. Krames, E.S. 1996. Intraspinal opioid therapy for chronic nonmalignant pain: current practice and clinical guidelines. *J. Pain Symptom. Manage.* **11:** 333–352.

47. Hassenbusch, S.J. *et al.* 2004. Polyanalgesic Consensus Conference 2003: an update on the management of pain by intraspinal drug delivery—report of an expert panel. *J. Pain Symptom. Manage.* **27:** 540–563.

48. Eisenach, J.C. *et al.* 1995. Epidural clonidine analgesia for intractable cancer pain. The epidural clonidine study group. *Pain* **61:** 391–399.

49. Coombs, D., L.H. Maurer, R.I. Saunders & M. Gaylor. 1984. Outcomes and complications of continuous intraspinal narcotic analgesia for cancer pain control. *J. Clin. Oncol.* **2:** 1414–1420.

50. Ackerman, L.L., K.A. Follett & R.W. Rosenquist. 2003. Long-term outcomes during treatment of chronic pain with intrathecal clonidine or clonidine/opioid combinations. *J. Pain Symptom. Manage.* **26:** 668–677.

51. Stearns, L. *et al.* 2005. Intrathecal drug delivery for the management of cancer pain: a multidisciplinary consensus of best clinical practices. *J. Support. Oncol.* **3:** 399–408.

52. Sjoberg, M. *et al.* 1994. Long-term intrathecal morphine and bupivacaine in patients with refractory cancer pain. Results from a morphine:bupivacaine dose regimen of 0.5:4.75 mg/ml. *Anesthesiology* **80:** 284–297.

53. Staats, P.S. *et al.* 2004. Intrathecal ziconotide in the treatment of refractory pain in patients with cancer or AIDS: a randomized controlled trial. *JAMA* **291:** 63–70.

54. Deer, T.K., E.S. Hassenbusch, *et al.* 2007. Polyanalgesic consensus conference 2007: recommendations for the management of pain by intrathecal (intraspinal) drug delivery: report of an interdisciplinary expert panel. *Neuromodulation* **10:** 301–328.

55. Elan Pharmaceuticals, I. 2005. Prialt (Ziconotide) Prescribing Information. Dublin.

56. Ridgeway, B., M. Wallace & A. Gerayli. 2000. Ziconotide for the treatment of severe spasticity after spinal cord injury. *Pain* **85:** 287–289.

57. Turner, J.A., J.M. Sears & J.D. Loeser. 2007. Programmable intrathecal opioid delivery systems for chronic noncancer pain: a systematic review of effectiveness and complications. *Clin. J. Pain.* **23:** 180–195.

58. de Lissovoy, G. *et al.* 1997. Cost-effectiveness of long-term intrathecal morphine therapy for pain associated with failed back surgery syndrome. *Clin. Ther.* **19:** 96–112; discussion 84–85.

59. Prager, J. & M. Jacobs. 2001. Evaluation of patients for implantable pain modalities: medical and behavioral assessment. *Clin. J. Pain* **17:** 206–214.

60. Hassenbusch, S.J. *et al.* 1995. Long-term intraspinal infusions of opioids in the treatment of neuropathic pain. *J. Pain. Symptom. Manage.* **10:** 527–543.

61. Devulder, J. *et al.* 1994. Spinal analgesia in terminal care: risk versus benefit. *J. Pain Symptom. Manage.* **9:** 75–81.

62. Onofrio, B.M. & T.L. Yaksh. 1990. Long-term pain relief produced by intrathecal morphine infusion in 53 patients. *J. Neurosurg.* **72:** 200–209.

63. Penn, R.D. & J.A. Paice. 1987. Chronic intrathecal morphine for intractable pain. *J. Neurosurg.* **67:** 182–186.

64. Meenan, D. *et al.* 1999. Managing intractable pain with an intrathecal catheter and injection port: technique and guidelines. *Am. Surg.* **65:** 1054–1060.

65. Ricci, V., A. Dalpane & E. Lolli. 1995. Continuous spinal analgesia in home care of oncologic pain. *Minerva. Med.* **86:** 409–414.

66. Schultheiss, R., J. Schramm & J. Neidhardt. 1992. Dose changes in long- and medium-term intrathecal morphine therapy of cancer pain. *Neurosurgery* **31:** 664–669; discussion 669–670.

67. Serlin, R.C. *et al.* 1995. When is cancer pain mild, moderate or severe? Grading pain severity by its interference with function. *Pain* **61:** 277–284.

68. Chochinov, H.M. *et al.* 1999. Will to live in the terminally ill. *Lancet* **354:** 816–819.

69. Lillemoe, K.D. *et al.* 1993. Chemical splanchnicectomy in patients with unresectable pancreatic cancer. A prospective randomized trial. *Ann. Surg.* **217:** 447–455; discussion 456–457.

70. Candido, K. & R.A. Stevens. 2003. Intrathecal neurolytic blocks for the relief of cancer pain. *Best. Pract. Res. Clin. Anaesthesiol.* **17:** 407–428.

71. Patt, R.B. 1993. *Cancer Pain.* Lippincott. Philadelphia, xxi, 650 p.

72. Cousins, M., B. Dwyer & D. Bigg. 1988. Chronic pain and neurolytic blockade. In *Neural Blockade in Clinical Anesthesia and Management of Pain*, 2 edn. M. Cousins & P.O. Bridenbaugh, Eds. JB Lippincott. Philadelphia.

73. Waxman, S. 2003. *Clinical Neuroanatomy.* Lange Medical Books/McGraw-Hill. New York.

74. Winnie, A. 1996. Subarachnoid neurolytic blocks. In *Interventional Pain Management*. W.A. Waldman, Ed., 401. WB Saunders. Philadephia.

75. Gerbershagen, H.U. 1981. Neurolysis. Subarachnoid neurolytic blockade. *Acta Anaesthesiol. Belg.* **32:** 45–57.

76. Bonica, J.B., F.P., G. Moricca, *et al.* 1990. Neurolytic blockade and hypophysectomy. In *The Management of Pain*, 2nd edn. J. Bonica, Ed. Lea & Febiger. Philadelphia, 1980.

77. Kappis, M. 1919. Sensibilitat und lokale anasthesie im chirurgischen gebeit der bauchkikle mit besonderer berucksichtigung der splanchnicusanasthesia. *Beitr. Klin. Chir.* **115:** 161–175.

78. Ischia, S. *et al.* 1998 Labat Lecture: the role of the neurolytic celiac plexus block in pancreatic cancer pain management: do we have the answers? *Reg. Anesth. Pain. Med.* **23:** 611–614.

79. Eisenberg, E., D.B. Carr & T.C. Chalmers. 1995. Neurolytic celiac plexus block for treatment of cancer pain: a meta-analysis. *Anesth. Analg.* **80:** 290–295.

80. Ischia, S. *et al.* 2000. Celiac block for the treatment of pancreatic pain. *Curr. Rev. Pain.* **4:** 127–133.

81. Ward, E.M. *et al.* 1979. The celiac ganglia in man: normal anatomic variations. *Anesth. Analg.* **58:** 461–465.

82. Singler, R.C. 1982. An improved technique for alcohol neurolysis of the celiac plexus. *Anesthesiology* **56:** 137–141.

83. Woodburne, R. 1973. *Essentials of Human Anatomy*, 5th edn. 450–454. Oxford University Press. Oxford, England.

84. Boas, R. 1978. Sympathetic blocks in clinical practice. *Int. Anesthesiol. Clin.* **16:** 149–182.

85. Moore, D. 1984. Intercostal nerve block and celiac plexus block for pain therapy. In *Advances in Pain Research and Therapy*, Vol. 7. C. Beneditti, *et al.*, Eds. 309–329. Raven Press. New York.

86. Mercadante, S. and F. Nicosia. 1998. Celiac plexus block: a reappraisal. *Reg. Anesth. Pain Med.* **23:** 37–48.

87. Moore, D.C., W.H. Bush & L.L. Burnett. 1981. Celiac plexus block: a roentgenographic, anatomic study of technique and spread of solution in patients and corpses. *Anesth. Analg.* **60:** 369–379.

88. Lieberman, R.P. & S.D. Waldman. 1990. Celiac plexus neurolysis with the modified transaortic approach. *Radiology* **175:** 274–276.

89. Brown, D.L. & D.C. Moore. 1988. The use of neurolytic celiac plexus block for pancreatic cancer: anatomy and technique. *J. Pain Symptom. Manage.* **3:** 206–209.

90. Rathmell, J.P. 2006. *Atlas of Image-Guided Intervention in Regional Anesthesia and Pain Medicine*, 1st edn. 128–129. Lippincott Williams & Wilkins. Philadelphia.

91. Ischia, S. *et al.* 1983. A new approach to the neurolytic block of the coeliac plexus: the transaortic technique. *Pain* **16:** 333–341.

92. Romanelli, D.F., C.F. Beckmann & F.W. Heiss. 1993. Celiac plexus block: efficacy and safety of the anterior approach. *Am. J. Roentgenol.* **160:** 497–500.

93. Davies, D.D. 1993. Incidence of major complications of neurolytic coeliac plexus block. *J. R. Soc. Med.* **86:** 264–266.

94. Lieberman, R., S.L. Lieberman, D.J. Cuka & G.B. Lund. 1988. Celiac plexus and splanchnic nerve block: a review. *Semin. Intervent. Radiol.* **5:** 257–266.

95. Wong, G. & Brown, D.L. 1995. Transient paraplegia following alcohol celiac plexus block. *Reg. Anesth.* **20:** 352–355.

96. Woodham, M.J. & M.H. Hanna. 1989. Paraplegia after coeliac plexus block. *Anaesthesia* **44:** 487–489.

97. Prasanna, A. 1996. Unilateral celiac plexus block. *J. Pain Symptom Manage* **11:** 154–157.

98. Ischia, S.P. 1999. Computed tomography eliminates paraplegia and/or death from neurolytic celiac plexus block. *Reg. Anesthesia Pain Med.* **24:** 484–486.

99. Moore, D.C. 1999. Computed tomography eliminates paraplegia and/or death from neurolytic celiac plexus block. *Reg. Anesthesia Pain Med.* **24:** 483.

100. Mercadante, S. 1993. Celiac plexus block versus analgesics in pancreatic cancer pain. *Pain* **52:** 187–192.

101. Polati, E. *et al.* 1998. Prospective randomized double-blind trial of neurolytic coeliac plexus block in patients with pancreatic cancer. *Br. J. Surg.* **5:** 199–201.

102. Weber, J.G. *et al.* 1996. Celiac plexus block. Retrocrural computed tomographic anatomy in patients with and without pancreatic cancer. *Reg. Anesth.* **21:** 407–413.

103. Iki, K. *et al.* 2003. Celiac plexus block: evaluation of injectate spread by three-dimensional computed tomography. *Abdom. Imaging.* **28:** 571–573.

104. Rosenberg, S.K. *et al.* 1998. Superior hypogastric plexus block successfully treats severe penile pain after transurethral resection of the prostate. *Reg. Anesth. Pain. Med.* **23:** 618–620.

105. de Leon-Casasola, O.A. 2000. Critical evaluation of chemical neurolysis of the sympathetic axis for cancer pain. *Cancer Control.* **7:** 142–148.

106. Mauroy, B. *et al.* 2003. The inferior hypogastric plexus (pelvic plexus): its importance in neural preservation techniques. *Surg. Radiol. Anat.* **25:** 6–15.

107. Plancarte, R. *et al.* 1990. Superior hypogastric plexus block for pelvic cancer pain. *Anesthesiology* **73:** 236–239.

108. de Leon-Casasola, O.A., E. Kent & M.J. Lema. 1993. Neurolytic superior hypogastric plexus block for chronic pelvic pain associated with cancer. *Pain* **54:** 145–151.

109. Wechsler, R.J. *et al.* 1995. Superior hypogastric plexus block for chronic pelvic pain in the presence of endometriosis: CT techniques and results. *Radiology* **196:** 103–106.

110. Cariati, M. *et al.* 2002. CT-guided superior hypogastric plexus block. *J. Comput. Assist. Tomogr.* **26:** 428–431.

111. Michalek, P. & J. Dutka. 2005. Computed tomography-guided anterior approach to the superior hypogastric plexus for noncancer pelvic pain: a report of two cases. *Clin. J. Pain.* **21:** 553–556.

112. de Oliveira, R., M.P. dos Reis & W.A. Prado. 2004. The effects of early or late neurolytic sympathetic plexus block on the management of abdominal or pelvic cancer pain. *Pain* **110:** 400–408.

113. Kitoh, T. *et al.* 2005. Combined neurolytic block of celiac, inferior mesenteric, and superior hypogastric plexuses for incapacitating abdominal and/or pelvic cancer pain. *J. Anesth.* **19:** 328–332.

114. Waldman, S.D., W.L. Wilson & R.D. Kreps. 1991. Superior hypogastric plexus block using a single needle and computed tomography guidance: description of a modified technique. *Reg. Anesth.* **16:** 286–287.

115. Erdine, S. *et al.* 2003. Transdiscal approach for hypogastric plexus block. *Reg. Anesth. Pain Med.* **28:** 304–308.

116. Kanazi, G.E. *et al.* 1999. New technique for superior hypogastric plexus block. *Reg. Anesth. Pain Med.* **24:** 473–476.

117. Soysal, M.E. *et al.* 2003. Laparoscopic presacral neurolysis for endometriosis-related pelvic pain. *Hum. Reprod.* **18:** 588–592.

118. Chen, F.P., T.S. Lo & Y.K. Soong. 1998. Management of chylous ascites following laparoscopic presacral neurectomy. *Hum. Reprod.* **13:** 880–883.

119. Kwok, A., A. Lam & R. Ford. 2001. Laparoscopic presacral neurectomy: a review. *Obstet. Gynecol. Surv.* **56:** 99–104.

120. Plancarte, R. *et al.* 1997. Neurolytic superior hypogastric plexus block for chronic pelvic pain associated with cancer. *Reg. Anesth.* **22:** 562–568.

121. Chan, W.S. *et al.* 1997. Computed tomography scan-guided neurolytic superior hypogastric block complicated by somatic nerve damage in a severely kyphoscoliotic patient. *Anesthesiology* **86:** 1429–1430.

122. Dutka, J.M. 2002. Neurological complications in neurolytic blocks in the visceral and pelvic regions. *Int. Monitor. Reg. Anesth.* **14:** 69.

123. Plancarte, R.A., R.B. Patt, *et al.* 1990. Presacral blockade of the ganglion of Walther (ganglion impar). *Anesthesiology* **73:** A751.

124. Foye, P.M. 2007. New approaches to ganglion impar blocks via coccygeal joints. *Reg. Anesthesia Pain Med.* **32:** 269.

125. Hong, J.H. & H.S. Jang. 2006. Block of the ganglion impar using a coccygeal joint approach. *Reg. Anesthesia Pain Med.* **31:** 583.

126. Munir, M.A., J. Zhang & M. Ahmad. 2004. A modified needle-inside-needle technique for the ganglion impar block: [Une technique modifiee pour le bloc du ganglion coccygien : une aiguille dans une aiguille]. *Can. J. Anesth.* **51:** 915–917.

127. Nebab, E.G. & I.M. Florence. 1997. An alternative needle geometry for interruption of the ganglion impar. *Anesthesiology* **86:** 1213–1214.

128. Loev, M.A. *et al.* 1998. Cryoablation: a novel approach to neurolysis of the ganglion impar. *Anesthesiology* **88:** 1391–1393.

129. Yeo, S.N. & J.L. Chong. 2001. A case report on the treatment of intractable anal pain from metastatic carcinoma of the cervix. *Ann. Acad. Med. Singapore* **30:** 632–635.

130. Oh, C.S. *et al.* 2004. Clinical implications of topographic anatomy on the ganglion impar. *Anesthesiology* **101:** 249–250.

131. Reig, E. *et al.* 2005. Thermocoagulation of the ganglion impar or ganglion of walther: description of a modified approach. Preliminary results in chronic, nononcological pain. *Pain Practice* **5:** 103–110.

132. de Leon-Casasola, O. 1997. Superior hypogastric plexus block and ganglion impar neurolysis for pain associated with cancer. *Tech. Reg. Anesth Pain Manag.* **1:** 27–31.

133. Wemm, K., Jr. & L. Saberski. 1995. Modified approach to block the ganglion impar (ganglion of Walther). *Reg. Anesth.* **20:** 544–545.

134. Huang, J.J. 2003. Another modified approach to the ganglion of Walther block (ganglion of impar). *J. Clin. Anesth.* **15:** 282–283.

135. de Leon-Casaola, O.A. 2001. Ganglion impar block: critical evaluation. *Tech. Reg. Anesth. Pain Manag.* **5:** 120–122.

136. Swofford, J.R. & D.M. Ratzman. 1998. A transarticular approach to blockade of the ganglion impar (ganglion of walther). *Reg. Anesth. Pain. Med.* **23:** 103.

Febrile Neutropenia

Evolving Strategies

Michael Ellis

Department of Medicine, Faculty of Medicine and Health Sciences, Tawam-Johns Hopkins and Al Ain Hospitals, Al Ain, United Arab Emirates

This review summarizes the current status and diagnostic-therapeutic challenges in febrile neutropenia. Patients with neutropenia-associated infections have a poor prognosis. A large meta-analysis of trials assessing prophylactic antibiotics has shown significant survival benefits; clinical significance of resistance is unclear. Administering broad-spectrum antibiotics to established febrile neutropenic patients has become selective, vancomycin is withheld unless absolutely necessary, and low-risk patients are identified with biological markers. Such patients are now managed with oral antibiotics at home or even without antibiotics. Protracted prolonged neutropenia is the setting par excellence for invasive fungal infections. Conventional amphotericin B administered to such risk patients reduces the incidence of fungal infections. New antifungal drugs have heightened efficacy and lowered toxicity. Novel antifungal diagnostic tests include imaging, particularly the CT "halo" sign (aspergillosis), and serology (glucan, galactomannan), and provide earlier diagnosis and treatment and better outcomes. Negative tests may indicate withholding antifungal therapy. High intermittent dosing of liposomal amphotericin B seems as safe and as effective as standard dosing regimens, but at half the drug acquisition cost. The use of nonantibiotic agents has offered alternative management strategies. Recombinant interleukin-11 reduces bacteremia, through a cytoprotective mechanism on the gut. rhIL-11 releases C-reactive protein and causes shedding of soluble TNF receptor-1, modulating the immunological milieu and the systemic inflammatory response. Other candidate molecules include RANTES and long-pentraxin 3. Recombinant growth factors reduce febrile episodes, permitting completion of chemotherapy, increase overall survival, and minimize infection mortality.

Key words: febrile; neutropenia; antifungal; antibiotics; CT halo; glucan; galactomannan; polyenes; RANTES; rhIL-11

Introduction

The single most significant advance in hematological cancer chemotherapy in the last 40 years has been increased availability and use of more potent and effective cytotoxic chemotherapeutics, which have optimized the chance of inducing remission and bringing increased long-term survival to an increased majority of patients with acute leukemia.[1,2] This success has been tempered by its inextricable linkage to the "innocent casualty" phenomenon of creating a highly immunocompromised milieu fruitful for establishing a wide profile of opportunistic infections, whose morbidity and mortality threaten the outcome of otherwise successful hematological treatment.[1] Several components of the immune system are affected by chemotherapy including immunoglobulin function, T lymphocytes, and macrophages, as well as the fixed anatomical skin and mucosal membrane barriers. The neutrophil, after the macrophage, is the most important part of the immune system to be affected,[2,3] and the consequences of neutropenia

Address for correspondence: Professor Michael Ellis, FRCP, FACP, Chairman, Department of Medicine, Faculty of Medicine & Health Sciences, UAE University, PO Box 17666, Al Ain, UAE. Voice: +971-3-7137656; fax: +971-7672995. michael.ellis@uaeu.ac.ae

Ann. N.Y. Acad. Sci. 1138: 329–350 (2008). © 2008 New York Academy of Sciences.
doi: 10.1196/annals.1414.035

are the major focus of this review. The symptom complex of febrile neutropenia (FN) will be addressed in some detail from key diagnostic and interventional aspects. Results of concluded and ongoing studies by this author will be included to illustrate some of the ongoing challenges and suggest novel strategies for the future.

Historical Perspective

An association between depletion of granulocytes, fever, toxicity, and severe pharyngitis (agranulocytic angina) first appeared definitively in the medical literature over 100 years ago ("Ein fall von extremer Leukopenie").[4] The statement by Schwarz that the course of this symptom complex is so dramatic "and the mortality so high that when a patient recovers it is sufficiently significant to merit a report"[4] presents us with an ageless truth testifying to the challenge that the neutropenic patient presents.

When granulocytopenia was first described in the literature, the cause was usually ascribed to arsenic or benzene poisoning or infection.[5–7] However the original cases more accurately suggest that infection was usually a consequence rather than a cause of the granulocytopenia. Although there is an etiological contribution from congenital and acquired causes (including some infections, such as Parvovirus, nutritional deficiencies, copper deficiency, and immune-mediated mechanisms), it is medications that play the largest role in causing neutropenia.[5] Among the more than 70 documented drug causes, chemotherapeutic agents are the commonest. The mechanism is usually to direct toxicity to the bone marrow progenitor cells.[5]

The 1960s saw the beginning of the modern era of identifying, describing, and understanding the occurrence, pathogenesis, and consequence of neutropenia in patients with hematological malignancy who receive chemotherapy. Bodey is credited with the first clear documentation of the link between infection and leukopenia.[8] He described the inverse relation between frequency of infection and the neutrophil (and lymphocyte) count, the particular association of infection with severe leukopenia ($<0.5 \times 10^9$cells/L) and the increased frequency with increased duration of leukopenia. He observed that the mortality of most patients who had infection and neutropenia was on the order of 90%, or 100% if there was failure of bone marrow recovery. This pivotal paper with its sentinel observations was to set the scene for the next 50 years (Fig. 1).

As cytotoxic therapy has evolved, the intensification and increased frequency of doses of the agents used, as well as the class of agent, preselect for certain infections. Other factors that contribute to the complex interactive etiology include the patient's environment, antibiotic use, and technological support devices. Consequently, the approach to managing the patient at risk from or encountering neutropenia, FN, or persistent FN is dynamic and involves a multifaceted approach including prophylaxis, diagnostics, antimicrobial therapy, immunomodulation, and supportive care.

Bacterial Pathogens

Bacteria have always been the predominant identified organisms; however, the predominant categories of pathogens have fluctuated with each decade in a phenomenon described as a "roller coaster" (Fig. 2). In the late 1950s/early 1960s Gram-positive organisms were the commonest, particularly *Staphylococcus aureus*. The late 1960s/early 1970s were typified by Gram-negative organisms of gastrointestinal tract origin, particularly *Escherichia coli*, *Klebsiella* spp, and *Pseudomonas* spp. By the 1990s *Staphylococcus* spp, including coagulase-negative organisms, *Streptococcus* spp, and *Enterococcus* spp were increasingly seen, as Gram-negatives diminished.[9,10] This cyclical profiling is of both great interest and alarm since organisms, such as the coagulase-negative staphylococci and *S. viridans*, had previously not been encountered as potent pathogens. In particular *S. viridans* was described as producing a toxic shock syndrome

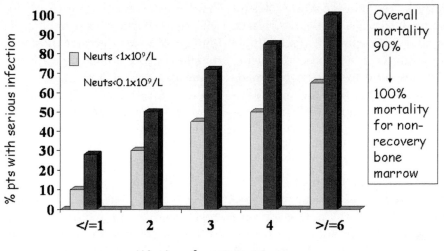

Weeks of neutropenia

From Bodey et al 1966, reference 8

Figure 1. Incidence of serious infection.

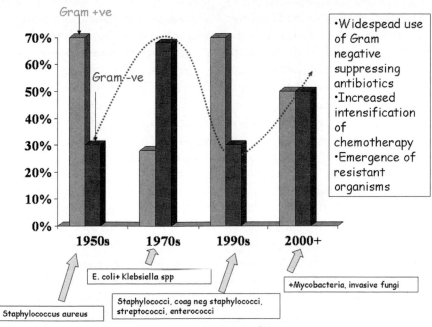

Figure 2. Changing pathogens in febrile neutropenia.

with hypotension, rash, skin desquamation, and adult respiratory distress—in association with a mortality of up to 30%.[11] Since the start of the second millennium Gram-negative organisms have reappeared as leading pathogens.[12] Many "new" bacteria have been documented in association with sepsis in the hematological patient. These have included vascular device–associated *Stomatococcus mucilaginosus, Leuconostic* spp, *Pediococcus* spp, and *Corynebacterium jeikeum* and the myonecrotic/severe mucositis agent *Clostridium septicum. Enterococcus faecalis* has been replaced by *E. faecium* as the lead in enterococcemia bloodstream infections associated with vancomycin resistance and mycobacterial bloodstream infections.[13] Of great concern is escalating antibiotic resistance, for example extended spectrum beta-lactamase–producing organisms, in response to overuse of broad-spectrum agents such as beta lactam antibiotics including the carbapenems.[14,15] Occasional situations have occurred in which no known antibiotic has been available to manage life-threatening septicemias.

Reasons advanced for the changing profile of bacterial organisms include increased chemotherapy intensification (more severe mucositis), use of prophylactic antibiotics (which suppress Gram-negatives at the expense of Gram-positives occupying the microbiological niche), and increased technological sophistication (which results in increased breach of the mechanical skin and mucosal barriers secondary to the plethora of invasive and intrusive devices).[11] Despite increasing efforts to contain opportunistic bacterial sepsis with infection-control policies including antibiotic restrictions, the rate of bacteremia among all febrile and neutropenic episodes has actually increased by around 25% to an incidence figure of 28% in recent years.[12]

Fungal Pathogens

Invasive fungal infections (IFI) are increasingly seen as contributing to the pathogen profile. Thus candidemia currently is the fourth commonest bloodstream infection in North America.[16] In the 1980s *Candida* spp were more frequent than *Aspergillus* spp, but as a result of widespread azole prophylactic use and other factors, *Aspergillus* has emerged as the lead fungal pathogen.[17–20] Over the last 5 years, however, molds other than *Aspergillus* spp, particularly the agents that cause mucormycosis make up 25% of all invasive mold infections,[21,22] raising susceptibility challenges in the area of antifungal drug management. Approximately 40% of patients who die with cancer have evidence of an IFI diagnosed at autopsy[23]—the fungal

burden in such patients is clearly high and our efforts to diagnose and treat in life are very limited. IFI carry greater mortality than bacterial infections; for example the mortality rate of invasive aspergillosis among bone marrow transplant recipients is 50%[24]; the presence of a non-*Candida* IFI after human peripheral stem allo-transplantation increases mortality three times. The apparent increase in prevalence of IFI is in part due to greater physician awareness and earlier and more accurate diagnostic techniques, but there maybe absolute factors including antimicrobially driven selection of fungal colonization preceding fungal invasion.[25] Similar to bacterial resistance, antimicrobial drug resistance is now common. The yeasts, in particular, show that overall the susceptibility of *C. albicans* to fluconazole has decreased[25] (though it is still possible to treat such infections with higher doses), and species other than *albicans*, such as *C. krusei*, with resistance to fluconazole have emerged. In some parts of Europe for example, *C. albicans* accounts for only 10% of bloodstream candidemias—a striking reversal of the situation less than 10 years ago[26,27] (Fig. 3). This emphasizes the importance of defining a particular institution's IFI profile. The widespread use of voriconazole (VRC), a "new generation" azole with excellent activity against *Aspergillus* infections, has been so active against this mold infection in several units that mucormycosis with inherent resistance to VRC has emerged.[28] *A. terreus* has become as frequent as *A. fumigatus* (normally the most frequent of the *Aspergillus* spp) in selected cancer units that have a higher proportion of more critically ill and more immunocompromised patients.[29] The importance of this particular epidemiological shift lies in the identifying the *Aspergillus* accurately to species level, since the gold-standard of treatment, amphotericin B, has no activity against *A. terreus*; in contrast VRC is the drug of choice and is best used as primary rather than salvage treatment, as mortality increases with delayed specific therapy with this azole. Finally, unusual molds have now established themselves within the possibilities

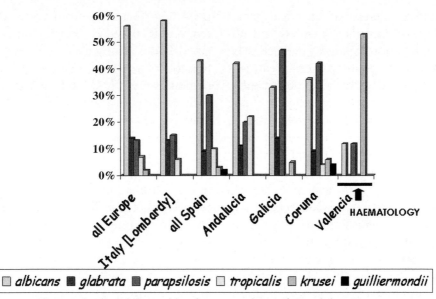

Figure 3. Variability in bloodstream isolates of *Candida* in Europe.

of fungal pathogens, including *Scedosporium* and *Fusarium*.[25]

Management of the Patient with Febrile Neutropenia of Acute Onset

Current Infectious Diseases Society of America (IDSA) guidelines[30] stipulate that at onset of fever in a neutropenic patient, a careful clinical evaluation including perineal and vascular access site inspection should be performed to exclude a focus for fever/infection, followed by immediate sampling of blood for culture from both the central lines and peripheral veins and (if no focal source) prompt institution of empirical broad-spectrum antibiotics intravenously. This approach has seen a dramatic reduction in bacteremia-associated mortality, to <5%, in such patients.[31] For coverage of the most likely pathogens an aminoglycoside (gentamicin) plus an antipseudomonal penicillin (piperacillin-tazobactam) or cephalosporin (ceftazidime) or carbapenem (imipenem) are recommended.[30] Vancomycin is only added for clinical or bacteriological evidence of a methicillin-resistant *S. aureus* (MRSA) infection, such as severe mucositis, catheter-related sepsis, and hypoten-

sion, since early combined use of vancomycin confers no advantage, drives resistance, and increases costs and the risk of adverse reactions.[30]

This "blundermycin" approach is highly cost ineffective since not all patients with FN require intravenous administrations, not all require such potent broad-spectrum agents, and many have fever of an origin other than infectious (such as thromboembolic disease).[31,32] Moreover, combination antibiotic treatment has been shown to be, in general, no more effective than monotherapy,[33] but the situation in immunocompromised patients is probably unique. Local factors, such as institution resistance data and economics, may also determine which antibiotic regimen should be used. Therefore, there has been considerable attention in recent years to risk stratification—that is to attempt to identify the subgroup of patients who might be safely managed with a more simplified and streamlined antibiotic regimen, for example on an outpatient monitored basis.[34] This concept however is not new; oral cotrimoxazole, ciprofloxacin, or perfloxacin with amoxicillin-clavulanate have been safely used in the 1980s and early 1990s.[30,35] Several meta-analyses of randomized controlled clinical studies comparing oral (quinolone-based) with intravenously administered empirical treatment for FN have confirmed the safety and efficacy of the oral option in patients deemed to be at low risk for not responding to oral treatment or developing a serious medical complication, such as sepsis-associated hypotension.[36,37] The challenge is to delineate those criteria used to define the low-risk patient. Two major models have been derived—the Talcott[38] and the Multinational Association for Supportive Care in Cancer (MASCC)[39] classifications. They utilize demographic and clinical data, such as age, clinical status, and medical history, to arrive at a numerical score, which determines a low-risk patient with less than a 10% chance of developing a severe complication. The MASCC model is more recent than the Talcott, and appears, in limited studies to date, to return a 71% sensitivity and 91% positive predictive value (PPV) to identify low-risk patients.[34] However, there are limitations including subjectivity in clinical assessment of some parameters, such as "disease burden," and rather limited validation data in the outpatient setting so far. Other clinical parameters have utilized expected duration of neutropenia, but this approach may be unreliable in some centers. The overriding factors in applying this risk-stratification approach include the need for patient compliance, the ability of the patient to self-determine clinical deterioration, and the availability of rapid transportation to the hospital if needed.[34,37]

There have been two further innovative developments in this area. The first is an evaluation of inflammatory markers and early-phase reactant proteins as adjunctive information in risk assessment. C-reactive protein (CRP) appears to be relatively nonspecific as a predictor of bacterial sepsis in an FN patient. IL-6, IL-8, and procalcitonin (PCT), however, are more hopeful candidate markers.[40,41] For example, Persson and colleagues showed that PCT levels rose within 2 days of onset of FN, and were sustained in those patients more likely to develop severe or unstable infection compared to those with no complications.[42,43] When compared to CRP, PCT could discriminate FN patients with bacteremia from those without bacteremia. IL-6 and IL-8 have also been investigated in this setting and high levels have been found to variably predict subsequent complications of FN.[40,42,44] The current status is that such markers are able to generate high negative predictive values (NPVs) but low PPVs for complications—that is they are most useful to identify patients at a low risk for complications, in whom it might be possible to modify antibiotic use. In this regard, a recent feasibility study investigated the effect of withholding antibiotics in FN patients using a two-step approach.[45] First, high-risk patients were identified using clinical and microbiological criteria—mainly positive blood cultures and hypotension. These patients were managed with standard intravenous antibiotic therapy. Second, those remaining patients classified at low/moderate risk had plasma IL-8 determinations. Patients in this group with low levels were hospitalized for a 12-h observation period and then discharged home on no antibiotics. The patients in this well-defined, low-risk group had no complications. This pilot study requires confirmation in a larger patient group. Clearly, however, the findings represent an important step forward in the rationalization of antibiotic treatment, offering the potential for cost savings, reduction in adverse drug events, decreasing resistance drive, reducing hospitalization, and improving quality of life.

Prophylactic Antibiotics

The current IDSA guidelines[30] speak strongly against the use of antibiotics to prevent fever in neutropenic patients. Although the frequency of febrile episodes and infections has been shown to be reduced ever since this approach, there has been no solid evidence of an impact on all-cause or infection-related mortality. Additionally concern has been mooted over the negating influence of toxicity, antibiotic resistance, and fungal overgrowth.

However many of these issues had previously eluded answers because the statistical power of clinical trials had been insufficient and the topic of resistance had been bypassed. The large meta-analysis by Gafter-Gvili and colleagues is therefore a significant advance.[46] Using a total population of 9283 highly immunocompromised predominantly hematological-malignancy patients accumulated from 95 high-quality clinical trials, the authors showed a highly significant reduction in all-cause as well as infection-related mortality with prophylactic antibiotics. The relative risk being 0.67 and 0.58, respectively, for these two major end points ($P < 0.001$). This phenomenon was more strongly seen when quinolones were specified—with RR of 0.52 and 0.38, respectively. Other infection event parameters, such as the proportion of clinical infections, febrile episodes, and microbiological infections (Gram-positive, Gram-negative, and bacteremias), were also highly significantly reduced by prophylactic antibiotics (Fig. 4). Although there were unsurprisingly more adverse drug events with antibiotics, none were life-threatening. Furthermore, there was no increase in fungal infections among patients receiving prophylaxis—an unanticipated finding.

At the same time as this publication, the results from two randomized controlled clinical trials assessing levofloxacin prophylaxis became available.[47,48] The "Significant" study used a cohort of severely neutropenic patients with solid tumors and demonstrated a reduction in the proportion of febrile episodes, probable infection, and hospitalization during the first as well as subsequent chemotherapy cycles, but there was no impact on infection deaths.[47] The Gimema study explored the use of levofloxacin prophylaxis in a severely neutropenic leukemic population.[48] The primary end point was subtly different from that used in the "Significant" study—neutropenic febrile episodes *requiring antibiotic treatment*. However this end point was also favorably influenced by prophylaxis with levofloxacin, as were the secondary end points of microbiological infections and bac-

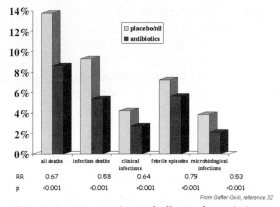

Figure 4. Meta-analysis of effects of prophylactic antibiotics.

teremias. This study showed a trend toward reduction in all-cause mortality but no effect on infection deaths. There was a reported observation of an increased proportion of emergent resistant isolates in the bacteremic patient subpopulation, which was not linked to mortality. A recent further meta-analysis by Gafter-Gvili and co-workers addressed specifically the resistance issue.[49] This analysis included 7878 patients from 56 trials. Those patients who received quinolone prophylaxis did not have an increased rate of colonization with resistant organisms nor an increased overall rate of infection with resistant organisms. However, when bacteremias were used as the denominator in the analysis there was a significant increase in bacteremias with organisms resistant to quinolones—but these did not appear to be associated with any increased risk of death. On the basis of these recent findings, antibiotic prophylaxis should probably now no longer be withheld from neutropenic patients.[50] Furthermore, there may be substantial cost savings in adopting a prophylactic approach compared to treating an FN episode. Some authorities remain cautious noting that there are inherent problems in the meta-analytical method, the two most recent studies failed to show significant survival advantages and hence balance the somewhat emotive statements that have been published over bioethics, trial end points are somewhat variable, and there needs to be more detailed analyses of microbial resistance that include survival outcomes.

Preventing Infection: Targeting the Enterocyte

The gastrointestinal tract is the primary reservoir of organisms, particularly yeasts and Gram-negative bacteria, which are the source of bacteremia in the neutropenic patient. These organisms translocate across the intestinal barrier, which has been rendered permeable due to cytotoxic chemotherapy-induced crypt cell apoptosis, cellular dysmorphism, and intercellular tight junction (TJ) opening.[51] This mechanism provides one explanation for bacteremia in patients with hematological malignancy. Invasive estimates of the damaged enterocytes, such as intestinal biopsy, are contra-indicated in such patients but may be documented semi-quantitatively by measuring the urinary ratio of lactulose to mannitol following oral administration.[51,52] Based on the differential route of absorption of these two inert sugars (lactulose paracellularly through the TJs and mannitol transcellularly), a ratio higher than 0.02 is indicative of abnormal permeability due to cellular damage. The enterocyte damage has been documented in animal models and by serial endoscopy sampling in human subjects.[51] Chemotherapy causes accelerated apoptosis within 24 h of the first dose and reduction in crypt size by 72 h. The fraction of open TJs increases from 4.4% to 20.1% over 5 days. Other permeability-testing agents, such as isotope probes, pegylated glycols, and intestinal fatty acid binding, have been used. Detailed electron microscopy analysis has shown anatomical changes to the cytoskeleton, specifically to actin. Furthermore the passage of *E. coli* and other pathogens across the damaged enterocyte barrier has been documented. In addition to the anatomical breach that occurs in these patients, other factors are contributory in the genesis of bacteremia of gut origin: intraluminal bacterial load, intestinal motility, macrophage dysfunction, hypogammaglobulinema A, malnutrition, trace element depletion, and nitric oxide–mediated endotoxin damage.[51] Knowledge of such mechanisms has provided some interesting prospects for intervention. These have included the use of selective inducible NO synthase inhibitors, immunonutrition via enteral feeding supplemented by glutamine, probiotic therapy with *Lactobacillus* spp, and hyperoxia.[51] Although these approaches have been effective in animal models and validated partially in critically ill burn patients, their action in the chemotherapy patient remains unknown.

However, several growth factors, such as growth hormone, transforming growth factor-β, and granulocyte colony stimulating factor, are known to have proliferative effects on the enterocyte. Among these, recombinant human interleukin-11 (rhIL-11) has been shown to have some exciting potential. This multifactorial, stromal-derived growth factor has a better known function of causing proliferation of megakaryocyte progenitor cells and has a use in alleviating chemotherapy-induced thrombocytopenia. However it has potent anti-apoptotic and antimucositis activity. In a recent double-blinded, placebo-controlled clinical trial,[53] when rhIL-11 was administered prophylactically to patients undergoing chemotherapy, it was found to prevent the increase in intestinal permeability that was documented in a matched control group that received placebo (Fig. 5A). Fifteen out of 20 patients (75%) receiving placebo developed abnormal L/M ratios compared to only 6/18 (33%) receiving rhIL-11 ($P = 0.02$). This observed effect of rhIL-11 on permeability was associated with a significant reduction in bacteremia, delayed onset of first bacteremic event, and reduced bacterial load. (Fig. 5B). This novel finding of a cytokine reducing the frequency of bacteremia through a shielding gastrointestinal cytoprotective mechanism offers an important alternative to antibiotics in managing infection in such patients.

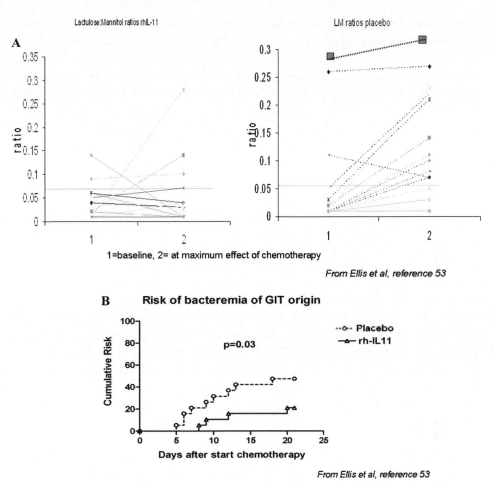

Figure 5. (A) Improvement in L/M ratios on rhIL-11 but not on placebo. **(B)** Reduction in bacteremia by rhIL-11.

Gut Decontamination

Selective digestive decontamination (SDD) is a term used to describe the approach of reducing infection by lowering intestinal bacterial load of pathogens while at the same time preserving anaerobic bacteria that are believed to prevent colonization and overgrowth of pathogens.[51] Initial attempts using co-trimoxazole were faulted because this antibiotic was not confined to the intestine but had systemic bioavailability, adverse drug events were frequent, there was no coverage against *Pseudomonas* spp, and antibiotic sensitivity was compromised. Other regimens have focused on truly nonadsorbable agents, such as neomycin plus oral amphotericin B, but again have sometimes combined this with a short intravenous systemic course, for example of cefotaxime.[54] An extensive meta-analysis, as well as some recent clinical studies among severely ill patients on an intensive care unit (ICU) (few of whom had underlying hematological malignancy), showed that SDD was effective in reducing subsequent ICU-associated pneumonia and mortality.[55] However SDD approaches have yet to be explored in the hematological patient.

Patients with Protracted Severe Neutropenia and Fever

This frequently encountered scenario, in which patients are not responding after 3–7 days of empirical broad-spectrum antibiotic therapy and have no microbiological or clinical evidence of focal infection (antibiotic unresponsive neutropenic fever, or AUNF), points to increased risk for the development of an IFI. Indeed the fever itself may be the first and only recognizable feature of the IFI at this stage. In the only prospective controlled clinical trial, the use of empirical antifungal therapy with conventional amphotericin B (CAB) was shown, to be significantly effective in improving the overall response and nonsignificantly improved the emergence of an IFI and reduced IFI related deaths.[56] On the basis of this study, conducted 20 years ago, as well as several uncontrolled observational studies, the use of CAB as empirical therapy has been widely accepted as "good" clinical practice and incorporated into the IDSA guidelines for managing the patient with AUNF.[30] Yet there are several problems with this generalized approach. First, 90% of the patients with AUNF who do not receive CAB do not develop an IFI, indicating a highly cost-ineffective policy. Second, CAB use has a high rate of adverse reactions, including chills and rigors but particularly nephrotoxicity, which occurs in one-third of patients directly causes increases in death rates, hospitalization, and health care costs in those patients given the drug. Third, CAB does not fully prevent later breakthrough IFIs, and its use is based on slender clinical evidence.

Available Antifungal Drugs for Treating AUNF

Some, but not all, lipid-associated amphotericin B products have demonstrated greatly improved efficacy and reduced toxicity. The relative aggregate efficacies have been reviewed by Ostrosky-Zeichner and associates.[57] The liposomal amphotericin B (LAB) product appears to have the least toxicity and most efficacy, though comparative studies are limited. However, animal data strongly support this clinical observation.[58,59] LAB has been compared to CAB for FN: LAB was significantly more effective than CAB in preventing breakthrough IFI, and nephrotoxicity was substantially reduced.[60] On the basis of this study LAB is the preferred polyene for this indication. LAB has been compared to VRC, and the overall composite performance score indicated that VRC did not meet predetermined noninferiority criteria.[61] Particularly there were more discontinuations of therapy with VRC for treatment failure issues. VRC is not licensed for treating FN. LAB has been compared with Caspofungin (CSP) for FN.[62] Although the overall success rates were identical, considerable concern has been raised over intrinsic design issues of this trial. For example, patients with established invasive pulmonary aspergillosis (IPA) had the lowest-ever recorded response rates to LAB, and 56% of patients were previously on azole prophylaxis, giving rise to a potential antagonistic antifungal drug effect in those patients randomized to amphotericin B, while those receiving CSP might have benefited from a synergistic action. The further concerns over the bacteriostatic activity of CSP[63] and its missing coverage for a number of the emerging new IFI, such as Mucor, have caused concern among clinicians, some of whom have not found such a favorable response[64] as Walsh and colleagues originally documented.[61]

A thorough review of all the published studies that compared two different drugs in FN suggests that the overall success rate is around 45%, irrespective of which drug is used.[65] However, there are trial issues of definitions for success that impact on the success rate of any particular trial. This results in success rates ranging from as low as 25% to over 80%. Studies which use defervescence as the only end point, therefore, artificially increase the success rate, while studies using a 5-point composite score tend to lower success rates as each component has to be

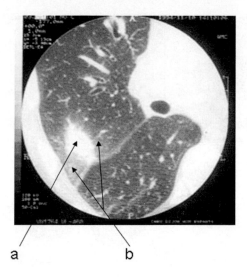
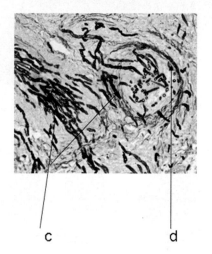

a   b   c   d

HRCT lung with central nodule (a) and surrounding halo (b)   Lung biopsy showing fungal hyphae (c) and blood vessel (d)

Figure 6. CT halo sign and corresponding histology in lung biopsy.

fulfilled, which may artificially lower the success rate. Despite the limitations imposed by such variable definitions of success, there remains the concern that too many patients with AUNF need to be treated to prevent relatively few IFI.

Selection of Patients for Empirical or Pre-emptive Antifungal Therapy

When CAB was first introduced into clinical practice, fungal diagnostics were insensitive, unspecific, and delayed, and so the late implementation of CAB was associated with extremely high mortality rates from established IFI. The current era of improved, more sensitive and specific fungal diagnostics coupled with less toxic antifungal therapy has had a major impact on empirical therapy management.

Current diagnostic emphasis has shifted away from invasive techniques—which provide samples to demonstrate fungal hyphal invasion (patients too ill or thrombocytopenic) or to culture the fungus (takes too long and requires expertise)—toward a variety of noninvasive non-culture-based methods, which are safe and rapidly performed.

The CT Halo Sign

Plain chest radiography is highly insensitive for specific and early IPA diagnosis. Patients with AUNF and IPA undergoing high-resolution CT (HRCT) scanning early will have detectable lesions of IPA at a median of 10 days of AUNF, though several will have positive scans as early as 1–3 days of AUNF.[66] A central nodule surrounded by a glow-blush of the administered IV contrast medium is called the "halo" sign.[66,67] This is virtually pathognomonic of IPA in the particular patient setting of AUNF.[68] This halo sign is the imagery manifestation of the angio-invasive pathological process (Fig. 6). Detection of early IPA in this way has been shown to substantially improve the outcome, provided early and effective antifungal therapy is given. Caillot and colleagues demonstrated that improved survival in IPA from 50% to 80% could be achieved using routine systematic CT scanning to guide the institution of early antifungal drug treatment.[67] It has been demonstrated that using repeated HRCT, starting as early as day 3 of AUNF, combined with a moderately high dose of LAB improved overall response, reduced all-cause

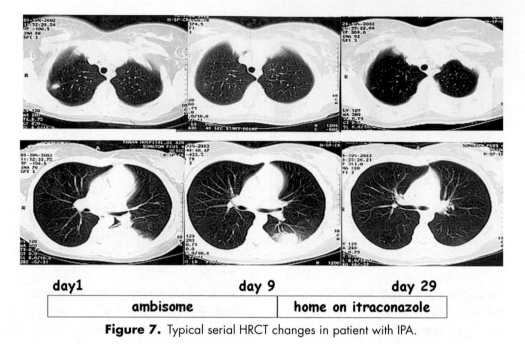

day1	day 9	day 29
ambisome		home on itraconazole

Figure 7. Typical serial HRCT changes in patient with IPA.

mortality, and reduced IPA-related death when compared to current literature reviews.[66,68,69] The current survival rate from IPA in Tawam Hospital's Hematology unit is 90% using this approach. A representative successful outcome is shown in Figure 7. In contrast, if antifungal therapy is delayed until more "classical" imaging features of IPA have become established, the mortality rate is higher due to the larger fungal burden, the difficulty in penetration of drugs to the site of the abscess-like lesions, and the danger from catastrophic bleeding. The recently developed definitions of an IFI as published by the European Organization for Research and Treatment of Cancer/Invasive Fungal Infections Cooperative Group and the National Institute of Allergy and Infectious Diseases Mycoses Study Group (EORTC/MSG)[70] present some confusion to the clinician.[71] Thus the therapy that is given when only a halo sign is present is termed "pre-emptive" rather than definitive, despite the wide consensus that the halo sign indicates already established IPA. This may appear to be squabbling semantics, but in fact it has an important bearing on entry criteria in clinical trials concerning efficacy definitions.

Blood and Serology Testing

There are several possible options for diagnosing an IFI using blood or serum. Detection of fungal antibodies, such as to *Candida mannan* or *Aspergillus*, are performed by enzyme immunoassay techniques or with immunofluorescence tags. Sensitivities around 60% are achievable. Detection of fungal nucleic acid by PCR is another evaluated approach, but again it is limited by both false positive and negative results. These assays are usually performed in association with antigen detection, in which case the performance is slightly better. Two relatively recent antigen detection tests have been evaluated in clinical practice.

β-D Glucan

The observation that the β-D glucan (BDG) component of fungal cell walls can activate the horseshoe crab's coagulation system has been captured to generate a spectrophotometric assay for BDG.[72] Two commercial kits are available—the Glucatell or Fungitell assay, which uses enzymes from *Limulus polyphemus* amebocytes, and the Fungitec-G assay

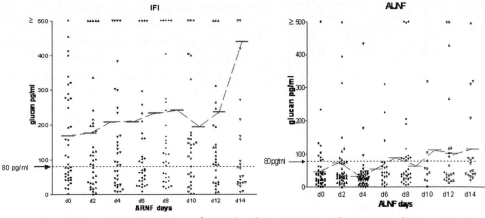

Figure 8. Comparison of BDG levels in patients with AUNF and IFI.

which uses *Tachypleus tridentatus* enzymes.[73–75] The Glucatell assay has 100% NPV and ≥96% specificity when defining a positive test as two sequential values of BDG of ≥60 pg/mL, in acute myelogenous leukemia subjects matched with healthy controls.[74] A recent large multicenter evaluation using just one sample per patient gave sensitivities, specificities, PPV, and NPV values of 69.9%, 87.1%, 83.8%, and 75.1%, respectively.[73]

The Glucatell assay was evaluated in Tawam Hospital recently in a population of 100 patients from the UAE with hematological malignancy undergoing chemotherapy and with anticipated neutropenia. Thirty-eight patients developed an IFI: 5 definite (3 candidemia, 1 hepatosplenic candidiasis (HSC), 1 IPA), 21 probable (14 IPA, 6 HSC, 1 disseminated candidiasis), and 12 possible (9 IPA, 1 invasive fungal sinusitis, 2 disseminated candidiasis). Forty-two patients had AUNF and 15 patients had NF less than 4 days duration. In five patients, insufficient sampling was performed. Alternate-day sampling was performed from the first day of AUNF (d0) for a capture period of 14 days. Using two consecutive values of BDG ≥80 pg/mL to define a positive result, our sensitivities, specificities, PPV, and NPV values were 86.8%, 76.2%, 76.7%, and 86.5%, respectively. The overall test accuracy was 81.3%. The mean and median values of BDG concentrations were significantly higher in the IFI group than in the AUNF alone group at d0 and at each time point over the first 8 days (Fig. 8). Ninety percent of the patients with an IFI had a positive result within the first 6 days of onset of AUNF. Stored samples of blood were available for further testing from the first day of neutropenia in 15 of the 38 patients with an IFI. Analysis of these samples indicated that the first positive test result occurred a mean of 5.3 ± 1.4 (1–15) days earlier than the first positive result from the AUNF phase, suggesting that antifungal therapy could be initiated several days earlier if testing was routinely done from the start of neutropenia rather than from the first day of AUNF. Sampling on a daily basis did not advance the timing to initiation of antifungal treatment by more than 1 day. Some of the patients with AUNF had persistently elevated high BDG concentrations. Eight of 11 such patients (72.7%) had either a positive blood culture and/or evidence of severe mucositis (on visual score of the oral cavity) or enterocolitis (on CT or ultrasound examination), compared to only 6/31 (19.4%) of patients who had BDG with sporadic or low BDG concentrations($P = 0.002$). One explanation could be the occurrence of glucanemia due to yeast translocation through the diseased gastrointestinal tract rather than an established tissue or bloodstream IFI.

Figure 9A is indicative of the usefulness of the BDG test. Note the first elevation of BDG

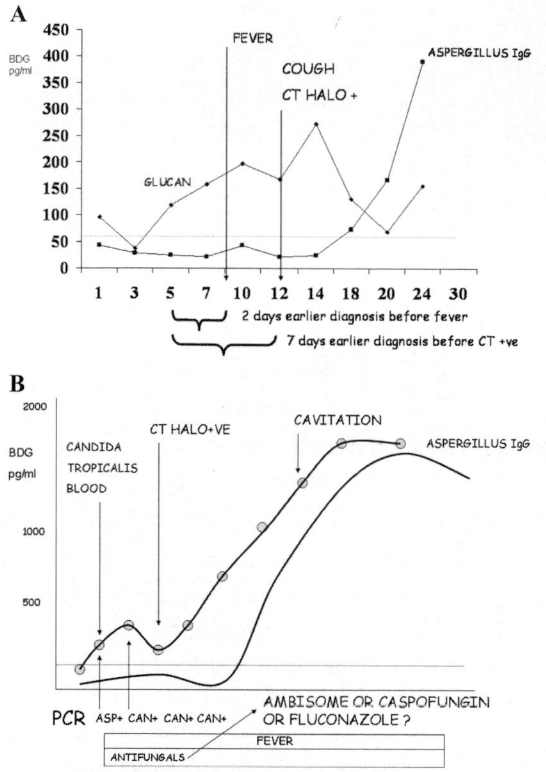

Figure 9. (A) Example of clinical applicability of serological marker monitoring. **(B)** Second example of clinical applicability of serological marker monitoring.

occurs 2 days prior to fever and 7 days prior to the first clinical/radiological evidence of IPA. Figure 9B in contrast illustrates a dilemma of testing. Note that the first BDG elevation occurs at the time that a blood culture is positive for *Candida* spp. The accompanying series of PCR results suggests an initial false positive test for *Aspergillus*. However, the patient does develop a second IFI with IPA. If a narrow-spectrum antifungal agent, such as fluconazole, had been used initially rather than a broad-spectrum agent, such as LAB, the outcome in this patient might have been unsuccessful.

Our own experience is that the BDG test may be a useful adjunctive tool for tailoring empirical antifungal treatment in the FN patient. A possible paradigm might be to screen all patients for BDG from onset of neutropenia (or from the first day of AUNF) and to give antifungal treatment only to those patients whose test was positive. The choice of antifungals might further be decided through results of HRCT scanning such that patients with early halo signs would receive LAB while those with normal scans could be given CSP or even fluconazole. Patients with spurious low-level glucan readings should not receive antifungals but continue with observation and other appropriate investigations. Limitations of the BDG test include its ability to detect "generic" fungi only, its inability to detect agents of mucormycosis and *Cryptococcus* spp, the possibility of false positive results with certain biologics, such as immunoglobulins and cellulose, and the need for further validation to determine reproducibility, define optimal sampling times, and investigate its potential in influencing the use of antifungal drugs safely.[73,74]

Galactomannan

In contrast to the pan-fungal BDG test, galactomannan (GM) is specific for *Aspergillus*.[75] The Platelia test is a double-sandwich ELISA that incorporates the B 1–5 galactofuranose-specific EBA2 monoclonal antibody and is FDA approved for invasive aspergillosis (IA) diagnosis. The first major publication was by Maertens and co-workers in 1999 with sensitivity, specificity, PPV, and NPV all >92%.[76] However, subsequent clinical validation studies, while confirming the very high specificity and NPV, have reported highly variable sensitivities, which have ranged from 0% to 90%, with several in the range of 50%. The meta-analysis by Pfeiffer and colleagues in 2006 was therefore timely.[77] Using data from 27 studies, the overall sensitivity was determined to be 71%, specificity 89%, and the Youden index and mean D and Q* indicated only moderate accuracy.[77] Several factors appear to influence the performance of the GM test: the cutoff values (which have been reduced from 1.5 to 0.5 ng/mL), the prevalence of IA in the studied population (the higher the prevalence the more reliable the test), the clinical stage at which IA presents (abscesses or cavities may not release GM into the circulation), the phase of the fungal growth (galf antigens are released during the log growth phase), and the use of antifungal drugs (which reduce detectable GM: Marr and colleagues showed that the sensitivity of the test was reduced from 87.5% when no drugs were used to 20% if antifungal drugs were used).[78] As with BDG testing, there are several false positive tests that require explanation and identification. The GM assay requires careful patient selection as described above to optimize its reliability in the clinical arena.[77] If such selection is optimal, then GM testing is reliable and could find a role in rationalizing empirical antifungal therapy. This was demonstrated in a recent publication by Maertens and associates.[79] One hundred seventeen NF episodes were prospectively followed, of which 41 (35%) developed AUNF. Under existing guidelines these patients would have received empirical treatment with an antifungal drug. However, through serial GM screening combined with HRCT scanning and broncho-alveolar lavage for GM, the number of patients who were actually given antifungal therapy was only 9 (7.7%). This approach was found to be safe and effective and returned substantial cost savings.

Alternative Dosing Schedules of Polyenes

Triggered by the inconsistency of thoroughly validated clinical studies of serological and blood testing techniques, empirical therapy will remain a treatment option for the foreseeable future. However, since the drug-acquisition cost of the newer antifungal agents is high, there is a need to explore alternative dosing approaches. The favorable performance of LAB—high C_{max}, elevated AUC, nonlinear kinetics, and rapid blood clearance to saturate the reticulo-endothelial system and other tissues—offers the possibility of intermittent dosing.[80] Animal experiments have shown that a single

high dose of LAB given immediately before a *Candida* challenge was very effective in reducing tissue fungal burden and could produce high levels in tissues 7 days after the dose.[59] The application of this was recently explored in Tawam Hospital in patients with hematological malignancy. In a randomized open clinical trial, patients with AUNF received either conventional dosing with LAB at 3 mg/kg/day for 14 days or 10 mg/kg on day 0 and 5 mg/kg on days 2 and 5. In this pilot feasibility study of 15 patients in each arm, there were no differences in adverse drug events or rises in creatinine, though there was a trend toward less hypokalemia in the intermittent high-dose arm. The overall success was similar as measured by a 5-point composite outcome score[62] (67% versus 66%), by time to defervescence (8.4 + 6.1 versus 8.8 ± 5.1 days), or by the proportion of patients developing a positive serological test by fungus by GM BGM or PCR (27% versus 28%). Using a 2-compartment model to fit the serum amphotericin B concentrations that were sampled on infusion days, very large blood space and peripheral organ space volumes were detected, as a result of the extended sampling time range that was used—up to 400 h—and suggested the existence of an hitherto unknown deep drug compartment. Although the AUC values were different in the two regimens the drug-dose AUCs were similar, suggesting the potential for lowered toxicity in the intermittent high-dose arm. The levels of amphotericin B in the bone marrow aspirate taken 1 day after the completion of the 14 days standard dosing and 7 days after the third dose of the intermittent high-dose regimen showed persistence of the drug in that tissue. The results therefore suggest that an intermittent high-dose regimen may be administered safely to patients with AUNF, without loss of efficacy, provides a bone marrow (and probably other tissues) deposition of the drug, and offers cost savings of 50%. A further possibility would be to combine this approach with serological testing and HRCT scanning to tailor the use of empirical antifungal treatment.

increases survival.[98] PTX3 is therefore an interesting possible adjunctive therapeutic candidate to use in patients at a very early stage of IPA or during antifungal therapy in which serological evidence with BDG or GM is also present.

The Neutrophil Itself

It is generally accepted that restoration of neutrophil quantity or quality is mandatory for successful outcome of FN, particularly when associated with a bacterial or fungal focus.[1,8] Delays in chemotherapy dose administration and/or dose reductions because of concerns for or actual FN directly increase mortality in patients with cancer.[99] Hence supporting the patients to permit successful completion of planned chemotherapy of a planned dose is crucial. Granulocyte/monocyte colony stimulating factors (GCSF) have been available for several years to achieve this goal. They increase both quantity and quality of neutrophils and other cells. Earlier studies showed some evidence for an impact on mortality, and a large meta-analysis has confirmed a possible influence of colony stimulating factors on infection mortality.[100] Thus, growth factors have a major impact on recovery of the neutrophil, reduce hospital stays, and, although they may not have any impact on overall mortality when analyzed by this means, they possibly reduce infection-related mortality.[100] There is no increase in leukemic disease relapse, which might be otherwise expected. In fact the use of growth factors as support is widely practiced. Guidelines have been produced by the two North American bodies, the American Society of Clinical Oncology[101] and the National Comprehensive Cancer Network.[102] The European Organization for Research and Treatment of Cancer has produced the most up-to-date guidelines.[103] Based on a comprehensive literature search using PUBMED, PreMED, EMBASE, and The Cochrane Library, the taskforce developed ranked levels of efficacy based on all eligible evidence collated from meta-analyses, controlled clinical trails (the strongest evidence), and case studies (the weakest). The summary conclusions are that, in the case of solid tumors or lymphoma, GCSF should be used routinely to prevent FN when the following are likely: 1) a predicted overall FN risk of $\geq$20%, 2) a predicted overall FN risk of 10–20% when other factors are present, such as age >65 years, previous FN, or advanced malignancy, 3) when dose density or dose intensification are crucial to uphold to optimize survival. Additionally growth factors should be used in established FN in those situations where severe sepsis/septic shock are established or where the patient is not responding to antibiotics.

Conclusion

Neutropenia presents a great hurdle to achieving overall success of chemotherapy or transplantation in the patient with hematological malignancy. The previous philosophy of treating every FN patient with antimicrobials or preventing all possible infections with prophylaxis has evolved to one commensurate with basic science findings of pathogenic molecular mechanisms and clinical observations. The current management of neutropenia attempts a logical, evidence-based approach to the complication of fever, utilizing diagnostic information from surrogate markers and specific fungal diagnostics as well as administering less toxic drugs in a more directed fashion to patients. Greater awareness of the need to restore the host immune system, particularly by correcting neutrophil deficiency has also had an impact on management. Finally, the emergence of widespread antimicrobial resistance has triggered investigations for novel approaches to prevention and management of infection in this patient population.

Conflicts of Interest

The author declares no conflicts of interest.

References

1. Vento, S. & F. Cainelli. 2003. Infections in patients with cancer undergoing chemotherapy: aetiology, prevention, and treatment. *Lancet. Oncol.* **4:** 595–604.

2. Crawford, J., D.C. Dale & G.H. Lyman. 2004. Chemotherapy-induced neutropenia: risks, consequences, and new directions for its management. *Cancer* **100:** 228–237.

3. Meza, L. *et al.* 2002. Incidence of febrile neutropenia (DSN) after myelosuppressive chemotherapy. *Proc. Am. Soc. Clin. Oncol.* **21:** 255b.

4. Schwarz, E., Mitt d. Gesellsch. F. inn. Med. U. Kinderh., 1904, iii, 190. Ein Fall von extremer Leukopenie.

5. Bhatt, V. & A. Saleem. 2004. Review: drug-induced neutropenia—pathophysiology, clinical features, and management. *Ann. Clin. Lab. Sci.* **34:** 131–137.

6. Kracke, R.R. 1931. Recurrent agranulocytosis. Report of an unusual case. *Am. J. Clin. Path.* **1:** 385–390.

7. Reznikoff, P. 1930. Nucleotide therapy in agranulocytosis. *J. Clin. Invest.* **9:** 381–391.

8. Bodey, G.P. *et al.* 1966. Quantitative relationships between circulating leukocytes and infection in patients with acute leukemia. *Ann. Intern. Med.* **64:** 328–340.

9. Schimpff, S.C. *et al.* 1978. Three antibiotic regimens in the treatment of infection in febrile granulocytopenic patients with cancer. The EORTC international antimicrobial therapy project group. *J. Infect. Dis.* **137:** 14–29.

10. Viscoli, C. & E. Castagnola. 1995. Factors predisposing cancer patients to infection. *Cancer Treat. Res.* **79:** 1–30.

11. Elting, L.S., G.P. Bodey & B.H. Keefe. 1992. Septicemia and shock syndrome due to viridans streptococci: a case-control study of predisposing factors. *Clin. Infect. Dis.* **14:** 1201–1207.

12. De Bock, R. *et al.* 2001. Incidence of single agent Gram-negative bacteremias (SAGNB) in neutropenic cancer patients (NCP) in EORTC-IATG trial of empirical therapy for febrile neutropenia [abstract L-773]. In *Program and Abstracts of the 41st Interscience Conference on Antimicrobial Agents and Chemotherapy (Chicago)*. American Society for Microbiology, Washington, DC. 445.

13. Cappellano, P. *et al.* 2003. Bloodstream infections (BSI) due to *Enterococcus* sp. In allogenic bone marrow transplantation (ALLOBMT) [abstract 11CD]. In *Scientific Program and Abstracts of the 6th International Symposium on Febrile Neutropenia (Brussels)*. Imedex, Alpharetta, GA.

14. Vahaboglu, H. *et al.* 2001. Clinical importance of extended-spectrum beta-lactamase (PER-1-type)-producing Acinetobacter spp. and Pseudomonas aeruginosa strains. *J. Med. Microbiol.* **50:** 642–645.

15. Vahaboglu, H. *et al.* 1997. Widespread detection of PER-1-type extended-spectrum beta-lactamases among nosocomial Acinetobacter and Pseudomonas aeruginosa isolates in Turkey: a nationwide multicenter study. *Antimicrob Agents Chemother.* **41:** 2265–2269.

16. Fridkin, S.K. 2005. The changing face of fungal infections in health care settings. *Clin. Infect. Dis.* **41:** 1455–1460.

17. Marr, K.A. *et al.* 2000. Prolonged fluconazole prophylaxis is associated with persistent protection against candidiasis-related death in allogeneic marrow transplant recipients: long-term follow-up of a randomized, placebo-controlled trial. *Blood* **96:** 2055–2061.

18. Marr, K.A. *et al.* 2000. Candidemia in allogeneic blood and marrow transplant recipients: evolution of risk factors after the adoption of prophylactic fluconazole. *J. Infect. Dis.* **181:** 309–316.

19. Marr, K.A. *et al.* 2002. Epidemiology and outcome of mould infections in hematopoietic stem cell transplant recipients. *Clin. Infect. Dis.* **34:** 909–917.

20. Marr, K.A. *et al.* 2002. Invasive aspergillosis in allogeneic stem cell transplant recipients: changes in epidemiology and risk factors. *Blood* **100:** 4358–4366.

21. Pagano, L. *et al.* 2001. Infections caused by filamentous fungi in patients with hematologic malignancies. A report of 391 cases by GIMEMA infection program. *Haematologica* **86:** 862–870.

22. Martino, R. & M. Subira. 2002. Invasive fungal infections in hematology: new trends. *Ann. Hematol.* **81:** 233–243.

23. Bodey, G. *et al.* 1992. Fungal infections in cancer patients: an international autopsy survey. *Eur. J. Clin. Microbiol. Infect. Dis.* **11:** 99–109.

24. Lin, S.J., J. Schranz & S.M. Teutsch. 2001. Aspergillosis case-fatality rate: systematic review of the literature. *Clin. Infect. Dis.* **32:** 358–366.

25. Richardson, M.D. 2005. Changing patterns and trends in systemic fungal infections. *J. Antimicrob. Chemother.* **56**(Suppl 1): i5–i11.

26. Diekema, D.J. *et al.* 2002. Epidemiology of candidemia: 3-year results from the emerging infections and the epidemiology of Iowa organisms study. *J. Clin. Microbiol.* **40:** 1298–1302.

27. Pfaller, M.A. & D.J. Diekema. 2007. Epidemiology of invasive candidiasis: a persistent public health problem. *Clin. Microbiol. Rev.* **20:** 133–163.

28. Kontoyiannis, D.P. & R.E. Lewis. 2006. Invasive zygomycosis: update on pathogenesis, clinical manifestations, and management. *Infect. Dis. Clin. North Am.* **20:** 581–607, vi.

82. Neth, O. *et al.* 2001. Deficiency of mannose-binding lectin and burden of infection in children with malignancy: a prospective study. *Lancet* **358:** 614–618.

83. Bajetto, A. *et al.* 2002. Characterization of chemokines and their receptors in the central nervous system: physiopathological implications. *J. Neurochem.* **82:** 1311–1329.

84. Ellis, M. *et al.* 2005. Significance of the CC chemokine RANTES in patients with haematological malignancy: results from a prospective observational study. *Br. J. Haematol.* **128:** 482–489.

85. Cavaillon, J.M. *et al.* 2003. Cytokine cascade in sepsis. *Scand. J. Infect. Dis.* **35:** 535–544.

86. Ellis, M. *et al.* 2005. Invasive fungal infections are associated with severe depletion of circulating RANTES. *J. Med. Microbiol.* 54(Pt 11): 1017–1022.

87. McDermott, M.F. *et al.* 1999. Germline mutations in the extracellular domains of the 55 kDa TNF receptor, TNFR1, define a family of dominantly inherited autoinflammatory syndromes. *Cell* **97:** 133–144.

88. Fisher, C.J. Jr. *et al.* 1996. Treatment of septic shock with the tumor necrosis factor receptor: Fc fusion protein. The soluble TNF receptor sepsis study group. *N. Engl. J. Med.* **334:** 1697–1702.

89. Annane, D. *et al.* 2002. Effect of treatment with low doses of hydrocortisone and fludrocortisone on mortality in patients with septic shock. *JAMA* **288:** 862–871.

90. Nguyen, H.B. *et al.* 2006. Severe sepsis and septic shock: review of the literature and emergency department management guidelines. *Ann. Emerg. Med.* **48:** 28–54.

91. Bernard, G.R. *et al.* 2001. Efficacy and safety of recombinant human activated protein C for severe sepsis. *N. Engl. J. Med.* **344:** 699–709.

92. Ellis, M. *et al.* 2006. Modulation of the systemic inflammatory response by recombinant human interleukin-11: a prospective randomized placebo controlled clinical study in patients with hematological malignancy. *Clin. Immunol.* **20:** 129–137.

93. Tilg, H. *et al.* 1993. Anti-inflammatory properties of hepatic acute phase proteins: preferential induction of interleukin 1 (IL-1) receptor antagonist over IL-1

beta synthesis by human peripheral blood mononuclear cells. *J. Exp. Med.* **178:** 1629–1636.

94. Mantovani, A., C. Garlanda & B. Bottazzi. 2003. Pentraxin 3, a non-redundant soluble pattern recognition receptor involved in innate immunity. *Vaccine* **21**(Suppl 2): S43–S47.

95. Mantovani, A., C. Garlanda & B. Bottazzi. 2003. Pentraxin 3, a non-redundant soluble pattern recognition receptor involved in innate immunity. *Vaccine* **21**(Suppl 2): S43–S47.

96. Muller, B. *et al.* 2001. Circulating levels of the long pentraxin PTX3 correlate with severity of infection in critically ill patients. *Crit. Care. Med.* **29:** 1404–1407.

97. Al-Ramadi, B.K. *et al.* 2004. Selective induction of pentraxin 3, a soluble innate immune pattern recognition receptor, in infectious episodes in patients with haematological malignancy. *Clin. Immunol.* **112:** 221–224.

98. Garlanda, C. *et al.* 2002. Non-redundant role of the long pentraxin PTX3 in anti-fungal innate immune response. *Nature* **420:** 182–186.

99. Mayers, C., T. Panzarella, & I.F. Tannock. 2001. Analysis of the prognostic effects of inclusion in a clinical trial and of myelosuppression on survival after adjuvant chemotherapy for breast carcinoma. *Cancer* **91:** 2246–2257.

100. Clark, O.A. *et al.* 2005. Colony-stimulating factors for chemotherapy-induced febrile neutropenia: a meta-analysis of randomized controlled trials. *J. Clin. Oncol.* **23:** 4198–4214.

101. Ozer, H. *et al.* 2000. 2000 update of recommendations for the use of hematopoietic colony-stimulating factors: evidence-based, clinical practice guidelines. American society of clinical oncology growth factors expert panel. *J. Clin. Oncol.* **18:** 3558–3585.

102. National Comprehensive Guidelines Network. 2005 Myeloid Growth Factors. Available from: http://www.nccn.org/ (accessed September 7 2005).

103. Aapro, M.S., D.A. Cameron. *et al.* (2006. EORTC guidelines for the use of granulocyte-colony stimulating factor to reduce the incidence of chemotherapy-induced febrile neutropenia in adult patients with lymphomas and solid tumours. *Eur. J. Cancer* **42:** 2433–2453.

Attenuated Bacteria as Effectors in Cancer Immunotherapy

Basel K. al-Ramadi,[a] **Maria J. Fernandez-Cabezudo,**[b] **Hussain El-Hasasna,**[a] **Suhail Al-Salam,**[c] **Samir Attoub,**[d] **Damo Xu,**[e] **and Salem Chouaib**[f]

Departments of [a]Microbiology & Immunology, [b]Biochemistry, [c]Pathology, and [d]Pharmacology, Faculty of Medicine and Health Sciences, UAE University, Al Ain, United Arab Emirates

[e]Department of Immunology, University of Glasgow, Western Infirmary, Glasgow, United Kingdom

[f]Institut National de la Sante et de la Recherche Medicale, Unite 487, Institut Gustave Roussy, Villejuif, France

Despite the great strides made in understanding the basic biology of cancer and the multiple approaches to cancer therapy that have been utilized, cancer remains a major cause of death worldwide. The two properties that define the most successful tumors are low antigenicity, enabling cancer cells to escape immune system recognition, and high tumorigenicity, allowing the cells to proliferate aggressively and metastasize to other tissues. The development of novel anticancer therapies is aimed at enhancing the antigenicity of tumors and/or increasing the functional efficiency of various effector immune system cells. The use of obligate/facultative anaerobic bacteria, which preferentially replicate within tumor tissue, as an oncolytic agent is one of the innovative approaches to cancer therapy. Over the past several years, we have studied the properties of attenuated strains of *Salmonella typhimurium*, a facultative anaerobe, genetically engineered to express murine cytokines. Previously, we demonstrated that cytokine-expressing strains have the capacity to modulate immunity to infection. Given the preferential tumor-homing properties of attenuated *Salmonella* bacteria, the potential capacity of a cytokine-encoding *Salmonella* strain to retard the growth of experimental melanomas was investigated. Mice pre-implanted with melanoma cells were treated with an attenuated strain of *S. typhimurium* or with one of its derivatives expressing IL-2. Our data demonstrate that IL-2-encoding *Salmonella* organisms were superior in suppressing tumor growth as compared to the parental noncytokine-expressing strain. This supports the notion of using cytokine-expressing attenuated *Salmonella* organisms in cancer therapy.

Key words: cancer; immunotherapy; low antigenicity; high tumorigenicity; IL-2-encoding *Salmonella*

Introduction

Despite the remarkable advances made over the past 50 years in understanding the basis of cancer development, and the increased availability of antitumor treatment modalities, the cancer-related death toll remains one of the highest among chronic human diseases. The success of tumor growth and metastasis owes much to the ineffectiveness of the host's immune system. As the nature of interactions between different types of tumors and the immune system began to be better understood at the cellular and molecular levels, so did our appreciation of the fact that tumor success is

Address for correspondence: Prof. Basel K. al-Ramadi, Department of Microbiology & Immunology, Faculty of Medicine and Health Sciences, UAE University, P.O. Box 17666, Al Ain, UAE. Voice: +9713-7137-529; fax: +9713-767-1966. ramadi.b@uaeu.ac.ae

Ann. N.Y. Acad. Sci. 1138: 351–357 (2008). © 2008 New York Academy of Sciences.
doi: 10.1196/annals.1414.036

mainly related to its ability to escape recognition by the immune system. Both central and peripheral immune tolerance mechanisms have been implicated in the failure of humans to mount antitumor immune responses. This fact has been a major obstacle in the development of effective tumor immunotherapy. Many approaches have been developed to induce immunity against cancer, and some have yielded remarkably potent antitumor-specific cytotoxic T cell responses.[1] Despite these effects, however, most *in vivo* tumors fail to regress even in the presence of circulating antitumor cytotoxic T cells.[2] Reasons for the failure of tumor-specific cytotoxic T cells to control tumor growth include restricted accessibility into the tumor mass, active inhibition of T cell function, or inability to recognize target tumor antigens due to downregulation of antigen or MHC molecules.[3–6] It is clear, therefore, that the immunosuppressive environment generated by the tumor can restrain the positive effects of potentiating the antitumor immune response.

Live Bacteria as Oncolytic Agents

Recent evidence suggests that it is possible to increase the visibility of the tumor by inducing an inflammatory state within the tumor microenvironment.[7,8] More than a century ago, it was realized that deliberate exposure of cancer patients to certain microbes could induce tumor regression and sometimes even eradication.[9] This gave rise to the notion of cancer immunotherapy as a potential treatment modality for some types of cancer. Currently, the only approved infection-based immunotherapy for human cancer is the use of Bacillus Calmette-Guérin (BCG) (*M. bovis* strain) for the treatment and prophylaxis of superficial transitional cell carcinoma of the urinary bladder.[10] Over the past 5–10 years, renewed interest in the potential use of facultative anaerobic bacteria as anticancer agents has re-emerged.[11,12] This has come about as a result of increased understanding of the tumor tissue microenvironment and growth properties of a number of anaerobic bacterial species, including *Salmonella*, *Bifidobacterium*, and *Clostridium* spp. These bacterial species have all been shown to preferentially home into, and replicate within, tumor tissue. This selective capacity leads to accumulation of bacterial organisms within tumors to concentrations exceeding 1000-fold their concentration in other target organs. A seminal study, published in 1997 by Pawelek and colleagues, demonstrated the capacity of attenuated *Salmonella typhimurium* strains to replicate preferentially within human and murine tumors, leading to an inhibition of tumor growth and enhanced animal survival.[13] It is now thought that multiple factors within the tumor tissue, such as the chaotic vascularization, regions of necrosis, and hypoxic conditions, combine to provide an ideal environment for the growth of anaerobic and facultative anaerobic bacteria.[14]

The mechanism by which bacterial administration, and subsequently their accumulation within the tumors, leads to an inhibition of tumor growth remains incompletely understood. *Salmonella* organisms have been shown to invade and cause the death of macrophages, their natural host target cells, via caspase-1-dependent, and independent, pathways.[15–18] Moreover, invasive *Salmonella* organisms have the capacity to infect nonphagocytic cells via the expression of a type III secretion system that enables them to penetrate a wide variety of cell types.[19] In the case of tumor cells, however, invasion-deficient strains of *S. typhimurium* retained their capacity to suppress tumor growth.[20] Furthermore, in comparison with their death-promoting influence on macrophages, invasive *Salmonella* organisms do not induce apoptosis in tumor cells.[21] This suggests that *Salmonella*-dependent invasion and apoptosis of target cancer cells is unlikely to be responsible for the suppression of tumor growth. It has been proposed that the antitumor effect of *Salmonella* is partly mediated by recognition and lysis of *Salmonella*-infected tumor cells by host CD8 T lymphocytes.[21] However, this requires concurrent vaccination with bacteria-pulsed dendritic cells for effective control of tumor growth. This is unlikely to represent the mechanism by which bacterial administration to tumor-bearing mice leads to inhibition of tumor growth.

The success of tumor immunotherapy using live bacteria in a number of animal studies quickly prompted investigators to attempt a similar protocol in a clinical trial. Low and colleagues developed an attenuated strain of *Salmonella* expressing a mutated lipid A, which rendered the strain nonpathogenic.[22] This strain retained the capacity to home in on and replicate in tumor tissue. However, in a phase I clinical trial, the strain proved to be ineffective in retarding tumor growth in patients with metastatic melanoma.[23] The inefficacy of treatment using this hyperattenuated *Salmonella* strain has been postulated to be related to its poor homing to tumor sites in humans.[23,24]

Cytokine-Expressing *Salmonella* Strains

Over the past few years, we have investigated the characteristics of attenuated *Salmonella* strains expressing eukaryotic cytokines under the control of bacterial promoters. A number of strains, each encoding the gene for a specific murine cytokine, such as IL-2, IFN-γ, or TNF-α, were derived by transfecting an expression plasmid containing the cloned cytokine gene under the control of the anaerobic growth-inducible promoter *nirB* into the *aroA⁻ aroD⁻* deletion mutant strain of *S. typhimurium*, designated BRD509.[25–27] One of the principal findings from these studies was the demonstration that *Salmonella*-expressed cytokines can influence, each cytokine-encoding bacterial strain in its own specific way, the ensuing anti-*Salmonella* immune response.[27,28] Moreover, as the activity of the *nirB* promoter is induced under hypoxic conditions, the level of cytokine synthesis by each of the strains was increased approximately 1000-fold when grown anaerobically.[27]

It is important to note that these transfected bacterial strains do not secrete cytokines extracellularly, but rather the cytokines are expressed within the bacterial cytosol (al-Ramadi *et al.*, unpublished data). Given that *Salmonella* organisms are invasive facultative intracellular pathogens, the use of the cytokine gene–transfected mutant strains represented an attractive means by which relatively high levels of potent immunoregulatory molecules can be delivered locally.

Much of our early attention was focused on a strain of *S. typhimurium* that encodes IL-2, designated GIDIL2,[26,27] which was found to dramatically enhance the ability of the host's immune system to resist infection.[29,30] This was achieved by the rapid induction of the host's innate immune response through the activation of macrophages and NK cells within as short as 2 h of entry into the host.[29–31] Importantly, the induction of this strong innate immune response proved physiologically significant as it afforded a high level of protection against a challenge with virulent *Salmonella* given within 24 h of GIDIL2 inoculation.[29] As expected, the observed protection was not antigen specific, as GIDIL2 administration could also protect murine hosts against a lethal challenge with *Listeria monocytogenes* (al-Ramadi *et al.*, unpublished data). We concluded that the expression of IL-2 by the bacterial vector enabled the induction of a strong host innate immune response which, independently of the slower-developing adaptive immune response, could efficiently bring under control homologous as well as heterologous lethal infections.

The observed immuno-enhancing properties of cytokine-encoding *Salmonella* strains, combined with the high levels cytokine expression achievable under anaerobic conditions, allowed us to hypothesize that these strains might well be desirable as tools for antitumor therapy. Furthermore, the expression of proinflammatory cytokines by these strains could well improve their homing efficiency to tumor tissue, as well as their antitumor activity, by influencing the local tumor vasculature.

In order to test this hypothesis, we selected the B16 melanoma syngeneic tumor model. Success of experimental intervention in this well-established model, known for its poor immunogenicity and high tumorigenicity, usually correlates with highly effective antitumor responses. Indeed, immunotherapeutic approaches with demonstrated efficacy in many tumor models are often ineffective in the B16 melanoma model because of the low immunogenicity of B16 melanoma cancer cells.[32]

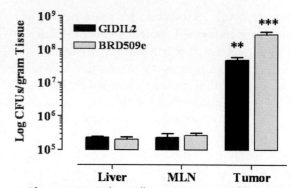

Figure 1. *Salmonella* organisms preferentially target tumor sites. Mice previously implanted with B16F1 melanoma were treated with a single i.p. injection of either BRD509e or GIDIL2 strain of *S. typhimurium*. On day 7 post treatment, mice were sacrificed and tissue homogenates were prepared from tumor, liver, and mesenteric lymph nodes (MLN). Bacterial colony forming units (CFUs) were determined after plating on T-soy agar plates. Each data point represents the mean ± SEM of 7 mice per group. Asterisks denote statistically significant differences between tumor CFUs in comparison with either liver or MLN CFUs of the same group (***$P < 0.001$; **$P < 0.01$).

IL-2-Expressing *Salmonella* in B16 Melanoma Model

In our experimental model, C57BL/6 mice were inoculated subcutaneously in the right flank with B16.F1 melanoma cells and staged to day 13, a time at which tumor growth becomes clearly visible. Tumor growth was followed by quantitative determination twice weekly of the volume of tumor tissue, measured as the product of the perpendicular diameters, according to the formula: volume $= L \times W^2/2$. On day 13 post inoculation, animals were injected i.p. with log-phase bacterial suspensions, prepared in pyrogen-free saline, in 0.5 mL volume at a dose of 5×10^5 CFUs per mouse. The two bacterial strains used in this study were the parental attenuated strain transfected with the empty vector, designated BRD509e,[31] or the IL-2-encoding strain, designated GIDIL2. Tumor volume and survival were then followed for another 3 weeks. In some experiments, bacterial load in various organs was determined at different time points post treatment.

Preferential Homing and Replication of IL-2-Expressing *Salmonella* in Tumors

To date, our findings indicate that the GIDIL2 strain exhibits a preferential homing capacity to, and survival in, melanoma tumor tissue (Fig. 1). There were 100- to

1000-fold more bacterial CFUs in tumor tissue in comparison with other target organs, including liver, mesenteric lymph nodes, and spleen (Fig. 1 and data not shown). This pattern of distribution was indistinguishable from that observed with the noncytokine-expressing BRD509e strain. Differences in bacterial numbers between the different tissues were observed as early as 3 days and continued for up to 21 days post treatment (data not shown). Collectively, these data demonstrate that *Salmonella* organisms, of either the BRD509e or GIDIL2 strain, home preferentially to, and survive in, tumor tissue *in vivo*.

Immunotherapy Using IL-2-Expressing *Salmonella* Bacteria

The potential of using the BRD509e and GIDIL2 *Salmonella* strains as tools for cancer immunotherapy was next investigated. Mice

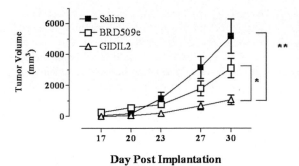

Figure 2. Suppression of tumor growth by attenuated *Salmonella* strains and superior efficacy of the IL-2-encoding strain. Tumor-bearing mice were treated with a single i.p. injection of either saline, BRD509e, or GIDIL2 strain of *S. typhimurium* on day 13 post implantation. Growth of tumor was followed up to day 30 post implantation. Each data point represents the mean ± SEM of 8 mice per group. Asterisks denote statistically significant differences between the saline control group, and GIDIL2 (**P < 0.01) and between BRD509e and GIDIL2 (*P < 0.05).

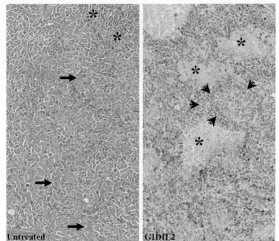

Figure 3. Increased tumor necrosis following administration of IL-2-expressing *Salmonella* strain. Mice (5 per group) implanted with B16.F1 cells on day 0 were treated with either saline (Untreated group) or GIDIL2 strain on day 13 post implantation. Fourteen days later, tumors were excised and processed for hematoxylin/eosin staining. *Arrows* point to blood vessels, which are more prevalent in untreated group. *Arrow heads* point to a ring of apoptotic cells in hypoxic regions of the tumor surrounding healthy tumor tissue. *Asterisks* indicate regions of necrosis, which are larger in size and more abundant in GIDIL2-treated mice. Original magnification ×100.

were implanted with B16.F1 melanoma cells and, on day 13, were inoculated i.p. with a single dose of either saline, BRD509e, or GIDIL2. Growth of tumor was followed up to day 30 post implantation. As shown in Figure 2, treatment with *Salmonella* resulted in a dramatic inhibition of tumor growth. On day 17 of treatment, mean tumor volume of the BRD509e-treated group was reduced by approximately 39% compared to the saline-treated group, although the difference was not statistically significant. In sharp contrast, the mean tumor volume of GIDIL2-treated mice was suppressed significantly by approximately 80% and 65% in comparison with the control and BRD509e-treated mice (*P* = 0.005 and 0.01), respectively. To gain some insight into the underlying reasons for the observed differences among the different experimental groups, histological sections of tumor tissue were prepared and stained with hematoxylin/eosin (Fig. 3). The superior retardation of tumor growth in GIDIL2-treated mice correlated directly with the extent of cellular necrosis seen in histological sections of tumor tissue (Fig. 3). This demonstrates that *Salmonella* or-

ganisms genetically engineered to encode IL-2 are potentially far more effective immunotherapeutic agents against even poorly immunogenic melanomas than the parental strain.

Summary

The above data demonstrate the potential of using cytokine-expressing *Salmonella* strains as antitumor therapeutic tools. Cytokine expression in the bacterial strains is regulated by the *nirB* promoter, whose activity is significantly enhanced under hypoxic conditions. This provides the advantage of specifically targeting cytokine delivery to within the tumor tissue. While the exact mechanism of antitumor effect of *Salmonella* organisms is unknown, the targeting of IL-2 to tumor sites may provide an immuno-enhancing stimulus to cells of the innate immune system with known roles in antitumor immunity, such as NK cells and macrophages. Consequently, the resulting local inflammatory response may well contribute to the enhanced tumor necrosis observed in *Salmonella*-treated animals. Additionally, there is a potential effect of treatment with IL-2-expressing bacteria on tumor angiogenesis, which is suggested by the observed changes in tumor vasculature. Taken together, the use of *nirB* promoter-regulated cytokines engineered in attenuated *Salmonella* strains may prove an attractive model for the utilization of live bacteria in cancer immunotherapy.

Acknowledgments

We thank Ms. Ghada Bashir and Mr. Mohamed Elwasila for excellent technical assistance. This work was supported by a grant from the Terry Fox Fund for Cancer Research.

Conflicts of Interest

The authors declare no conflicts of interest.

References

1. Finn, O.J. 2003. Cancer vaccines: between the idea and the reality. *Nat. Rev. Immunol.* **3:** 630–641.
2. Marincola, F.M. *et al.* 2003. Tumors as elusive targets of T-cell-based active immunotherapy. *Trends Immunol.* **24:** 335–342.
3. Khong, H.T. & N.P. Restifo. 2002. Natural selection of tumor variants in the generation of "tumor escape" phenotypes. *Nat. Immunol.* **3:** 999–1005.
4. Mortarini, R. *et al.* 2003. Lack of terminally differentiated tumor-specific CD8+ T cells at tumor site in spite of antitumor immunity to self-antigens in human metastatic melanoma. *Cancer Res.* **63:** 2535–2545.
5. Garcia-Lora, A., I. Algarra & F. Garrido. 2003. MHC class I antigens, immune surveillance, and tumor immune escape. *J. Cell Physiol.* **195:** 346–355.
6. Kaufman, H.L. & M.L. Disis. 2004. Immune system versus tumor: shifting the balance in favor of DCs and effective immunity. *J. Clin. Invest.* **113:** 664–667.
7. Dang, L.H. *et al.* 2001. Combination bacteriolytic therapy for the treatment of experimental tumors. *Proc. Natl. Acad. Sci. U.S.A.* **98:** 15155–15160.
8. Ganss, R. *et al.* 2002. Combination of T-cell therapy and trigger of inflammation induces remodeling of the vasculature and tumor eradication. *Cancer Res.* **62:** 1462–1470.
9. Thomas-Tikhonenko, A. & C.A. Hunter. 2003. Infection and cancer: the common vein. *Cytokine & Growth Factor Reviews* **14:** 67–77.
10. Alexanderoff, A.B. *et al.* 1999. BCG immunotherapy of bladder cancer: 20 years on. *Lancet* **353:** 1689–1694.
11. Jain, R.K. & N.S. Forbes. 2001. Can engineered bacteria help control cancer? *Proc. Natl. Acad. Sci. USA* **98:** 14748–14750.
12. Pawelek, J.M., K.B. Low & D. Bermudes. 2003. Bacteria as tumor-targeting vectors. *Lancet Oncol.* **4:** 548–556.
13. Pawelek, J.M., K.B. Low & D. Bermudes. 1997. Tumor-targeted *Salmonella* as a novel anticancer vector. *Cancer Res.* **57:** 4537–4544.
14. Forbes, N.S. *et al.* 2003. Sparse initial entrapment of systemically injected *Salmonella typhimurium* leads to heterogeneous accumulation within tumors. *Cancer Res.* **63:** 5188–5193.
15. Chen, L.M., K. Kaniga & J.E. Galan. 1996. *Salmonella* spp. are cytotoxic for cultured macrophages. *Mol. Microbiol.* **21:** 1101–1115.
16. Monack, D.M. *et al.* 1996. *Salmonella typhimurium* invasion induces apoptosis in infected macrophages. *Proc. Natl. Acad. Sci. USA* **93:** 9833–9838.
17. Monack, D.M., W.W. Navarre & S. Falkow. 2001. *Salmonella*-induced macrophage death: the role of caspase-1 in death and inflammation. *Microbes. Infect.* **3:** 1201–1212.
18. Hernandez, L.D. *et al.* 2003. A Salmonella protein causes macrophage cell death by inducing autophagy. *J. Cell. Biol.* **163:** 1123–1131.
19. Galan, J.E. 2001. *Salmonella* interactions with host cells: type III secretion at work. *Annu. Rev. Cell. Biol.* **17:** 53-.
20. Pawelek, J.M. *et al.* 2002. *Salmonella* pathogenicity island-2 and anticancer activity in mice. *Cancer Gene. Ther.* **9:** 813–818.
21. Avogadri, F. *et al.* 2005. Cancer immunotherapy based on killing of *Salmonella*-infected tumor cells. *Cancer Res.* **65:** 3920–3927.
22. Low, K.B. *et al.* 1999. Lipid A mutant *Salmonella* with suppressed virulence and TNF alpha induction retain tumor targeting in vivo. *Nat. Biotechnol.* **17:** 37–41.
23. Toso, J.F. *et al.* 2002. Phase I study of the intravenous administration of attenuated *Salmonella typhimurium* to patients with metastatic melanoma. *J. Clin. Oncol.* **20:** 142–152.

24. Rosenberg, S.A., P.J. Spiess & D.E. Kleiner. 2002. Antitumor effects in mice of the intravenous injection of attenuated *Salmonella typhimurium*. *J. Immunother.* **25:** 218–225.

25. Strugnell, R. *et al.* 1992. Characterization of a *Salmonella typhimurium aro* vaccine strain expressing the P.69 antigen of *Bordetella pertussis*. *Infect. Immun.* **60:** 3994–4002.

26. Xu, D. *et al.* 1998. Protective effect on *Leishmania major* infection of migration inhibitory factor, TNF-α, and IFN-γ administered orally via attenuated *Salmonella typhimurium*. *J. Immunol.* **160:** 1285–1289.

27. al-Ramadi, B.K. *et al.* 2001. Influence of vector-encoded cytokines on anti-*Salmonella* immunity: divergent effects of interkeukin-2 and tumor necrosis factor alpha. *Infect. Immun.* **69:** 3980–3988.

28. al-Ramadi, B.K. *et al.* 2002. Cytokine expression by attenuated intracellular bacteria regulates the immune response to infections: the *Salmonella* model. *Mol. Immunol.* **38:** 931–940.

29. al-Ramadi, B.K. *et al.* 2003. Induction of innate immunity by IL-2-expressing *Salmonella* confers protection against lethal infection. *Mol. Immunol.* **39:** 763–770.

30. al-Ramadi, B.K. *et al.* 2004. Activation of innate immune responses by IL-2-expressing *Salmonella typhimurium* is independent of Toll-like receptor 4. *Mol. Immunol.* **40:** 671–679.

31. al-Ramadi, B.K. *et al.* 2004. Poor survival but high immunogenicity of IL-2-expressing *Salmonella typhimurium* in inherently resistant mice. *Microbes Infect.* **6:** 350–359.

32. Furumoto, K. *et al.* 2004. Induction of potent antitumor immunity by in situ targeting of intratumoral DCs. *J. Clin. Invest.* **113:** 774–783.

In Vitro Effects of Tea Polyphenols on Redox Metabolism, Oxidative Stress, and Apoptosis in PC12 Cells

Haider Raza and Annie John

Department of Biochemistry, Faculty of Medicine and Health Sciences, UAE University, Al Ain, United Arab Emirates

Tea polyphenols, especially catechins, have been reported to be potent antioxidants and beneficial in oxidative stress–related diseases including cancer. Numerous animal and cell culture models demonstrate anticancer effects of tea catechins. Experimental and epidemiological evidence suggests the use of black tea polyphenols (BTP), green tea catechins (especially epigallocatechin gallate [EGCG]), and other polyphenols in preventing the progression of cancer both in animal and human populations. In the present study, we have demonstrated alterations in oxidative stress and redox metabolism using an isolated cell-free system and also in PC12 cancer cells after treatment with EGCG and BTP. We have demonstrated that tea catechins, alter the production of reactive oxygen species, glutathione metabolism, lipid peroxidation, and protein oxidation under *in vitro* conditions. We have also demonstrated that EGCG and BTP affect redox metabolism under cell culture conditions. Induction of apoptosis was observed, after the treatment with tea polyphenols, as shown by increased DNA breakdown and activation of the apoptotic markers, cytochrome c, caspase 3, and poly-(ADP-ribose) polymerase. These results may have implications in determining the chemopreventive and therapeutic use of tea catechins *in vivo*.

Key words: black tea polyphenols; EGCG; oxidative stress; GSH metabolism; apoptosis

Introduction

Green tea, a processed form of tea (*Camellia sinensis*) leaves, has strong antioxidant activity and acts as a scavenger of reactive oxygen species (ROS).[1–3] The major green tea polyphenols are epicatechin (EC), epigallocatechin (EGC), epicatechin gallate (ECG), and epigallocatechin gallate (EGCG). Black tea polyphenols (BTP) are rich in theaflavins, catechins, and other polyphenols. Catechins are also found in high concentrations in fruits and other plants and constitute about 30–40% of the solid green tea extract (dry weight).[4] Following oral ingestion, catechins are found in the blood and tissues in high concentrations.[4,5] Tea polyphenols also stimulate cellular antioxidant defense metabolisms and activate redox-regulated transcription factors.[4–6] It was found that tea catechins have radical scavenging activity greater than vitamin C in sparing vitamin E under physiological and experimental conditions.[7] Tea polyphenols have also been implicated in cell cycle regulation and apoptosis preferentially in cancer cells. EGCG, the most potent catechin, has been associated with reduced risks of cancer, diabetes, and cardiovascular diseases.[8,9] On the contrary, *in vitro* studies have linked EGCG and other catechins to the production of ROS and subsequent cell death.[9,10] This property may, however, differ in different cell types and in different cellular compartments due to the varying nature of metabolism and the antioxidant pool.

Address for correspondence: Prof. Haider Raza, Department of Biochemistry, Faculty of Medicine and Health Sciences, UAE University, P.O. Box 17666, Al Ain, UAE. Voice: +97137137506; fax: +97137672033. h.raza@uaeu.ac.ae

Ann. N.Y. Acad. Sci. 1138: 358–365 (2008). © 2008 New York Academy of Sciences.
doi: 10.1196/annals.1414.037

The primary sites of ROS interaction in the cells are the macromolecules and membrane structures located in the near vicinity of ROS production, namely, the mitochondria, the plasma membrane, and the endoplasmic reticulum. Under physiological conditions, ROS are eliminated by enzymatic and nonenzymatic antioxidant defense systems mainly by glutathione (GSH) scavenging mechanisms. However, recent studies[11] have clearly demonstrated that the dietary administration of EGCG (up to 500 mg/kg) to rats for several weeks was not found to be toxic. We therefore investigated the effect of EGCG and BTP on $NADPH/Fe^{+2}$-induced microsomal membrane lipid peroxidation (LPO), GSH metabolizing enzymes, protein carbonylation induced by 4-hydroxynonenal (4-HNE; a product of LPO under oxidative stress conditions), and ROS formation, using isolated cell-free systems *in vitro* as well as PC12 cells in culture. In this study, we have shown that both EGCG and BTP exert significant alteration on subcellular oxidative stress related to GSH metabolism and ROS productions in the cells. In addition, we have demonstrated the protection of oxidative stress–induced lipid and protein degradations by the tea polyphenols under *in vitro* conditions.

Materials and Methods

Chemicals

BTP, 1-chloro 2,4-dinitrobenzene (CDNB), cumene hydroperoxide, hydrogen peroxide, thiobarbituric acid (TBA), malonaldehyde (MDA), GSH, NADPH, dinitrophenylhydrazine (DNPH), lucigenin and anti-dinitrophenol antibody were purchased from Sigma-Aldrich Fine Chemicals (St. Louis, MO). 4-HNE was purchased from Oxis International Inc. (Portland, OR). Apoptosis detection kits for TUNEL assay were purchased from Serologicals Corp. (Temecula, CA). PC12 cells were purchased from American Type Culture Collection (Manassas, VA). Antibodies

against cytochrome c, caspase 3, poly-(ADP-ribose) polymerase (PARP), and β-actin were purchased from Santa Cruz Biotechnology Inc. (Santa Cruz, CA).

Preparation of Sub Cellular Fractions

Adult male Wistar rats ($n = 3$, 200–220 g) were obtained from the animal house facility of the Faculty of Medicine and Health Sciences, UAE University. Rats were fasted overnight and sacrificed according to the approved institutional guidelines. Livers were removed, perfused with ice-cold saline, and homogenized (10% w/v) in 0.1 M potassium phosphate buffer pH 7.4 containing 0.1 mM ethylene diamine tetra acetic acid (EDTA), 0.1 mM phenylmethylsulfonylfluoride (PMSF), and 0.15 M KCl. Cellular fractions were prepared by ultracentrifugation as described before.[12] Protein concentration was measured by the method of Bradford.[13]

PC12 Cell Culture, Treatment, and Cellular Fractionation

PC12 cells were grown in poly-L-lysine-coated 75 cm^2 flasks ($\sim$2.0–2.5 × 10^6 cells/mL) in Roswell Park Memorial Institute (RPMI) 1640 medium which is supplemented with 2 mM glutamine, 5% heat inactivated horse serum, and 10% heat inactivated fetal bovine serum, in the presence of 5% CO2–95% air at 37°C, as described before.[12] Cells were treated with 100 μM 4-HNE dissolved in ethanol (final concentration less than 0.2%) for 2 h, EGCG (100 μM for 16 h), or BTP (5 μg and 10 μg for 16 h). Control cells were treated with vehicle alone. The selection of doses of tea polyphenols was based on our cell viability assay and published reports.[12] After the desired time of treatment, cells were harvested, washed with PBS (pH 7.4), and homogenized in 10 mM phosphate buffer pH 7.4 containing 0.15 M KCl, 0.1 mM EDTA, 1 mM dithiothreitol (DTT), and 0.1 mM PMSF.[12,14]

Effect of Tea Catechins on ROS Production

Freshly prepared PC12 extract was used to measure the effect of tea catechins on 4-HNE-induced ROS production. The NADPH oxidase-dependent lucigenin-enhanced chemiluminescence method of Li and colleagues,[15] which detects mainly superoxide formation, was used to measure ROS production using a Turner Design TD-20/20 luminometer (Sunnyvale, CA), as described recently.[12,14,16] Appropriate controls were used and blank readings were subtracted from the final values expressed.

Effect of Tea Catechins on Microsomal LPO

Microsomal LPO was induced by NADPH/$FeSO_4$, and TBA reactive substances (TBARS) were measured using MDA as standard, as described before.[16]

GSH Metabolism in Rat Liver Cytosol and PC12 Cell Extract

Activity of the GSH metabolizing enzymes, glutathione S-transferase (GST), glutathioneperoxidase (GSH-Px), and glutathione reductase (GSSG-reductase) was measured in the presence of EGCG or BTP in rat liver cytosol and PC12 cell extract using CDNB, cumene hydroperoxide, or hydrogen peroxide and GSSG/NADPH, respectively, as substrates using standard methods as described before.[12,14,16]

Effect of Tea Catechins on Protein Carbonylation

4-HNE, a physiological stable product of LPO, was used to induce protein carbonylation in the presence or absence of EGCG (100 μM) and BTP (5 μg and 10 μg). The carbonylated proteins were then measured as DNPH-derived protein spectrophotometrically at 370 nm, as described by Reznick and Packer.[17] The values reported were obtained after subtracting the values of protein oxidation in the presence of tea polyphenols alone measured against appropriate blanks.

Analysis of Apoptosis by TUNEL and DNA Fragmentation Assays

PC12 cells were seeded onto 35 mm diameter culture dishes containing 22 mm^2 sterile cover slips. After allowing 24 h for attachment, cells were treated with 100 μM EGCG or 5 μg and 10 μg BTP for 16 h. TUNEL assay, as determined by DNA fragmentation using digoxigenin reactive ApopTag peroxidase kit (Millipore Corp., Billerica, MA), performed essentially as described previously.[12] Apoptotic cells (brown cells) against the blue viable cells were counted under the light microscope. DNA fragmentation was assayed by UV transillumination after staining the electrophoretically separated fragments with 0.5 μg/mL ethidium bromide as previously described.[14]

SDS-PAGE and Western Blot Analysis

Proteins (50 μg) from the PC12 cell extract of control and treated cells and from the DNPH-derived carbonylated and control rat liver microsomes were separated on 12% sodium dodecyl sulfate polyacrylamide gel electrophoresis (SDS-PAGE) and electrophoretically transferred onto nitrocellulose paper by Western blotting using standard procedures as described before.[12,14] The immunoreacting protein bands were visualized after interacting with primary antibodies against cytochrome c, caspase 3, PARP, β-actin, and DNPH.

Statistical Analysis

All the values shown are expressed as mean ± SEM of three determinations. Statistical significance of the data was assessed by analysis of variance followed by Dunnett analysis

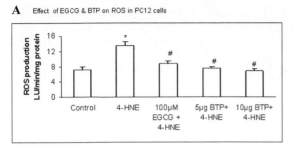

A Effect of EGCG & BTP on ROS in PC12 cells

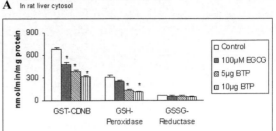

Effect of EGCG & BTP on GSH metabolism
A In rat liver cytosol

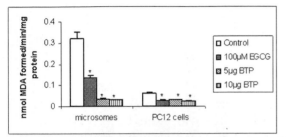

B Effect of EGCG & BTP on LPO in rat liver microsomes & in PC12 cells

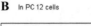

B In PC 12 cells

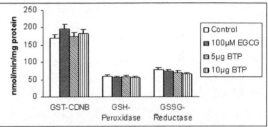

Figure 1. (A) Effect of EGCG and BTP on ROS production. PC12 cells cultured (~2.5 × 10^6 cells/mL) in RPMI medium, treated with 100 μM EGCG or 5 μg and 10 μg BTP for 16 h were homogenized after harvesting and analyzed for ROS as described in the Materials and Methods section. The values are mean ± SEM of 3 experiments. (*$P \leq$ 0.05 compared with control; #$P \leq$ 0.05 compared with 4-HNE treated values.) **(B)** Effect of EGCG and BTP on LPO *in vitro* and in PC12 cells. Rat liver microsomes were prepared by ultracentrifugation and the rate of NADPH/Fe^{+2}-supported LPO was measured, using 50–100 μg protein/mL as TBARS, using MDA as standard. 100 μM EGCG or 5 μg and 10 μg BTP were added just before the addition of NADPH/Fe^{+2}, and the reaction was continued for 1 h. Values are mean + SEM of 3 experiments. (* $P \leq$ 0.05 compared with control.) PC12 cells were cultured, treated, and harvested as described in the legend of Figure 1A and analyzed for LPO as TBARS, using MDA as standard.

and *P* values ≤0.05 were considered statistically significant.

Results

Effects on ROS and LPO

An increase (~two-fold) in ROS production was observed after the treatment of cells with 4-HNE, which was decreased significantly (35–50%) after the treatment with EGCG and BTP

Figure 2. (A) Effect of EGCG and BTP on GSH metabolism *in vitro*. Cytosolic (100 μg protein) GSH-metabolizing enzymes, GST, GSH-Px, and GSSG-reductase activities were measured after the addition of 100 μM EGCG or 5 μg and 10 μg BTP, as described in the Materials and Methods section. Values are expressed as mean ± SEM of 3 determinations. Asterisks indicate significant difference (P ≤ 0.05) from control values. **(B)** PC12 cells (~2.5 × 10^6 cells/mL) were cultured in RPMI medium, treated with 100 μM EGCG or 5 μg and 10 μg BTP for 16 h, homogenized after harvesting, and analyzed for the GSH-metabolizing enzymes, as described in the Materials and Methods section.

(Fig. 1A). Tea polyphenols were inhibitory in the presence of 4-HNE, indicating the ROS scavenging activity of tea polyphenols under oxidative stress conditions. LPO, both in PC12 cells and liver microsomes, was also markedly inhibited by EGCG and BTP treatments (Fig. 1B), and this effect was more profound under *in vitro* conditions.

Effects on GSH Metabolism

Cytosolic GST activity, *in vitro*, was significantly inhibited (30–55%) by the tea polyphenols, while a marked inhibition of GSH-peroxidase activity was observed mainly with the BTP (57–64%). GSSG-reductase, on the other hand, showed no significant change (Fig. 2A). In PC12 cells, a marginal increase in GST activity was observed (Fig. 2B). GSH-peroxidase and GSSG-reductase activities, in contrast, showed no appreciable change.

Effects on Protein Carbonylation

Oxidative stress–induced protein carbonylation in the isolated microsomes, as assayed by DNPH coupling, exhibited an increase (two–fold) of protein carbonylation after 4-HNE treatment. Tea polyphenols treatment, however, caused significant inhibition (65–80%) of protein carbonylation (Fig. 3A). We have demonstrated that protein bands in the range of 55–65 kDA were carbonylated by 4-HNE treatments and that the tea polyphenols have inhibited the oxidative breakdown of the proteins (Fig. 3B).

Effects on Apoptosis and DNA Fragmentation

Treatment with EGCG and BTP induced apoptosis and DNA fragmentation as shown in Figure 4A and B, respectively.

Effects of EGCG and BTP on the Expression of Apoptotic Markers

As shown in Figure 5, the expression of the apoptotic marker proteins cytochrome c, caspase 3, and PARP was significantly increased after tea polyphenol treatments, which compliments the observation made by TUNEL apoptosis and DNA fragmentation assays.

Discussion

Imbalances in redox metabolism and altered mitochondrial oxygen utilization have been implicated in the increased production of ROS.[18,19] ROS-induced formation of lipid peroxides is thought to play an important role

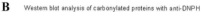

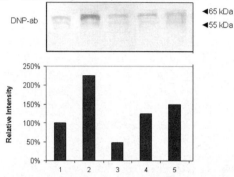

Figure 3. (A) Effect of EGCG and BTP on 4-HNE-induced protein carbonylation *in vitro*. Rat liver microsomes (100 μg protein) were used for 4-HNE (100 μM) induced carbonylation studies using DNPH, as described in the Materials and Methods section. Values are expressed as mean ± SEM of 3 determinations. Asterisks indicate significant difference from control (**$P \leq 0.01$). # indicates a significant difference from 4-HNE-treated values ($P \leq 0.05$). **(B)** The DNPH-coupled carbonylated proteins (100 μg) mentioned in the legend of Figure 3A, were then separated by 12% SDS-PAGE and immunoblotted with antibody against DNPH-coupled protein. The molecular mass of the proteins was determined using Bio-Rad (Hercules, CA) protein molecular weight standard. The results shown represents a typical blot from 3 experiments. Lane 1, microsome alone; lane 2, microsome + 4-HNE; lane 3, as in lane 2 + 100 μM EGCG; lane 4, as in lane 2 + 5 μg BTP; lane 5, as in lane 2 + 10 μg BTP. The quantitation of the major 65 kDa protein was performed and shown as percent of control bars under the corresponding lanes.

in the etiology and pathogenesis of a number of oxidative stress–related diseases, including cancer. As a result of LPO, a number of toxic metabolites, such as 4-HNE, are produced from cellular molecules.[20] In oxidative stress–induced toxicity, 4-HNE concentrations as high as 10 nmol/g have been reported, and being a strong electrophile, 4-HNE readily reacts with

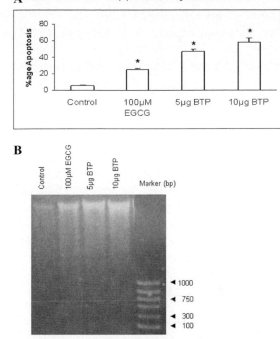

A Effects of EGCG & BTP on apoptosis & DNA fragmentation in PC12 cells

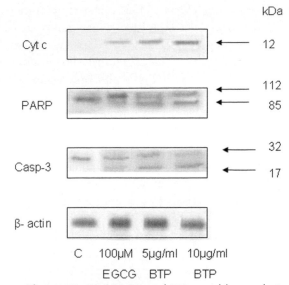

Figure 4. Effect of EGCG and BTP on apoptosis and DNA fragmentation in PC12 cells. PC12 cell cultures grown on cover-slips were treated with 100 μM EGCG and 5 μg and 10 μg BTP for 16 h. Following the treatment, cells were fixed with 4% buffered paraformaldehyde, and immunocytochemical localization of TUNEL positive cells (per 10 fields) were visualized using ApopTag peroxidase apoptosis kit. **(A)** The results are expressed as the percentage of apoptotic nuclei in a single slide from 3 different experiments. Asterisk indicates a significant difference ($P \leq 0.05$) from control values. **(B)** DNA isolated from controls and from the cells treated with 100 μM EGCG or 5 μg and 10 μg BTP were separated by 1.5% agarose gel electrophoresis, and the DNA was visualized using ethidium bromide. A small base pairs DNA ladder was used as a marker.

Figure 5. SDS-PAGE and Western blot analysis of apoptotic marker proteins. PC12 cells were cultured in the presence of 100 μM EGCG or 5 μg and 10 μg BTP for 16 h. Proteins from the postmitochondrial fractions (50 μg) were analyzed by 12% SDS-PAGE and transferred on to nitrocellulose membrane by Western blotting and immunochemically characterized using antibodies against cytochrome c, PARP, and caspase 3. Apparent molecular mass (kDa) was calculated using Bio-Rad protein molecular weight standard. β-actin was used as a loading control.

nucleophilic biomolecules and alters cell signaling and gene expression.[21–24] Dietary polyphenols, especially catechins, are known to protect oxidation of biomolecules against oxidant species by preventing LPO.[8,25] In this study, using EGCG and purified BTP, we have observed a marked inhibition of NADPH/Fe^{+2}-induced LPO in rat liver microsomes. Interestingly, inhibition of membrane LPO was also observed when tea catechins were added in the medium of PC12 cells in culture.

Increased oxidative stress is also known to cause oxidative protein carbonylation.[20] We have investigated the extent of protein carbonylation under increased oxidative stress conditions in isolated rat liver microsomes treated with 4-HNE. Oxidative modification of proteins, assessed as DNPH-reactive, protein-bound carbonyls, was markedly increased after 4-HNE treatment. EGCG and BTP treatments have protected the protein modifications by 4-HNE. We could not precisely identify individual proteins modified under these conditions. However, proteins in the range of 55–65 kDa molecular mass appeared to have been modified more effectively. Our preliminary studies have, however, shown that after 4-HNE treatment, one of the major carbonylated proteins in microsomes co-immunoprecipitated with the polyclonal antibody against cytochrome P450

2E1 (data not shown). This effect is presumably associated with the ROS scavenging activity of tea polyphenols, as CYP2E1 is known to produce ROS.[12,14] The protein-binding ability of tea polyphenols helps in the protection of cellular proteins against oxidative damage by the reactive oxygen and nitrogen species.[26,27] Increased carbonylation and oxidative damage of cellular proteins have been reported in many oxidative stress–related diseases. The inhibition of this reaction by tea polyphenols may have significant implications in preventing the toxicity and disease complications.[26,28]

GSH metabolism was also affected when tea polyphenols were added in the catalytic reaction mixture to measure the GSH metabolizing enzyme activities. EGCG and BTP inhibited GST activity significantly (30–55%), and a marked inhibition (57–64%) was observed with the BTP, however GSH-Px activity was only slightly inhibited (20%) by EGCG. On the other hand, GSSG-reductase activity was not significantly inhibited. Thus it appears that redox cycling of GSH was not affected by tea catechins under *in vitro* conditions. However, in PC12 cells, a marginal increase in GST activity and a slight inhibition of GSSG-reductase activity were observed with almost no change in GSH-Px activity.

The use of tea polyphenols as antitumor agents has greater significance as there appear to be discriminating effects in normal and cancer cells. Variations in cell signaling and cell cycle regulation, oxidative stress environment, antioxidant metabolism, and induction and/or suppression of apoptosis are considered to be involved in these discriminating effects of tea polyphenolsl.[1–6] Our results have shown increased apoptosis, as indicated by TUNEL assay, DNA laddering, and activation of apoptotic signals after treatment with the tea polyphenols.

In summary, we have clearly demonstrated that both green tea EGCG and BTP exhibit strong inhibitory activity on the free radical–induced oxidation of membrane lipid and proteins, which correlate well with their antioxidant potentials *in vivo*.[29] Cancer and other degenerative disorders, under a compromised antioxidant mechanism, are likely to have increased oxidative stress due to the increased production of ROS. The etiological and pathological complications in cancer cells, under these conditions, may therefore, be attributed to the perturbations in cellular redox metabolisms. Antioxidants and plant polyphenols are being tried as chemopreventive agents to prevent the progression of cancer. Our study has attempted to provide a mechanistic approach to understanding the molecular mechanism of action of oxidants and antioxidants on cancer cells, which would, in turn, help in designing the appropriate therapeutic strategies to increase the efficacy of chemotherapy in cancer patients.

Acknowledgments

We wish to acknowledge support from Terry Fox Cancer Research Fund, UAE and grant support from the Research Committee, Faculty of Medicine and Health Sciences, UAE University.

Conflicts of Interest

The authors declare no conflicts of interest.

References

1. Rice-Evans, C.A. 1995. Plant polyphenols: free radical scavengers or chain-breaking antioxidants? *Biochem. Soc. Sym.* **61:** 103–116.
2. Yang, C.S., P. Maliakal & X. Meng. 2002. Inhibition of carcinogenesis by tea. *Ann. Rev. Pharmacol. Toxicol.* **42:** 25–54.
3. Ahmad, N., D.K. Feyes, A.L. Nieminen, *et al.* 1997. Green tea constituent epigallocatechin-3-gallate and induction of apoptosis and cell cycle arrest in human carcinoma cells. *J. Natl. Cancer Inst.* **89:** 1881–1886.
4. Wang, Z.Y., M.T. Huang, Y.R. Lou, *et al.* 1994. Inhibitory effects of black tea, green tea, decaffeinated black tea, and decaffeinated green tea on ultraviolet B light-induced skin carcinogenesis in 7, 12 dimethylbenz[a]anthracene-initiated SKH-1 mice. *Cancer Res.* **54:** 3428–3435.

5. Lee, M.-J., Z.Y. Wang, H. Li, *et al.* 1995. Analysis of plasma and urinary tea polyphenols in human subjects. *Cancer Epidemiol. Biomarkers Prev.* **4:** 393–399.

6. Elbling, L., R.M. Weiss, O. Teufelhofer, *et al.* 2005. Green tea extract and (−)-epigallocatechin-3-gallate, the major tea catechin, exert oxidant but lack antioxidant activities. *FASEB J.* **19:** 807–829.

7. Bors, W., W. Heller, C. Michel & M. Saran. 1990. Flavonoids as antioxidants: determination of radical-scavenging efficiencies. *Methods Enzymol.* **186:** 343–355.

8. Guo, Q., B. Zhao, M. Li, *et al.* 1996. Studies on protective mechanisms of four components of green tea polyphenols against lipid peroxidation in synaptosomes. *Biochim. Biophys. Acta* **1304:** 210–222.

9. Halliwell, B., J. Rafter & A. Jenner. 2005. Health promotion by flavonoids, tocopherols, tocotrienols, and other phenols: direct or indirect effects? Antioxidant or not? *Am. J. Clin. Nutr.* **81:** 268S–276S.

10. Higdon, J.V. & B. Frei. 2003. Tea catechins and polyphenols: health effects, metabolism, and antioxidant functions. *Crit. Rev. Food Sci. Nutr.* **43:** 89–143.

11. Isbrucker, R.A., J.A. Edwards, E. Wolz, *et al.* 2006. Safety studies on epigallocatechin gallate (EGCG) preparations. Part 2: dermal, acute and short term toxicity studies. *Food Chem. Toxicol.* **44:** 636–650.

12. Raza, H. & A. John. 2005. Green tea polyphenol epigallocatechin-3-gallate differentially modulates oxidative stress in PC12 cell compartments. *Toxicol. Appl. Pharmacol.* **207:** 212–220.

13. Bradford, M.M. 1976. A rapid and sensitive method for the quantitation of protein utilizing the principle of protein-dye binding. *Anal. Biochem.* **72:** 248–254.

14. Raza, H. & A. John. 2006. 4-Hydroxynonenal induces mitochondrial oxidative stress, apoptosis and expression of glutathione S-transferase A4-4 and cytochrome P450 2E1 in PC12 cells. *Toxicol. Appl. Pharmacol.* **216:** 309–318.

15. Li, Y., H. Zhu, P. Kuppusamy, *et al.* 1998. Validation of lucigenin (bis-N-methylacrydium) as a chemiluminogenic probe for detecting superoxide anion radical production by enzymatic and cellular systems. *J. Biol. Chem.* **273:** 2015–2023.

16. Raza, H. & A. John. 2007. In vitro protection of reactive oxygen species-induced degradation of lipids, proteins and 2-deoxyribose by tea catechins. *Food Chem. Toxicol.* **45:** 1814–1820.

17. Reznick, A.Z. & L. Packer. 1994. Oxidative damage to proteins: spectrophotometric method for carbonyl assay. *Methods Enzymol.* **233:** 357–363.

18. Whiteside, M.A., D.C. Heimburger & G.L. Johanning. 2004. Micronutrients and cancer therapy. *Nutr. Rev.* **62:** 142–147.

19. Fariss, M.W., C.B. Chan, M. Patel, *et al.* 2005. Role of mitochondria in toxic oxidative stress. *Mol. Inter.* **5:** 94–111.

20. Enns, G.M. 2003. The contribution of mitochondria to common disorders. *Mol. Gen. Metab.* **80:** 11–26.

21. Esterbauer, H., R.J. Schaur & H. Zollner. 1991. Chemistry and biochemistry of 4-hydroxynonenal, malonaldehyde and related aldehydes. *Free Radic. Biol. Med.* **11:** 81–128.

22. Awasthi, Y.C., G.A. Ansari & S. Awasthi. 2005. Regulation of 4-hydroxynonenal mediated signaling by glutathione S-transferases. *Methods Enzymol* **401:** 379–407.

23. Nakashima, I., W. Liu, A.A. Akhand, *et al.* 2003. 4-Hydroxynonenal triggers multistep signal transduction cascades for suppression of cellular functions. *Mol. Aspects Med.* **24:** 231–238.

24. Uchida, K., M. Shiraishi, Y. Naito, *et al.* 1999. Activation of stress signaling pathways by the end product of lipid peroxidation: 4-hydroxy-2-nonenal is a potential inducer of intracellular peroxide production. *J. Biol. Chem.* **274:** 2234–2242.

25. West, J.D. & L.J. Marnett. 2005. Alterations in gene expression induced by the lipid peroxidation product, 4-hydroxy-2-nonenal. *Chem. Res. Toxicol.* **18:** 1642–1653.

26. Steffen, Y., T. Schewe & H. Sies. 2005. Epicatechin protects endothelial cells against oxidized LDL and maintains NO synthase. *Biochem. Biophys. Res. Commun.* **331:** 1277–1283.

27. Hagerman, A.E., R.T. Dean & M.J. Davies. 2003. Radical chemistry of epigallocatechin gallate and its relevance to protein damage. *Arch. Biochem. Biophys.* **414:** 115–120.

28. Stanner, S.A., J. Hughes, C.N. Kelly & J. Buttris. 2004. A review of the epidemiological evidence for the "antioxidant hypothesis". *Pub. Hlth. Nut.* **7:** 407–422.

29. Erba, D., P. Riso, A. Bordoni, *et al.* 2005. Effectiveness of moderate green tea consumption on antioxidative status and plasma lipid profile in humans. *J. Nut. Biochem.* **16:** 144–149.

The Swi2/Snf2 Bromodomain Is Important for the Full Binding and Remodeling Activity of the SWI/SNF Complex on H3- and H4-acetylated Nucleosomes

Salma Awad and Ahmed H. Hassan

Faculty of Medicine and Health Sciences, Department of Biochemistry, UAE University, Al Ain, United Arab Emirates

The SWI/SNF chromatin-remodeling complex contains a bromodomain in its Swi2/Snf2 subunit that helps tether it to acetylated promoter nucleosomes. To study the importance of this bromodomain in the SWI/SNF complex, we have compared the nucleosome-binding and the chromatin-remodeling activities of the SWI/SNF to a mutant complex that lacks the Swi2/Snf2 bromodomain. Here we show that the SWI/SNF complex deleted of the Swi2/Snf2 bromodomain cannot bind to SAGA- or NuA4-acetylated nucleosomes as well as the wild-type complex. Moreover, we show that this reduced binding leads to partial remodeling of these acetylated nucleosome templates by the Δbromodomain SWI/SNF complex. These results demonstrate that the Swi2/Snf2 bromodomain is required for the full binding and functional activity of the SWI/SNF complex on H3- and H4-acetylated nucleosomes.

Key words: bromodomain; SWI/SNF; acetylation; chromatin

Introduction

The packaging of eukaryotic DNA into chromatin inhibits the access of transcription or replication machinery to its binding sites and thus results in the repression of these very important cellular processes. Numerous conserved protein complexes whose function is to modulate the access of these factors to regulatory regions of genes have been described in recent years.[1–13] Their actions result in relieving the repressive effects of chromatin and include ATP-dependent chromatin remodeling enzymes, such as the yeast SWI/SNF complex, as well as enzymes that post-translationally modify the N-terminal histone tails by acetylation, methylation, phosphorylation, Sumoy-

lation, ubiquitination, and ADP-ribosylation. The yeast SWI/SNF is a 1.15-MDa complex composed of 12 subunits, which uses the energy of ATP hydrolysis to remodel chromatin by sliding nucleosomes *in cis* and/or displacing nucleosomes *in trans* (octamer transfer), leading to changes in the expression of a subset of yeast genes.[4–6] The yeast Spt7, Ada2, Gen5 acetyltransferase (SAGA) and Nucleosome Acetyltransferase on histone H4 (NuA4) histone acetyltransferases preferentially acetylate histones H3 and H4, respectively, leading to transcription stimulation *in vitro* and *in vivo*.[2,7,8,14–18] The SWI/SNF remodeling complex as well as the SAGA and NuA4 histone acetyltransferase complexes are recruited to these gene promoters by sequence-specific DNA binding transcription activators.[18–29]

We have previously shown that acetylation of nucleosomal array templates can stabilize SWI/SNF binding to promoter nucleosomes after the dissociation of the activator.[30]

Address for correspondence: Ahmed H. Hassan, Department of Biochemistry, Faculty of Medicine and Health Sciences, UAE University, P.O. Box 17666, Al Ain, UAE. Voice: +971-3-713-7478; fax: +971-3-767-2033. E-mail: ahmedh@uaeu.ac.ae

Ann. N.Y. Acad. Sci. 1138: 366–375 (2008). © 2008 New York Academy of Sciences.
doi: 10.1196/annals.1414.038

One evolutionarily conserved motif found in many transcriptional co-activators, including the chromatin remodeling complex SWI/SNF, is the bromodomain. It is a small domain that has been shown to interact with acetylated lysine residues in N-terminal tails of histones H3 and H4 *in vitro*.[31-40] In studies looking into functional interactions between the histone acetyltransferases and the SWI/SNF complex, we have shown that the Swi2/Snf2 bromodomain was necessary for the anchoring of the SWI/SNF to acetylated promoters.[30,41] We observed that the deletion of the Swi2/Snf2 bromodomain resulted in the dissociation of the SWI/SNF complex from acetylated nucleosomal arrays upon activator removal. Consistent with these *in vitro* experiments, we found that the Swi2/Snf2 bromodomain was required for SWI/SNF presence at the SUC2 promoter *in vivo*.[41] More recently, we have shown the displacement of SAGA histone acetyltransferase by the SWI/SNF complex on acetylated nucleosomes and the requirement of the Swi2/Snf2 bromodomain for this activity.[42] Furthermore, using GST-pulldown assay, we have demonstrated that bromodomains show selective recognition of acetylated peptides and histones.[43]

It seems that bromodomains act as targeting modules for the anchoring of chromatin-modifying proteins, such as SWI/SNF, to promoters to regulate gene expression. The recruitment and binding of the SWI/SNF to acetylated histones is possibly as a result of the recognition of the "histone code" by the bromodomain. To determine the role of the Swi2/Snf2 bromodomain in the function of the SWI/SNF complex, we have purified a SWI/SNF complex lacking the Swi2/Snf2 bromodomain and tested its functional activity comparing it to that of the wild type. In this study, we show that the Swi2/Snf2 bromodomain is necessary for the full binding and functional activity of the complex on H3- or H4-acetylated nucleosomal templates. We observed that while the loss of the Swi2/Snf2 bromodomain has no effect on the remodeling activity of unmodified nucleosomes, the bromodomain-deleted (∆bromodomain) SWI/SNF was not able to bind or remodel H3- or H4-acetylated nucleosomes as efficiently as the wild type. These results demonstrate the requirement of the Swi2/Snf2 bromodomain for the full activity of the complex on acetylated promoter nucleosomes.

Experimental Procedures

Purification of Wild-type and Mutant SWI/SNF Complexes

The endogenous ∆bromodomain Swi2/Snf2, Snf6-TAP strain was generated using the Cre-Lox recombination system. Wild-type and ∆bromodomain SWI//SNF complexes were purified from yeast whole-cell extract by the tandem affinity purification (TAP) method using Snf6-TAP strains over two affinity columns, as described previously.[44-47] Briefly, whole-cell extracts were prepared from 6 L of yeast cells grown in Yeast extract, Peptone, Dextrose (YPD) media and added to IgG resin (Amersham Biosciences, Uppsala, Sweden). The complexes were eluted from the beads by Tobacco Etch Virus (TEV) Protease (Invitrogen, Carlsbad, CA) cleavage in a buffer containing 10 mM Tris (pH 8), 150 mM NaCl, 0.5 M ethylenediamine tetraacetic acid (EDTA), 0.1% Nonidet P-40, 10% (v/v) glycerol, 1 mM phenylmethylsulphonyl fluoride (PMSF), 2 µg/mL leupeptin, 1 µg/mL pepstatinA, and 1 mM Dithiothreito (DTT). Following binding to calmodulin resin (Amersham Biosciences), the complexes were eluted using a buffer containing 10 mM Tris (pH 8), 150 mM NaCl, 1 mM MgAc, 1 mM imidazole, 2 mM ethylene glycol tetraacetic acid (EGTA), 0.1% Nonidet P-40, 10% (v/v) glycerol, 1 mM PMSF, 2 µg/mL leupeptin, 1 µg/mL pepstatinA, and 0.5 mM DTT. Purification was monitored by western blot analysis using anti-TAP antibody (Open Biosystems, Huntsville, AL) as well as silver staining. The same amounts of the wild-type and the Δbromodomain SWI/SNF complexes were used in both the immobilized template binding and the restriction enzyme accessibility assays after normalization of the amounts of purified protein.

Immobilized Template Binding Assay

pG5E4–5S containing a dinucleosome length G5E4 fragment flanked on both sides by 5S sequences was prepared as described.[48,49] The G5E4–5S fragments were produced by digesting pG5E4–5S with *Asp*718 and end-labeling with biotin-14-dATP using Klenow. The 2.5 kb end-labeled G5E4–5S fragments were then gel purified away from the backbone by digesting with *Cla*I and *Eae*I. This array was then reconstituted by step dilution with histones as described previously.[30,41] The nucleosomal arrays were then bound to para-magnetic beads coupled to streptavidin (Dynabeads streptavidin; Invitrogen Corporation, Carlsbad, CA), as described before.[30,41,42] After acetylation of the template by either the H3-specific histone acetyltransferase SAGA or the H4-specific histone acetyltransferase NuA4 for 1 h at 30°C, about 4 nM of either the wild-type or the mutant SWI/SNF was added to 200 ng of the above template in 20 μL binding buffer and incubated for an additional 1 h at 30°C. The templates were then concentrated on a magnet, the supernatant was removed, and the beads were washed twice before performing western blot analysis. The blots were probed with antibodies against the tag (anti-TAP antibodies). Graphical representation of the percentage SWI/SNF bound to the template with standard deviation is shown after quantification of three independent experiments determined by scanning the gels and using the signal intensities of the western blots.

Restriction Enzyme Accessibility Assay

In this assay, we used a 183 bp pGAL4-USF BEND (GUB) fragment as the DNA template generated by PCR using a radio-labeled 5′ primer and the pGALUSFBEND plasmid.[20,27,50] This DNA fragment was reconstituted into a nucleosome using short oligonucleosomes. The assay was performed as described previously.[27,42] Briefly, after acetylating the templates with either the H3-specific histone acetyltransferase SAGA or the H4-specific histone acetyltransferase NuA4 for 1 h at 30°C, wild-type or Δbromodomain mutant SWI/SNF complexes were added to approximately 10 ng of the ^{32}P-labeled GUB template in a binding buffer [10 mM HEPES (pH 7.8), 50 mM potassium chloride (KCl), 5 mM DTT, 5 mM PMSF, 5% glycerol, 0.25 mg/mL bovine serum albumin (BSA), and 2 mM MgCl$_2$] in the presence or absence of 2 mM ATP. After incubation for 1 h at 30°C, the binding reactions were treated with 10 units of *Sal*I for 30 min at 30°C. An equal volume of stop buffer [20 mM Tris-HCl (pH 7.5), 50 mM EDTA, 2% sodium dodecyl sulfate (SDS), 0.2 mg/mL proteinase K, 1 mg/mL glycogen] was added to the reactions, and incubated at 50°C for 1 h. Deproteinized samples were precipitated with 200 mM NaCl and 3 volumes of ethanol, and the pellet resuspended in 5 μL of the formamide dye [95% formamide, 10 mM EDTA, 0.1% xylene cyanol, 0.1% bromophenol blue]. After heat denaturation, the samples were resolved on a 6% acrylamide (19:1 acrylamide to bis-acrylamide), 8 M urea sequencing gel at 150 volts for 3 h and visualized by autoradiography. Graphical representation (Fig. 2C) of percent cleavage with standard deviation is shown after quantification of three independent experiments determined by scanning the gels and using the signal intensities.

Results

The Bromodomain-deleted SWI/SNF Complex Has Reduced Affinity for H3- or H4-acetylated Nucleosomes

Previous studies have shown that the SWI/SNF complex is recruited to promoters by

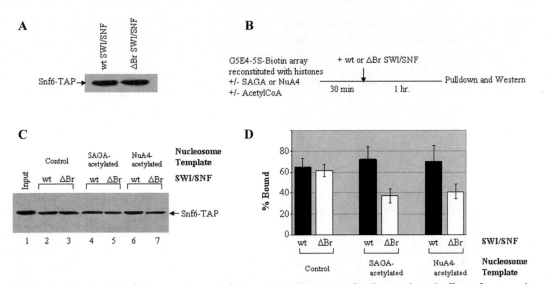

Figure 1. The Swi2/Snf2 bromodomain deletion SWI/SNF complex has reduced affinity for acetylated nucleosome. **(A)** Normalization of the TAP-purified wild-type SWI/SNF and the Δbromodomain SWI/SNF by western blotting using anti-TAP antibody on the Snf6 subunit of the SWI/SNF complex. The purified complexes were run on a 10% SDS gel, transferred to a nitrocellulose membrane and probed with the antibody. Equal amounts of the two complexes (wild-type and the mutant) were used in subsequent experiments. **(B)** Diagram of the immobilized template-binding experiment. Biotinylated G5E4–5S was reconstituted with histones and bound to paramagnetic beads (Dynabeads) coupled to streptavidin as described previously.[30,41,42] Following an acetylation step with either SAGA or NuA4 and the addition of the wild-type and Δbromodomain SWI/SNF complexes, the beads were separated from the supernatants and western blotting was performed using anti-TAP antibody as described in Refs. 41,42. **(C)** Immobilized template-binding assay shows that the Δbromodomain SWI/SNF complex has a lower affinity for SAGA- or NuA4-acetylated templates compared to the wild-type SWI/SNF complex (lanes 4–7). In contrast, both the wild-type and the Δbromodomain SWI/SNF complex bound equally well to the control template (lanes 2 and 3). **(D)** The quantification of three independent experiments is shown as the percent SWI/SNF bound (relative to the input) to the template (with standard deviation) determined by scanning the gels and using the signal intensities of the western blots for control, SAGA-acetylated, and NuA4-acetylated histones.

yeast transcriptional activators[18–29] and is stabilized to acetylated nucleosomes through its Swi2/Snf2 bromodomain.[30,41,42] Moreover, the bromodomain of Swi2/Snf2 participates in the functions of this protein complex *in vivo*.[41] We have recently shown that various bromodomains from co-activator complexes have higher affinity for hyperacetylated histones.[43] In GST-pulldown assays, the Swi2/Snf2 bromodomain had the highest increase in binding to hyperacetylated histones compared to unacetylated histone templates. Indeed, higher affinity for total histones when acetylated was observed by all bromodomains tested. In general, the increased affinity of the GST-bromodomains for hyperacetylated histones confirms the importance of the bromodomain

as an acetylated binding domain within co-activator proteins. These results led us to investigate the role of the Swi2/Snf2 bromodomain in binding to and remodeling of H3- and H4-acetylated nucleosomes. To directly test whether this bromodomain contributes to the binding and the functional activity of the complex on nucleosomes, we purified wild-type SWI/SNF as well as SWI/SNF from a strain lacking the Swi2/Snf2 bromodomain (Δbromodomain SWI/SNF), and tested them in histone-binding as well as chromatin-remodeling assays. For all of these experiments, we used wild-type and mutant SWI//SNF complexes that had been highly purified over two affinity columns using the TAP method. The loss of the Swi2/Snf2 bromodomain does not affect complex integrity as detected by silver staining (data not shown). The same amounts of the wild-type and the Δbromodomain SWI/SNF complexes were used in these assays based on the normalization of the amounts of purified protein after western blotting (Fig. 1A).

To investigate the binding abilities of the wild-type and the Δbromodomain SWI/SNF complexes to nucleosomes, we utilized an immobilized nucleosomal array template, pG5E4, which contains five Gal4 binding sites and an E4 promoter flanked on both sides by 5S rDNA nucleosome positioning sequences.[48,49] Figure 1B shows the outline of the experiment. Briefly, the template was first biotinylated and reconstituted with histones, followed by the addition of either the H3-specific SAGA histone acetyltransferase or the H4-specific NuA4 histone acetyltransferase in the presence or absence of acetyl-CoA. After acetylation, wild-type or the Δbromodomain SWI/SNF complex was added followed by pull-down. The binding of the SWI/SNF complexes (wild-type versus mutant) to nucleosome arrays was detected by western blot analysis using an anti-TAP antibody (Fig. 1C), testing the ability of the Swi2/Snf2 bromodomain to bind to acetylated nucleosomes. While both the wild-type and the mutant bind equally well to the control template (Fig. 1C, lanes 2 and 3), the Δbromodomain SWI/SNF complex had a reduced affinity for both SAGA- and NuA4-acetylated nucleosomal templates (Fig. 1C, lanes 4–7). Figure 1D shows a graphical representation of the percent SWI/SNF bound (relative to the input template) for three independent immobilized binding experiments, with standard deviations. Again these results confirmed that both the wild-type and the Δbromodomain SWI/SNF complex bound equally well to the control unacetylated templates. Thus, the binding of the SWI/SNF complex to unmodified nucleosomes did not depend on the Swi2/Snf2 bromodomain of the SWI/SNF complex. However, while the wild-type SWI/SNF complex

did not have a reduced affinity for H3- or H4-acetylated templates, the binding of the mutant SWI/SNF complex was reduced on these templates. These results show that while both an intact SWI/SNF complex and a complex that lacked the Swi2/Snf2 bromodomain can bind to unmodified promoter nucleosomes, the bromodomain-containing SWI/SNF complex binds with a greater affinity to the acetylated nucleosomes. The data clearly illustrate the importance of the Swi2/Snf2 bromodomain in the efficient binding and anchoring of the SWI/SNF complex to these acetylated templates, which could lead to chromatin remodeling and subsequent gene activation.

The Bromodomain-deleted SWI/SNF Complex Has Reduced Remodeling Activity on H3- or H4-acetylated Nucleosomes

In previous studies, we demonstrated that acetylation of nucleosomes prior to addition of the SWI/SNF complex helps stabilize this remodeling complex on the template.[30] Moreover, the importance of the Swi2/Snf2 bromodomain in this retention has been observed.[41] These data have led us to investigate the role of the Swi2/Snf2 bromodomain in remodeling of acetylated nucleosomes. A restriction enzyme digestion assay was performed to directly test: (1) the affects of the reduced binding of the Δbromodomain SWI/SNF complex to both SAGA- and NuA4-acetylated nucleosomes on the function of the SWI/SNF complex, and (2) whether the bromodomain within the Swi2/Snf2 subunit of the complex contributes to the remodeling activity of the complex on acetylated nucleosomes. Here, we compared the activities of both the wild-type and the Δbromodomain mutant SWI/SNF complex on templates that are acetylated with the SAGA or NuA4 complex in a restriction enzyme digestion assay. The DNA used here is the 183 bp GUB fragment generated by PCR using a radiolabeled 5′ primer and

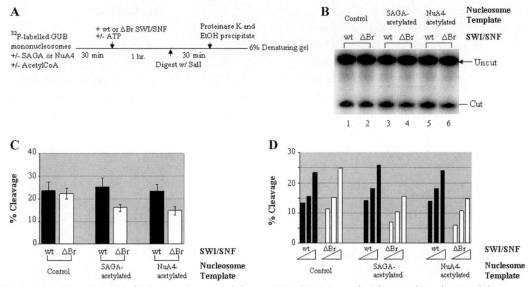

Figure 2. The Swi2/Snf2 bromodomain deletion SWI/SNF complex has reduced remodeling activity on acetylated nucleosomes. **(A)** Diagram of the restriction enzyme accessibility assay. Briefly, ^{32}P-labeled GUB fragment (10 ng) reconstituted into mononucleosomes was incubated in the presence or absence of SAGA or NuA4 and acetyl-CoA for 30 min at 30°C, followed by the addition of equal amount of wild-type and Δbromodomain SWI/SNF in the presence or absence of ATP for 1 h at 30°C. The binding reactions were then treated with 10 units of *Sal*I for 30 min at 30°C. After stopping the digestion reaction and ethanol precipitation, the DNA was resuspended in the formamide dye, heat denatured, and resolved on a 6% acrylamide-8 M urea sequencing gel at 150 volts for 3 h. The gels were dried and visualized by autoradiography or exposed to phosphoimager and quantified. **(B)** Restriction enzyme accessibility assay showed reduced activity on acetylated nucleosomes when the Swi2/Snf2 bromodomain was deleted. The positions of the cut and uncut GUB fragments are shown. **(C)** The quantification of three independent restriction enzyme accessibility experiments is shown as percentage cleavage of the template relative to the total input template. The remodeling activities of wild-type and Δbromodomain SWI/SNF complexes on control (unmodified) or pre-acetylated (by SAGA or NuA4) templates are shown, with standard deviations. The figure shows reduced activity on both SAGA- and NuA4-acetylated nucleosomes when the Swi2/Snf2 bromodomain is deleted. **(D)** The quantification (shown as percentage cleavage) of restriction enzyme accessibility assay on acetylated nucleosomes with a titration of the amounts of the wild-type and Δbromodomain SWI/SNF complexes. The titration shows increased digestion activity with increasing concentration for both the wild-type and the mutant complex, while there is reduced overall activity when the Swi2/Snf2 bromodomain is deleted (on pre-acetylated templates) at all concentrations compared to the wild-type.

the pGALUSFBEND plasmid as the template. The outline of the experiment (Fig. 2A) shows that the radio-labeled GUB template is reconstituted into a nucleosome template by octamer transfer and then incubated with either the SAGA or the NuA4 complex in the presence or absence of acetyl-CoA, followed by the remodeling reaction and digestion by the restriction enzyme *Sal*I. We analyzed the ability of the *Sal*I restriction enzyme to digest its site in about the middle of the 183 bp GUB nucleosomal DNA with the wild-type and the

Δbromodomain SWI/SNF complexes in the presence of ATP. Digestion of the naked DNA template by *Sal*I was not affected by acetylation with the either of the histone acetyltransferases (data not shown). The activities of the wild-type and the bromodomain-deleted SWI/SNF complexes were then compared on unmodified nucleosomes. Both of these complexes increased the accessibility of the restriction enzyme *Sal*I to its site on the control nucleosomal DNA in an ATP-dependent manner (Fig. 2B, lanes 1 and 2). While there was no obvious difference in amount of nucleosomal template cleaved with the wild-type versus the mutant complex on unmodified nucleosomes (Fig. 2B, lanes 1 and 2), there was a decrease in the cleavage when the bromodomain-deleted SWI/SNF complex was used on either SAGA- or NuA4-acetylated nucleosomes (Fig. 2B, lanes 3–6). These results show that the bromodomain within the Swi2/Snf2 subunit of the SWI/SNF complex is important for the efficient remodeling activity of the complex on acetylated nucleosome templates. Quantification of three independent restriction accessibility experiments with standard deviations (Fig. 2C) confirmed these results and showed that the deletion of the bromodomains in the Swi2/Snf2 subunit of the SWI/SNF complex did not significantly affect its remodeling activity on control (unmodified) histone templates. However, when the template was acetylated by either the SAGA or NuA4 histone acetyltransferases (in the presence of acetyl-CoA), reduced digestion by the *Sal*I restriction enzyme was observed with the mutant SWI/SNF complex. On the other hand, the activity of the wild-type SWI/SNF did not change on these acetylated nucleosomes, suggesting that pre-acetylation of nucleosomes by the SAGA or NuA4 complex has no significant effect on the remodeling activity of the wild-type SWI/SNF. In addition, using a titration of concentrations of the wild-type and the mutant SWI/SNF complexes, we have confirmed these results (Fig. 2D). Three different concentrations of the SWI/SNF wild type and the mutant complex were compared in their remodeling activity of both SAGA- and NuA4-acetylated nucleosomes. Quantification of the results in Figure 2D shows that using the same concentrations of the two complexes, the Swi2/Snf2 bromodomain-deleted complex has a reduced remodeling activity (about 1/2) on SAGA- and NuA4-acetylated nucleosomes compared to the wild-type complex, demonstrating the importance of the Swi2/Snf2 bromodomain within the SWI/SNF complex in efficient remodeling of H3- or H4-acetylated nucleosomes.

Discussion

In this report, we have examined the effect of the Swi2/Snf2 bromodomain in the yeast SWI/SNF on the binding to and the activity of this chromatin remodeling complex on H3- and H4-acetylated promoter nucleosomes. We show that even though SWI/SNF purified from a Swi2/Snf2 bromodomain deletion strain bound to unacetylated nucleosome templates as well as did the wild-type complex, it could only partially bind to acetylated nucleosomes. The remodeling activity of the bromodomain-deleted SWI/SNF mutant complex was similarly impaired on acetylated nucleosomes. These data illustrate the requirement for the Swi2/Snf2 bromodomain in anchoring the complex on acetylated templates prior to any remodeling. We have previously shown that the Swi2/Snf2 bromodomain deletion reduces occupancy of the SWI/SNF complex at the *SUC2* promoter under derepressing conditions.[41] In addition, we have shown the displacement of the SAGA complex by the SWI/SNF complex from acetylated nucleosomes and the role of the Swi2/Snf2 bromodomain in this competition.[42] Since both the SWI/SNF and the SAGA complex (but not the NuA4 complex) contain bromodomains, they can both recognize and bind to the same acetylated patterns and perhaps co-occupy the same acetylated promoter for some time before the SAGA complex is displaced. These are consistent with our data here that the bromodomain-deleted SWI/SNF complex cannot efficiently bind and remodel acetylated promoter nucleosomes. These data together show the importance of the Swi2/Snf2 bromodomain within SWI/SNF in the binding and activity of the complex on promoter nucleosomes. Investigating the remodeling of nucleosomes at the SWI/SNF-specific promoters such as the *SUC2* or *PHO8* promoters in the bromodomains-deleted strain would also give us important information on the requirements of these promoters on the Swi2/Snf2 bromodomain.

The ATP-dependent reduced remodeling of SAGA- and NuA4-acetylated nucleosomes by the bromodomain-deleted SWI/SNF complex demonstrates the importance of this domain in the full functional activity of the complex on acetylated promoters. Thus, nucleosomes that are pre-acetylated require the Swi2/Snf2 bromodomain for complete remodeling prior to any gene activation. Together, all these results show that the deletion of the bromodomain significantly reduced the binding as well as the functional activity of the SWI/SNF to remodel acetylated (both H3 and H4) nucleosome templates. In conclusion, acetylation by SAGA or NuA4, leading to localized or broad patterns of acetylation, respectively, can stabilize bromodomain-containing SWI/SNF on acetylated nucleosomes in order to remodel them. Thus, nucleosome acetylation by histone acetyltransferases, such as the SAGA or the NuA4 complex can generate a high-affinity docking site for bromodomain-containing protein complexes, including the SWI/SNF and SAGA, as well as others such as Remodels the structure of Chromatin (RSC) and Transcription Factor IID (TFIID). Thus, it is possible to envision acetylated nucleosomes serving as substrates for sequential and ordered binding of these bromodomain-containing proteins to the promoter leading to an enhanced transcription activity of some genes.

Acknowledgments

We are grateful to Philip Prochasson and Jerry L. Workman for many helpful comments during this study. This work was supported by a Grant (NP/05/15) from the Faculty of Medicine and Health Sciences at the UAE University.

Conflicts of Interest

The authors declare no conflicts of interest.

References

1. Workman, J.L. & R.E. Kingston. 1998. Alteration of nucleosome structure as a mechanism of transcriptional regulation. *Annu. Rev. Biochem.* **67:** 545–579.
2. Brown, C.E., T. Lechner, L. Howe & J.L. Workman. 2000. The many HATs of transcription coactivators. *Trends. Biochem. Sci.* **25:** 15–19.
3. Peterson, C.L. & J.L. Workman. 2000. Promoter targeting and chromatin remodeling by the SWI/SNF complex. *Curr. Opin. Genet. Dev.* **10:** 187–192.
4. Vignali, M., A.H. Hassan, K.E. Neely & J.L. Workman. 2000. ATP-dependent chromatin-remodeling complexes. *Mol. Cell. Biol.* **20:** 1899–1910.
5. Wang, W. 2003. The SWI/SNF family of ATP-dependent chromatin remodelers: similar mechanisms for diverse functions. *Curr. Top. Microbiol. Immunol.* **274:** 143–169.
6. Johnson, C.N., N.L. Adkins & P. Georgel. 2005. Chromatin remodeling complexes. ATP-dependent machines in action. *Biochem. Cell Biol.* **83:** 405–417.
7. Strahl, B.D. & C.D. Allis. 2000. The language of covalent histone modifications. *Nature* **403:** 41–45.
8. Jenuwein, T. & C.D. Allis. 2001. Translating the histone code. *Science* **293:** 1074–1080.
9. Gill, G. 2005. Something about SUMO inhibits transcription. *Curr. Opin. Genet. Dev.* **15:** 536–541.
10. Kimura, A., K. Matsubara & M. Horikoshi. 2005. A decade of histone acetylation: marking eukaryotic chromosomes with specific codes. *J. Biochem. (Tokyo)* **138:** 647–662.
11. Martin, C. & Y. Zhang. 2005. The diverse functions of histone lysine methylation. *Nat. Rev. Mol. Cell Biol.* **6:** 838–849.
12. Santos-Rosa, H. & C. Caldas. 2005. Chromatin modifier enzymes, the histone code and cancer. *Eur. J. Cancer* **41:** 2381–2402.
13. Shilatifard, A. 2006. Chromatin modifications by methylation and ubiquitination: Implications in the regulation of gene expression. *Annu. Rev. Biochem.* **75:** 243–269.
14. Grant, P.A., D.E. Sterner, L.J. Duggan, *et al.* 1998. The SAGA unfolds: convergence of transcription regulators in chromatin-modifying complexes. *Trends Cell Biol.* **8:** 193–197.
15. Sterner, D.E. & S.L. Berger. 2000. Acetylation of histones and transcription-related factors. *Microbiol. Mol. Biol. Rev.* **64:** 435–459.
16. Timmers, H.T. & L. Tora. 2005. SAGA unveiled. *Trends Biochem. Sci.* **30:** 7–10.
17. Pollard, K.J. & C.L. Peterson. 1997. Role for ADA/GCN5 products in antagonizing

chromatin-mediated transcriptional repression. *Mol. Cell Biol.* **17:** 6212–6222.

18. Utley, R.T., K. Ikeda, P.A. Grant, *et al.* 1998. Transcriptional activators direct histone acetyltransferase complexes to nucleosomes. *Nature* **394:** 498–502.

19. Natarajan, K., B.M. Jackson, H. Zhou, *et al.* 1999. Transcriptional activation by Gcn4p involves independent interactions with the SWI/SNF complex and the SRB/mediator. *Mol. Cell.* **4:** 657–664.

20. Neely, K.E., A.H. Hassan, A.E. Wallberg, *et al.* 1999. Activation domain-mediated targeting of the SWI/SNF complex to promoters stimulates transcription from nucleosome arrays. *Mol. Cell* **4:** 649–655.

21. Yudkovsky, N., C. Logie, S. Hahn & C.L. Peterson. 1999. Recruitment of the SWI/SNF chromatin remodeling complex by transcriptional activators. *Genes Dev.* **13:** 2369–2374.

22. Vignali, M., D.J. Steger, K.E. Neely & J.L. Workman. 2000. Distribution of acetylated histones resulting from Gal4-VP16 recruitment of SAGA and NuA4 complexes. *EMBO J.* **19:** 2629–2640.

23. Wallberg, A.E., K.E. Neely, A.H. Hassan, *et al.* 2000. Recruitment of the SWI-SNF chromatin remodeling complex as a mechanism of gene activation by the glucocorticoid receptor t1 activation domain. *Mol. Cell Biol.* **20:** 2004–2013.

24. Brown, C.E., L. Howe, K. Sousa, *et al.* 2001. Recruitment of HAT complexes by direct activator interactions with the ATM-related Tra1 subunit. *Science* **292:** 2333–2337.

25. Hassan, A.H., K.E. Neely, M. Vignali, *et al.* 2001. Promoter targeting of chromatin-modifying complexes. *Front. Biosci.* **6:** 1054–1064.

26. Neely, K.E., A.H. Hassan, C.E. Brown, *et al.* 2002. Transcription activator interactions with multiple SWI/SNF subunits. *Mol. Cell Biol.* **22:** 1615–1625.

27. Prochasson, P., K.E. Neely, A.H. Hassan, *et al.* 2003. Targeting activity is required for SWI/SNF function in vivo and is accomplished through two partially redundant activator-interaction domains. *Mol. Cell.* **12:** 983–990.

28. Swanson, M.J., H. Qiu, L. Sumibcay, *et al.* 2003. A multiplicity of coactivators is required by Gcn4p at individual promoters in vivo. *Mol. Cell Biol.* **23:** 2800–2820.

29. Cosma, M.P., T. Tanaka & K. Nasmyth. 1999. Ordered recruitment of transcription and chromatin remodeling factors to a cell cycle- and developmentally regulated promoter. *Cell* **97:** 299–311.

30. Hassan, A.H., K.E. Neely & J.L. Workman. 2001. Histone acetyltransferase complexes stabilize swi/snf binding to promoter nucleosomes. *Cell* **104:** 817–827.

31. Dhalluin, C., J.E. Carlson, L. Zeng, *et al.* 1999. Structure and ligand of a histone acetyltransferase bromodomain. *Nature* **399:** 491–496.

32. Ornaghi, P., P. Ballario, A.M. Lena, *et al.* 1999. The bromodomain of Gcn5p interacts in vitro with specific residues in the N terminus of histone H4. *J. Mol. Biol.* **287:** 1–7.

33. Hudson, B.P., M.A. Martinez-Yamout, H.J. Dyson & P.E. Wright. 2000. Solution structure and acetyllysine binding activity of the GCN5 bromodomain. *J. Mol. Biol.* **304:** 355–370.

34. Jacobson, R.H., A.G. Ladurner, D.S. King & R. Tjian. 2000. Structure and function of a human TAFII250 double bromodomain module. *Science* **288:** 1422–1425.

35. Owen, D.J., P. Ornaghi, J.C. Yang, *et al.* 2000. The structural basis for the recognition of acetylated histone H4 by the bromodomain of histone acetyltransferase gcn5p. *EMBO J.* **19:** 6141–6149.

36. Ladurner, A.G., C. Inouye, R. Jain & R. Tjian. 2003. Bromodomains mediate an acetyl-histone encoded antisilencing function at heterochromatin boundaries. *Mol. Cell.* **11:** 365–376.

37. Matangkasombut, O. & S. Buratowski. 2003. Different sensitivities of bromodomain factors 1 and 2 to histone H4 acetylation. *Mol. Cell.* **11:** 353–363.

38. Loyola, A. & G. Almouzni. 2004. Bromodomains in living cells participate in deciphering the histone code. *Trends Cell Biol.* **14:** 279–281.

39. Martinez-Campa, C., P. Politis, J.L. Moreau, *et al.* 2004. Precise nucleosome positioning and the TATA box dictate requirements for the histone H4 tail and the bromodomain factor Bdf1. *Mol Cell.* **15:** 69–81.

40. Yang, X.J. 2004. Lysine acetylation and the bromodomain: a new partnership for signaling. *Bioessays* **26:** 1076–1087.

41. Hassan, A.H., P. Prochasson, K.E. Neely, *et al.* 2002. Function and selectivity of bromodomains in anchoring chromatin-modifying complexes to promoter nucleosomes. *Cell* **111:** 369–379.

42. Hassan, A.H., S. Awad & P. Prochasson. 2006. The Swi2/Snf2 bromodomain is required for the displacement of saga and the octamer transfer of saga-acetylated nucleosomes. *J. Biol. Chem.* **281:** 18126–18134.

43. Hassan, A.H., S. Awad, Z. Al-Natour, *et al.* 2007. Selective recognition of acetylated histones by bromodomains in transcriptional co-activators. *Biochem. J.* **402:** 125–133.

44. Rigaut, G., A. Shevchenko, B. Rutz, *et al.* 1999. A generic protein purification method for protein

complex characterization and proteome exploration. *Nat. Biotechnol.* **17:** 1030–1032.

45. Puig, O., F. Caspary, G. Rigaut, *et al.* 2001. The tandem affinity purification (TAP) method: a general procedure of protein complex purification. *Methods* **24:** 218–229.

46. Graumann, J., L.A. Dunipace, J.H. Seol, *et al.* 2004. Applicability of tandem affinity purification MudPIT to pathway proteomics in yeast. *Mol. Cell Proteomics* **3:** 226–237.

47. Lee, K.K., P. Prochasson, L. Florens, *et al.* 2004. Proteomic analysis of chromatin-modifying complexes in Saccharomyces cerevisiae identifies novel subunits. *Biochem. Soc. Trans.* **32:** 899–903.

48. Ikeda, K., D.J. Steger, A. Eberharter & J.L. Workman. 1999. Activation domain-specific and general transcription stimulation by native histone acetyltransferase complexes. *Mol. Cell Biol.* **19:** 855–863.

49. Carrozza, M.J., A.H. Hassan & J.L. Workman. 2003. Assay of activator recruitment of chromatin-modifying complexes. *Methods Enzymol.* **371:** 536–544.

50. Juan, L.J., R.T. Utley, C.C. Adams, *et al.* 1994. Differential repression of transcription factor binding by histone H1 is regulated by the core histone amino termini. *EMBO J.* **13:** 6031–6040.

Investigation of Heat Stress Response in the Camel Fibroblast Cell Line Dubca

Faisal Thayyullathil,[a] Shahanas Chathoth,[a] Abdulkader Hago,[a] Ulli Wernery,[b] Mahendra Patel,[a] and Sehamuddin Galadari[a]

[a]Department of Biochemistry, Faculty of Medicine and Health Sciences, UAE University, Al Ain, United Arab Emirates

[b]Central Veterinary Research Laboratory, Dubai, United Arab Emirates

We have used a camel cell line model (Dubca) to investigate the effect of heat stress on cell survival. The mechanism(s) of such survival response are very important not only for normal physiological function, but also, in pathological conditions, such as cancer. Those cells that have escaped the normal response to heat are an important model in helping us better understand the intricate signaling change(s) that might have occurred in changing a cell's phenotype from normal to cancerous. Our findings in this study indicate that unlike comparative fibroblast cells (L929), Dubca cells are quite resistant and survive the 42°C heat stress in a time-dependent manner; indeed, the cells even show growth on par with those cells that are kept at the control temperature of 37°C. Expression levels of Akt, an important prosurvival kinase, are uniform, and irrespective of the experimental or control temperature, show basal control levels. In other words, there is no loss of Akt protein level following heat stress at 42°C. Similarly, no significant change in HSP70 expression level is observed. In contrast, the stress transcription factor c-Jun, and the stress activated kinase (Jnk) were induced during this heat-shock condition. This is in line with the fact that suppression of stress kinase Jnk renders cells thermoresistant. On the other hand, acquired tolerance to severe heat shock is associated with downregulation of Jnk.

Key words: heat stress; Akt; camel fibroblast; cell line Dubca; heat-shock protein; Jnk; c-Jun

Introduction

Cancer cells evade apoptotic signals and cell clearance through overexpressing prosurvival signals or effectors and/or inhibition of pro-apoptotic signals that may control cell death and tumor formation. Similarly, exposure of cells to elevated temperatures switches on several signaling pathways, some facilitating cell survival and some initiating apoptosis.[1] Therefore, cancer may be viewed as a state of cellular stress, to which cancerous cells have developed a state of tolerance. This tolerance is the result of either prevalence of the prosurvival signaling pathway and/or the attenuation of the death pathway. The camel (*Camelus dromedarius*) is a homothermic organism perfectly adapted to extreme conditions of arid zones and is capable of tolerating extreme heat accompanied by a significant elevation of the whole body temperature.[2] Therefore, cameloids must have developed signaling pathways that allow their survival; making them an ideal model in studying signaling pathways involved in stress tolerance.

The first discovered survival pathway activated by heat was the heat-shock response. Heat-shock response is characterized by transcriptional activation and accumulation of

Address for correspondence: Sehamuddin Galadari, Cell Signaling Laboratory, Department of Biochemistry, Faculty of Medicine and Health Sciences, UAE University, PO Box 17666, Al Ain, UAE. Voice: +97137137507; fax: +97137672033. sehamuddin@uaeu.ac.ae

Ann. N.Y. Acad. Sci. 1138: 376–384 (2008). © 2008 New York Academy of Sciences.
doi: 10.1196/annals.1414.039

heat-shock proteins, such as heat-shock protein 70 (Hsp70), that are responsible for the provision of a state of temperature resistance to the cell.[3] Like many other stressors, heat shock induces specific and tightly regulated signaling networks that either initiate cell death or facilitate cellular survival.[1,4]

Akt (PKB) is a serine/threonine kinase, belonging to the cAMP-dependent protein kinase A/ protein kinase G/protein kinase C (AGC) super family of protein kinases. These kinases share structural homology within their catalytic domain and have similar activation mechanism that when deregulated lead to human diseases including cancer.[5] Akt is a downstream target of phosphatidylinositol 3-kinase (PI3-kinase) in cytokine and growth factor signaling pathways.[6] There are three highly homologous members of the Akt kinase family, known as Akt1, 2, and 3. All Akt isoforms, except Akt 3 splice variant, contain two regulatory phosphorylation sites, Thr308 and Ser473, in the C-terminal regulatory domain that are important for full activation of the enzyme.[7]

It has been reported that the most potent inducers of c-Jun (one of the constituents of the activator protein 1 (AP-1) early response transcription factor) activation are agents associated with cellular stress, such as thermal shock, inflammatory cytokines, ultraviolet radiation, and metabolic poisons, suggesting a major role for this transcription factor in mediating repair or protection against cellular injury.[8] Hence, regulators of this protein are important in the process of repair and/or protection against environmental stress. One such group of regulators is the stress-activated protein kinases (SAPKs), a subfamily of the MAP kinase signaling pathway. Jnk is a member of SAPK family, and its pathway is generally considered pro-apoptotic.[9] It has been shown that Jnk mediates cell-death signals by a variety of stressors, including heat shock.[10] Under these stressors, Jnk activation may cause cytochrome c efflux from mitochondria, either via the inactivation of the anti-apoptotic proteins, Bcl-2 and Bcl-

x, or the cleavage and activation of the pro-apoptotic protein, Bid, leading to the execution of the apoptotic cascade triggered by activated caspases.[11]

In this study, we have used the camel fibroblast cell line Dubca, a representative model of tolerance to stress, as a model system in order to investigate the effect of heat stress on the induction of signaling proteins important to cell survival. Our knowledge of signaling pathways responsible for cell survival under stress is still rudimentary. Identifying and understanding these important signaling pathways is of utmost importance to a better understanding of disease situations, such as cancer.

Materials and Methods

Materials

Modified Eagle's medium (MEM), fetal calf serum (FCS), phosphate-buffered saline (PBS), and trypsin-2-[2-(Bis(carboxymethyl)amino) ethyl-(carboxymethyl)amino]acetic acid (Trypsin-EDTA) were from GIBCO-Invitrogen Corp. (Carlsbad, CA). Tissue culture dish and flasks from Nunc (Roskilde, Denmark). sodium dodecyl sulfate polyacrylamide gel electrophoresis (SDS-PAGE) chemicals from BioRad (Hercules, CA). Anti-Akt were from Cell Signaling Inc. (Danvers, MA), and anti-Hsp70, anti-PARP, anti-Jnk1, and anti-actin antibodies were from Santa Cruz Biotechnology Inc. (Santa Cruz, CA). Anti-rabbit IgG, anti-mouse IgG, 3-[4,5- dimethylthiazol-2-yl]-2,5-diphenyl tetrazolium bromide (MTT), and all other chemicals were purchased from Sigma (St. Louis, MO).

Cell Culture

Dubca cells were maintained in MEM containing heat-inactivated 10% FCS at 37°C in 5% CO_2. Cells that were 70% confluent were used for experiments. Control cells were kept at 37°C and experimental plates were placed at 42°C for heat-shock studies in 5% CO_2

incubator for different times for the heat-stress studies, or for 3 h only for the heat-shock studies. The heat-shocked plates were then replaced at 37°C for recovery and followed for the time course 0, 1, 2, 6, 12, 24, and 48 h or as otherwise indicated.

MTT Assay

Cytotoxicity assays were carried out as described elsewhere with slight modifications.[12] Cells grown in 96-well microtiter plates (10,000 cells/well) were incubated for 24 h. Experimental treatments, either heat stress or heat shocked at 42°C for 3 h, were placed into a preheated, humidified 5% CO_2 incubator. After each time point, heat-shocked/stressed plates were treated with 25 μL MTT (5 mg/mL in PBS). The cells were then incubated at 37°C for 3 h. The formazan crystals that formed were solubilized in 200 μL of dimethyl sulfoxide (DMSO). Once the color was developed, quantification was done at 570 nm, using an Anthos Labtec HT2 plate reader (Cambridge, UK).

Cell Preparation and SDS-PAGE and Western Blot Analysis

Following the different experiments, cells were washed twice with cold PBS, pH 7.4, and lysed with lysis buffer [50 mM Tris HCl (pH 7.4), 10% NP-40, 40 mM NaF, 10 mM NaCl, 10 mM Na_3VO_4, 1 mM freshly prepared phenylmethylsufonyl fluoride (PMSF), and 10 mM dithiothreitol (DTT), containing protease inhibitors 10 mg/mL leupeptin, 10 mg/mL aprotinin, 10 mg/mL trypsin, and 1 mg/mL pepstatin A]. The lysates were centrifuged at 15,000 rpm for 10 min at 4°C. An aliquot of the supernatant was kept for protein determination by BioRad protein assay kit, and the rest of the lysate was immediately boiled for 3 min with 6X SDS-PAGE sample buffer containing 0.05% bromophenol blue, 10% glycerol, and 2% beta mercaptoethanol. Samples were stored at −80°C. When needed, samples were boiled again and equal amounts of protein from cell lysates were subjected to electrophoresis on SDS-PAGE.

The cell lysates (40 μg protein) were resolved by SDS-PAGE, and the separated proteins were transferred on to nitrocellulose membrane by wet transfer method using the Bio-Rad electrotransfer apparatus. After blocking with 5% nonfat milk in Tris Buffer Saline (TBS) containing 0.1% Tween 20, the membrane was incubated with primary antibodies followed by secondary antibody-conjugated horseradish peroxidase. Proteins were visualized by the enhanced chemiluminescence system (Pierce Biotech, Rockford, IL).

Cleavage of Poly (ADP-ribose) Polymerase

In order to examine the cleavage of poly (ADP-ribose) polymerase (PARP), 30 μg whole-cell extract was resolved on 8% SDS polyacrylamide gel and subjected to PAGE. The resolved protein was transferred to nitrocellulose membrane blocked with 5% nonfat milk protein, and probed with PARP antibodies; bands were detected by the enhanced chemiluminescence system (Pierce Biotech) as described above.

Results

Heat Resistance of Dubca Cells

Cellular responses to stress are important in survival and recovery. The mechanism(s) of such survival response are very important not only for normal physiological function, but also in pathological conditions, such as cancer. Heat is one such stress condition, in that it causes numerous intracellular changes that may lead a cell to survive or die. We have used a camel cell line model to investigate heat-stress responses. The effect of heat stress on the camel fibroblast cell line Dubca was investigated by stressing Dubca cells at 42°C during a 48 h time course. As can be seen in Figure 1A, Dubca cells were

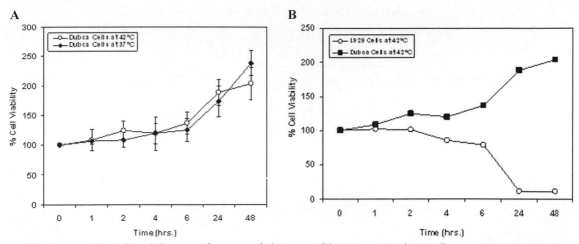

Figure 1. (A) Cell viability as a function of duration of heat stress. Dubca cells are grown at 37°C or 42°C, and cell growth is monitored over time. **(B)** Cell viability as a function of duration of heat stress. Dubca cells and L929 cells are grown at 42°C, and cell growth is monitored over time.

quite resistant to the 42°C heat stress, indeed, the cells even showed growth on a par with cells that were kept at control temperature of 37°C. This is not a normal phenomenon, since, when the murine fibroblast cell line, L929 cells, was subjected to the same stress condition as Dubca cells, the cells were almost totally dead by 24 h of stress, as seen in Figure 1B. While, L929 cell viability attenuated after only a couple of hours of heat stress, Dubca cells actually continued to grow. The divergence in cell viability between Dubca cells and L929 cells after 2 h of heat stress is seen in Figure 1B.

Effect of Heat Stress on Akt and Hsp70 in Dubca Cells

One possibility for the observed heat resistance in Dubca cells may be an over-induction of the survival kinase Akt. In order to investigate this possibility, Dubca cells were heat stressed and at the indicated times were lysed. The cells lysate was then subjected to SDS-PAGE/western blot analysis, and Akt protein levels were detected through chemiluminescence. As can be seen in Figure 2A, Akt protein expression levels were uniform and, irrespective of the experimental or control temperature, showed basal control levels. In other words,

there was no loss of Akt protein level following heat stress at 42°C.

Interestingly, when Hsp70 protein induction was measured in Dubca cells following heat stress, the protein levels were almost the same as control cells (Fig. 2B). Nevertheless, after 4 h of heat stress, a slight increase was seen and a second band of protein began to appear, which was not present in the time-matched control cells, as can be seen in Figure 2B. Therefore, no change in Akt or Hsp70 was observed following heat stress.

Heat-Shock Recovery and Protein Induction

Following the observed lack of effect of heat stress on Akt and Hsp70 protein level and the resistance of Dubca cells to prolonged heat stress, it was imperative to test the effect of heat shock on Dubca cells in comparison to the mouse fibroblast cells, L929. In this experiment, Dubca cells (as well as L929 cells) were subjected to a 3-h heat shock at 42°C. Dubca cells were then transferred to the ambient normal temperature of 37°C, and cell viability was monitored by using the MTT assay. Figure 3 illustrates the comparative relationship of cell viability and heat on Dubca and L929 cells. It can

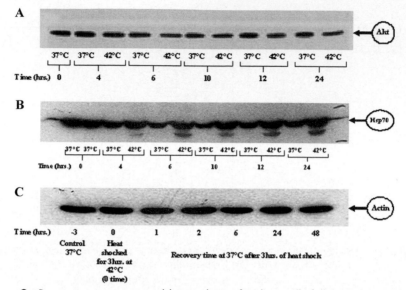

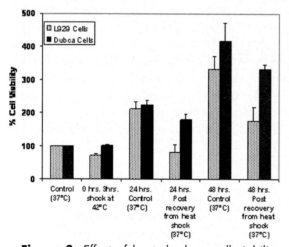

Figure 2. Representative western blot analysis of Dubca cells following growth at 37°C and 42°C. **(A)** Expression level of Akt protein, **(B)** expression level of Hsp70, and **(C)** actin expression level.

Figure 3. Effect of heat shock on cell viability. Dubca and L929 cells were grown at 37°C and at 42°C. After 3 h at 42°C, the cells were transferred to 37°C, which is referred to as time 0; thereafter the time indicates the time of cell recovery at 37°C. Time-matched controls are indicated at 24 h and 48 h of recovery for both Dubca and L929 cells.

be seen that L929 cell viability was attenuated, while Dubca cell viability remained as control following 3 h of heat shock. At 24 h post–heat-shock recovery, L929 cells were almost at the control viability level, whereas Dubca cells had doubled in percent viability, indicating that not

only Dubca cells were resistant to heat stress, but also that they were capable of normal cell growth following 24 h of recovery from 3 h of heat shock. Indeed, it was only after 48 h of recovery from heat shock that L929 cells showed normal cell growth as can be seen in Figure 3.

Akt was seen to be resistant to heat stress in Dubca cells up to 24 h. Therefore, the effect of 3 h of heat shock on Akt protein level was examined in Dubca cells. Figure 4A illustrates Akt protein expression level in Dubca cells following 3 h of heat shock. As expected, Akt protein was not affected at all by heat shock, and Akt expression level was similar to control, whether during the heat shock or during the recovery period (Fig. 4A). Unlike Akt, Hsp70 was over-expressed following 3 h of heat shock, and it was maintained at the elevated level up to at least 6 h postrecovery. At 24 h postrecovery, Hsp70 protein level decreased, as can be observed in Figure 4B. Given that Dubca cells did not undergo apoptosis following heat stress or during heat shock, as expected, there was no PARP cleavage in Dubca cells, as seen in Figure 4C.

It is noteworthy that the stress transcription factor c-Jun and the stress-activated kinase (Jnk) were induced during this heat-shock condition,

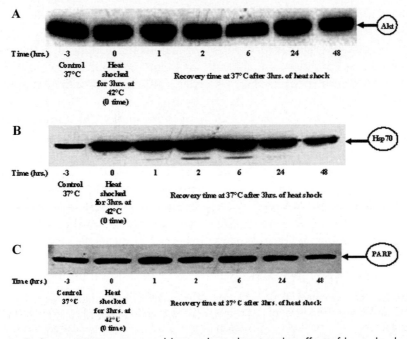

Figure 4. Representative western blot analysis showing the effect of heat shock at 42°C and recovery at 37°C on Dubca cells. **(A)** Akt protein, **(B)** Hsp70 protein, and **(C)** PARP protein.

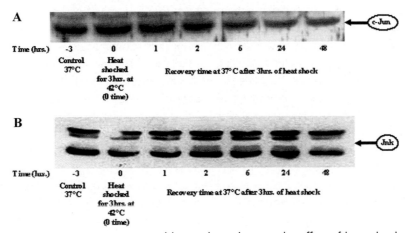

Figure 5. Representative western blot analysis showing the effect of heat shock at 42°C and recovery at 37°C on Dubca cells. **(A)** c-Jun protein, and **(B)** Jnk protein.

as can be seen in Figures 5A and 5B. The transcription factor c-Jun was expressed following the heat shock, reaching a maximum at 1 h postrecovery, and returning to normal background level by 6 h, as seen in Figure 5A. Similarly, Jnk was attenuated somewhat but it then was overexpressed slightly during the recovery period, as observed in Figure 5B.

Discussion

We have used a camel cell line model (Dubca) to investigate the effect of heat stress on cell survival. Our data indicate that Dubca cells are quite resistant and survive the 42°C heat stress in a time-dependent manner, indeed, the cells even show growth on a par with cells that are kept at the control temperature of 37°C (Fig. 1A). However, cells of another fibroblast cell line, L929 (of mouse origin), when subjected to the same stress condition, are almost totally dead after 24 h of heat stress (Fig. 1A and B). Clearly, Dubca cells are extremely heat resistant. While, L929 cells viability start to attenuate after only a few hours of heat stress, Dubca cells actually continue to grow. Cellular responses to stress are important in survival and recovery. It has been reported that treatment of primary human fibroblasts with severe heat shock (45°C, 75 min) causes cell death.[13] This cell-death process is accompanied by strong activation of Akt, extracellular signal-regulated kinase 1 (ERK1) and ERK2, p38, and c-Jun N-terminal (Jnk) kinases. Suppression of Akt kinase increases cell thermosensitivity.[13] As can be seen in Figure 2A, Akt protein expression levels in Dubca cells are uniform, and irrespective of the experimental or control temperature show basal control levels. In other words, there is no loss of Akt protein level following heat stress at 42°C. Akt is an important player in the cell-survival signaling pathway. We have shown that Akt depletion is a prerequisite for L929 cell death following heat stress (later in this volume), and it is possible that the lack of depletion of Akt following heat shock may be a reason for Dubca cell survival.

The first discovered survival pathway activated by heat is the heat-shock response. Heat-shock response is characterized by transcriptional activation and accumulation of heat-shock proteins, such as Hsp70, that are responsible for the provision of a state of temperature resistance to the cell.[3] Interestingly, when Hsp70 protein induction is measured in Dubca cells following heat stress, the protein level is almost the same as in control cells (Fig. 2B). Although, after 4 h of heat stress, a slight increase is seen and a second band of protein begins to appear, which is not present in the time-matched control cells (Fig. 2B). The expected significant increase in Hsp70 protein induction, as is the case with L929 cells (see

Ref. 14), is lacking. However, the second band that appears following 4 h of heat stress might be significant, it may represent lower molecular weight heat-shock proteins present in camel cells. This can be confirmed only by a detailed investigation of cameloid heat-shock proteins.

On examining the comparative relationship of cell viability and heat on Dubca and L929 cells, it is observed that L929 cell viability is attenuated, while Dubca cell viability remains similar to control following 3 h of heat shock (Fig. 3). At 24 h post–heat-shock recovery, L929 cells are almost at the control viability level, whereas, Dubca cells have doubled in percentage viability, indicating not only that Dubca cells were resistant to heat stress, but that they were capable of normal cell growth. Indeed, it is only after 48 h of recovery from heat shock that L929 cells show normal cell growth, as can be seen in Figure 3. This implies that Dubca cells have a better response in returning to normal cell growth following the removal of heat shock. It has been reported that cells exposed to nonlethal elevated temperatures develop resistance to a subsequent severe heat stress, a phenomenon referred to as acquired thermotolerance.[13] Thermotolerant cells also become more resistant to some other stressful treatments, such as ethanol, UV irradiation, doxorubicin (Adriamycin), or tumor necrosis factor-α.[15,16]

When the effect of Akt protein expression level in Dubca cells following 3 h of heat shock is examined, no change is observed, and Akt expression level is as in controls, whether during the heat shock or during the recovery period (Fig. 4A). Therefore, Akt is constitutively expressed in Dubca cells and this expression is protective against cell death. Unlike Akt, Hsp70 level is enhanced following the 3 h heat shock, and it is maintained at the elevated level up to at least 6 h postrecovery. At 24 h postrecovery, Hsp70 protein level decreases, as illustrated in Figure 4B. It may well be that this initial phase of Hsp70 increase, together with the unaffected level of Akt protein in response to heat shock, is important in the maintenance of Dubca cell survival during the stress period. Furthermore, given that Dubca cells do not undergo apoptosis following heat stress or during heat shock, as expected, there is no PARP cleavage in Dubca cells as seen in Figure 4C. Once the stress is removed Hsp70 returns to normal level. It is possible that Hsp70 expression is required in the maintenance of Akt and cell survival, and Akt expression alone is then enough to sustain growth (Fig. 3).

As mentioned earlier, it has been shown that suppression of Akt increases cell thermosensitivity. In contrast, suppression of stress kinase Jnk renders cells thermoresistant. On the other hand, acquired tolerance to severe heat shock is associated with downregulation of Jnk.[13] Hence, it is noteworthy that the stress transcription factor c-Jun, and the stress activated kinase (Jnk) were induced during this heat shock condition (Fig. 5A and B). The transcription factor c-Jun is expressed following the heat shock, reaching a maximum at 1 h postrecovery from heat shock, returning to normal background level by 6 h (Fig. 5A). Similarly, Jnk is attenuated somewhat, but it then is overexpressed slightly during the recovery period (Fig. 5B), implying that a decrease in Jnk expression level has an important function in promotion of the growth signaling.

In conclusion, cellular responses to stress are important in survival and recovery. The mechanism(s) of such survival response are very important not only for normal physiological function, but also, in pathological conditions, such as cancer. Those cells that have escaped the normal response to heat are an important model in helping us better understand the intricate signaling change(s) that might have occurred in changing cell phenotype from normal to cancerous.

Acknowledgment

This work was supported by a grant from the Sheikh Hamdan Award for Medical Sciences (MRG14-2003-2004).

Conflicts of Interest

The authors declare no conflicts of interest.

References

1. Gabai, V.L. & M.Y. Sherman. 2002. Molecular biology of thermoregulation: interplay between molecular chaperones and signaling pathways in survival of heat shock. *J. Appl. Physiol.* **92:** 1743–1748.
2. Schmidt-Nilsen, K. 1972. *Animals of the Deserts*, pp 308–310. Nauka. Moscow.
3. Lindquist, S. 1986. The heat-shock response. *Ann. Rev. Biochem.* **55:** 1151–1191.
4. Nadeau, S.I. & J. Landry. 2007. Mechanism of activation and regulation of the heat shock-sensitive signaling pathways. In *Molecular Aspects of the Stress Response; Chaperones, Membranes and Networks.* P. Csermely & L. Vigh, Eds.: Chapter 10, 100 113. Springer. Berlin, Germany.
5. Nicholson, K.M. & N.G. Anderson. 2002. The Akt/PKB signaling pathway in human malignancy. *Cell Signal.* **14:** 381–395.
6. Burgering, B.M. & P.J. Coffer. 1995. Protein kinase B (c-Akt) in phosphatidylinositol-3-OH kinase signal transduction. *Nature* **376:** 599–602.
7. Brazil, D.P. & B.A. Hemmings. 2001. Ten years of protein kinase B signaling: a hard Akt to follow. *Trends Biochem. Sci.* **26:** 657–664.
8. Kyriakis, J.M., P. Banerjee, E. Nikolakaki, *et al.* 1994. The stress-activated protein kinase subfamily of c-Jun kinases. *Nature* **369:** 156–160.
9. Sluss, H.K., T. Barrett, B. Dérijard, *et al.* 1994. Signal transduction by tumour necrosis factor mediated by JNK protein kinases. *Mol. Cell. Biol.* **14:** 8376–8384.
10. Enomoto, A., N. Suzuki, C. Liu, *et al.* 2001. Involvement of c-Jun NH2-terminal kinase 1 in heat-induced apoptotic cell death of human monoblastic leukaemia U937 cells. *Int. J. Radiat. Biol.* **77:** 867–874.
11. Deng, Y., X. Ren, L. Yang, *et al.* 2003. Jnk-dependent pathway is required for TNFα-induced apoptosis. *Cell* **115:** 61–70.
12. Denizot, F. & R. Lang. 1986. Rapid colorimetric assay for cell growth and survival: modifications to the tetrazolium dye procedure giving improved sensitivity and reliability. *J. Immunol. Methods* **89:** 271–277.
13. Gabai, V.L., J.A. Yaglom, V. Volloch, *et al.* 2000. Hsp72-Mediated suppression of c-Jun N-terminal kinase is implicated in development of tolerance to caspase-independent cell death. *Mol. Cell Biol.* **20:** 6826–6836.

14. Galadari, S., F. Thayyullathil, A. Hago, *et al.* 2008. Akt depletion is an important determinant of L929 cell death following heat stress. *Ann. N. Y. Acad Sci.* Recent Advances in Clinical Oncology. In press.

15. Gabai, V.L., I.V. Zamulaeva, A.F. Mosin, *et al.* 1995. Resistance of Ehrlich tumor cells to apoptosis can be due to accumulation of heat shock proteins. *FEBS Lett.* **375:** 21–26.

16. Gabai, V.L., A.B. Meriin, J.A. Yaglom, *et al.* 1998. Role of Hsp70 in regulation of stress-kinase JNK: implication in apoptosis and aging. *FEBS Lett.* **438:** 1–4.

Akt Depletion Is an Important Determinant of L929 Cell Death following Heat Stress

Sehamuddin Galadari, Faisal Thayyullathil, Abdulkader Hago, Mahendra Patel, and Shahanas Chathoth

Department of Biochemistry, Faculty of Medicine and Health Sciences, UAE University, Al Ain, United Arab Emirates

Exposure of mammalian cells to heat stress causes impairment of numerous physiological functions and activates a number of signaling pathways. Some of these pathways, such as induction of heat-shock proteins and activation of Akt, enhance the ability of cells to survive heat stress. On the other hand, heat stress can trigger cell-death signaling via activation of the stress-activated protein kinase/c-Jun NH2-terminal kinase (SAPK/Jnk). Recently, it has been shown that kinases activated by heat stress can regulate synthesis and functioning of the molecular chaperones, and these chaperones modulate the activity of the cell death and survival pathways. We have found that Akt plays a central role in determining the fate of L929 fibroblast cells exposed to heat stress. In our experiments heat stress causes Akt depletion and L929 cells to undergo cell death. Heat-shock protein 70 (Hsp70) is known to prevent stress-induced cell death by interfering with the SAPK/Jnk signaling pathway. In our study, there is a very high level of induction of Hsp70, yet this is not sufficient to rescue Akt depletion and L929 from cell death. The Akt depletion is specific, since actin protein level does not change during the heat stress. Moreover, our studies show that L929 cells can recover from a short-term heat shock, whereby, Akt level is returned to normal following recovery from heat shock. Therefore, it appears that the fate of the prolonged heat-stressed fibroblast cells is determined by Akt level, and that return of Akt protein level to normal prevents cell death.

Key words: heat-stress response; AKT depletion; L929 cell death

Introduction

Heat-shock response is characterized by transcriptional activation and accumulation of heat-shock proteins, such as heat-shock protein 70 (Hsp70), that are responsible for the provision of a state of temperature resistance to the cell.[1] In fact the first survival pathway activated by heat shock is the heat-shock response. Like many other stressors, heat shock induces a specific and tightly regulated signaling network that either initiates cell death or facilitates cellular survival.[2,3] Indeed, following heat shock and within minutes, an array of signal transducing kinases, such as Akt and c-Jun N-terminal kinase (Jnk) are activated.[4,5]

Akt, also known as PKB or Rac kinase, is a serine/threonine kinase, belonging to the cAMP-dependent protein kinase A/protein kinase G/protein kinase C (AGC) super family of protein kinases. These kinases share structural homology within their catalytic domain and have similar activation mechanisms that when deregulated lead to human diseases including cancer.[6] Akt is a downstream target of phosphatidylinositol 3-kinase (PI3-kinase) in cytokine and growth factor signaling pathways.[7] There are three highly homologous members of Akt kinase known as Akt 1, 2, and 3. All Akt

Address for correspondence: Sehamuddin Galadari, Cell Signaling Laboratory, Department of Biochemistry, Faculty of Medicine and Health Sciences, UAE University, PO Box 17666, Al Ain, UAE. Voice: +97137137507; fax: +97137672033. sehamuddin@uaeu.ac.ae

Ann. N.Y. Acad. Sci. 1138: 385–392 (2008). © 2008 New York Academy of Sciences.
doi: 10.1196/annals.1414.040

isoforms except the Akt 3 splice variant contain two regulatory phosphorylation sites, Thr308 and Ser473, in the C-terminal regulatory domain that are important for full activation of the enzyme.[8]

It has been reported that the most potent inducers of c-Jun activation are agents associated with cellular stress, such as thermal shock, inflammatory cytokines, UV radiation, and metabolic poisons, suggesting a major role for this transcription factor in mediating repair or protection against cellular injury.[9] Hence, regulators of this protein are important in the process of repair and/or protection against environmental stress. One such group of regulators is the stress-activated protein kinases (SAPKs), a subfamily of the MAP kinase signaling pathway that is activated following stress. Jnk is a member of SAPK family, and its pathway is generally considered a pro-apoptotic.[10] It has been shown that Jnk mediates cell-death signals by a variety of stressors including heat shock.[11] Under these stressors, Jnk activation may cause cytochrome c efflux from mitochondria, either via the inactivation of the anti-apoptotic proteins, Bcl-2 and Bcl-x, or the cleavage and activation of the pro-apoptotic protein, Bid, leading to the execution of the apoptotic cascade triggered by activated caspases.[12]

In this study, we investigated the effect of heat stress on the induction of signaling proteins important to L929 cell survival and cell death. Identifying and understanding the important players in cell survival and cell-death balance is of utmost importance to better understanding disease situations, such as cancer, where this balance is derailed.

Materials and Methods

Materials

Dulbecco-modified Eagle's medium (DMEM), fetal calf serum (FCS), phosphate-buffered saline (PBS) and trypsin-2-[2-(Bis(carboxymethyl)amino)ethyl-(carboxymethyl)amino]acetic acid (Trypsin-EDTA) were from GIBCO-Invitrogen Corp. (Carlsbad, CA). Tissue culture dish and flasks from Nunc (Roskilde, Denmark). SDS-PAGE chemicals from Bio-Rad (Hercules, CA). Anti-Akt were from Cell Signaling Inc. (Danvers, MA) and anti-Hsp70, anti-PARP, anti-Jnk1, and anti-actin antibodies were from Santa Cruz Biotechnology Inc. (Santa Cruz, CA). Anti-rabbit IgG, anti-mouse IgG, 3-[4,5-dimethylthiazol-2-yl]-2,5-diphenyl tetrazolium bromide (MTT), and all other chemicals were purchased from Sigma (St. Louis, MO).

Cell Culture

L929 cells were maintained in DMEM supplemented with heat-inactivated 10% fetal calf serum (FCS) without antibiotics at 37°C in 5% CO_2. 70% confluent cells were used for the experiment. Control cells were kept at 37°C, and experimental plates were placed at 42°C for heat-shock studies in 5% CO_2 for different times for the heat-stress studies, or for 3 h only for the heat-shock studies. The heat-shocked plates were then placed at 37°C for recovery and followed for the time course 0, 1, 2, 6, 12, 24, and 48 h or as otherwise indicated.

MTT Assay

Cytotoxicity assays were carried out as described elsewhere with slight modifications.[13] Cells grown in 96-well microtiter plates (10,000 cells/well) were incubated for 24 h. Experimental plates, either heat stress or heat-shocked at 42°C for 3 h, were placed into a preheated humidified 5% CO_2 incubator. After each time point, heat shocked/stressed plates were treated with 25 μL MTT (5 mg/mL in PBS). The cells were then incubated at 37°C for 3 h. The formazan crystals that formed were solubilized in 200 μL of dimethyl sulfoxide (DMSO). Once the color was developed, quantification was done at 570 nm using an Anthos Labtec HT2 plate reader (Cambridge, UK).

Cell Preparation and SDS-PAGE and Western Blot Analysis

Following the different experiments, cells were washed twice with cold PBS, pH 7.4 and lysed with lysis buffer [50 mM Tris HCl (pH 7.4), 10% NP-40, 40 mM NaF, 10 mM NaCl, 10 mM Na_3VO_4, 1 mM freshly prepared phenylmethylsufonyl fluoride (PMSF), 10 mM dithiothreitol (DTT), containing protease inhibitors 10 mg/mL leupeptin, 10 mg/mL aprotinin, 10 mg/mL trypsin and 1 mg/mL pepstatin A]. The lysates were centrifuged at 15,000 rpm for 10 minutes at 4°C. An aliquot of the supernatant was kept for protein determination by BioRad protein assay kit, and the rest of the lysate was immediately boiled for 3 min with 6X SDS-PAGE sample buffer containing 0.05% bromophenol blue, 10% glycerol, and 2% beta mercaptoethanol. Samples were stored at −80°C. When needed, samples were boiled again and equal amounts of protein from cell lysates were subjected to electrophoresis on SDS-PAGE.

The cell lysates (40 μg protein) were resolved by SDS-PAGE, and the separated proteins were transferred onto nitrocellulose membrane by the wet transfer method using the Bio-Rad electrotransfer apparatus. After blocking with 5% nonfat milk in Tris buffer saline containing 0.1% Tween 20, the membrane was incubated with primary antibodies followed by secondary antibody-conjugated horseradish peroxidase. Proteins were visualized by the enhanced chemiluminescence system (Pierce Biotech, Rockford, IL).

Cleavage of Poly (ADP-ribose) Polymerase

In order to examine the cleavage of poly (ADP-ribose) polymerase (PARP), 30 μg whole-cell extracts were resolved on 8% SDS polyacrylamide gel and subjected to PAGE. The resolved protein was transferred to nitrocellulose membrane blocked with 5% nonfat milk pro-

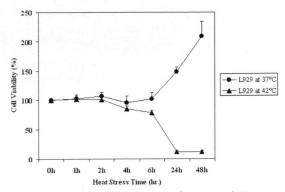

Figure 1. Cell viability as a function of duration of heat stress. L929 cells were grown at 37°C or 42°C and cell growth was monitored over time.

tein, and probed with PARP antibodies. Bands were detected by the enhanced chemiluminescence system (Pierce Biotech) as described above.

Results

Effect of Continued Heat Stress on L929 Cell Viability

In order to study the effect of heat stress on cell viability, mouse fibroblasts from cell line L929 were subjected to continued heat treatment at 42°C. The results of this treatment on L929 cell viability are shown in Figure 1. Cells that were kept at 37°C followed a normal cell-growth curve. During the first hour no significant difference was observed between cells growing at the control temperature and cells that were heat stressed at 42°C. However, the cell viability rates began to diverge by 2 h, and tat 42°C L929 cell viability began to decline. This decline was further abrogated at 6 h, when the viability declined sharply to almost zero by 24 h. In comparison, the control cells that were kept at 37°C continued to grow and show a normal growth pattern.

Effect of Continued Heat Stress on Protein Induction Level

Figure 2A illustrates the effect of heat stress on Akt protein level. L929 cells were kept

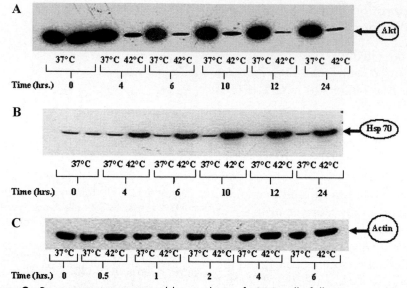

Figure 2. Representative western blot analysis of L929 cells following growth at 37°C and 42°C. **(A)** Expression level of Akt protein, **(B)** expression level of Hsp70, and **(C)** actin expression level.

either at 42°C or 37°C and Akt levels were measured by western blot analysis. Initially, Akt protein levels were the same in both groups at time 0. However, as early as 4 h Akt level was attenuated in cells that were stressed at 42°C, while cells at 37°C maintained the control level of Akt protein for up to 24 h. Next, the effect of heat stress on the chaperone protein Hsp70 was investigated. As can be seen in Figure 2B, Hsp70 was at a basal level in both groups cells, while by 4 h Hsp70 was highly induced in cells that were stressed at 42°C, and it was continuously induced up to 24 h. It can be observed from Figure 2C that actin protein level remained unchanged irrespective of whether the cells were at 37°C or 42°C.

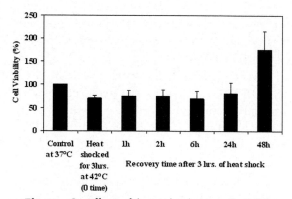

Figure 3. Effect of heat shock on cell viability. L929 cells were grown at 37°C and at 42°C. After 3 h at 42°C L929 cells were transferred to 37°C, which is referred to as time 0, thereafter the time indicates the time of recovery at 37°C.

Heat-Shock Recovery and Cell Viability

As observed in Figure 1, cell viability began to diverge at around 2 h, and it was hypothesized that around this time the fate of stressed cells is decided at the molecular level. In order to investigate this, L929 cells were heat treated at 42°C for 3 h, after which (designated time 0) the cells were transferred and allowed to re-

cover at 37°C. As shown in Figure 3, at time 0 the heat-shocked cells were at approximately 75% viability, indicating that 25% cell death had occurred during the 3 h of heat shock. L929 cells were then followed up during the recovery period up to 48 h. It is observable in Figure 3 that no significant change occurred with respect to cell viability during recovery at 37°C up to 24 h. However, by 48 h cells had almost doubled in viability. Interestingly, cells

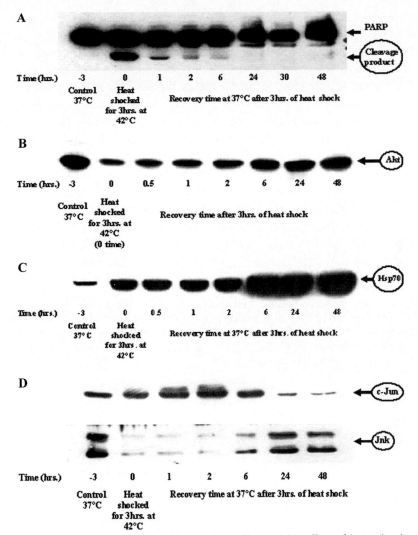

Figure 4. Representative western blot analysis showing the effect of heat shock at 42°C and recovery at 37°C on L929 cells. **(A)** PARP and its cleavage fragment, **(B)** Akt protein, **(C)** Hsp70, and **(D)** c-Jun and Jnk expression levels.

only started to proliferate after the initial 24-h recovery period.

Effect of Heat Shock on Protein Level

In order to test whether the 25% loss in cell viability observed in heat-shocked L929 cells was the result of apoptosis, the levels of poly (ADP-ribose) polymerase (PARP) cleavage, which is indicative of caspase 3 activation, were examined. In control cells that were not heat shocked and that were kept at 37°C (−3 h), no PARP cleavage was observed. However, in cells that were subjected to 3 h of heat shock at 42°C, PARP was cleaved, indicating caspase 3 activation as seen at time 0 in Figure 4A. Moreover, after moving the heat-shocked cells to 37°C for 1 h, a reduction in PARP cleavage was observed (Fig. 4A). There was a continuous reduction in PARP cleavage following recovery up to 6 h. By 24 h there were no signs of PARP cleavage, implying the loss of caspase 3 activity (Fig. 4A).

Interestingly, as can be observed in Figure 4B, as early as 30 min Akt protein level was enhanced following the replacement of

L929 cells to 37°C from 42°C. This increment in Akt protein levels seemed to continue with time up to 48 h. On the other hand the effect of heat shock on Hsp70 appeared to be biphasic, as can be seen in Figure 4C. At control (37°C) Hsp70 level was almost background. Following heat shock an elevation in Hsp70 levels occurred that was characteristically the same even after moving the cells to the recovery temperature (37°C) for 2 h. However, at 6 h, the expression level of Hsp70 was significantly enhanced, and this induction continued for 48 h. This Hsp70 induction occurred despite the fact that the cells were at the control temperature of 37°C, as seen in Figure 4C.

We further examined the effect of stress-activated MAP kinase pathway (SAPK) by looking at the expression levels of the transcription factor c-Jun and the stress-activated protein kinase Jnk. As shown in Figure 4D, there appeared to be an inverse relationship between Jnk and c-Jun. At control temperature, Jnk was present, and following heat-shock Jnk level was almost undetectable. This reduction in Jnk protein level continued even after 2 h at a recovery temperature of 37°C, as seen in Figure 4D. It was only after 6 h at recovery that the level of Jnk began to increase with time and did so up to 48 h. Although, c-Jun was expressed in control cells, after 3 h of heat shock, c-Jun level was further enhanced. This enhancement of c-Jun level was further increased up to 2 h following the transfer of cells from 42°C to the 37°C recovery temperature, as seen in Figure 4D. At 6 h c-Jun level was reduced, and by 24–48 h it was almost undetectable, as can be seen in Figure 4D.

Discussion

In this study we have demonstrated that Akt depletion is a prelude to cell death following heat stress, and that Hsp70 induction was not sufficient to prevent L929 cell death. It is apparent from our studies that the inactivation of the survival pathway is a prerequisite for the initiation of cell death. One such survival pathway is the Akt signaling pathway.[14] Akt resides in a central position controlling many important signaling proteins involved in survival and metabolism.[8] Therefore, Akt regulation is important in regulating survival and death pathways. Previous studies have focused on the role of Akt phosphorylation level as a means of regulating heat stress.[14] We have attempted to understand the role of protein induction, or its absence, as a possible means of regulation of the heat-shock response. We can see from Figure 1 that cell viability was dramatically reduced after 6 h of heat stress. This dramatic change appears to have been initiated earlier by a specific reduction in Akt protein level (Fig. 2A), since actin level did not change during the same heat-stress period (Fig. 2C). Interestingly, Hsp70 induction (Fig. 2B) does not relieve Akt protein depletion and it is not able to carry out its protective role, and the L929 cells undergo apoptosis (Figs. 1 and 4A). Clearly, Akt depletion is an important determinant of L929 cell death when cells are exposed continuously to heat. This is in line with previous studies in which it was reported that Akt inhibition augments drastically apoptosis of heat-shocked cells and enhances their susceptibility to cell death.[3,14,15]

It is noteworthy to observe that L929 cells are likely to have been primed for cell death early following heat shock. In order to investigate the effect of a relatively short heat stress (heat shock), L929 cells were heat shocked for 3 h and then allowed to recover at 37°C. Cell viability, although initially slightly reduced (75% of control), remained constant until 24 h postrecovery. Indeed, by 48 h postrecovery, the cells had actually continued to proliferate (Fig. 3). It is clear from Figure 4A that 3 h at 42°C was sufficient to reach the execution state of apoptosis, that is caspase 3 activation, and hence PARP cleavage, a hallmark of caspase activation. However, at 1 h recovery this cleavage level is reduced tremendously, and by 24 h no PARP cleavage is observed, indicating that this process is very tightly controlled in heat shock, and that recovery is possible following shock in L929 cells. Though Akt is degraded following 3 h of heat shock as early as 30 min at recovery temperature (37°C) Akt protein level has somewhat recovered. In fact, by 6 h, Akt protein levels were almost the same as controls (Fig. 4B). Since Akt is known to inhibit many proteins closely implicated in apoptosis, its induction during the recovery time is likely to attenuate many pro-apoptotic mechanisms in order to shut down cell death and initiate the survival signaling pathway(s).[3]

Hsp 70 was examined during the heat shock and recovery experiment. The protein level was at basal level at 37°C, and by 3 h heat shock Hsp70 was induced (Fig. 4C). However, following transfer and recovery at 37°C Hsp70 level was still induced for up to 2 h and did not return to basal level. Moreover, Hsp70 shows a second phase of protein induction, which occurs around 6 h into recovery and continues until 48 h postrecovery, indicating that this second phase of protein increase is important to the concomitant proliferation and growth of L929 cells (Figs. 3 and 4C). Hence, this implicates a possible proproliferative role for Hsp70 given that previous reports have indicated that Hsp70 may inhibit the apoptotic pathway by preventing activation of caspase 9 via direct binding to Apaf-1.[2,16]

Jnk is a member of SAPK, and its pathway is generally considered pro-apoptotic.[10,12,17] It has been shown that Jnk mediates cell-death signals by a variety of stressors including heat shock.[11] Therefore, we were interested to investigate the role of the Jnk pathway in the heat-shock recovery experiment. It is observed that Jnk protein, although present at normal temperatures, is attenuated following heat shock and it does not recover until 6 h of recovery, after which, induction occurs and Jnk level is raised back to control (37°C) levels (Fig. 4D). On the other hand, c-Jun is overexpressed during heat shock and returns to basal levels at about 6 h. It has been reported that in some cells blocking Jnk activation during heat shock is sufficient for protection and that this blocking is likely to be carried out by Hsp70.[18] This

might explain the second phase of Hsp70 induction at 6 h postrecovery, which seems to be concurrent with that of Jnk level. However, these suppositions need to be confirmed by further experiments.

In conclusion, we have investigated the role of important signal transduction pathways in heat-stress–induced cell death, and our findings underscore the important role that Akt plays in maintaining cell survival. These findings shed some light on possible prerequirement for Akt depletion prior to cell death during heat stress. Moreover, our findings implicate Hsp70 in an important signaling role in proliferation.

Acknowledgments

This work was supported by grants from the Terry Fox Foundation for Cancer Research, the Sheikh Hamdan Awards for Medical Research, and the Faculty of Medicine and Health Sciences at UAE University.

Conflicts of Interest

The authors declare no conflicts of interest.

References

1. Lindquist, S. 1986. The heat-shock response. *Ann. Rev. Biochem.* **55:** 1151–1191.
2. Gabai, V.L. & M.Y. Sherman. 2002. Molecular biology of thermoregulation: interplay between molecular chaperones and signaling pathways in survival of heat shock. *J. Appl. Physiol.* **92:** 1743–1748.
3. Nadeau, S.I. & J. Landry. 2007. Mechanism of activation and regulation of the heat shock-sensitive signaling pathways. In *Molecular Aspects of the Stress Response; Chaperones, Membranes and Networks.* P. Csermely & L. Vigh, Eds.: Chapter 10, 100–113. Springer. Berlin, Germany.
4. Ider, V., A. Schaffer, J. Kim, *et al.* 1995. UV irradiation and heat shock mediate JNK activation via alternate pathways. *J. Biol. Chem.* **270:** 26071–26077.
5. Konishi, H., H. Matsuzaki, M. Tanaka, *et al.* 1996. Activation of RAC protein kinase by heat shock and hyperosmolarity stress through a pathway independent of phosphatidylinositol 3-kinase. *Proc. Natl. Acad. Sci. USA* **93:** 7639–7643.

6. Nicholson, K.M. & N.G. Anderson. 2002. The Akt/PKB signaling pathway in human malignancy. *Cell Signal.* **14:** 381–395.

7. Burgering, B.M. & P.J. Coffer. 1995. Protein kinase B (c-Akt) in phosphatidylinositol-3-OH kinase signal transduction. *Nature* **376:** 599–602.

8. Brazil, D.P. & B.A. Hemmings. 2001. Ten years of protein kinase B signaling: a hard Akt to follow. *Trends Biochem. Sci.* **26:** 657–664.

9. Kyriakis, J.M., P. Banerjee, E. Nikolakaki, *et al.* 1994. The stress-activated protein kinase subfamily of c-Jun kinases. *Nature* **369:** 156–160.

10. Sluss, H.K., T Barrett, B. Dérijard, *et al.* 1994. Signal transduction by tumour necrosis factor mediated by JNK protein kinases. *Mol. Cell. Biol.* **14:** 8376–8384.

11. Enomoto, A., N. Suzuki, C. Liu, *et al.* 2001. Involvement of c-Jun NH2-terminal kinase 1 in heat-induced apoptotic cell death of human monoblastic leukaemia U937 cells. *Int. J. Radiat. Biol.* **77:** 867–874.

12. Deng, Y., X. Ren, L. Yang, *et al.* 2003. Jnk-dependent pathway is required for TNF alpha-induced apoptosis. *Cell* **115:** 61–70.

13. Denizot, F. & R. Lang. 1986. Rapid colorimetric assay for cell growth and survival: modifications to the tetrazolium dye procedure giving improved sensitivity and reliability. *J. Immunol. Methods* **89:** 271–277.

14. Bang, O-S., B-G. Ha, E.K. Park, *et al.* 2000. Activation of Akt is induced by heat shock and involved in suppression of heat-shock-induced apoptosis of NIH3T3 cells. *Biochem. Biophys. Res. Comm.* **278:** 306–311.

15. Ma, N., J. Jin, F. Lu, *et al.* 2001. The role of protein kinase B (PKB) in modulating heat sensitivity in a human breast cancer cell line. *Int. J. Radiat. Oncol. Bio. Phys.* **50:** 1041–1050.

16. Beer, H., B. Wolf, K. Cain, *et al.* 2000. Heat shock protein 70 inhibits apoptosis by preventing recruitment of pro-caspase 9 to the Apaf-1 apoptosome. *Nat. Cell Biol.* **2:** 469–475.

17. Tournier, C., P. Hess, D.D. Yang, *et al.* 2000. Requirement of JNK for stress-induced activation of the cytochrome c-mediated death pathway. *Science* **288:** 870–874.

18. Gabai, V.L., A.B. Meriin, D.D. Mosser, *et al.* 1997. Hsp70 prevents activation of stress kinases. A novel pathway of cellular thermotolerance. *J. Biol. Chem.* **272:** 18033–18037.

Potential Inhibition of PDK1/Akt Signaling by Phenothiazines Suppresses Cancer Cell Proliferation and Survival

Jang Hyun Choi,[a] Yong Ryoul Yang,[a] Seul Ki Lee,[a]
Sun-Hee Kim,[a] Yun-Hee Kim,[a] Joo-Young Cha,[b] Se-Woong Oh,[b]
Jong-Ryul Ha,[b] Sung Ho Ryu,[a] and Pann-Ghill Suh[a]

[a]Department of Life Science, Pohang University of Science and Technology,
Pohang, Kyungbuk, Republic of Korea

[b]Central Research Institute, Choongwae Pharma Corporation, Annyung-dong,
Hwasung, Kyunggi-do, Republic of Korea

3'-Phosphoinositide-dependent kinase-1 (PDK1) has been identified for its ability to phosphorylate and activate Akt. Accumulated studies have shown that the activation of the PDK1/Akt pathway plays a pivotal role in cell survival, proliferation, and tumorigenesis. Therefore, the PDK1/Akt pathway is believed to be a critical target for cancer intervention. In this paper, we report the discovery of a new function of phenothiazines, widely known as antipsychotics, inhibiting PDK1/Akt pathway. Upon epidermal growth factor (EGF) stimulation, phenothiazines specifically suppressed the kinase activity of PDK1 and the phosphorylation level of Akt. The inhibition of PDK1/Akt kinase resulted in suppression of EGF-induced cell growth and induction of apoptosis in human ovary cancer cells. In particular, phenothiazines were highly selective for downstream targets of PDK1/Akt and did not inhibit the activation of phosphatidylinositol 3-kinase (PI3K), EGFR, or extracellular signal-regulated kinase 1/2 (ERK1/2). In particular, phenothiazines effectively suppressed tumor growth in nude mice of human cancer cells. Taken together, these findings provide strong evidence for novel function of phenothiazines, pharmacologically targeting PDK1/Akt for anticancer drug discovery.

Key words: phenothiazines; PDK1; Akt; cancer cells; apoptosis; proliferation

Introduction

The phosphoinositide-3-kinase (PI3K)/Akt-mediated signaling pathway is activated by a variety of cellular stimuli that can regulate fundamental biological functions, such as proliferation, survival, and migration.[1] Activation of PI3K results in the generation of a second messenger phosphatidylinositol-3,4,5-triphosphate (PIP3), and subsequent recruitment of 3'-phosphoinositide-dependent kinase 1 (PDK1) and Akt to plasma membrane.[2]

Plasma membrane–bound PDK1 can phosphorylate Akt at Thr[308], which results in activation of Akt.[3] Furthermore, Akt can be fully activated when it is phosphorylated at Ser[473] by PDK2, integrin-linked kinase, or via autophosphorylation.[4,5] Once activated, Akt promotes cell growth, proliferation, and survival through the phosphorylation of downstream substrates, such as p70S6K, glycogen synthase kinase (GSK)-3β, Bad, and the Forkhead family of transcription factors (FKHRL1).[6–9]

It is well known that the PI3K/PDK1/Akt signaling pathway can promote transformation, tumorigenesis, and tumor growth. In many types of human cancer, Akt has been highly amplified.[10] Ectopic expression of constitutively active Akt induces cell survival and

Address for correspondence: Pann-Ghill Suh, Department of Life Science, Pohang University of Science and Technology, San 31, Hyojadong Pohang, Kyungbuk, 790-784, Republic of Korea. Voice: +82-54-279-2293; fax: +82-54-279-2199. pgs@postech.ac.kr

Ann. N.Y. Acad. Sci. 1138: 393–403 (2008). © 2008 New York Academy of Sciences.
doi: 10.1196/annals.1414.041

malignant transformation, whereas inhibition of Akt activation promotes apoptosis in a variety of mammalian cells.[11,12] In addition, Akt has been implicated in tumor formation in transgenic mice.[13,14] Taken together, these studies suggest that the specific inhibitors of PDK1/Akt-mediated signaling would be effective therapeutic agents for cancer treatment either alone or in combination with other oncogene-specific inhibitors, such as tyrosine kinase–specific inhibitors.

Phenothiazines and their related compounds are widely used as psychotropics in clinical practice.[15] By inhibiting the interaction between dopamine and its receptors, specifically the D2 receptor, phenothiazines have prompted their widespread use for the treatment of such mental disorders as anxiety, depression, and psychosis. However, some of these agents also possess non-neuronal activity in cellular proliferation and differentiation. Phenothiazines including trifluoperazine (TFP) and chlorpromazine (CPZ) inhibited DNA polymerase activity in rat kidney cells, arresting the cells in the S phase of the cell cycle.[16] Moreover, perphenazine and TFP inhibited the proliferation of osteoblasts and affected their alkaline phosphatase activity *in vitro* and *in vivo*.[17] It has been reported that phenothiazines exert antiproliferative effects in many tumor cells. CPZ and TFP inhibited the proliferation and clonogenicity of leukemic cells.[18] Glass-Marmor and colleagues have shown that thioridazine (TRDZ) inhibits B16 melanoma cell proliferation.[19] In other studies, CPZ and TFP inhibited the proliferation of small lung cancer cells, most likely due to the inhibition of protein kinase C (PKC) activity.[20] However, these studies have mostly been achieved at high pharmacological concentrations of phenothiazines, and the exact target proteins for phenothiazines in normal and cancer cells have not been characterized.

In this study, we demonstrate that phenothiazines directly inhibit PDK1 and suppress its downstream signaling pathways, such as Akt, without interfering with other kinases upstream of PDK1. Furthermore, we show that phenothiazines potentially inhibit cancer cell proliferation and induce apoptosis in cancer cell lines. From these results, we propose the approach of selectively targeting PDK1 to treat human cancers, and identify phenothiazines as small-molecule PDK1 inhibitors.

Materials and Methods

General Materials

Phenothiazines, haloperidol (HAL), and daunorubicin were purchased from Sigma-Aldrich (St. Louis, MO). BAPTA-AM, W7, LY294002, and etoposide were purchased from Calbiochem (San Diego, CA). Epidermal growth factor (EGF) and Dulbecco's modified Eagle's medium (DMEM) were purchased from Invitrogen (Carlsbad, CA). Fetal bovine serum (FBS) was obtained from HyClone (Logan, UT). All phospho-specific antibodies were purchased from Cell Signaling Technology, Inc. (Danvers, MA) and nonphospho antibodies were from Santa Cruz Biotechnology, Inc. (Santa Cruz, CA).

Cell Culture, Immunoprecipitation, and Immunoblot Assay

Human ovarian carcinoma cell line (OVCAR-3) cells were maintained in Dulbecco's Modified Eagle's Medium (DMEM) medium supplemented with 10% (v/v) FBS at 37°C in a humidified, CO_2-controlled (5%) incubator. Cells were plated on a 6- or 10-cm tissue culture dish, and grown for 2 days until they reached 50–80% confluency. Cells were then placed in serum-free DMEM for 12–18 h before pretreatment of the cells with chemicals for 20 min, then treated with 100 ng/mL of EGF for 10 min. Cells were washed with phosphate-buffered saline (PBS) and lysed with lysis buffer (1% Triton X-100, 150 mM NaCl, 20 mM Tris-HCl, pH 7.4, 20 mM NaF, 1 mM sodium orthovanadate, 1 mM phenylmethylsulphonyl fluoride (PMSF), 1 μg/mL leupeptin, 5 μg/mL aprotinin and 2 μM pepstatin A). Immunoprecipitation and immunoblotting were performed as previously described.[21]

In Vitro Kinase Assay

PI3K assays were carried out essentially as previously described.[21] PDK1 kinase assay was conducted using kinase assay kit from Upstate USA, Inc. (Chicago, IL).

Cell Viability and Apoptosis Assay

To determine the effect of various chemicals on cell viability, cells were seeded in 96-well microtiter plates. After 24 h, cells were treated with the chemicals at the indicated concentrations. After treatment with the chemicals, MTT [3-(4,5-dimethylthiazol-2-yl)-2,5-diphenyltetrazolium bromide, 0.5 mg/mL] was added, and cells were incubated for 2 h in a CO_2 incubator. After centrifuging at 2000 rpm for 10 min, supernatant was carefully removed and DMSO (100 μL) was added to each well. Absorbance was measured at 570 nm in a microplate reader. Morphological changes in the nuclear chromatin of cells were detected by staining with 2 μg/mL Hoechst 33342 fluorochrome (Invitrogen), followed by examination under a fluorescence microscope. For DNA ploidy analysis, cells were suspended in PBS containing 5 mM EDTA and fixed by adding 100% ethanol. RNase A (2 μg/mL) was added to the suspended cells, and the cells were incubated at room temperature for 30 min. Then, propidium iodide (50 μg/mL) was added before reading. DNA contents of the cells were analyzed on a FACScan flow cytometer (Becton Dickinson, Franklin Lakes, NJ), which was also used to determine the percentage of cells in the different phases of the cell cycle.

Measurement of Cancer Growth In Vitro and In Vivo

Thymidine incorporation assay was conducted as previously described.[21] Various human cancer cells [SK-MLE-28 (melanoma); HT-29, Colo205, SW480, and HCT116 (colorectal); and MCF7 (breast)] were seeded in 96-well culture plates and incubated with test drugs for 48 h. Cell proliferation was assessed using CellTiter 96 Aqueous One Solution (#G3581; Promega, Madison, WI). Absorbance at 490 nm of each well was determined with a microplate reader (Molecular Devices, Sunnyvale, CA) and 50% growth inhibition concentration (GI_{50}) was calculated with software (Prism 3.0, San Diego, CA).

Mice Xenograft Model

The antitumor effect of phenothiazine drugs was investigated in the OVCAR-3 mouse xenograft model. Female 5-to-6-week-old athymic BALB/c nude mice (Charles River Japan Inc., Kanakawa, Japan) were transplanted with OVCAR-3 (ATCC, Manassas, VA) human ovarian cancer cells (1.5×10^7) subcutaneously in the right axillary region. Tumor size was measured using digital calipers (Mitutoyo Corp., Kanakawa, Japan), and tumor volume was estimated according to the following formula: tumor volume $(mm^3) = L \times W \times H \times 0.5$, where L is the length, W is the width, and H is the height. When the mean tumor volume in mice had reached 70 mm^3, six mice were allocated into each group after randomization. Test drugs were dissolved in sterile saline and administered intraperitoneally at the dose of 10 mg/kg, once daily, 5 days a week, for 2 weeks (Days 1–5 and Days 8–12). A control group received saline only. Mice injected with a dose of 16 mg/kg taxol served as positive control. Data are expressed as means ± SD of each group.

Results

Phenothiazines Inhibited EGF-induced OVCAR-3 Cell Growth

To observe the biological roles of phenothiazines, we investigated the effect of

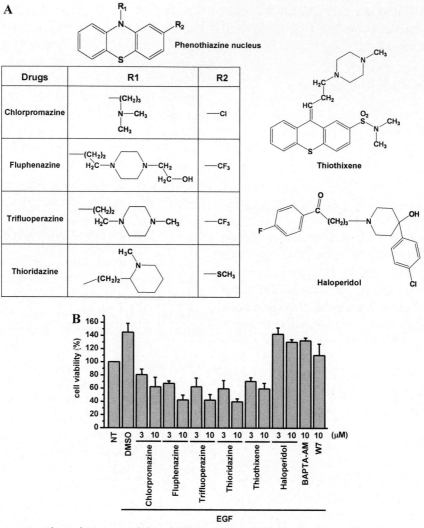

Figure 1. Phenothiazines inhibited EGF-induced OVCAR-3 cell growth. **(A)** Representative chemical structures of phenothiazines and haloperidol. **(B)** OVCAR-3 cells treated with various concentrations of chemicals, and cell viability determined by MTT assay. These results are representative of three independent experiments.

phenothiazines on the viability of OVCAR-3 cells, progressive adenocarcinoma of the ovary.[22] The chemical structures of phenothiazines including CPZ, fluphenazine (FPZ), TFP, TRDZ, and thiothixene (TTX) are shown in Figure 1A. In addition, we used HAL, which has potent antipsychotic activity, as the negative control. After treating with phenothiazines, we found that they selectively inhibited OVCAR-3 cell growth in a dose-dependent manner (Fig. 1B). Under same conditions, phenothiazines also suppressed SKOV-3 cancer cell

(ovarian adenocarcinoma) growth (data not shown). On the other hand, HAL did not suppress cell viability, indicating that among antipsychotic drugs phenothiazines specifically inhibit cancer cell growth.

It has been reported that these phenothiazines inhibited calmodulin (CaM) in addition to dopamine receptors.[23] Furthermore, reducing intracellular Ca^{2+} levels or inhibiting CaM leads to the inactivation of Akt.[24] We therefore investigated the effect of W-7, a specific CaM inhibitor and BAPTA-AM, a chelator of intracellular Ca^{2+}. Interestingly, neither W7 nor BAPTA-AM inhibited cell growth (Fig. 1B). These results strongly indicate that specific inhibition of cell growth by phenothiazines is not due to targeting CaM.

Phenothiazines Induced Dephosphorylation and Inactivation of Akt

It has been well established that the PI3K/Akt signaling pathway promotes cancer cell survival through direct phosphorylation of downstream signaling proteins.[1] Thus, we first investigated the effect of phenothiazines on activation of Akt in OVCAR-3 cells. As shown in Figure 2A, phenothiazines inhibited EGF-induced phosphorylation of Akt on both Thr^{308} and Ser^{473} in a dose-dependent manner. Specifically, FPZ, TFP, and TRDZ had more potent activity on the inhibition of Akt than CPZ and TTX. Moreover, HAL did not inhibit Akt phosphorylation, and BAPTA-AM and W7 had little effect on the phosphorylation of Akt, suggesting that phenothiazines specifically suppress Akt phosphorylation without secondary effects. Next, we conducted additional studies to determine IC_{50}s of Akt inhibition by FPZ and TRDZ. As shown in Figure 2B, the calculated IC_{50}s for FPZ and TRDZ in OVCAR-3 cells were 3.84 and 2.48 μM, respectively, indicating that phenothiazines inhibited Akt within minutes at low micromolar concentrations.

To investigate the inhibitory role of phenothiazines on Akt activation, we used activation state–specific antibodies against other downstream signaling substrates in immunoblotting experiments. As expected, treatment of OVCAR-3 cells with phenothiazines significantly inhibited the phosphorylations of p70S6K, mTOR, GSK-3β, and PKC-δ (Fig. 2C). Especially, pretreatment of BAPTA-AM considerably abrogated the phosphorylation of p70S6K and PKC-δ, not mTOR and GSK-3β. However, W7 did not affect the phosphorylation of these proteins, suggesting that phenothiazines directly regulate Akt-mediated

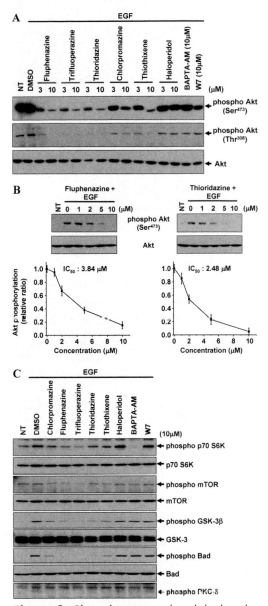

Figure 2. Phenothiazines induced dephosphorylation and inactivation of Akt. **(A)** OVCAR-3 cells were stimulated with chemicals for the indicated doses. Cell lysates were immunoreacted with antiphospho (Ser^{473}, Thr^{308}) Akt antibodies. **(B)** Cells were treated with fluphenazine and thioridazine for the indicated doses, and lysates were analyzed by immunoblotting with phospho-Akt (Ser^{473}) and Akt antibodies. The graph represents mean ± SD for Akt phosphorylation of triplicate determinations. **(C)** Cells were treated with chemicals, and lysates were immunoreacted with antiphospho p70S6K (Thr^{389}), mTOR (Ser^{2448}), GSK-3 (Ser^9), Bad (Ser^{136}), and PKC-δ (Thr^{505}). The protein expressions of each protein were estimated with direct antibodies.

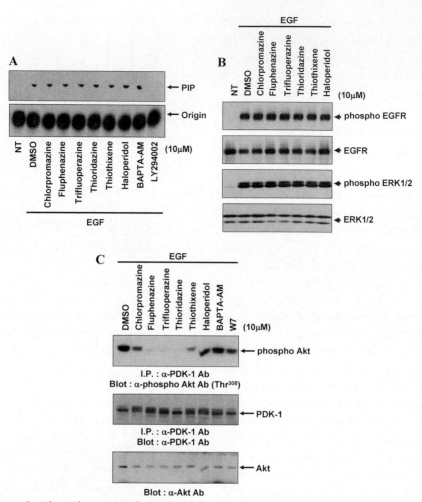

Figure 3. Phenothiazines selectively inhibited PDK1. **(A)** PI3K assays were performed as described in Materials and Methods. **(B)** OVCAR-3 cells were stimulated with chemicals for the indicated doses. Cell lysates were immunoreacted with antiphospho EGFR (Tyr[1068]) and ERK1/2 (Thr[202]/Tyr[204]) antibodies. The protein expressions of each protein were estimated with direct antibodies. **(C)** PDK1 kinase assay was performed as described in Materials and Methods. The amount of immunoprecipitated PDK1 was confirmed by immunoblotting with anti-PDK1 antibody.

signaling, not through CaM-mediated signaling pathway.

Phenothiazines Selectively Inhibited PDK1

It is well known that Akt is activated by EGFR and intracellular signaling molecules through a PI3K-dependent manner.[1] Therefore, the inhibition of Akt by phenothiazines can result from targeting upstream molecules of Akt. Thus, we tried to examine the change of EGF-induced EGFR or PI3K activation after phenothiazine treatment. As shown in Figure 3A, the EGF-induced PI3K activity was inhibited by LY294002 but not by phenothiazines. In addition, phosphorylations of EGFR or ERK1/2 were not inhibited by phenothiazines (Fig. 3B), indicating that neither EGFR nor PI3K is a target for phenothiazines.

Next, we examined the change of PDK1 kinase activity by phenothiazines. As shown in Figure 3C, we found that phenothiazines suppressed PDK1 kinase activity. However, HAL had no effects on PDK1 kinase activity. Interestingly, FPZ, TFP, and TRDZ significantly abrogated PDK1 kinase activity, but CPZ and TTX had mild effects on PDK1 kinase activity. These results are consistent with previous results about the inhibition of EGF-induced Akt phosphorylation (Fig. 2A). Taken together, these results indicate that PDK1 is a target of phenothiazines and PDK1 inhibition is involved in phenothiazine-mediated Akt dephosphorylation and inactivation.

Phenothiazines Induced Apoptotic Cell Death

Because phenothiazines were shown to inactivate Akt signaling by inhibiting PDK1, with the result of a significant reduction in cell growth, we surveyed phenothiazine-induced apoptotic cell death. After staining by Hoechst 33342, the large population of phenothiazine-treated cells displayed chromatin condensation (Fig. 4A). In addition, cell counts in $subG_0$ phase (defined as the population of apoptotic cell death) were determined to 10.3% for control and 20.1% and 34.9% for treatment with FPZ and TRDZ, respectively (Fig. 4B). The result from the DNA content analysis correlates well with that from the MTT assay (Fig. 1B). Specifically, FPZ and TRDZ increased oligonucleosomal cleavage of genomic DNA in a dose-dependent manner (Fig. 4C). Furthermore, cleavage of the caspase substrate poly adenosine diphosphate ribose was observed in FPZ- and TRDZ-treated cells, not in HAL-treated cells (Fig. 4D). Taken together, these results suggest that phenothiazines induced caspase-dependent apoptotic cell death.

Phenothiazines Inhibited Tumor Growth *In Vitro* and *In Vivo*

Since phenothiazines can promote cancer cell apoptosis, we further examined the effect of phenothiazines on EGF-induced cancer cell proliferation. As shown in Figure 5A, phenothiazines were effective in suppressing OVCAR-3 cell proliferation. In addition, we applied phenothiazines to several cancer cell lines, including melanoma (SK-MEL-28), colon cancers (HT29, Colo205, SW480, and HCT116) and breast cancer (MCF7), and measured the half inhibition concentration of cancer growth (GI_{50}) for 48 h. Many of these cell lines were responsive to the growth inhibitory effect of phenothiazines at concentrations as low as 3–7 µM (Fig. 5B), indicating that the effects of phenothiazines are not restricted to ovarian cancer, but are extant in other cancers, such as breast and colon cancers. Because phenothiazines inhibited colon cancer growth *in vitro* (Fig. 5B), we subcutaneously implanted OVCAR-3 cells into nude mice. When the tumors reached an average size of 70 mm^3, mice were treated intraperitoneally with saline, taxol, or phenothiazines (Fig. 5C). As shown in Figure 5C, CPZ, TFZ, and TRDZ suppressed tumor growth by 64%, 46%, and 26%, respectively, compared with control, indicating that phenothiazines selectively inhibit the growth of tumors by targeting PDK1. However, FPZ injected-mice died due to toxicity after 5 days.

Discussion

Based on the significant roles of PDK1/Akt signaling in cancer cell survival and proliferation,[3,11] this signaling cascade represents a therapeutic target for anticancer drugs. In the present study, we characterized phenothiazines for their ability to inhibit PDK1 activity and to induce apoptosis in cancer cell lines. Treatment of ovarian cancer cells with phenothiazines suppressed PDK1/Akt signaling without inhibitory effects on other oncogenic kinases including EGFR, PI3K, and ERK1/2. In addition, compared with HAL, phenothiazines selectively abrogated EGF-induced PDK1 signaling, indicating that phenothiazines play two distinct role—both antipsychotic and anticancer activity.

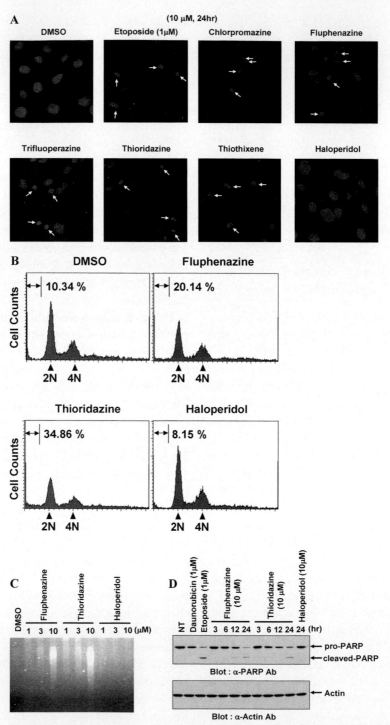

Figure 4. Phenothiazines induced apoptotic cell death. After treatment of OVCAR-3 cells with chemicals for 48 h, chromatin condensation and sub-G_0 population of cells were monitored by Hoechst 33342 staining **(A)** and flow cytometric analyses **(B)**, respectively. **(C)** Prepared from OVCAR-3 cells after treating chemicals for the indicated doses, genomic DNA was analyzed by agarose gel electrophoresis. **(D)** Cells were treated with chemicals for the indicated times, cell lysates were analyzed by immunoblotting with anti-PARP and actin antibodies. (In color in *Annals* online.)

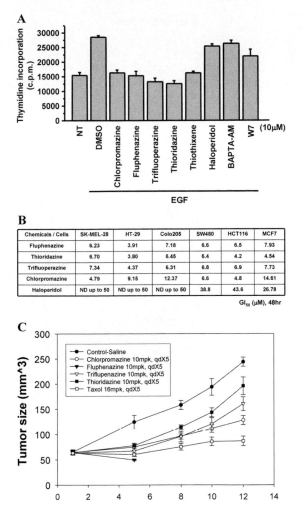

Figure 5. Phenothiazines inhibited tumor growth *in vitro* and *in vivo*. **(A)** Cell proliferation was measured by thymidine incorporation assay as described in Materials and Methods. **(B)** Various cancer cells were plated in 96-well plates and treated with phenothiazines. Fifty percent growth inhibition concentration (GI$_{50}$) was calculated with software (Prism 3.0). ND, not detected. **(C)** The antitumor effect of phenothiazines was analyzed in the OVCAR-3 mouse xenograft model as described in Materials and Methods.

Phenothiazines cause the inhibition of ovarian cancer cell growth associated with decreased Akt phosphorylation, assessed by decreased Thr^{308} and Ser^{473} phosphorylation. It is now clear that PDK1 plays a central role in the activation of the AGC superfamily of protein kinases including Akt.[3] In the present study,

several lines of evidence suggest that phenothiazines can directly inhibit PDK1. First, the inhibition of PDK1/Akt signaling by phenothiazines was dose- or time-dependent. Among these, the IC$_{50}$s for FPZ and TRDZ were in the low micromolar range, which might be achievable *in vivo*. Second, the potency of inhibiting PDK1 by phenothiazines was closely correlated with the suppression of EGF-induced phosphorylation of Akt or its downstream signaling proteins. Finally, the inhibition of PDK1 by phenothiazines was not due to suppression of upstream kinases such as EGFR or PI3K. Taken together, these results strongly indicated that phenothiazines selectively targeted PDK1 and inhibited PDK1-mediated signaling pathways.

It is well known that phenothiazines including TFP function as dopamine receptor antagonists and CaM inhibitors.[22] While phenothiazines suppressed Akt-mediated Forkhead box class O family 1a (FOXO1a) phosphorylation and translocation, structurally unrelated dopamine receptor antagonists, such as HAL or clozapine, did not.[25] In addition, other CaM inhibitors including W-13 and calmidazolium inhibited FOXO1a translocation. These results indicate that CaM may be a regulator of Akt-mediated FOXO1a activation. Consistent with these results, it has been reported that inhibition of intracellular Ca^{2+} or CaM can lead to the suppression of Akt and that W-13 decreased Akt activation in a PI3K-independent manner.[26] However, we demonstrated that neither W-7, specific CaM inhibitor, nor BAPTA-AM inhibited EGF-induced PDK1/Akt activation. In addition, EGF-induced cancer cell growth was not affected. Typically, BAPTA-AM significantly inhibited EGF-induced p70S6K because intracellular Ca^{2+} is an essential factor for the activation of p70S6K.[27] Together, these results suggest that specific inhibition of PDK1/Akt and cancer cell growth by phenothiazines is not due to other secondary effects.

The activated PDK1/Akt was reported to suppress apoptosis by phosphorylating the proapoptotic Bcl-2 family member Bad at

Ser^{136}.[8] In addition, PDK1/Akt directly or indirectly phosphorylates and inhibits GSK-3β.[7] Our flow cytometric analysis experiments showed that phenothiazines significantly reduced the cell population of G_0-G_1 phase and increased the apoptotic population of sub-G_0 phase. Furthermore, cancer cells treated with phenothiazines displayed distorted chromatin condensation and showed DNA fragmentation comparable to that of the control cells. Consistent with these data, cleavage of PARP was induced by phenothiazines. These results suggest that the inhibition of PDK1/Akt-dependent GSK-3β or Bad activation by phenothiazines can result in cancer cell apoptosis and eventually suppress cell proliferation.

In recent years, many biotechnology companies have focused on drug repositioning, presenting existing drugs for new uses.[28] Repositioned drugs can enter clinical testing more rapidly, reducing time and risk otherwise required in *de novo* drug discovery. In this study, we demonstrated that phenothiazines perform antitumor activity in several cancer cell lines. In the tumor xenograft mouse model, we observed an antitumor effect of phenothiazine drugs. Among the phenothiazines, CPZ potently suppressed tumor growth by 64%, compared with control. However, we could not find a strong correlation between the *in vitro* and *in vivo* effect of CPZ on tumor growth. TFP and TRDZ also exhibited antiproliferative effects *in vivo* against human ovarian cancer cell.

These results suggest that phenothiazines at low dose can achieve antitumor effect, and that phenothiazines can be repositioned from an antipsychotic drug against the D2 receptor to an anticancer drug against PDK1. Further investigations will be required to determine the exact region in phenothiazines critical for the inhibition of PDK1 activity so that we can minimize the side effects of phenothiazine therapy.

Conflicts of Interest

The authors declare no conflicts of interest.

References

1. Vivanco, I. & C.L. Sawyers. 2002. The phosphoinositol 3-kinase Akt pathway in human cancer. *Nat. Rev. Can.* **2:** 489–501.
2. Fruman, D.A., R.E. Meyers & L.C. Cantley. 1998. Phosphoinositide kinases. *Annu. Rev. Biochem.* **67:** 481–507.
3. Toker, A. & A.C. Newton. 2000. Cellular signaling: pivoting around PDK1. *Cell* **103:** 185–188.
4. Downward, J. 1998. Mechanisms and consequences of activation of protein kinase B/Akt. *Curr. Opin. Cell Biol.* **10:** 262–267.
5. Franke, T.F. *et al.* 1997. Direct regulation of the Akt proto-oncogene product by phosphatidylinositol-3,4-bisphosphate. *Science* **275:** 665–668.
6. Harada, H. *et al.* 2001. p70S6 kinase signals cell survival as well as growth, inactivating the pro-apoptotic molecule BAD. *Proc. Natl. Acad. Sci. USA* **98:** 9666–9670.
7. Cross, D.A. *et al.* 1995. Inhibition of glycogen synthase kinase-3 by insulin mediated by protein kinase B. *Nature* **378:** 785–789.
8. Datta, S.R. *et al.* 1997. Akt phosphorylation of BAD couples survival signals to the cell-intrinsic death machinery. *Cell* **91:** 231–241.
9. Biggs, W.H. III. *et al.* 1999. Protein kinase B/Akt-mediated phosphorylation promotes nuclear exclusion of the winged helix transcription factor FKHR1. *Proc. Natl. Acad. Sci. USA* **96:** 7421–7426.
10. Staal, S.P. 1987. Molecular cloning of the akt oncogene and its human homologues AKT1 and AKT2: amplification of AKT1 in a primary human gastric adenocarcinoma. *Proc. Natl. Acad. Sci. USA* **84:** 5034–5037.
11. Datta, S.R., A. Brunet & M.E. Greenberg. 1999. Cellular survival: a play in three Akts. *Genes Dev.* **13:** 2905–2927.
12. Sun, M. *et al.* 2001. AKT1/PKB kinase is frequently elevated in human cancers and its constitutive activation is required for oncogenic transformation in NIH3T3 cells. *Am. J. Pathol.* **159:** 431–437.
13. Holland, E.C. *et al.* 2000. Combined activation of Ras and Akt in neural progenitors induces glioblastoma formation in mice. *Nat. Genet.* **25:** 55–57.
14. Malstrom, S. *et al.* 2001. Tumor induction by an Lck-MyrAkt transgene is delayed by mechanisms controlling the size of the thymus. *Proc. Natl. Acad. Sci. USA* **98:** 14967–14972.
15. Baldessarini, R.J. & F.I. Tarazi. 2001. Drugs and the treatment of psychiatric disorders. In *The Pharmacological Basis of Therapeutics.* J.G. Hardman & L.E. Limbird, Eds.: 971–1002. McGraw Hill. New York, NY.

16. Lopez-Girona, A. *et al.* 1992. Calmodulin regulates DNA polymerase a activity during proliferative activation of NRK cells. *Biochem. Biophys. Res. Commun.* **184:** 1517–1523.

17. Komoda, T. *et al.* 1985. Inhibitory effect of phenothiazine derivatives on bone in vivo and osteoblastic cells in vitro. *Biochem. Pharmacol.* **34:** 3885–3889.

18. Schleuning, M., V. Brumme & W. Wilmanns. 1993. Growth inhibition of human leukemic cell lines by the phenothiazine derivative fluphenazine. *Anticancer Res.* **13:** 599–602.

19. Glass-Marmor, L., H. Morgenstern & R. Beitner. 1996. Calmodulin antagonists decrease glucose 1,6-bisphosphate, fructose 1,6-bisphosphate, ATP and viability of melanoma cells. *Eur. J. Pharmacol.* **313:** 265–271.

20. Zhu, H.G. *et al.* 1991. Different susceptibility of lung cell lines to inhibitors of tumor promotion and inducers of differentiation. *J. Biol. Regul. Homeost. Agents* **5:** 52–58.

21. Choi, J.H. *et al.* 2006. Phospholipase Cgamma1 negatively regulates growth hormone signalling by forming a ternary complex with Jak2 and protein tyrosine phosphatase-1B. *Nat. Cell Biol.* **8:** 1389–1397.

22. Hamilton, T.C. *et al.* 1984. Induction of progesterone receptor with 17beta-estradiol in human ovarian cancer. *J. Clin. Endocrinol. Metab.* **59:** 561–563.

23. Levin, R.M. & B. Weiss. 1977. Binding of trifluoperazine to the calcium-dependent activator of cyclic nucleotide phosphodiesterase. *Mol. Pharmacol.* **13:** 690–697.

24. Egea, J. *et al.* 2001. Neuronal survival induced by neurotrophins requires calmodulin. *J. Cell Biol.* **154:** 585–597.

25. Kau, T.R. *et al.* 2003. A chemical genetic screen identifies inhibitors of regulated nuclear export of a Forkhead transcription factor in PTEN-deficient tumor cells. *Cancer Cell.* **4:** 463–476.

26. Yang, C. *et al.* 2000. Calmodulin antagonists inhibit insulin-stimulated GLUT4 (glucose transporter 4) translocation by preventing the formation of phosphatidylinositol 3,4,5-trisphosphate in 3T3L1 adipocytes. *Mol. Endocrinol.* **14:** 317–326.

27. Graves, L.M. *et al.* 1997. An intracellular calcium signal activates p70 but not p90 ribosomal S6 kinase in liver epithelial cells. *J. Biol. Chem.* **272:** 1920–1928.

28. Ashburn, T.T. & K.B. Thor. 2004. Drug repositioning: identifying and developing new uses for existing drugs. *Nat. Rev. Drug Disc.* **3:** 673–683.

Index of Contributors